HENRI DE ROTHSCHILD, 1872–1947

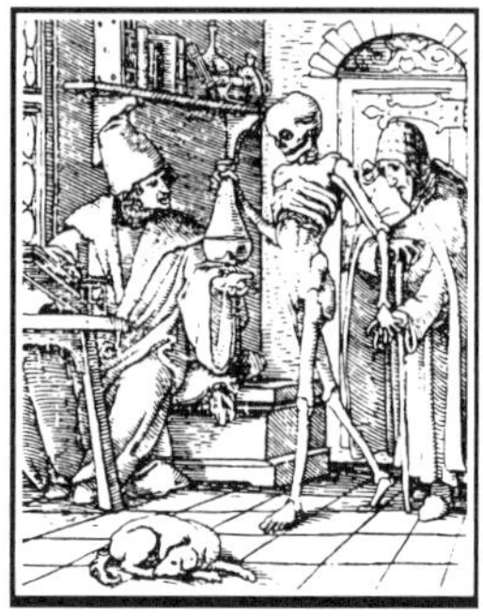

The History of Medicine in Context

Series Editors: Andrew Cunningham and Ole Peter Grell

Department of History and Philosophy of Science
University of Cambridge

Department of History
Open University

Titles in this series include

Centres of Medical Excellence?
Medical Travel and Education in Europe, 1500–1789
Edited by Ole Peter Grell, Andrew Cunningham and Jon Arrizabalaga

The Anatomist Anatomis'd
An Experimental Discipline in Enlightenment Europe
Andrew Cunningham

Crafting Immunity
Working Histories of Clinical Immunology
Edited by Kenton Kroker, Jennifer Keelan and Pauline M.H. Mazumdar

Before My Helpless Sight
Suffering, Dying and Military Medicine on the Western Front, 1914–1918
Leo van Bergen

Negotiating the French Pox in Early Modern Germany
Claudia Stein

Ireland and Medicine in the Seventeenth and Eighteenth Centuries
Edited by James Kelly and Fiona Clark

Henri de Rothschild, 1872–1947
Medicine and Theater

HARRY W. PAUL
University of Florida, USA

ASHGATE

Published by
Ashgate Publishing Limited
Wey Court East
Union Road
Farnham
Surrey, GU9 7PT
England

Ashgate Publishing Company
Suite 420
101 Cherry Street
Burlington
VT 05401-4405
USA

www.ashgate.com

British Library Cataloguing in Publication Data
Paul, Harry W.
Henri de Rothschild, 1872–1947: Medicine and Theater. – (The History of Medicine in Context)
1. Rothschild, Henri de, 1872–1947 – Career in medicine. 2. Rothschild, Henri de, 1872–1947--Dramatic works. 3. Rothschild, Henri de, 1872–1947 – Family.
4. Pascal, Andre, 1872–1947 – Criticism and interpretation. 5. Physicians – France – Biography. 6. Medical innovations – France – History – 20th century. 7. Physicians in literature. 8. Medicine in literature. 9. French drama – 20th century – History and criticism. 10. Paris (France) – Intellectual life – 20th century.
I. Title II. Series
610.9'2–dc22

Library of Congress Cataloging-in-Publication Data
Paul, Harry W.
Henri de Rothschild, 1872–1947: Medicine and Theater / Harry W. Paul.
p. ; cm. – (History of Medicine in Context)
Includes bibliographical references and index.
1. Rothschild, Henri de, 1872–1947. 2. Physicians – France – Biography. 3. Pediatricians – France – Biography. 4. Philanthropists – France – Biography. 5. Dramatists – France – Biography. I. Title. II. Series: History of medicine in context.
[DNLM: 1. Rothschild, Henri de, 1872–1947. 2. Physicians – France – Biography. 3. Gift Giving – France – Biography. 4. Health Facilities – history – France--Biography. 5. History, 19th Century – France – Biography. 6. History, 20th Century – France – Biography. 7. Pediatrics – history – France – Biography. WZ 100]
R507.R67P38 2010
610.92–dc22
[B] 2010041850

ISBN 9781409405153 (hbk)

MIX
Paper from responsible sources
FSC www.fsc.org
FSC® C018575

Printed and bound in Great Britain by the MPG Books Group, UK

Contents

List of Figures

Acknowledgements

For assistance in resurrecting Henri de Rothschild, M.D., I thank Melanie Aspey and the staff at The Rothschild Archive London and the personnel of the Archives de Paris, the Archives Nationales (Centre des archives du monde, Roubaix), the Archives de l'Assistance publique-Hôpitaux de Paris, the Service historique de la défense – Centre historique des archives, and the Bibliothèque nationale de France. Eric de Rothschild kindly gave me permission to consult the Rothschild documents in French archives. It has been a pleasure working with Emily Yates, commissioning editor, history, and Kirsten Weissenberg, senior editor, at Ashgate Publishing, as well as with my copyeditor, Diane Wardle. Lisa Scholey compiled the index. And for help and advice over the years, I thank Claire Orologas, Director of Education and Public Programs, Freer Gallery of Art and Arthur M. Sackler Gallery, Smithsonian Institution, Washington, D. C.

I remind everyone, including those I carelessly failed to thank, of La Rochefoucauld's canny observation that gratitude is a secret hope for future favors.

Introduction
Resurrecting Baron Henri de Rothschild, M.D.

.. A rare instance of the heir to wealth who has devoted his whole energy to science and philanthropy .. [1]

Henri de Rothschild (1872–1947) was the great grandson of the founding father of the French Rothschild enterprise, James Mayer (1792–1868), who settled in France in 1811. James Mayer established the first Rothschild hospital in Paris; it was later expanded and modernized by his son Edmond (1845–1934), an enthusiastic supporter of scientific research. Henri's paternal grandfather, Nathaniel (1812–70), was the son of Nathan Mayer (1777–1836), who established the Rothschild business and bank in London. Nathaniel came to the Paris bank at the invitation of his uncle, James Mayer, married the artistic and socially prominent Charlotte (1825–99), James Mayer's only daughter, and became a partner in the bank. James Edouard (1844–81), their son, married Laura Thérèse (1847–1931), one of the daughters of the Frankfurt Rothschilds, who were also seriously involved in medical activities.[2] In the 1870s James Edouard set up an important medical establishment at Berck-sur-Mer; the hospital was lovingly tended and developed by his widow. Thérèse's uncle Adolphe and aunt Julie later established an ophthalmological hospital in the northeast (19th arrondissement) of Paris. Deep in his medical studies, Henri escaped from his mother's Paris compound in 1895 by marrying Mathilde de Weisweiller (1874–1926), daughter of the financier Georges de Weisweiller. Mathilde managed to integrate her fantastic social life with considerable charitable work and medical activity. The context of great wealth, closeness to political

---

1 Cecil Roth, *The Jewish Contribution to Civilization* (1938; New York, 1940), 340.

2 The authoritative guide to all this begetting is *The Rothschild Family Tree* (London, 2000). Interesting and sometimes unreliable is Henri de Rothschild [HR], *La Lignée française de la famille Rothschild 1792–1942. Etude historique et biographique* (Oporto, 1942). Henri's connection with the English branch of the family was further solidified in the marriage of his maternal aunt, Emma Louisa (1844–1935), to Nathaniel Mayer (1840–1915), the first Lord Rothschild. On intermarriages of Jewish business and banking dynasties, see Abigail Green, "Rethinking Sir Moses Montefiore: Religion, Nationhood, and International Philanthropy in the Nineteenth Century," *American Historical Review* 110 (June 2005): 631–58.

power, family patronage of elite culture, and medical philanthropy makes up an important part of the social world into which Henri was born.

In a superb study of the house of Rothschild as the world's banker, Niall Ferguson does not have to spend much time on Henri de Rothschild, a French "sleeping" partner in the bank. Henri is damned with faint praise as "another of the fifth generation's scientists." Classifying him as a "misanthropic" doctor, Ferguson notes that Henri "published extensively on ... infant nutrition" and took an interest in "the medical use of radium."[3] All of this is not enough for Henri to escape the dreadful label of dabbler.[4] "He also dabbled in the theater, as a sponsor of the famous 1909 tour by Diaghilev's *Ballet russe* [sic], and as an amateur playwright using the *nom de plume* 'André Pascal'."[5] In 1909 Serge Diaghilev (1872–1929) took a troupe of Russian dancers to Paris, where their dynamic performance at the Châtelet theater created a sensation. The troupe was then baptized as the *Ballets russes* company. It is misleading to say that Henri, the author of many successful plays, dabbled in the theater. One mid-nineteenth-century line of propaganda about Jews was dangerously flattering: "Today [c. 1885] the barons of Israel represent luxury … charity … the arts … the smart set … fashion's latest style."[6] In the Belle Epoque it appears difficult to find many figures more deserving than Henri of this bigoted praise. Ferguson does not mention Henri's successful novel *Un crime à St. Solaire* or his even more successful biography of the notorious murderer Pranzini. And fortunately his work on philately – stamp collecting is a fertile source of bad jokes – goes unnoticed. Although Henri was only being a typical Rothschild in building his "château" at La Muette (a superb long-term real-estate investment, now the home of the OECD), in Paris and a "mock-Tudor Villa" (now named the Villa Strassburger) in Deauville as well as enjoying a yacht, Ferguson sums up this rich man's activities with the dour judgment that "Henri tried not to make money but to spend it." Worse, he managed to lose money when he tried to make it. "His various attempts at entrepreneurship (he tried at various times to manufacture cars, mustard, soap and canned pheasant) were commercial

---

[3] Niall Ferguson, *The House of Rothschild. The World's Banker 1449–1999* (2 vols, New York: 1999), II, 444. According to the publication *Nos docteurs. Répertoire photo-biographique et annuaire du corps médical* (7th year, Paris, n.d.), Henri's surgery hours at 33 rue du Faubourg Saint-Honoré were one to three on Tuesdays and Thursdays. Jean-Pierre Camilleri, *L'Institut Curie, son histoire, ses valeurs. Un siècle de cooperation entre chercheurs et médecins* (Paris, 2003), mentioned Henri at least twice; see also Jean-Pierre Camilleri and Jean Coursaget, *Les pionniers de la radiothérapie* (Les Ulis, 2005).

[4] An idea emphasized by Henri's son Philippe in Joan Littlewood, *Baron Philippe. The Very Candid Autobiography of Baron Philippe de Rothschild* (New York, 1986). Originally published with the droll title of *Milady Vine* in London (1984).

[5] Ferguson, *The House of Rothschild*, 444–5.

[6] Cited in Eugen Weber, *France, Fin de siècle* (Cambridge, Mass., 1986), 131; see Paula E. Hyman, "Acculturation of the Jews in Nineteenth-Century France," in *The Emergence of Jewish Artists in Nineteenth-Century Europe* (New York, 2001), 31–9.

failures."[7] Château Mouton-Rothschild gets no notice in this catalog; nor do his great collections of art, manuscripts, and books get any attention.[8] Henri's life can be misleadingly represented as a sort of Chekhovian drama, with no action, no subject, just a mixture of the meaningful and the insignificant, the sublime and the ridiculous.[9]

During most of the nineteenth century, the "multinational partnership" of N. M. Rothschild & Sons "was easily the biggest bank in the world," and "strictly in terms of their combined capital, the Rothschilds were in a league of their own until, at the earliest, the 1880s."[10] In his social history of London, Roy Porter gives a few lines to the Rothschild bankers because of their immense wealth and because they "outstripped" the other bankers. "When Baron Lionel Rothschild died in 1879, his personal estate was valued at some £2,700,000."[11] The Rothschild bank in Paris was certainly among the leading houses, if not number one, of *la haute banque* in the city down to 1905 or perhaps even 1914.[12] In the Paris bank the death in 1905 of Alphonse, James Mayer's oldest son, can be taken as a convenient if not evident hiatus. Accounting appearances can be deceiving: though after Alphonse's death the capital of the bank was low compared to some other banks, family capital contributions made it effectively much higher. Secrecy took its toll. After 1898, because of its refusal to show its accounts to the tax authorities, the firm could not act directly on the Paris stock exchange.

Not that continuing to manage investments made in the nineteenth century was a losing proposition – far from it, in areas like railroad transport, electricity, petroleum, and insurance, for example. Nor did having some prestigious if stuffy clients such as Vatican officials and members of the British royal family hurt business.[13] At the bank Edmond seems to have been keen on investing in businesses based on recent discoveries in mining and in the application of electricity; he suggested to Alphonse that electrical energy was a profitable avenue of investment, at least in the future. Edmond supported Marcel Deprez, a pioneer in solving the problem of how to transport electricity long distances and co-inventor of the Deprez-d'Arsonval galvanometer. The bank employed

---

7 Ferguson, *The House of Rothschild*, II, 445.

8 Harry W. Paul, "Collecting Chardins: Charlotte and Henri de Rothschild," *The Rothschild Archive* ("Review of the year April 2004 to March 2005"), 21–6.

9 Fabrienne Darge, "La tragi-comédie du docteur Tchekhow," *Le Monde* (26 mars 2004).

10 Ferguson, *The House of Rothschild*, I, 3.

11 Roy Porter, *London. A Social History* (London, 1994), 203.

12 Jean-Marc Dreyfus, *Pillages sur ordonnances. Aryanisation et restitution des banques en France 1940–1953* (Paris, 2003), 214.

13 Dreyfus, *Pillages sur ordonnances*, 215. Dreyfus says that after 1905 the capital of the Paris bank was fifty million francs. For the year 1904 Ferguson, *The House of Rothschild*, II, 505, perhaps including the family capital contributions, gives a figure of £21,086,000, which was about 527,150,000 francs.

two engineers (Jules Aron and Théophile Weill) to give advice on its industry-related business.[14] One of the important Rothschild investments was in the Baku Elektrische Kraft Company, organized by Russian and German companies with the primary aim of supplying electricity to the naphtha industry in Baku as well as to Transcaucasia. Edmond was the key decision maker in this investment, with Jules Aron playing an important advisory role in his contacts with the Deutsche Bank and the Allgemeine-Elektricitäts-Gesellschaft, big players in the Baku Company. By about 1900 Russian oil production, which accounted for about one-half of the world's crude oil production, was practically controlled by the Nobel and the Rothschild groups.

Describing Henri as a Rothschild who knew how to spend and invest badly, risks overlooking why he was able to spend and lose money on various businesses and still stay rich. Henri himself tells us the general secret. The period 1895–1926 favored him, along with many others, with thirty years of prosperity because industrial stocks rose considerably in value; Henri was thinking particularly of investments in oil and electrical industries. The Rothschilds were the largest shareholders in Royal Dutch and Shell. He could also have mentioned investment in non-ferrous metals and precious stones. Selling some shares could easily compensate for a low rate of dividend income. Henri did not believe that drawing on bank capital was as important as some historians later concluded, for the rise in value of his portfolio more than adequately compensated for the withdrawals.[15] In the period 1911–12 because of strikes, instability, and anti-Semitism in Russia, the Rothschilds abandoned the Russian oil business, selling out to Royal Dutch. After the Great War Henri remained rich enough to continue building in Paris, including renovating his hospital. But, as Dreyfus points out, the myth of the bank and of the rule of the plutocracy masked a striking hard fact, namely that, from the viewpoint of world finance, by the end of the 1930s there was only one really important Jewish bank in France, Lazard, whose Paris branch had 170 employees, with a balance sheet of 1.83 billion francs and business activity of nearly thirty-seven billion.[16]

In 1948, the year after Henri de Rothschild died, he received a few lines of appreciation in *La Presse médicale*: thirty-seven lines on a three-column page.[17] The pediatrician Henri Diriart gave a brief survey of Henri's medical career and activities and followed up with the opinion that Henri's medical colleagues owed a final homage to a man whose sustained effort and disinterested generosity had made

---

[14] François Caron and Fabienne Cardot (eds), *Histoire générale de l'électricité en France; vol. 1: Espoirs et conquêtes 1881–1918*, 322, 755, note 2 (Paris, 1991).

[15] HR (André Pascal), *Une dame d'autrefois. La baronne Mathilde de Rothschild 1872–1926* (Lausanne, 1946), 34–5, and Ferguson, *The House of Rothschild*, II, 355–6.

[16] Dreyfus, *Pillages sur ordonnances*, 227; gross profits were 23.7 and net profits 5.2 million francs.

[17] Henri Diriart, "Henri de Rothschild (1872–1947)," *La Presse médicale* 34 (56th year, 12 juin 1948), 414. Diriart became president of the Comité national de l'enfance.

a large contribution to charitable work as well as to the social progress of his epoch. This good advice seems to have fallen mostly on deaf ears. There was a surprising, somewhat erroneous, and slightly amusing though woefully incomplete entry in a recent historical dictionary.[18] What was worth recording about Henri in a historical dictionary dealing with doctors at the end of the twentieth century? Of primary importance was the fact that he was the grandson of Nathaniel, astute purchaser of Château Brane-Mouton (now Mouton Rothschild) in 1853 for somewhat less than the 1,200,000 francs the seller had paid for it in 1830. His father, James Edouard, was ignored. Theater got good mention: Henri, disguised as André Pascal (his most common theatrical pseudonym), wrote "boulevard plays" or light comedy, but expiated this frothy sin by building the Pigalle theater. His thespian genes were passed on: his granddaughter enjoyed the footlights as Philippine Pascal. He made gifts to museums – his fabulous gifts to the Bibliothèque nationale are not mentioned. An exciting titbit gets maximum exposure: in the 1920s Henri organized pleasure cruises on his yacht *Eros* – mention of Colette on board is usually obligatory here – and gave sumptuous receptions on the Côte d'Azur. Henri did get credit for establishing the modern hospital named for Mathilde and himself. He did not play any role in Parisian Jewish life comparable to that of Alphonse and Robert, presidents of the *Consistoire de Paris* between 1871 and 1940, or of Edouard, president of the *Consistoire central*, the organization symbolizing the position of Paris as the center of French Judaism. Fame, Emily Dickinson sang, is a bee, with a song, a sting, and a wing.

In some publications Henri was established as a prominent citizen, benefactor, and author. Under the entry for "dramatic authors" in the *Annuaire orange* for 1931 there is a lapidary entry flattering him as the author of several plays that had enjoyed some fame in their time.[19] The *Annuaire* hailed the protean Henri as financier, medical doctor, theater owner, author of some major plays, one of the directors of the *Chemin de fer du Nord*, and officer of the Legion of Honor. More titles and honors could have been listed, for such "bagatelles flattered his

---

18 Michel Dupont, *Dictionnaire historique des médecins dans et hors de la médecine* (Paris, 1999). The date of death is erroneously given as 1942; it was 1947. Henri would also have been disappointed to find his address given as the earlier one at rue du Fg. St. Honoré instead of his favorite and final abode in Paris, Château de La Muette, rue André Pascal. Henri was a stickler for accuracy in the dissemination of social information and distinctions, especially that broadcast by sources on the social elite. He made sure that the entries in the *Livre d'or* for himself and his sons (James and Philippe) were correct and complete. Corrections noted: James had a racing stable and a hunting *équipage*. Henri was a Commander of the Legion of Honor *and* of the Mérite Agricole, a member of the Automobile Club, the Aéro Club, Golf de Paris, Polo, the Société Hippique, and the Yacht Club de France. James, whose wife, née Claude Dupont, was la baronne James, also belonged to most of these groups. Philippe, keen racer of automobiles and yachts, listed his sailing yacht.

19 "Auteurs dramatiques," *Annuaire orange. Arts, lettres, sciences ...* (Paris, 1931), 103.

vanity."[20] In December 1929 his magnificently equipped modern theater of 1100 seats had opened at 10–12 rue Pigalle (9th arrondissement). In 1925 Henri had bought and demolished the fine building in which Eugène Scribe lived and died (1861). Four years later his sixty-million-franc theater, full of the latest technical marvels, opened but only to live a mediocre existence, not attracting either the plays or audiences it deserved. The theater might be regarded as Philippe's folly; his son's influence may also explain why it eschewed medical drama, including Henri's.[21]

For a considerable time Henri, a medical doctor, was a figure of some significance in Parisian medicine. According to Philippe, quoted in the unreliable Joan Littlewood gospel, his father "hated the thought of practicing medicine and, except during the war, never did."[22] This is nonsense, but it might be said that Henri, like Chekhov, regarded medicine as his lawful wife and literature as his mistress.[23] More consonant with all other evidence is Henri's own statement that for over thirty years he went to his polyclinic in the rue Marcadet in the north of Paris (18th arrondissement) to examine and treat patients. He returned home at about one p. m. Two interns did the evening rounds, but if a patient were seriously ill, Henri would show up at the hospital before dinner. There was always the possibility that he would be called in before a patient underwent an operation. He could always be reached by telephone, and sometimes he was called at early hours.[24] Henri did not spend much of his life sleeping.

An enthusiastic physician declared infant feeding to be one of the great issues of the day (1890s), with intellectuals worried about depopulation and doctors debating breastfeeding. A new children's crusade had begun, this time to reduce infant mortality.[25] Responding to "a pressing request" of one of his former medical professors, Pierre Budin, Henri early turned his attention to milk, a liquid that inspired him with scientific and charitable passion. (Lacking any passionate interest in wine production, he sent his son Philippe to run the Mouton estate in 1922, and for a certain historical period at least, the son's success made him better known than the father. They had certain common interests: science, the theater,

[20] Henri lists them at the end of *La Lignée*. Légion d'Honneur: Croix de chevalier, 1904; officier, 1914; commandeur, 1924. Médaille d'or des épidemies (Assistance publique de Paris). Rosette d'officier de l'Instruction publique. Cravate de commandeur de Mérite Agricole. Grand collier de Saint Jacques de l'Epée, bestowed by the king of Portugal in 1905. The quotation is from Ben Rogers, *A. J. Ayer. A Life* (1999; New York, 2000), 299, and is the judgment of Rogers on Ayer.

[21] Philippe Chauveau, *Les Théâtres parisiens disparus 1402–1986* (Paris, 1999), 298, 467–71.

[22] Littlewood, *Baron Philippe*, 8.

[23] Ernest J. Simmons, *Chekhov – A Biography* (1962; Chicago, 1970), 158.

[24] HR, *La Lignée*, 84.

[25] Madame Bronislas Dluski, *Contribution à l'étude de l'allaitement maternel* (thesis, Paris Faculty of Medicine, 1894), 4.

and literature.) Budin's research at the *Consultation de nourrissons* of the *Hôpital de la Charité* showed that the high infant mortality in artificially or bottle-fed babies was largely due to bad milk sold by a variety of merchants. On the urging of Budin, in 1896 Henri began the difficult task of organizing the distribution of pure milk in the working-class quarters of Paris. (Budin was an ardent advocate of breastfeeding, when possible.) On the Rothschild property in the rue de Picpus (12th arrondissement) Henri organized one of the very first "clinics" for nurslings (*consultations de nourrissons*), with the distribution of sterilized milk. The heavily medical period of Henri's life was a happy one, or at least he seems to have had a consistent purpose manifested in his work. Bertrand Russell pointed out that although "consistent purpose is not enough to make life happy, ... it is an almost indispensable condition of a happy life. And consistent purpose embodies itself mainly in work."[26] *Concordia, integritas, industria* –"Unity, integrity, diligence" – are the three words on the Rothschild shield, and Henri emphasized that the word *industria* in the family motto referred to the Roman virtue of hard work.[27]

During the ten or so years after becoming a physician, Henri studied the different methods of treating milk that was intended for feeding infants (up to three months of age). He was looking for the best processes for the treatment of milk and for the apparatuses that were the most practical and the easiest to get accepted by mothers. The industrial establishments then being created in response to the demands of pediatric specialists also had to be consulted. Henri experimented on the nurslings who came to the rue de Picpus by feeding them different kinds of milk prepared according to French and foreign methods. The results of the experiments, some of which were done by Henri alone and some with young collaborators supported by his foundation, were communicated to French and foreign scientific societies. He became the treasurer of the *Ligue contre la mortalité infantile* and in 1902 founded the *Revue d'hygiène et de médecine infantiles*.

Henri appeared on the public scene in a major way in 1901, a couple of years before his press coverage as the founder of a modern children's hospital. Appearing as Dr Henri de Rothschild, he gave a series of lectures at the Pasteur Institute on milk.[28] In 1900 milk was a more exciting and potentially deadly liquid than wine, though it must be admitted that there was also a lot of adulterated wine served in Paris. Henri first dealt with Pasteur's theories applied to the milk industry. In his work on food products, Pasteur had stuck pretty much to problems in the production of beer, vinegar, and, above all, wine. In two successive talks, Henri

---

26 Bertrand Russell, *The Conquest of Happiness* (London, 1930), 218.

27 J. B. Rietstop, *Armorial general* (2 vols, London, 1965; reproduced from the 2nd edn, 1887), II, 616, has the following entry for Rothschild: "Nob. Autricienne, 23 mars 1817. Eagle, ... tenant 5 flèches d'argent, les pointes en bas. Barons autriciens, 29 sept. 1822. ...lion de guerre. ... une étoile d'or... . lion.... Une licorne d'arg. D: Concordia, integritas, industria." See also F. Edward Hulme, *The History, Principles and Practice of Heraldry* (New York, 1969 [1892]).

28 HR, *Le Lait* (Paris, 1903). Lecture four was entitled "Falsification du lait."

trod on safe ground: the subjects of pasteurization and sterilization, followed by a dissection of the methods of milk analysis. The audience received the last talk (on the adulteration of milk) with typical scientific placidity, though listeners were perhaps surprised by the extent of the problem. Out of some 600,000 liters of milk that were consumed daily in Paris, 575,000 liters could be considered bad, that is, the milk contained harmful bacteria. Most of the French press, including the big Parisian papers, reported the shocking news but emphasized that the milk was made safe by pasteurization or sterilization. *L'Industrie laitière* (20 Jan. 1901), voice of the milk industry, ran a long article on the lectures, emphasizing the remedy: pasteurization at seventy degrees centigrade, which made the milk safe for twenty-four hours; or sterilization at 120 degrees centigrade to kill the bacteria and the spores, thus making milk hermetically sealed in sterilized bottles safe for an indefinite period. The publication did not note the difficulty of implementing these procedures.

The foreign press was less forgiving and more amusing. Some American papers lived up to their reputations. The *Chicago Chronicle* (10 Feb. 1901) warned of "deadly milk in Paris"; and the *New York Herald* (9 Jan. 1901) screamed "poisonous milk" before going on to summarize a scientific lecture that "interested but horrified [the] audience." The *Mexican Herald* took the bland approach: "all Paris is astir over unpleasant revelations regarding … café au lait."[29] Across the channel, the *Westminster Gazette* (14 Jan. 1901) also lamented the blow striking a French institution, "le petit déjeuner with café au lait." A serious approach was clear in the *Daily Telegraph* (12 Jan. 1901), whose headline "Milk and Microbes" hinted at the paper's good coverage of the lectures while also warning people to consume only sterilized milk in Paris. The *Telegraph* made an interesting scientific observation to the effect that some doctors were not so optimistic as Henri and the dairy industry concerning the impossibility for humans to catch tuberculosis from consuming milk and beef products coming from infected cattle. This storm of press coverage extended to Tunis, where *Le Promeneur* (14 Jan. 1901) indulged in a short ironic commentary on the excitement caused by the lectures of "le jeune milliardiare sémite." Back to Jews and billions, nearly always the sinister subtext in such narratives.[30]

The inauguration of Rothschild's Paris polyclinic in 1902 was an impressive media event for the young doctor. The fact that Henri was only thirty years old was nearly as interesting to some journalists as his status of multimillionaire. In addition to the eulogies in the French press, including medical publications, there was flattering foreign coverage. Some articles were brief; some were impressively long, such as that in *Le Petit Parisien* with the touching headline "Pour les enfants." *Le Progrès medical* supported this popular view: the polyclinic was a true children's hospital. Most of the articles appear similar enough to have

29 Undated clipping.

30 Book of press clippings entitled "Comptes rendus de Conférences 1900–01," in Archives de Paris, Perotin/8Roth/77/1 100.

issued from news central, namely the *Agence nationale* for the French press. The *Archive israélite* welcomed Henri's philanthropic creation in a way he might not have found in good taste, but it was proud to make a point in the anti-Semitic climate of the day. "Parisian Judaism can only applaud," for the charitable work showed once again "the truth of the Talmudic adage *Rachmanim b'né Rachmanim* – Jews are a merciful people descended from a merciful people."[31] The *Berliner Tagblatt* carried a picture of "Rothschild's Automobil Ambulanze," which was praised elsewhere as a marvelous electric vehicle; *Le Monde Illustré* also carried a picture of the ambulance. A figure of some minor importance in the history of the automobile, including manufacturing and racing the machine, Henri must have been pleased though not surprised to find coverage in *Auto-vélo*. It is doubtful that Mathilde was thrilled by an article in Marguerite Durand's *La Fronde*, a feminist paper perhaps supported by Rothschild money. Rumor – especially right wing – had it that Gustave de Rothschild was her lover and gave her seven million francs to make her paper a supporter of Dreyfus.[32] Although it was good to have the news in a women's paper, most of the poor women who came to the Rothschild hospitals were not readers of the feminist press; indeed, many probably did not read at all. A Spanish medical publication provided a suitable prose epithalamium for this union of medicine and philanthropy. "A supremely active man, highly cultivated, possessing a heart of inexhaustible generosity, H. Rothschild has put his sharp mind and a large part of his fortune in the service of the poor."[33] On a more prosaic level, Charles Maygrier, *professeur agrégé* and accoucheur at the Charité hospital, praised Henri's "magnificent establishment" in the rue Marcadet.[34]

The opening of the polyclinic, an event grabbing the attention of *le tout Paris* for a moment, put Henri in the company of doctors in the news – "les médecins dont on parle."[35] If you don't get an internship, it is comforting to be able to fall back on becoming medical director of your own spanking new hospital, publicly recognized for its therapeutic modernity and good patient care. Henri could boast of a silver medal from the faculty of medicine, and he could advertise his status as an *Officier d'académie* and a *Chevalier du mérite agricole*. He was also prominent in a standard professional way as a member of the *Société d'obstétrique de Paris*

[31] Undated clipping.

[32] Mary Louise Roberts, "Acting Up: The Feminist Theatrics of Marguerite Durand," in Jo Burr Margadant (ed.), *The New Biography. Performing Femininity in Nineteenth-Century France* (Berkeley, 2000), 212.

[33] Book of press clippings in Archives de Paris, Perotin/8Roth/77/1 100. On 19 October 1902 articles appeared in all the big papers such as *Le Figaro*, *Le Temps*, *Le Soir*, and *Le Journal des Débats*. Foreign coverage included the *New York Herald*, the *Chicago Tribune*, *La Stampa*, and *El Porvenir*. The medical press included *La Gazette médicale* (27 Oct.), *La Médecine française* (1 Jan. 1903), *La Vie médicale* (Jan. 1903), and the *Boletín de la Revista de medicina y cirugia practicas* (28 Oct. 1903).

[34] Charles Maygrier, *Les Consultations de nourrissons* (Paris, 1903), 7.

[35] *La Vie médicale* (Jan. 1903), in Archives de Paris, Perotin/8/Roth/77/1 100.

(1898), an editor at the *Progrès médicale*, and co-editor (1902) of the *Bibliographia medica*, a publication headed by Charles Richet and Marcel Baudoin. Last but not least from a professional viewpoint, Henri was one of the leading experts on infant feeding, widely interpreted, and on setting up organizations to help nursing mothers.[36] So in March 1903 Henri lectured the *Société médicale de Monaco*, presided over by his friend Prince Albert I, on "the question of milk" – the question was multiple, involving the product's safety along with infant feeding. Two days after this talk he gave a warmly applauded talk in Montpellier on the fight against infant mortality, a topic much in the news. By December he was on the stage in the Paris banlieue (Saint-Mandé) to speak at a section of the *Société Républicaine des conférences populaires*: he entertained about 300 people with an account of "genuine diseases." Such a menu would probably include infant diarrhea, tuberculosis, and syphilis – just to name some prevalent Parisian plagues.

In October 1903 Henri stirred up considerable media interest in his report to the Academy of Medicine on a possible cure for infant diarrhea, the great killer of Parisian babies.[37] How to end this Parisian tragedy was the medico-political question of the day – the question was, of course, also a national issue. In an academy session classified as "extra-rapide," Henri reported on an experiment inspired by the work of Ilya Mechnikov and Henri Tissier on milk ferments and intestinal microbes. (Tissier's reputation in medicine has been damaged by the fact that the artist Henri Bellery-Desfontaines (1867–1909) died from typhoid fever caught from oysters slurped chez Dr Tissier.) Floundering around in experimental desperation for a way to increase the human lifespan, Mechnikov finally came up with recommending the consumption of pure cultures of lactic acid bacteria in skim milk products. After Pasteur's classic experiment on lactic acid fermentation, the bacteria aroused considerable scientific and even some medical interest; the bacteria later went on to enological fame as the agent of malolactic fermentation, a subject curiously of little scientific interest to Henri. Georges Hayem and Adolphe Lesage had administered lactic acid ferments to cure certain types of infant diarrhea. Henri's originality was to feed sick infants fat-free milk containing ten percent of pure cultures of lactic acid.

The young Dr Rothschild could boast of his modest success in treating all fourteen of the infants by feeding them the acidified milk. He admitted that this was not a sufficient number of cases to be sure that the cure really worked, and the academy appointed a group to pursue the experiment. Up to that time Henri's other treatments for infant diarrhea were chiefly of a standard antiseptic sort, with a cure rate of about fifty percent. The optimistic Rothschild experimenter enjoyed a long article in *Le Figaro* (14 Oct. 1903) on his "new" treatment. Limited success

---

36 HR, *Les Gouttes de lait. Organisation d'une "Goutte de lait" et d'une "Consultation de nourrissons,"* from the *Revue d'Hygiène et de Médecine infantiles* 1 (1902).

37 *Académie de médecine*, session of 13 octobre 1903; report in the *Gazette des hôpitaux* (15 octobre 1903).

turns out to be the right description for this cure of what is often an infection of the intestines caused by bacteria, viruses, or parasites. Later devotees of lactobacillus, the chief part of the lactic acid bacteria, may see the treatment as a step in the right direction. At the Pasteur Institute after 1888, Mechnikov shared the Nobel Prize (physiology or medicine) in 1908 with Paul Ehrlich, the scientist whose clinical work would excite Henri because it promised a cure for syphilis.[38] In the Third Republic alcohol may have been perceived as "a new social and medical scourge responsible for the defeat [Franco-Prussian war], the Commune and much more," but syphilis was not far behind, at least as a "frightening disease" fraught with potential national disaster.[39]

People who make notable scientific advances are often rewarded with prizes. It is assumed that prizes stimulate research. Sharing this assumption, Henri established two prizes in milk-related research, both of which were awarded by the *Société scientifique d'hygiène alimentaire et d'alimentation rationnelle de l'homme*, founded in 1904. This scientific organization "had as its aim the study and popularization of the best methods of feeding man scientifically and economically as well as the determination of the rules of food hygiene."[40] The interests of the society in food contamination and adulteration along with the connection between nutrition and disease coincided perfectly with Henri's interest in pediatrics. The first prize was for the best work on infant feeding from birth to the age of two years; the second was for the best study on the provisioning of milk in a large city, including hygiene, technology, transport, legislation and regulation, sale, and social economy. In 1905 Henri was the logical choice for rapporteur of the first international congress (Paris) on milk supply and dairy farms.

Medical care was only part of the charitable work Henri supported for working-class Paris. About 1910 he established a *Restaurant populaire économique* in the rue Damrémont (18th arrondissement), near his new hospital. Between 1905 and 1919 the restaurant, housed in a vast shack, served more than four million meals, at forty to ninety centimes each, to construction workers and low-paid employees of the 17th and 18th arrondissements. Later Henri said that the aim of the restaurant was to help the construction workers who were transforming Montmartre into "a modern and elegant quarter."[41] For one franc fifty centimes, a lunch or dinner offered a choice of roast meat, stew, fish, and vegetables with dessert. Wine (not Mouton-Rothschild) sold for thirty centimes a half-liter, half the cost to the restaurant, which gave a profit of up to three hundred francs daily to pay for expenses. Between four and five hundred meals were served daily to workers and low-level employees. The participation of the bank allowed a monthly distribution

---

38 See http://nobelprize.org/nobel_prizes/medicine/laureates/1908/.

39 Quotations from Bertrand Taithe, *Defeated Flesh. Welfare, Warfare and the Making of Modern France* (Manchester, 1999), 238, 208–32.

40 Harry W. Paul, *Bacchic Medicine. Wine and Alcohol Therapies from Napoleon to the French Paradox* (Amsterdam, 2001), 244–5, note 4.

41 HR, *La Lignée*, 85.

of soup with bread and a piece of meat to 25,000 women and old people; Henri vastly increased the distribution number. Coturier ran the restaurant; he came with a recommendation by Duval, the owner-manager of the popular restaurants *Bouillons Duval*. Henri had friends everywhere to give him free advice, good or bad. Free coupons for meals were available in the *mairies* during the Great War, which meant that 674,333 free meals were served during the war in addition to the low-cost meals served. By 1925 the area's new buildings were finished, the workers went off to work in the "fortification" areas recovered by the city after the war, and the restaurant closed. Henri's promotion of adult nutrition continued when he established popular cooperatives selling subsidized meat and fish to workers in Montrouge and automobile workers in Puteaux, who found life expensive at the end of the war. Coturier ran these very successful organizations, which lasted until food prices returned to normal and retailers were forced to follow guidelines established by the Seine *Préfecture de police*.[42]

Henri de Rothschild was a lifelong traveler and travel-writer. In his early professional life some of these trips, his *voyages scientifiques*, were medical investigations, often carried out with governmental approval. One of his most interesting trips was a tour of pediatric establishments in Berlin, St. Petersburg, Moscow, Vienna, and Budapest. Henri's pediatric patron, Budin, head accoucheur at the venerable hospital *La Maternité*, seems to have come up with the idea of the trip. As dean of the faculty of medicine in Paris, Paul Brouardel was able to get Henri sent on an "official mission" by the minister of the interior, thus facilitating the trip by providing a governmental umbrella to cover the information gathering. On his return to Paris, Henri published (1897) what he modestly called his notes on the public health and protection of children in the cities he visited. The notes are a marvelous medical document that tells us a great deal about different medical systems and pediatric practices at the end of the nineteenth century.[43]

In reflecting on the hospital establishments he visited in Germany, Russia, and the Habsburg Empire, Henri concluded that they differed in three essential ways. First, in the area of internal organization of the hospitals and hospices, St. Petersburg and Moscow were the leaders to be imitated. From a scientific point of view, Berlin and Vienna were leading, but Berlin beat out Vienna because the medical facilities in Berlin were more up to date, better integrated, and better laid out for teaching. None of the sites visited came up to snuff in the artificial feeding of infants, though Berlin and Vienna were more successful than the Russian cities in reducing infant mortality rates. Henri hoped that the spread of the proper use

42 HR, *La Lignée*, 87.

43 HR, Notes *sur l'hygiène et la protection de l'enfance d'après des études faites à Berlin, Saint-Petersbourg, Moscou, Vienne et Budapest* (Paris, 1897). Henri reprinted as an appendix the preface to Karl Rauchfuss (1835–1915), *Die Kinderheilanstalten* (Tübingen, 1882) with a reference to Gerhardt, *Handbuch fuer Kinderheilkunde und Hygiene*; I can find reference only to Carl Gerhardt, *Handbuch der Kinderkrankheiten* (6 vols, Tübingen, 1877–89).

of both sterilized and "maternalized" milk (processed to resemble mother's milk) would reduce death rates. Russia was the most backward in this area; its emphasis on a system of wet nurses was all very well, but it needed the complement of an artificial feeding system, much like the model found in *La Maternité* in Paris. Nearly a century later a historian of public health in Russia noted that "At the beginning of the twentieth century, the Russian Empire was an extremely unhealthy place in which to live … This was especially true of European Russia." When asked the question "What is the sanitary state of Russia?", Professor N. A. Veliaminov, chief physician of the imperial household, replied "dismal."[44] Henri gave more benign answers concerning the health of a potential French ally against the Second Reich.

Biography may be patchwork, tacking "together pieces of stuff with torn edges," but the medical biographer hopes to trim the edges and give the reader a satisfactory treatment of a major part of the subject's life.[45] I believe that Henri is the most important figure in Rothschild medical history. In addition to following the family's tradition of medical philanthropy, Henri took a unique step in becoming a physician. After his father's death in 1881, his mother steered him towards a medical career, particularly by immersing him in doctors' routines and having him observe the practices of her children's hospital at Berck-sur-Mer. Henri's influence on medicine in Paris lay chiefly in the establishment of a modern hospital in the north of Paris. His prolific output of written work and promotion of good infant care established him as a significant figure in the development of pediatrics, even if he remained outside the faculty medical establishment. Like his mother and wife, Henri did his duty in the Great War. In the radically changed post-war world he kept his medical career alive, in particular in maintaining and expanding his Paris hospital. Nor did he neglect his theatrical activities, some of which had earlier stirred up controversy as a result of his treatment of hot topics like women doctors and medical ethics.

We have recently come to recognize the close interaction at many levels of medicine and literature. The Third Republic in the late nineteenth and early twentieth centuries provides us with a striking period of Hippocratic theater. Unlike Jules Romains' perennial favorite *Knock* (1923), Henri's plays have not survived on the stage, but in their day they were notorious enough to attract good audiences and get excellent press coverage. And the issues he dealt with are, mutatis mutandis, still with us. In the 1930s Henri thought he could definitively move away from the influence of medicine on his writing. He was wrong. In the play *Circé* he found that creating an emotionally flawed character required more medicine rather than less.

---

44 John F. Hutchinson, *Politics and Public Health in Revolutionary Russia, 1890–1918* (Baltimore, 1990), 5.

45 Quotation from Lucasta Miller, "Missing Pieces," *The Times Literary Supplement* (26 June 2009), 4, in which Virginia Woolf's idea of biography as patchwork is mentioned.

Henri's last decade was ruined by illness and wartime exile from France. To get some relief from the boredom of *la dolce vita* in Portugal during World War II, he concocted a family history, which never ceased to fascinate him. Being a major figure of Rothschild medicine in France, he took an obsessive interest in its history. It began with James, "le grand baron."

PART I
The Rothschild Family Medical Tradition

Chapter 1
The Hospital that James Mayer ("le grand baron") Built

> *Tsedaqah* can be performed only with one's material possessions, *gemilut hasadim* both in kind and in personal service.[1]

The Rothschilds have a distinguished reputation in the establishment of medical facilities for the needy, particularly in building clinics and hospitals in Jerusalem, Frankfurt, Vienna, London, Berck-sur-Mer, and Paris.[2] James Mayer, Adolphe, and Henri make up the trinity of great Rothschild medical providers in Paris. On 26 May 1852, a colorful and newsworthy event took place in the somber rue de Picpus (now in the 12th arrondissement), in the east of Paris; the event attracted a crowd of upper crust Parisians who would not usually be found in that part of the city. Among the powerful males present were the minister of public works, the prefect of the Seine, members of the Paris municipal council, the mayor of the 8th arrondissement – before 1860 it included the Picpus quarter – and distinguished representatives of French Jewry. A publication devoted to the critical discussion of important institutions for the poor, the *Annales de la charité*, devoted a full article to the occasion.[3] The festive and also solemnly religious occasion was the opening of another Parisian hospital, but not just any hospital: it was a private hospital, odd enough in Paris, and, even more odd, a Jewish hospital. The founder was James Mayer de Rothschild, a baron after 1822, thanks to his support for Metternich, and often referred to as "le grand baron."

The Rothschild family was adored – nearly in the Catholic sense – for its charitable foundations helping Parisian Jews: aid to women having babies, clothing for poor school children and others in need, placement of young boys

---

1 R. J. Werblowsky and Geoffrey Wigoder (eds), *The Oxford Dictionary of the Jewish Religion* (New York, 1997), 154. The Hebrew word *tsedaqah*, derived from the word for justice, refers to any kind of righteous conduct and in the Talmud it is limited to the giving of alms or assistance (material gifts) to the poor. *Tsedaqah* is a duty, not optional charity.

2 Michael Graetz, *Les Juifs en France au XIX*^e^ *siècle. De la Révolution française à l'Alliance Israélite Universelle* (Paris, 1989), 112–51. Translated from the Hebrew by Salomon Malka. In Vienna the Bettina Frauenspital dates from 1892, but the hospital funded by Anselm goes back to 1869, as does the Evelina Children's hospital in Southwark, funded by Ferdinand.

3 Emile Leguay, "Inauguration de l'hôpital Israélite à Paris," *Annales de la charité*, 8th year (1852): 375–81.

and girls in apprenticeship, with provision of dowries for the girls, and payment of rent for those who needed help. The Rothschild hospital, noted for its big garden and old trees, was located to serve the Jewish immigrants of what are now the 11th, 12th, and 20th arrondissements of eastern Paris. Between 1880 and 1925 about 100,000 Jewish immigrants arrived in France.[4] Given the fact that there were about a quarter of a million foreigners in France by 1911, Jews made up a substantial part of the foreign population. (By 1914 the population of Paris had reached about three million.) The big building, the facade of which faced the rue de Picpus, soon complemented by other structures, replaced the old house of the Jewish community on the rue des Trois-Bornes (11th arrondissement), which was unable to shelter the sick and needy who came asking for help. Originally planned for the installation of 100 beds, by the 1860s the hospital had 150 beds, increasing to 284 by 1885.

The three-storied structure was divided into three pavilions, separated by a transversal building containing the lobby and oratory. The central pavilion housed the administration and the living quarters of the director, the rabbi, and the head doctor. Traditional religious practice prescribed the separation of sexes. The right pavilion was reserved for women: on the ground floor, baths; on the second floor, separate rooms for the treatment of special diseases or for use by paying patients; on the third floor, rooms for ordinary sick women. Men were assigned to the left pavilion, which housed the hospital kitchen and appurtenances on the ground floor, six rooms for special diseases on the second floor, and a dormitory for service personnel on the third floor. A reservoir for 80,000 gallons of water shared the left pavilion. Defining the hospital as modern necessarily included its laboratory and pharmacy. New schemes were introduced to ensure the circulation of air, thereby eliminating potentially toxic miasmas. Care was given to the general distribution of water, including its outside drainage. The interior setup allowed for constant supervision of all services for the sick as well as for the vigilant supervision of the hospital. Even looking at greenery possibly speeds healing, and so it is interesting that older hospitals often included gardens. The hospital on the rue de Picpus included a large garden for patients. The whole of the arrangements designed by the architect could, L. Rosier argued, be fruitfully applied to the big hospitals of Paris. A model institution.[5]

When Rosier wrote his account in 1852 he noted that the hospital did not have its own revenues and was waiting for benefactors. It seemed unwise to leave an establishment of this importance dependent on the caprice of individual donors. An optimistic Rosier thought that Jewish charity was inexhaustible: in Paris alone there were about thirty charitable organizations which were mutual societies but did not limit their generosity to members. A consistorial committee

[4] See Nancy L. Green, *The Pletzl of Paris. Jewish Immigrant Workers in the Belle Epoque* (New York, 1986).

[5] L. Rosier, "Hospice israélite de Paris," *L'Illustration, Journal Universel* (29 mai 1852), 363–4.

provided food, money, and medical care for the poor. It also gave aid to school children, encouraged children who did well in public school, helped parents whose children were apprentices, cared for women delivering babies, looked after old people, orphans, and abandoned children, helped workers, and chipped in for burials. Cradle to the grave care, if you needed it and could get it. Gambling helped. A lottery organized every year by the leading Jewish families supplied about 20,000 francs. So Rosier believed that the hospital would prosper from gifts. Not that there was much chance of the hospital going bankrupt: James Mayer de Rothschild's name was part of the institution, and that was the greatest guarantee of security for the poor needing free medical care. One estimate of the cost of the land, building, and furnishings was about 400,000 francs.[6] And according to one report, "le grand baron" paid approximately 1,300,000 francs annually to ensure the smooth running of the hospital.[7]

A foundation had been set up in 1852 to offer other services to Parisian Jews. It included a homeless shelter with fifty beds and a home for old folks, placed under the director of the hospital. A Rothschild orphanage for 200 persons existed on the nearby rue Lamblardie, in the 12th arrondissement. (After World War II baroness Edouard de Rothschild, who had considerable interest and expertise in dealing with the trials and tribulations of childhood, took control of this institution, which was transferred to the Château de la Guette in Villeneuve-Saint-Denis in 1947.) The foundation supplied the new funds needed to support this growing medical and social welfare enterprise. The French state and the city of Paris smiled appreciatively at this private generosity paying for services which, given a low basis of taxation on the rich and the growing cost of imperial and military dreams, governments could ill-afford. In 1886 the Conseil d'Etat recognized the "public utility" of the Rothschild foundation with its charitable activities. The new wave of immigration in the 1880s made the foundation's work all the more important for the social wellbeing – an optimistic phrase here – of eastern Paris.[8]

A comparison of the inauguration ceremony of James's hospital in 1852 with that of Henri's hospital opening in 1902 and especially the latter's rebuilt and expanded institution in 1929 reveals a striking public religious presence in James's institution that was absent in Henri's. No doubt part of the change can be explained by the role that religion still played in private and public life in the mid-nineteenth century and perhaps some of the change by the nature of the religious beliefs on the part of the principals themselves. Naipaul offers a psychological insight on charitable motives: "[Indar] felt that money had made him holy. All rich people

[6] Rosier, *L'Illustration*, 363–4.

[7] Marine Lefèvre, *Rothschild. Chronique d'un hôpital pas comme les autres, 1743–1999* (Paris, 1999). See also Nicolas Delalande, *La genèse d'un parcours philanthropique: les Rothschild et le cas de l'hôpital israélite (1852–1914)*, "Mémoire de maîtrise, histoire contemporaine," Paris I Panthéon-Sorbonne, 2003.

[8] *La Fondation de Rothschild, 1852–1952* (Paris, 1952).

are like that, I suppose," reflects a morose Kareisha.[9] In 1852 after a religious service in the oratory, with the participation of the chief rabbi, the Consistory of Paris, and representatives of the Central Consistory of Jews of France, and the administration of the Temple, the gathering in the garden enjoyed some further religious discourse by *le grand rabbin*, who emphasized the importance of religion in the healing process. And in this hospital the patient would be comforted by his own religion, by a familiar language, and by the beautiful prayer of the *Schema* that had greeted his entrance into the world. The hospital provided lodgings for a rabbi and an oratory. Albert Cohn, treasurer of the Jewish consistorial aid committee and long the agent for distributing charity from the Rothschild family, added to his inevitable praise of James some praise for the work of the baroness James (Betty), "la première juive de notre époque."[10] Further major discourses would have been anti-climatic, and so heavenly voices chanted the *Hallel*.

The founder himself was immortalized in a marble bust, carved by the well-known chisel of Adam Salomon, and put in the vestibule. Jewish aid societies paid for the bust to show their gratitude to the founder of the hospital. The president of the Paris Consistory, joined by the chief rabbi, presented James with a gold medal on behalf of the Jewish community of Paris. James expressed his gratitude in a few words; the minister of commerce also spoke briefly, and the young poet Eugène Dorville recited some poetry. The sick expressed their gratitude through the director of the hospital, Benoist Cohen, who also led important people on a tour of the hospital, an impressive establishment in size and quality for its day. During the tour people entered their names on an annual list to contribute to the maintenance of the building: conspicuous entries included the Rothschilds for 5600 francs. With the opening of this hospital the tradition of *tsedaqah* had produced one of the most remarkable creative events in the history of French Jews. The public was finally admitted to admire this fine creation of the architect Jean-Alexandre Thierry (1810–90), who had also designed the Temple in Paris.[11]

In his article in *L'Illustration* on the hospital, Rosier dealt with the general significance of this type of charity, including its lack of suitability for French Jews. Charity was, of course, a good thing and had to be defended against cynics: generosity implied magnanimity incompatible with the lower passions, an addiction of the lower classes. The Rothschild name was usually associated with works intended to improve and support the morals of the poor, who were particularly needy in times of public disasters. So far, so good, but what about the sick poor? The Frankfurt Rothschilds built a hospital in their city. In 1795 the

---

9 V. S. Naipaul, *A Bend in the River* (New York, 1979), 242.

10 Graetz, *Les Juifs en France au XIXe siècle*, 143, identifies Albert Cohn as "James's man of confidence ... and his advisor in all Jewish affairs."

11 The entry in E. Bénézit, *Dictionnaire critique et documentaire des peintres, sculpteurs, dessinateurs et graveurs* ..., (new edn, Paris, 1999), 586, identifies Thierry as a "peintre d'architecture, aquarelliste. Architecte, il construit entre autres l'hôtel de Rothschild, avenue Foch à Paris en 1859."

Goldsmid brothers in London opened subscriptions for building a Jews' Hospital (Nevek Zedek), which finally opened in 1807. Salomon Heine established a hospital in Hamburg, and the Berlin municipal council established a hospital for poor Jews. Rosier thought that the establishment of all of these hospitals was a good idea, except for the Parisian Rothschild hospital, which lacked real usefulness in certain regards. This sounds curious. What did he mean? It was understandable that these restricted hospitals existed where Jews did not enjoy civil liberties; forming a people apart, they needed such facilities. In France Jews did not have the same reasons for perpetuating their separation. Other religions in France had their private works but they did not have the exclusive character of the Jewish works. (Before the separation of churches and state in 1905 it was difficult to escape the identification of Catholicism and national identity.) Rosier dismissed as wild exaggerations the stories of deathbed conversions of Jews to Christianity in hospitals. The organization of hospitals, with the domination by doctors, neutralized religious influence, thus making patients confident that their souls were secure in the faith of their fathers.[12]

Rosier regretted that outside France the "race malheureuse et résignée" of Jews did not enjoy the civil and religious freedom they had in France. What he wanted was a complete and genuine fusion of the Jewish race with the great French family. Enlightened Jews had to work towards this goal, which was not encouraged by the founding of institutions like the Rothschild hospital. To maintain a separation between the Jewish community and Christian society justified the existence and perpetuation of the old Jewish condition of exclusion. So Rosier did not welcome the founding of the hospital, the old people's home, and the annex of the hospice. It would have been better for the Paris *Assistance publique* to take control of sick and old Jews. (The Parisian *Assistance publique* came into existence in 1849 as successor to the *Conseil général des hospices*. The *Assistance publique* was the administrative authority for Parisian hospitals, asylums, orphanages, and the home care bureaux; it also had non-public sources of income from gifts and urban and rural properties. Its mission included social aid and public health service on a vast scale. Its director was named by the minister of the interior on a proposition of the prefect of the Seine.[13]) Christians and Jews suffering together would provide evidence of the intimate union of the Jewish community with the nation. Rosier admitted that though the general concept was defective, the hospital would serve French Jews well; and few establishments were so well endowed.

---

[12] Perhaps the Catholic nursing sisters were more concerned with maintaining their own power than in converting Jews. See Jan Goldstein, *Console and Classify. The French Psychiatric Profession in the Nineteenth Century* (Cambridge, 1987), 216–25.

[13] Nathalie Plazanet, *Inventaire des archives de la Guerre 1914–1918* (AP-HP, 603 Foss, Feb. 1989), 2, and Paul Weindling, "From Isolation to Therapy: Children's Hospitals and Diphtheria in Fin de Siècle Paris, London and Berlin," in Roger Cooter (ed.), *In the Name of the Child. Health and Welfare, 1880–1940*, (London and New York, 1992), 127.

By the early twentieth century the hospital of 1852, which had been so carefully furnished with the latest in medical science as well as with the old religious comforts, had become obsolete and far too small to serve its base community. So Edmond de Rothschild, James's youngest son, hired Lucien Bechmann to build a big new hospital (400 beds) on a large piece of property at the angle of the streets Picpus and Santerre.[14] This new paragon of medical science, consecrated by the chief rabbi of France, opened in 1914 under the leadership of Léon Zadoc-Kahn, who, along with Emile Emery, Gaston Picot, and Pierre Ehrhardt, had been among Henri's "camarades d'hôpital." In the Great War the hospital became auxiliary military hospital number 1; in 1915 the hospital was divided into one part of 115 beds for general surgery and a second part to care for soldiers whose faces had been mutilated (*les gueules cassées*). This second part of the hospital was directed by Monestin, a specialist in maxillofacial surgery.[15] The old hospital became a hospice for old people, who were the sole occupants of 76 rue de Picpus after 1919; in 1928 half the edifice was demolished and rebuilt. In 1930 thirteen doctors were in service at the hospital. Toby Gelfand notes that the hospital "gave access to internships to gifted Jewish medical students who faced discrimination in competition for prestigious posts in the Paris hospital network."[16]

During the period 1941–44 the Rothschild establishments were used as places of detention for the old and sick of the concentration camp of Drancy and Jewish patients of public hospitals. Large numbers were deported along with medical and hospital personnel. Zadoc-Kahn, the head doctor at the hospital for thirty-four years, died in the Franco-German deportation of 1942. In 1943 Robert Debré, the only member of the hospital foundation's council remaining in Paris, assumed a sort of general responsibility as administrator of the hospital until he had to flee Paris. The hospital came under close German surveillance.[17] After World War II the hospice had the same financial problems as the hospital, whose budget had risen to 350 millions francs by 1952, when running the four establishments cost the foundation 514,332,000 francs annually. It was time for the public purse to assume a charge that had become too much of a burden for the family, and so the hospital became part of the vast medical empire of the *Assistance publique*. Leading Rothschild family members had carried on the work begun by James in 1852: Alphonse, Edmond, Edmond's wife, Adelaide (1853–1934), Robert

[14] Bechmann (1880–1968), later known for his role in developing the *Cité universitaire*, was the advisory architect of the University of Paris from 1923 to 1953.

[15] See Sophie Delaporte, *Les Gueules Cassées: les blessés de la face de la Grande Guerre* (Paris, 1996) and "Une exposition virtuelle de la Bibliothèque Interuniversitaire de Médecine de Paris," www.bium.univ.paris5.fr. This branch of medicine in World War I is at the core of the film *La Chambre des Officiers* (2001), directed by François Dupeyron.

[16] Toby Gelfand, "25,000 Medical Students: The Medical Thesis in the 19th Century," unpublished paper, 2.

[17] Robert Debré, *L'honneur de vivre. Témoignage* (Paris, 1974), 345.

(1880–1946), and Edouard (1868–1949).[18] In 1954 Guy de Rothschild accepted the symbolic one franc signaling the end of a remarkable chapter in the Rothschild medical adventure in Paris.[19]

Henri was familiar with the establishment and personnel on the rue de Picpus, where he had set up a *Consultation de lait/Consultation de nourrissons* to help mothers and their babies. The hospital itself had a considerable maternity section, which provided some interesting contrasts to the other maternity institutions in Paris. In the late 1920s the maternity section admitted an average of 1400 women with less than 1000 deliveries annually. During World War I this section was the only department to carry on its normal functions, delivering an annual average of 436 babies. Other services were devoted to handling the inexhaustible supply of wounded soldiers. Non-Jewish women made up less than two percent of the patients. Hospital regulations permitted admission of any Jews in Paris and the near suburbs as well as non-Jews in the hospital's circumscription or arrondissement. By 1930 the number of women admitted was up to 1433, which included 981 births, with 943 babies surviving – 19 of the 38 deaths occurred during labor; there were 81 spontaneous abortions, one of which was "therapeutic." Five mothers died.[20] Not a great record but respectable for the period and in comparison with similar patient populations of other institutions in Paris.

Doctors who had been at the hospital for some time before World War I and remained after the war were surprised at the difference in the behavior of most of the women who delivered before 1914 and those who delivered in the 1920s. The origin of patients changed significantly. Before the Great War most of the patients came from pre-1871 Alsace, which had been integrated into the Second Reich. Some patients were from families that had lived in France for generations. Some patients of course came from North Africa, the Balkans, and Turkey. The post-World War I immigrants, most of whom settled in Paris, came from Poland, Russia, Hungary, Rumania, and Salonika. Although the children were rapidly Frenchified, the more recent arrivals seem to have slowed up the process of cultural assimilation endured by their predecessors. Henri A. Victor regretted that one of the major differences evident in the latest group was that they had a "different perception of

---

18 *Paris charitable, bienfaisant et social* (new edn, 1936) carried the following entry: Hôpital-Fondation de Rothschild, 15 rue de Santerre, XIIe arrondissement. Gratuit pour malades israélites de Paris et malades indigents du voisinage. Médecine générale, chirurgie, maternité.

19 The number of people treated and cared for in the different Rothschild institutions for the entire period up to 1951 are given in *La Fondation de Rothschild, 1852–1952*:

Hospital: sick hospitalized in 100 years — 213,761

Hospice: *pensionnaires* in 100 years – 4565

Orphanage: orphans after1874 – 1853

Sanatorium: sick treated – 1482.

20 Henri-A. Victor, *La maternité de l'hôpital de Rothschild. Son fonctionnement jusqu'en 1930* (thesis, Paris Faculty of Medicine, 1931).

pain." He thought that French women supported pain better than Slavic women. The more Frenchified the woman, the more courageously she supported the pain of childbirth. Perhaps the degree of assimilation of Jewish women determined the degree to which they adopted French endurance or remained anchored to "Slavic and Eastern pusillanimity."

Moving to a different order of ideas, Victor wondered if these emigrants "represent the Semitic type at its most pure." He did not think so, meaning that their different perception of pain was not Jewish but was rather characteristic of the "Slavic race"; Jews and Slavs had interbred, it seemed. The conclusion of this reasoning was that it was medically difficult to prove that "the Semitic race does not conform to the typical data of obstetrics." Victor believed that the reason for the different behavior of recent immigrants was to be found in their social situation, in their difficult lives, dominated by a poverty that left them in a weak state of resistance. So their physiological wretchedness explained why they were unable to hold up during labor, that is, unable to keep "pushing" until the end of the birth process, thus forcing the doctor to use forceps. And statistics comparing the Rothschild hospital with the maternity departments of Baudelocque and Boucicaut did show much higher Rothschild use of forceps: in 8.15 percent of the deliveries for the period 1915–30, compared with 4.71 percent for Baudelocque during 1921–27 and 3.48 percent for Boucicaut during 1924–28.[21] Purists might complain about the lack of agreement of periods, but doctors could argue that the figures supported what they knew from long experience.

One surgical procedure provided by the Rothschild hospital not generally found in other hospitals was circumcision of male babies, which was done on the eighth day if the baby weighed at least 3000 grams and had no health problems. An additional 254 circumcisions were done on babies not born in the hospital; the mothers of these babies stayed with them in the hospital for twenty-four hours. There is no record of the deliverance of certificates of female virginity, a procedure that was not much more than a reasonable guess on the part of the doctor, though this parental fantasy was still around in the early twentieth century.[22]

Other figures were roughly the same for the three Parisian maternity departments, though with a considerably lower rate of syphilis and albuminuria (proteinuria) at Rothschild. There were also fewer cesareans over a five-year period in the late twenties. Since abortion was illegal, the treatment of women who had aborted their fetuses made doctors a bit uneasy. Victor thought that it was generally difficult to provide evidence of the cause and to get women to confess to a criminal abortion: in fact, less than two percent of the cases. Most cases aroused the suspicions of doctors, and at the other two maternity institutions it was claimed that the cause was established in about twenty-five per cent of the

[21] Victor, *La maternité de l'hôpital de Rothschild*, 81–2.

[22] Victor, *La maternité de l'hôpital de Rothschild*, 11–12. On the medical difficulty of certifying virginity, see "Sur la délivrance des certificats de virginité," *Annales d'hygiène publique et de médecine légale*, 4th series, 6 (1906): 181–2.

cases. The social-legal difficulty created for doctors (and women) by the anti-abortion legislation would remain a permanent feature of French life until well into the Fifth Republic.[23]

Sometimes forgotten in accounts of Rothschild medical enterprises are the institution founded by the baroness Adelheid (Addy), wife of Edmond, and the eye hospital founded by Adolphe de Rothschild. In 1926 Adelaide established a sanatorium for women suffering from pulmonary tuberculosis, initially seventy-five in number, at Hauteville in the Ain. Tuberculosis was one of the big killers of the poor, especially immigrants.[24] Adolphe, after having had a piece of metal removed from an eye by a doctor in Geneva, decided to build a small hospital in the 19th arrondissement (near the Parc des Buttes-Chaumont), devoted to ophthalmology.[25] In 1894 the sum of 1.5 million francs was established for construction, with 250,000 francs for maintenance, which required 10 million in capital. Though he died early in 1900, Adolphe's will provided for the building of the hospital; and the baroness Julie faithfully carried out the mission of creating a model medical establishment, which opened in 1905, two years before she died.[26] Desmarres would have been the director had he not died; A. Trousseau got the job. The architects made an effort to implement Adolphe's original ideas about incorporating what had been learned in medical practice into a building that functioned according to the latest advances in ophthalmology. Insofar as possible, Chatenay and Rouyre sacrificed their architectural egotism to medical needs. Devotees of medical architectural classicism were surprised by the abundance of light and air and the suppression of the classic dark room. Economy was also the rule, so that the money intended to

---

23 Medicalized abortion became legal on 17 January 1975, thanks in large part to the efforts of the minister of health, Simone Veil, a survivor of Auschwitz.

24 The first French sanatorium opened in 1896, and before long there were about thirty establishments for the treatment of tuberculosis, including five big ones on Mannian magic mountains, treating 2500 patients. See *La Fondation de Rothschild, 1852–1952*, and Pierre Baudin and Dr. L. Nass, *La Rançon du progress* (Paris, 1909), 4e partie, I, "La tuberculose, maladie sociale." Green, *The Pletzl of Paris*, 127–8, noted that TB was "the most common work-related disease." There were 120,000 workers in the clothing industry.

25 *Fondation ophtalmologique Adolphe de Rothschild*, 29 rue Manin, 19th arrondissement, sometimes referred to as *L'Institut ophtalmologique des Buttes-Chaumont.* Entry in *Paris charitable, bienfaisant et social* (published by *L'Office central des œuvres de bienfaisance*, new edn, 1936).

26 "Legs d'Adolphe de Rothschild," *La revue philanthropique* 7 (1900): 250–1; 8 (1900–01): 751–2; see also "Le testament de Mme Adolphe de Rothschild," *La revue philanthropique* 22 (1905): 397–8. Her bequests totaled 8,000,000 francs, including 2,000,000 for the *Comité israélite de bienfaisance* (Paris). The early 1900s (1901–06) were a bonanza period in French philanthropy, with about 380 million francs being given to public institutions and establishments of "public utility." The biggest gifts were those of Mme Hirsch (23,000,000) in 1901, M Galien (8,250,000), and M de Pierrecourt (5,4000,000), both in 1903. Female religious orders also received nearly 6,000,000 francs between 1901 and 1906. See *La revue philanthropique* 22 (1907–08): 357–63.

serve the sick would not be wasted on architectural frivolities. There were sixty-two beds and a bacteriological laboratory, installed as a diagnostic room that could also serve as a research laboratory. A library contained the chief works and journals in ophthalmology. Moulage was not neglected: a collection of wax models showed serious eye diseases as they really looked. The operating room boasted of having the big Volkmann electromagnet, and the annex sterilization room ended in a cul-de-sac. The hospital was open to everyone suffering from curable eye diseases, regardless of their religion or nationality, if they could prove their need or their poverty. Paying patients were not accepted.[27] Edmond, a victim of blindness after his mid-seventies, was a strong supporter of this hospital.

France has an excellent reputation for providing free medical and social aid for mothers and babies. The Rothschild hospitals were always keenly aware of the social importance of this kind of aid. An *Œuvre d'assistance médico-sociale* with two assistants was provided by an annex of James's hospital; this charitable society communicated with the hospital's *Dispensaire anti-tuberculeux* in the case of tubercular mothers and babies. Mothers could be sent to the sanatorium *L'Espérance* at Hauteville with their babies taken care of by the *Placement familial des tout petits* and the *Œuvre Grancher*. Fuchs notes that the Rothschild hospital before the 1880s was one of only three Parisian institutions to house single pregnant women; its sixteen beds for indigent Jewish women did not distinguish between single and married states.[28] The *Œuvre des femmes en couches* handled all problems connected with infant feeding; if the feeding were not free, the parents were found to be more interested in their children. And a cradle with layette was available from the *Comité français de secours aux enfants*, if the woman was particularly deserving of such help. *Crèches*, *asiles*, and *garderies* existed to take care of babies when their mothers were sick.[29] In 1893 the *Assistance publique* received a "magnificent gift" of one (some sources say one and a half) million francs in the name of Bettina de Rothschild (1858–92), the daughter of Mayer Alphonse (1827–1905). Bettina had married Salomon Albert (1844–1911) in 1876. This money allowed the *Assistance publique* to distribute 36,000 francs annually in sums of 10 to 50 francs to single women leaving the maternity wards with babies. No religious, social, civil, or any other requirement had to be fulfilled. If needed, governmental and charitable care from cradle to crèche was provided for children, and mothers were not so badly cared for either. Henri's father, James Edouard, pioneered in providing medical care for sick Parisian children; Henri dedicated his medical thesis to his memory as "founder of the Rothschild hospital at Berck-sur-Mer."

---

27 A. Trousseau, *La Fondation ophtalmologique Adolphe de Rothschild* (Paris, 1905).

28 Rachel Ginnis Fuchs, *Poor and Pregnant in Paris: Strategies for Survival in the Nineteenth Century* (New Brunswick, NJ, 1992), 106.

29 Victor, *La maternité de l'hôpital de Rothschild*, 84–6.

Chapter 2
The Rothschild Children's Hospital at Berck-sur-Mer

> All those canes, braces and crutches, and not a single glass eye, wooden leg or toupee.
>
> George Bernard Shaw, after observing cast-off objects in Lourdes.[1]

Like alcohol, water has always had a therapeutic role in medicine: marine hydrotherapy and balneotherapy (spa baths in water with high mineral content) have been in western medicine since time immemorial. Taking the waters became big business in Europe, to the profit of spas, hotels, and doctors. The big revival of marine hydrotherapy or seaside cures took place in eighteenth-century England. The nineteenth-century word thalassotherapy describes the therapeutic use of seawater in a beach climate. Giving a treatment a Latin or especially a Greek name enhances its medical, financial, and, possibly, its therapeutic value. In 1791 John Coakley Lettsom founded the General Sea Bathing Infirmary in Margate, on the Isle of Thanet. Doctors scribbled learned treatises, the most famous being by Richard Russell (1687–1759), "the booster of Brighton," as Roy Porter called him. Relying on the universal medical dogma of "no pain, no gain," the doctrines of hydropathy became popular with the English elite.[2] In Jane Austen's novel *Persuasion*, "Dr Shirley, after his illness … declares … that coming to Lyme [Regis] for a month, did him more good than all the medicines he took; and that

---

[1] Of the thousands of sick people who go annually to Lourdes, there are only about fifty who are declared cured. A medical bureau has inquired into thousands of cases to find 2000 cases of unexplained cures and sixty-six miracles (decided by kosher Catholic authorities). Henri Trinc, "Toutes les douleurs mènent à Lourdes," *Le Monde* (14 August 2004).

[2] Roy Porter, *The Greatest Benefit to Mankind. A Medical History of Humanity* (New York, 1998), 267–8, 392–3. Hydropathy was the new version of medical healing waters introduced by the Austrian Vincent Priessnitz (1799–1851) and imported into nineteenth-century England by Drs James Gully and James Wilson; Wilson published the very successful *The Water Cure in Chronic Disease* (1848). Dr A. B. Granville was a prolific scribbler on spas and such: *The Spas of England, and principal sea-bathing places* (London, 1841); *The Spas of Germany* (London, 1839); and *The Mineral Springs of Vichy* (London, 1859). Gwen Robyns, *The Mystery of Agatha Christie* (New York, 1978), 31, notes the fact that ill health had long been big business in Torquay; Dr Charles Radclyffe-Hall praised the climate's beneficial effect on consumptives.

being by the sea, always makes him feel young again."[3] The Germans had their establishments in the Baltic. In the second half of the nineteenth century marine cures spread in some Italian states and in France. Between 1847 and 1878 about 9000 persons were treated at a small hospital in Cette (Sète) in the Hérault. Forges and Saint-Malo also enjoyed the profits of marine cures, but it was Berck-sur-Mer in the Pas-de-Calais that rose to thalasso-therapeutic fame.[4]

The Healing Waters of Berck

The town of Berck-sur-Mer had become so famous by the early twentieth century that it earned several columns in that great work of collective genius *La Grande Encyclopédie*. The article on Berck was signed by one of the great republican physician-politicians of the day, Désiré-Magloire Bourneville.[5] The first *Guide Michelin* (1900) gave the population of Berck-sur-Mer as 5787. Known for its winter herring- fishing industry, Berck was also a seaside resort, with Berck-Plage (two km from Berck) attracting lots of swimmers in the summer, though the beach, offering sixteen km of fine sand, struck Bourneville as sad and monotonous. But Berck enjoyed an advantage over most other beaches: it was, as the popular phrase put it, a place for "miraculous cures" of people suffering from various forms of non-pulmonary tuberculosis. Two "variants of the tubercle bacillus … commonly parasitize man (*Mycobacterium tuberculosis hominis* and *bovis*). It [the bacillus] can involve almost any organ or tissue of the body…" Young American and European children suffered from a higher proportion of bone and joint tuberculosis and of tubercular meningitis than adults.[6] The rational explanation of Berck's healing powers took note of the salubrity of the sea air, constantly refreshed by an eternally blowing southwest wind. The sun was not ignored: heliotherapy required patients to lie nude on beds in the "galeries de cure maritime."

There were sanatoria at different points on the northern coast – Hendaye, Saint-Pol, and Roscoff, for example; so what explained the superiority of Berck, advertised as an international winter and summer station for adults and children?

---

[3] Jane Austen, *Persuasion* (1817; New York, 2003), 99.

[4] Caron Lise, *L'hôpital maritime de Berck-sur-Mer: des origines à 1914*. ("Mémoire de maîtrise," institution not listed, 2000/01), 9, 193–209 (sources).

[5] Albin Rousselet also collaborated on the article, *La Grande Encyclopédie* (3rd edn, n.d. [1886–1902]), 6: 277–80; On Bourneville, see Jan Goldstein, *Console and Classify. The French Psychiatric Profession in the Nineteenth Century* (Cambridge, 1987), 361–7. On Berck see also Marcel Fosseyeux, *Les grands travaux hospitaliers ,1903–1911. Hôpital maritime de Berck-sur-Mer, 1861–1911* (Paris, 1911), and Michèle and Guy Crépin, *Un hôpital crée une ville. L'hôpital maritime de Berck-sur-Mer, Assistance publique – Hôpitaux de Paris de sa création jusqu'en 1920* (Berck, 1999).

[6] John Walton and others (eds), *The Oxford Medical Companion* (Oxford, 1994), 977.

Why did doctors of the hospital empire of the Parisian *Assistance publique* and, eventually, doctors of all of France and other parts of the world, send their patients suffering from scrofula, anemia, lymphadenitis (inflammation of the lymph nodes), coxalgia, Pott's disease, rickets, osteitis, or cysts to Berck-sur-Mer? François Calot, exuding the confidence resulting from years of successful practice in most of the medical establishments of Berck, noted that nature had created the ideal environment for the treatment and cure of the most seriously ill patients.[7] The marine cure at Berck was superior because of the salt particles in the air. Armand Gautier, the chemist who could answer nearly any question, did an analysis finding a beneficial trace of sea salt in the air. And, added an informed Calot, the salt, ionized by its recent drying, was endowed with electrical properties making its therapeutic action more powerful as it penetrated the bronchial tubes and blood of those breathing the air. Some doctors advocated drinking about half a glass of seawater daily; others just settled for the seawater to be used in making bread or cooking shrimp. Two physicists declared the air of Berck-sur-Mer to be twice as pure as forest air and ten times as pure as mountain air. Add to this marine power the increased strength of the sun on the beach: the intense sunshine, reflected by the water and white sand, was rich in ultra-violet waves, powerful destroyer of pathogens. The physicists found only four bacteria per cubic meter of air on Berck beach, whereas they found eight in the forest at Fontainebleau, forty in Chamonix (mountain), and who could count them in Paris, where the number varied according to the time of day from 172,000 to 9 million. According to Calot, it was well known that scrofula was rarer in the Pas-de-Calais than anywhere else in France: 118/100,000 as compared with 2809/100,000 in the Nord, an adjoining department.[8] Not that a physician would give all the credit for miraculous cures to nature, and Calot noted the important role of medical expertise in good establishments, including hospitals, lodgings, and entertainment. The doctors were also specialists in treating the diseases of the patients who came to Berck. Calot argued that the methods by which they obtained superior results were also less invasive and gentler than the methods used by ordinary doctors. (Calot, who now appears in texts as a great specialist in surgery with a conservative approach, created his own

[7] F. Calot, *Berck. Ses méthodes de traitement et son climat idéal pour les malades* (Paris, 1914; 4th edn, 1929; 5th edn, 1933). Talks at Dusseldorf, Congress of Rome, and Congress of Saint Sebastian. Pott's disease, tuberculosis of the spine, which can lead to deformities if not treated, is transmitted in cow's milk; coxalgia describes pain in the (tubercular) hip joint.

[8] Scrofula: a word whose meaning has changed with the understanding of the nature of tuberculosis itself; at Berck the meaning also changed but generally referred to tuberculosis of the bones and joints, lymph nodes, and skin (scrofuloderma); now, according to *The New Shorter Oxford Dictionary*, scrofula refers to tuberculosis of the lymph nodes, particularly in the neck, giving rise to abscesses. See Henri Cazin, *De l'influence des bains de mer sur la scrofula des enfants* (Paris, 1885); the work won the *Prix Capuron* of the *Académie de médecine*.

hospital in 1901.) Any doubters could always be silenced by quoting from one of the German authorities who had visited Berck. Georg Joachimstal, professor in Berlin, declared: "What is being done in France at Berck for the treatment of sick children is quite simply admirable."[9]

Part of the explanation why Berck developed a large-scale government hospital, where thousands of children were treated over the years, and a smaller Rothschild establishment is that Berck was easily accessible from Paris in the railway age. (Berck is about 230 km from Paris.) The low cost of transport of patients was important for the *Assistance publique*. The history of the hospital may be divided, Caron Lise argues, into two big periods: 1856–91, an empirical period emphasizing the cure of sun and salt (helio-marine) under the pioneers Paul Perrochaud and Henri Cazin; and after 1891, when a surgical and orthopedic school developed under Calot and Victor Ménard. With the *Assistance publique* committed to supporting its Berck establishment as a model, the hospital enjoyed the introduction of such modern conveniences as running water, electricity, and telephone service. As procrustean chronologies go, this is as good as any. From the medical viewpoint, it is of some importance that the doctors of Berck discovered that there is a long cycle in the evolution of tuberculosis in bones and ganglions – invasion, destruction, and repair of tissues – which must occur before a cure takes place or, rather, before the doctor guides the evolution of the disease in the direction of a cure. Along with the growth of the hospital, the town itself grew from 2703 inhabitants in 1861 to 8813 in 1911. A real hospital-city.[10]

In a circuit lecture, "Twenty five years of practice at Berck," Calot advertised Berck as a "cité sanitaire," the equal of the Mayo clinic in Rochester, "the last [American] word in the industrialization of surgery." Long before Rochester's growth, Berck was "a true city of the sick," meaning "a city of cures." At the *Hôpital des Enfants-Malades* in Paris a monthly consultation of personnel decided which children to send to Berck. Doctors everywhere appreciated the "Ecole de Berck." Having this "national treasure" gave France a good reputation. Medical students who trained at Berck produced twenty-four works, including theses. (There is one woman in the list: Mlle Kohan.) Dr François Regnault praised Calot for his thirty years of labor in keeping the French school of orthopedics in the first rank. Much orthopedic work came to be done without surgery. Among the courses and books coming out of the Berck school, the most famous was Calot's indispensable *L'Orthopédie*, in a ninth edition by 1929 and translated into five languages. So instead of always singing the praises of rich American foundations,

---

[9] Quoted on the title page of Calot, *Berck. Ses méthodes de traitement et son climat idéal pour les maladies*. With Dr Dollinger, Georg Joachimstal was the author of the canonical *Handbuch der orthopädischen Chirurgie* (4 vols, Jena, 1905–07).

[10] Lise, *L'hôpital maritime de Berck-sur-Mer*, 46–7, 179.

which appeared on the scene much later than the Berck school, writers should pay more attention to the Berckian Wellville.[11]

For the unfortunate sick Parisians who could not get to Berck, there was the *Clinique de Paris* on the Quai d'Orsay, well enough known for medical bigwigs to tour its facilities during the meetings of medical congresses. Cases of pulmonary tuberculosis, especially patients with fever, were not accepted at Berck because they deteriorated in the very conditions good for the treatment of other diseases. These patients could go to a magic mountain, the Mediterranean, or places like Arcachon (Aquitaine). The *Clinique d'Angelès-Gazost* (Hautes-Pyrénées), with its baths of sulfurous waters, was excellent for lymphatic patients and patients with chests sensitive to infection. One germ could produce many medical specialities, and few parts of France did not possess their own version of Wellville.

The Maritime Hospital of the City of Paris

In 1931, when Berck received the sixth international congress of thalassotherapy, Berck-Plage had become a widely known ocean cure station with an impressive medical establishment. The politicians eagerly promoted this medical version of Lourdes by the sea.[12] How had this wild, isolated, desolate area been transformed into a paradise worthy of Asclepius? How did a large hospital of the *Assistance publique* get established at Berck for the poor, sick, and often crippled children of Paris, who were brought to the beach and were often transformed into more or less healthy creatures, at least until they returned home? The hospital was exclusively for the treatment of children suffering from chronic diseases such as scrofula and rickets, with a special aim of submitting the tubercular children of Paris to the famous maritime treatment. According to Bourneville, the idea of this special application of the maritime cure came from Dr Lhoste in Saint-Malo, who in 1846 asked the general council of Paris hospitals (*Assistance publique*) to send him ten boys and ten girls for treatment. A successful experiment permitted the cured children to return to Paris after three months. Nothing much more seems to have happened until 1857, when Paul Perrochaud (1816–79), doctor of the hospice *Enfants-Assistés* at Montreuil-sur-Mer (*Assistance publique*), renewed the experiment by sending some seriously afflicted children to the widow Duhamel

---

[11] Calot, *Berck. Ses méthodes de traitement et son climat idéal pour les malades*, 87–92.

[12] According to a brochure, written with the help of the doctors of Berck, put out by the Syndicat d'initiative de Berck-Plage, *Berck-Plage. Station orthopédique internationale d'hiver et d'été (8000 lits)*, in 1929 patients with the following diseases were treated in Berck: Pott's disease, 1775; coxalgia, 1070; cervical adenopathy, 700. The city of Paris hospital had 1100 beds for children and treated 400 adult patients in another Berck establishment. The town could handle about 3300 patients in its hospitals and sanatoria; every year 7000 new patients showed up.

(Marie-Anne Marseille, died in 1860), who took care of the children, transporting them twice a day from Groffliers for bathing and changing of dressings. Perrochaud concluded after trials at Sète and Saint-Malo that there would be benefits from marine therapy. In 1857 he and Dr Frère sent the good news to Henri Davenne (1789–1869), director of the *Assistance publique*, 1849–59. A doctor of the *Bureau de Bienfaisance* (Hôtel-Dieu hospital), Perrochaud became head of "the little wooden hospital" and went to Berck three times weekly while continuing to live at Montreuil-sur-Mer. During renovations at the Hôtel-Dieu he sent some patients to Berck for Paul Longavesne to take care of; he called the attention of colleagues to the good results. Perrochaud, brother-in-law of Cazin, a local doctor, became the supervising physician and moved to the big hospital when it opened in 1869. Cazin came to assist him in 1872.[13] Suffering from terrible gout, "papa Pocho" died in 1879, and Cazin took over as director.

The two doctors had been amazed and puzzled by the cures they saw, especially of those children in the care of Madame Duhamel. Perrochaud was satisfied with the progress of some seriously afflicted children turned over to Duhamel in 1856. Madame or the widow Brillard, Marie-Anne Bouville ("la célèbre Marianne-toute-seule") took over in 1859 (or 1858, according to Lise). Her salary was 240 francs a month per child, sixteen times the reimbursement of Duhamel, which indicates the growing importance of Berck to the *Assistance publique*. Seventy-six percent of the seventy-two children treated in 1860–1 were reported as cured.[14] After Perrochaud reported on results, Armand Husson, the director (1859–70) of the *Assistance publique*, sent three nursing sisters to Berck in 1860 to take charge of a medical service installed in a private house. The *Assistance publique*, accepting the "quasi-miracles" and hoping to produce more, bought three hectares of land in 1860 for 6000 francs and put up some wooden barracks or huts that came to be called "Le petit Berck." This small hospital at Berck-Plage, inaugurated on 8 July 1861, had fifty beds for boys and fifty for girls. Perrochaud became head of the miracle machine. It was the first marine sanatorium in France. Between 1861 and 1868, 549 children were sent to Berck-sur-Mer and 529 were hospitalized; in 1867 alone the number treated was 190, dropping to 181 in 1868. Over 87 percent of the 549 were eventually released as cured. In December 1865 the two children's hospitals in Paris sent 380 scrofulous children. News of the success of the "marine treatments" had reached the Empress Eugénie, who perhaps had as much interest in the medical part of the cures as in their possibly miraculous implications. She feared that the prince imperial was showing the first signs of coxalgia. As a result

[13] Cazin's father, a military surgeon, settled as a doctor at Boulogne-sur-Mer. Cazin replaced his father at Boulogne and married Amélie Perrochaud in 1864. Cazin won the Hugier prize in 1890 for his work on women's diseases. He was a poet and, like Henri de Rothschild, a playwright.

[14] Lise, *L'hôpital maritime de Berck-sur-Mer*, 188.

of her interest, two medical pashas of Paris arrived at Berck in 1861 to check out the reports sent to the *Assistance publique* by Perrochaud.

Their favorable medical report impressed Eugénie so much that she visited Berck in 1864.[15] More important for Berck was her support of the efforts of the city of Paris to expand the hospital. Several hundred beds were added to the small original establishment of the *Assistance publique*. At the end of 1869 the *Hôpital Maritime*, capable of admitting 700 children, was inaugurated with the empress present. The visit (July 1869) of the empress with her entourage (including Haussmann, prefect of the Seine, who had to approve the project) and *le petit prince*, for the inauguration of the *Hôpital Napoléon* with a well- lubricated banquet, held in one of the hospital gymnasiums, cost 4500 francs plus transport.

Another medical success? Yes, and that gave rise to a serious problem. Bourneville declared that the results gave the administration (*Assistance publique*) the unfortunate idea of buying nine hectares on which to erect a solid brick building, designed by the architect Emile Lavezzari. In 1869 an impressive hospital of 584 beds opened at a cost of over three and a quarter million francs.[16] (The *Assistance publique* eventually bought thirty-five hectares and twenty-seven ares of land for 141,084 francs.) A monument illustrating the pharaonic mentality of the *Assistance publique*? Monumental, expensive, and mediocre? Yes, lamented the critics. One of the finest jewels of the *Assistance publique*? Was money to help the sick poor and children well spent? Yes, sang the chorus of official defenders and some others. In spite of the warnings of locals and of maritime engineers, the hospital was built on an unstable part of the beach; in the period 1869–77 the sea advanced sixty meters onto the land, leaving only twenty-five meters between the building and high tide. Very expensive measures had to be taken to fend off an aggressive sea. This meant that the price per bed went up from the initial cost of 5500 to 6500 francs by 1878, when it was estimated that another quarter of a million francs was needed for protection.

Bourneville thought that economically and materially the building was not worth saving, though he noted the great importance of the establishment for the sick children of Paris. Between 1869 and 1882, doctors treated 5847 children, of whom 4602 were classified as tuberculous and 1482 as scrofulous; of the rest, 776 had osteitis, 619 coxalgia, and 554 Pott's disease. The rate of cure was 75 percent, with an average stay of over a year; with about 70 percent leaving as cured after about a year. Bourneville noted that there were "only" 339 deaths compared with 3321 cures; he noted not the death rate but the cure rate of 70.7 percent – the

15 Jules Bergeron and René Marjolin, *Rapport sur les résultats obtenus dans le traitement des enfants scrofuleux à l'hôpital de Berck-sur-Mer* (Paris, 1866).

16 Among the works of Emile Lavezzari (died 1887) were the hospital and a chalet at Berck-sur-Mer, a hospital in Abbeville, a distillerie in Maison-Alfort, the Gare maritime in Boulogne-sur-Mer, and a hôtel particulier at 58 rue du Rocher (8th arrondissement). See Anne Dugast and Isabelle Parizet, *Dictionnaire par noms d'architectes des constructions élevées à Paris aux XIXe et XX*e *siècles* (3 vols, Paris, n.d.), III.

Rothschild hospital claimed a cure rate of 94.9 percent. Each patient stayed an average of 423 days. The budget of 1888 had money (335,800 francs) for 104 beds for Petit-Berck (1861) and 606 beds for Grand-Berck (1869) as the two institutions were now called; boys and girls had an equal number of beds. In 1887 mortality was 21 boys and 11 girls; 358 boys and 308 girls were admitted; 235 boys and 230 girls were cured, with 107 of both sexes improved or released on demand; 14 children remained in the same state. Scabies afflicted 140 children.[17] The medical industry in Berck would flourish as long as Paris produced sick children. A rosy future then, back in 1869 and also in 1900.

In the beginning the wives of fishermen would wheel the sick children, most of whom were Parisian wards of the *Assistance publique*, onto the beach, where they would be left stretched out on the sand to enjoy sun and sea breezes. Henri de Rothschild described these women as secular sisters of charity who had volunteered without pay to take care of the sick children and did their job with zeal and devotion. When the miracles were institutionalized, medical personnel took over. In the Second Empire this meant the heavy presence of nursing sisters (Franciscan nuns); sisters with the proper diplomas also ran the schools for the invalid children. This was not to Bourneville's liking at all. As an aggressive anti-clerical politician and Paris municipal councilor, Bourneville led the fight to kick the nursing sisters out of Parisian medical institutions and replace them with lay nurses; the program was more or less completed in 1883 and much less successfully extended to the national scene.[18]

Among the reforms Bourneville advocated for Berck were the jettisoning of the chaplain and the replacing of nursing sisters and nuns by laypersons in both medical and educational areas. In 1892 the "maritime hospital" replaced the Franciscan sisters, some of whom certainly had no medical expertise, with lay personnel, at triple the salary of the sisters. The pariah nuns then created a hospital (*Institut Cazin-Perrochaud*) to give patients an alternative to the increasingly secular facilities of the *Assistance publique*. Henri says that his mother, a solid

[17] One finds lots of variations in the figures given for number of patients, perhaps because some of the numbers apply to adults, some to children, some to one hospital, some to the two, and so on. Loze says that in the period 1872–83, 315 patients came to the *Assistance Publique* maritime hospital: 229 (72.7 percent) were cured and 70 (22.2 percent) improved; 1 died, and that in the period 1883–1907 there were 4182 patients, of whom 1919 (45.8 percent) were cured and 1979 (47.3 percent) improved; 14 died. Henry Loze, *L'Hôpital Nathaniel de Rothschild à Berck-sur-Mer* (Paris, 1908), and François-Jean Calot, *L'hôpital de Henri de Rothschild à Berck-sur-Mer* (Paris, 1900). See also H. Cazin, *Les établissements hôspitaliers à Berck-sur-Mer* (Paris, 1885), 119. Cazin's book is dedicated to the memory of his brother-in-law, Dr Paul Perrochaud.

[18] See Goldstein, *Console and Classify*, chapter 9. The *Bureau central des infirmières* (within the *Office national de l'hygiène sociale*), responsible for such things as supervision, diplomas, and placement, did not come into existence until 1924.

supporter of Catholic charity, played a large role in founding the "*hôpital Cazin*."[19] Bourneville noted that there was only one doctor (Cazin) with two interns for the hospital, a bad situation made worse by the existence of two *Maisons des Enfants assistés de la Seine*, each having 150 children, with another 150–200 *enfants assistés* spread around in addition to 20 or so epileptics, all of whom were under the supervision of the medical personnel. Adding another doctor or two would also give Bourneville the opportunity to get a solid anti-clerical republican physician on the staff. Religion was incompatible with the development of sound minds. This program fitted into a rationalization scheme for the production of healthy minds and bodies. Ever vigilant also concerning the production of good food, Bourneville noted that there should be a serious use of wastewater to fertilize gardens to produce food for the hospital, as numerous comparable foreign establishments did. In 1909 a radiology laboratory and "salle de spectacle" were installed in the chapel. (X-rays became a key part of practice: in 1910 Dr Calvé x-rayed 691 children, some several times.) Secularization and practical science (not always benign) were twin pillars of any republican establishment.

In his article on Berck in *La Grande Encyclopédie*, Bourneville – who also wrote an appreciation of the Parisian good works of Henri, a fellow physician, after all – noted the presence of the Berck Rothschild hospital, with its sixty beds, for tubercular Jewish children. Shortly after the new century began, the hospital dropped the ethnic-religious requirement for admission, perhaps because the medical needs of the new immigrants were no longer pressing as their living conditions improved and also because the immigrants became aware of the availability of state and municipal resources.

The Rothschild Hospital

Among the various medical institutions established and supported by the Rothschilds, none was more loved and pampered by Henri's parents than the Rothschild Hospital at Berck, which was inaugurated on 24 May 1872.[20] There are at least two stories, more complementary than contradictory, explaining the origin of the Berck hospital, named for Nathaniel, Henri's paternal grandfather. One is given by Henry Loze, a doctor in the Rothschild hospital and separate dispensary.[21] His narrative was stimulated by the inauguration of the *Assistance publique* hospital. One of France's most famous if socially elusive citizens, James Edouard de Rothschild, Henri's father, was invited to attend the opening ceremony in 1869, an occasion for enthusiastic promotion of the medical industry by the director of

[19] André Pascal (Henri de Rothschild [HR]), *Une dame d'autrefois. La Baronne Mathilde-Henri de Rothschild 1872–1926* (Lausanne, 1946).

[20] For a mini-history of the hospital, see HR, *Conférence faite au VIe congrès de thalassothérapie à Berck-sur-Mer (Pas-de Calais) le 26 mai 1931* (Paris, n.d.).

[21] See Loze, *L'Hôpital Nathaniel de Rothschild à Berck-sur-Mer*, 9–12.

the *Assistance publique*: all the chief cities in France should imitate Paris. The project and the location impressed James Edouard and set him thinking about the rundown and scrofulous-appearing students he had seen on his visits to the Jewish schools in the Marais quarter of Paris. So he conceived the idea of a hospital reserved exclusively for these unfortunates. On 24 May 1871 the chief rabbi of France came from Paris to participate in an imposing ceremony and to consecrate, on a beautiful beach, this new temple of charity, a superb building whose Parisian architect (Lavezzari) had planned the Berck hospital of the *Assistance publique*. Cazin also waxed eloquent on the building as the most elegant and best organized of maritime establishments. Though obviously using some of the ideas embodied in the *Assistance publique* hospital, Lavezzari radically put the rooms for patients parallel with the sea instead of reserving the space for the administration.

Another founding story has James Edouard stumble onto the medical miracle of Berck-Plage by accident in 1869. This narrative makes Dr Cazin a fellow hero in the foundation story. James Edouard was twenty years old, a lawyer and a bibliophile, little interested in Parisian frivolities. Henri painted a Rousseauistic portrait: "d'un caractère assez sauvage, et peu mondain." All part of the mythic status one invents for a father with its kernel of truth. In order to get away from it all during the summer, James Edouard chose a quiet watering place in Boulogne-sur-Mer, which was served by the *Chemin de fer du Nord*, "the Rothschild company par excellence."[22] He would take the train once or twice a week from Paris, often visiting his relatives over from England before returning to his modest hotel room to relax. Idyllic, until one day he slipped on the platform of the railway station in Boulogne and broke a leg. Back at the hotel, the only surgeon in the area, Dr Cazin, set the leg and looked after him for six weeks. Since James Edouard had a great interest in forensic medicine, doctor and patient got along famously. One of the subjects Cazin mentioned was the "quasi-miraculous cures," as Henri generously called them, which Cazin had seen at the Berck beach, about thirty kilometers from Boulogne.

James Edouard asked Cazin to take him to the "pays des miracles." On the beach near the hospital built by the city of Paris they found children in shelters, on mattresses, and on wooden platforms, while some convalescing children played in the sand or waded in the water. Cazin examined the children and complemented the women's explanations with some technical information on the children's diseases. The group included children with coxalgia, scrofula, humped backs, and rickets. Cazin diagnosed also a benign knee tumor and a case of spina ventosa or tubercular dactylitis. Looking at the convalescents, Cazin found the scars of battle: earlier traces of lesions in various forms: articular ankylosis, ulcerations, and scarified fistulas. No one who saw what went on at Berck-Plage could fail to wonder about the nature of disease and of healing.

---

[22] François Caron, *Histoire des chemins de fer en France, I: 1740–1883* (Paris, 1997), I, 180.

Cazin also told his patient about the political ramifications of medical events at Berck. After the tour James Edouard told Cazin that he too would found a hospital at Berck for a group of sick Parisian children. The memory of the rickety and the scrofulous children pursued James Edouard back to Boulogne and then to Paris, where his younger brother, Arthur, joined him in the project. In December 1869 they bought 15,000 square meters of land in Berck and retained the architect Lavezzari. After their father died, the sons decided to name their Berck foundation the Nathaniel de Rothschild hospital in his memory. Soon there were two marble plaques at the entrance to the central pavilion, one to the memory of Nathaniel and the other to the memory of James Edouard, who died unexpectedly in 1881.[23] Cazin became the medical director. His brother-in-law, Perrochaud, was the surgeon at the Berck *Assistance publique* hospital. The Rothschild hospital catered to a special clientele. The foundation's rules supporting the hospital stipulated that the small sick children (rundown or anemic) sent to Berck were to be recruited in Jewish schools in Paris and among the children of employees of the *Chemin de fer du Nord*. Non-Jewish patients could be admitted. Admission was possible through registering at the Rothschild hospital on the rue Picpus in Paris, where the director (Mlle Fanny Weill) and Dr Leven judged the cases; later a patient could also get admitted through correspondence with the baroness James (Thérèse). But the first patients to be admitted to the partially finished hospital in 1870 were soldiers wounded in the Franco-Prussian war. Only in 1872 did sick children come for treatment, which was similar to that at the hospital of the *Assistance publique*. Cazin visited regularly at one o'clock on Tuesday and Friday, and daily if required. The interns of the *Assistance publique* hospital were present when he did operations. Like any institution with scientific ambitions, the hospital produced a significant medical literature as well as a good success rate in curing patients.

The food was very good at the Rothschild hospital. Mlle Weill supervised the kitchen for over a quarter of a century. As at the hospital on the rue Picpus, a kosher diet was required. Meat came in from Boulogne every day during summer and twice a week in winter. The Rothschild connection with Bordeaux is perhaps seen in the fact that children got a daily allowance of twenty centiliters of red bordeaux cut with water. Beer was more likely to be served in the *Assistance publique* establishment, though that diet did include wine as well as beer.

Man does not live by bread alone; this platitude seems especially relevant to the life of agony lived by hospital patients. The Rothschild hospital was infused with a moral outlook distinguishing it from the *Assistance publique* hospital, though it followed James Edouard's tolerant views in not imposing a religious test for patients.[24] The Rothschild hospital tried to cure the sick body while educating

---

[23] Nathaniel: "Les justes, même morts, sont toujours vivants, leurs oeuvres perpétuent leur souvenir." James: "Le souvenir de celui qui a répandu ses bienfaits sur les pauvres subsistera éternellement." Loze, *L'Hôpital Nathaniel de Rothschild à Berck-sur-Mer*, 14–15.

[24] B.-E. Susan, *Un bibliophile contemporain* (Paris, 1881), 15.

the child intellectually and morally.[25] Among the most important advice given to the hospital's new nurses was that they should encourage higher sentiments in the patients and also develop in them the idea of the good and the habit of doing one's duty. As Loze put it, the difference in this hospital was that the patient was not a number without a personality. Children were welcomed as members of a big family, in which moral and intellectual upbringing was as important as the relief and cure of their physical ills.[26]

Family history and vicissitudes heavily influenced the development of the Rothschild institution, built on a part of the beach one km from the *Assistance publique* hospital but never threatened by the sea. For a while the brothers James Edouard and Arthur funded the operation at Berck; and after James Edouard married his German cousin Thérèse in 1871, he supported it alone. In 1872 James Edouard built the *Chalet des Oyats*, a "Norwegian-style" villa (a few hundred meters away from the hospital) suitable for a family stay in August. It was 1878 before the six-year-old Henri and his four-year-old sister were taken to Berck. While indulging in the austere pleasures of Berck for a few weeks every summer, Thérèse got to know the doctors and the director of the hospital, Mme Katz, who ran the institution efficiently for more than thirty years. As custom and power dictated, the baroness got to know the local establishment, including the mayor, the druggist, the teacher, and the priest. Thérèse soon became an important source of charity for nearly everything in town. Over the years her activities in Berck increased considerably, perhaps excessively from the viewpoint of the directors of the hospital and the hospital dispensary – Katz, Bloch, Hirschmann, and Hutter, all women. She also asked for detailed information about the other institutions she supported in Berck. A regular correspondence between Berck and Paris ensured her intelligence when she was not in Berck. She even made the rounds to buy all sorts of supplies for these institutions until shortly before she died at the age of eighty-four in April 1931.

Thérèse personally read all of the numerous requests that were addressed to her. On New Year's Day her secretary would make a speech to the personnel and patients and Calot would reply. Then the children would get the gifts they had asked for, no matter how expensive or bizarre. During the weeks that she spent in Berck there would be a goodly number of parties for the children, providing an occasion for her to visit and inquire about their convalescence. She did this on an individual basis, calling each child by name. She would often be present at the evening meal, which the patients probably enjoyed because there was always something special on such occasions.[27]

---

[25] Sabrina Faux, *Aspects médicaux et sociaux du traitement de la tuberculose à Berck-sur-Mer, 1880–1940*, (University of Paris VII, "Mémoire maîtrise Histoire", 1992), 93.

[26] Loze, *L'Hôpital Nathaniel de Rothschild à Berck-sur-Mer*, 12, 29.

[27] Loze, *L'Hôpital Nathaniel de Rothschild à Berck-sur-Mer*, 30–1.

In his memoirs Henri speculates on the genesis of his mother's charitable drive.[28] Although weakened by "painful crises" – presumably nervous attacks – and tormented by "religious scruples," Thérèse was dominated by the urge to practice charity. Henri seems reluctant to see her religion as a source of her charitable activities. After the death of James Edouard in 1881, Thérèse made the hospital one of her major projects. Henri admitted that the good side of his mother's obsession was that 100 or so sick children were cared for. Her concern for them resulted in some well-deserved coddling. Head of the funding foundation, Thérèse showed her administrative skills. No doubt her experience in running a large household was vital to her success. Henri believed that his mother's desire to have an experienced, competent administrator running the hospital was partly responsible for her directing him towards science and for giving him a taste for medicine. Cazin was amused at the young Henri's coming to the Rothschild hospital to supervise the distribution of portions of food, carve at table, and serve the small boarders.

Just before James Edouard died he charged his wife with the responsibility for the hospital. Thérèse soon got the financial support of her mother-in-law (baroness Nathaniel) and her brother-in-law (Arthur) for the construction of a second wing of the hospital, which was finished in August 1883. Increasing the capacity of the hospital to 100 beds, she transformed it into an impressive monument in memory of her husband. James Edouard had died before setting up the capital for the foundation and the payment of expenses, which amounted to 90,000 francs annually in the period 1871–81, rising to 500,000 by 1910.[29] In 1892 the hospital became hers legally, when, with the agreement of Arthur, the surrogate guardian of Henri and his sister Jeanne, she became the sole owner of the hospital with its seven hectares of land. In 1930, after Henri's sister died, the mother gave a considerably expanded establishment back to Henri as a gift. James Edouard had supported medical care for small children in Paris, where he also helped maintain and educate many young people. Though few people knew the precise nature of his charitable work, James Edouard had a reputation for delivering charity in an efficient manner when and where it was needed. Vicomte de Falloux du Coudray had sadly noted that in Catholic circles the love of humanity was on every tongue but charitable acts and sacrifice were rare.[30] James Edouard could have easily agreed with this Catholic politician and extended the judgment beyond Catholic circles.

The Rothschild presence in Berck stimulated growth. Thérèse operated on a personal level in encouraging commercial activity in town and on a political

28 André Pascal (HR), *Croisière autour des mes souvenirs* (Paris, 1932), I, 43.

29 Hyppolite Lévy, "Un hôpital israélite modèle," *Archives israélites* 35 (28 août 1890), lavished praise on an establishment with 85 beds, 800 children hospitalized (by 1885), and an annual budget of 50,000 francs.

30 Emile Leguay, "Inauguration de l'hôpital israélite à Paris," 461, quoting from the *Annales de la charité* 8 (1852): 375–81.

level in listening to municipal and departmental authorities relate their hopes and fears. Her business and family connections in Paris were not without a powerful influence, according to Henri, in getting Berck linked to the major rail line of Paris–Boulogne–Calais and in the opening of a post office. She promoted schools, run by nuns, for boys and for girls in Berck-ville; the municipality paid part of the expenses. One church to which she contributed was decorated by Albert Besnard, who painted frescoes in thanks for the cure of one of his children. She made a large contribution to the building of the church of Berck-Plage. She helped the town's first *maisons de santé* (asylums or nursing homes), even paying for the board and medical care of the sick children. By 1931 Berck had become a true town, and for Henri this meant that it even had a casino and a racetrack. The main industry remained the one based on disease: over 100 *maisons de santé* and hospitals in a town with a population of 35,000 people, swelling to over 120,000 in July and August. The cool summer sea coupled with a mini-Lourdes reputation was a winning formula for urban development.

With its flourishing hospital-based economy, Berck attracted good doctors. Dr Cazin and Thérèse got along well from the first time they met. He advised her on charitable work while she reciprocated with a Rothschild smile and more for his daughter and relatives, including the painter Jean Charles Cazin. Dr Cazin's daughter-in-law, a Perrochaud, later became director of Henri's hospital in Paris. Among the interns at the Berck hospital, a few stood out, at least in Henri's mind: Page, who became surgeon at Saint-Malo, his wife, Dr Ducroquet (née Cohan), who acquired a good reputation in orthopedics, and Loze, who stayed on at the hospital. Thérèse called on her friend Charles Périer for advice on medical staffing. Chief physician of the *Chemin de fer du Nord* and surgeon of the Lariboisière hospital, he had no trouble discovering that Calot, one of his students, assistant in anatomy in the Paris Faculty of Medicine, was perfect for the job. But Cazin, a diabetic, died in 1891, opening up the position at the City of Paris maritime hospital. Administrative rules required that the position of chief physician at the *Assistance publique* hospital in Berck be offered to a surgeon in Paris. No one was interested, and so the position was opened up to a *concours*. Calot, who now had eighteen years of experience in the medical-surgical treatment of illnesses benefiting from the "maritime cure," thought he would win. Victor Ménard won instead. In the competition Calot lost by only one point (97 versus 98), but Ménard won the vote of jury by 5 to 2. Calot was ready to return to Paris when Thérèse and Henri convinced him to stay in Berck to direct the Nathaniel de Rothschild hospital. Given the medical boom underway there, it was not a bad decision for Calot to make, even with two young active surgeons in town. There were patients in abundance for both public and private facilities. And both hospital and Calot had a big enough reputation to attract doctors from Paris for their *internat* or residency.[31]

[31] See, e.g., Dr Lévy-Klotz, *Du traitement des tuberculoses locales en générale et de la coxalgie fistuleuse en particulier* (thesis, Paris Faculty of Medicine, 1896). He spent

The sick were no longer limited to the poor children of Paris. Patients now arrived from all over France, the rest of Europe, and even from across the Atlantic. To house the sick children of royalty, English and American millionaires, big financiers, known artists, and famous scientists – Henri's honor roll of "the privileged of fortune" – villas and impressive chalets were built, while others enjoyed modest accommodations. Whatever the social class of the patients, they were there to be cured of the great white plague, tuberculosis. Back in the Franco-Prussian war, the medical installations at Berck were put to good military use. In World War I the Rothschild hospital in Berck was among the first to receive sick military personnel. Most other medical facilities were put at the disposition of the *Société de Secours aux Blessés militaires* to take care of the maimed and wounded. During the war some of the militarized institutions received patients suffering from Pott's disease and coxalgia. According to Henri, these diseases could and did appear in healthy people after they had been overworked or spent a prolonged period in cold, humid places. They improved while at Berck; some were even cured. Soon male and female patients with tuberculosis of the bone and joints became conspicuous at Berck. The place appeared on the map as a quasi-miraculous source of cures. In little over half a century Berck became an ersatz magic mountain for children and adults with a medical establishment of over forty physicians, surgeons, radiologists, and so on permanently installed in town. The permanence of the medical personnel distinguished Berck from most thermal and marine establishments, which generally operated on a medical level only a few months during the year.

Up to World War II surgery played an important role in the treatment of tuberculosis. The surgeons of Berck (Calot, Ménard, and Etienne Sorrel) developed reputations partly based on their surgical techniques in operating on bones and joints deformed by the disease and in devising orthopedic measures and prostheses for inherited and acquired deformations. Ambitious and skilled doctors, the medical men of Berck published canonical treatises and manuals and communicated the results of their work to scientific and medical societies. Berck was put on the medical map. After 1900 Berck developed considerably, attracting new doctors and a bigger clientele, perhaps partly because of the success of the treatments along with the popularity of balneotherapy and thalassotherapy. Henri waxed eloquent about "the magnificent results that could be obtained at Berck, when the chemical and physical effects of air, sun, and sea were joined to a surgical technique that had become less interventionist and more and more conservative." These results represented "one of the great victories of thalassotherapy," according to Henri's optimistic description of the new lease of life offered to the adult sufferers from

thirteen months in Berck as an *interne* at the Rothschild hospital and Henri's dispensary. Both Thérèse and Henri's wife (Mathilde) have the thesis dedicated to them; la baronne James receives his "Hommage respectueux ... profonde reconnaissance." A major dedication is reserved for Calot, "chirurgien de l'hôpital Nathaniel de Rothschild et de l'hôpital Cazin-Perrochaud."

Pott's disease and coxalgia, all of whom used to be abandoned in asylums for the incurable. Given the potential medical boom in treating adults aged 25 to 35, the *Assistance publique* added 400 beds for them outside the *Hôpital maritime de la ville de Paris*, which reserved its 1100 beds for children.

So what were the results obtained by these splendid establishments in the treatment of those invaded by the bacillus *Mycobacterium tuberculosis*? In 1885 Cazin said that all medical establishments in Berck had treated about 800 children; good statistics supposedly showed the hospitals' superiority to establishments in other countries. Observers like Henri believed that public and private medical establishments had carried out a sort of "war on tuberculosis" through the creation of sanitoria, preventoria, and *colonies scolaires*, as well as through slum clearance, the organization of family hygiene, propaganda lectures, and educational cinema.[32] After the Great War, pulmonary tuberculosis seemed less prevalent than before. The number of cases of tuberculosis of the bones and joints clearly dropped during the 1920s. More good news could be spun from the fact that the deformation of bones and joints had become much less serious and less mutilating than before. Henri did not speculate whether this was due to a less virulent bacillus or earlier and better treatment for patients. The chief surgeon at the Paris Maritime Hospital drew on his ten years of experience to establish the statistical conclusion that Henri cited to make his case.[33] The 1100 beds of the Maritime Hospital always used to be full, at least before 1920; by 1931 the *Assistance publique* was unable to fill them. In the decade of the 1920s, when Sorrel replaced Ménard, there was a considerable drop in major surgery, including articular resections, and amputations. With the decline in TB surgical cases, Sorrel's knife was less busy than Ménard's.[34]

The Rothschild Dispensary

Henri made his own special personal contribution to medical care in Berck-sur-Mer after 1892 with the development of the Henri de Rothschild Dispensary, which Thérèse had founded to offer some urgent care for the poor. She funded the entire operation until her death in 1931, when the institution closed. By 1900 the annual expense was about 28,000 francs for giving 20 to 25 free daily consultations with

[32] See Laura Lee Downs, *Childhood in the Promised Land: Working-Class Movements and the Colonies de Vacances in France, 1880–1960* (Durham, NC, 2002).

[33] Etienne Sorrel, *la Presse médicale*, numbers 38 and 40.

[34] Etienne Sorrel (1882–1965), second in his promotion, began his internat at Berck under Ménard. Seriously wounded in the Great War, he was made a hospital surgeon in 1919, *chef de service* of the maritime hospital of Berck in 1920, and head of the *grand service d'enfants* of the Trousseau hospital in 1932. He spent time in the United States learning orthopedic surgical techniques. He married Mademoiselle Déjerine-Klumpke in 1921. Marcel Fèvre, "Etienne Sorrel (1882–1965)," *Bulletin de l'Académie de Médecine* 151 (1967): 38–46.

treatment if needed. During World War I the dispensary cared for 9 wounded soldiers at a time; in the period 1914–18 it treated 305 military personnel as well as many civilians; it boasted of giving a total of 905 consultations and doing 2000 dressings. Three doctors were on call, including Calot, who had not been conscripted, and, in surgery, Joseph Fouchou-Lapeyrade, who is also remembered for having sacrificed his right arm, amputated because of damage from x-rays.[35] During the war years other doctors also did duty in the dispensary.[36] In 1895 Henri and Calot wrote a mini-history of the origin and evolution of the dispensary; they hoped to enlighten people who were interested in free medical care, one of the hot medical topics of the day.[37] Calot and Henri believed that the history of the dispensary could demonstrate the best way of solving the problem posed by the difficulty the poor had in obtaining free medical care in small towns and the countryside. More important, philanthropists and doctors would certainly be impressed by the range of services that could be offered by a modest establishment functioning so simply, and perhaps they would open similar establishments.

What exactly was the medical problem outside larger towns and cities? The poor of Paris were medically well off, as least in statistical comparison with the other groups. There was help available when they were sick and unable to work. Forty-eight million francs went for "welfare" in Paris, and though it was not enough by any means, there was a good chance that a person in serious need would be able to get by because welfare was supplemented by aid from charitable institutions. Henri and Calot thought that the agricultural population was relatively well off compared to miners, industrial workers, and those living in maritime areas. Poor sailors made up a really needy group in towns of 4000 to 6000 people. There was usually no hospital, and the welfare office was able to serve only about one twentieth of the needy. The situation in Berck-sur-Mer was a particularly sad one. Out of the native population of about 7000, half were sailors, who could not support their families when rough weather kept them ashore. Owning land was of little help, for the soil was unproductive. No place in France seemed to have

---

35 Fouchou-Lapeyrade spent years at the *Institut orthopédique* (later *Institut Calot*) *de Berck-sur-Mer*, headed by Calot, where he interned and then ran the radiography service. See Joseph Fouchou-Lapeyrade, *Contribution à l'étude de la coxalgie par la radiographie* (thesis, Paris Faculty of Medicine, 1906).

36 Baronne James de Rothschild, *Souvenirs de la grande guerre (1914–1918)* (Mâcon, 1925), 167.

37 Information on the dispensary is found in F. Calot and H. de Rothschild, *Essai sur l'assistance médicale et chirurgicale gratuite dans les petites villes et dans les campagnes* (Paris, 1895), and HR, *Exposé des titres et travaux scientifiques du Docteur Henri de Rothschild* (Saint-Ouen, 1929), 49–50. The forty-six page *Essai* was dedicated to the memory of Henri's father, James Edouard de Rothschild, "who created the first charity work in Berck and which we [Henri] have devotedly followed the example." Calot's titles in 1895 included "chriurgien en chef de l'Hôpital Nathaniel de Rothschild, de l'Hôpital Cazin-Perrochaud et du Dispensaire Henri de Rothschild."

fewer resources and so little social help for such a number of people. The annual amount available for all of the social needs (including medical) of poor families was a paltry 3–4000 francs. If the population of Berck had received the same help as the sick of Paris, the town's welfare budget would have been 145,000 francs annually. Berck had 6 hospitals treating 2000 patients, but none of the hospitals admitted any of the nearly half of the local population needing medical help at sometime or other. This was where private charity played a role in making up for governmental neglect.

Henri's mother was the first to provide free medical help for the sick poor of Berck and its surroundings. Not only the clearly sick needed help. Thérèse's friend, the painter Francis Tattegrin, one of the first "Berckois" painters, gave her the idea of establishing a maritime asylum for homeless people in Berck.[38] Though he had not finished his medical education, Henri was keenly aware of the lacuna in the services offered by the family's twenty-five-year-old hospital at Berck-sur-Mer. The establishment had no external consultation, and it accepted only children sent from Paris, as stipulated in its regulations. Like the other hospitals in the area, it was closed to local sick children. Henri decided in 1892 to hire a nurse who would give home care. Soon swamped with work, she was given a small house in Berck-Plage, which was transformed into a dispensary under a head nurse, Caroline Hutter. This free external consultation was a complement to the family hospital. Sick Berckois children were seen a couple of times a week. When the dispensary opened its doors to adults as well as children, it took in seven or eight sick Berckois day and night.

The use of the word *dispensaire* as a name for the institution is somewhat curious.[39] Henri explained that it was impossible to find a more popular word, though the dispensary in Berck did not imitate Parisian dispensaries, which generally gave free medical care to sick children who came or were brought to the place. Henri's dispensary in Berck was open to every sick person: those who came in could get free medical and surgical care, dressings, and medications. In addition, the dispensary offered medical care to people who could not travel because of being disabled or seriously ill. A unique organization, Henri boasted, which did not exclude a single poor, sick person from its charitable program. But most of Henri's sick could walk into the building, conveniently located right in town, near the church and market, only 300 to 400 meters from the train station and the sea. The building was simple. No need, Henri noted, for an expensive

[38] See Emile Delignières, *L'asile maritime de Berck et les portraits de ses pensionnaires par M. Francis Tattegrain* (Montreuil-sur-Meer, 1904).

[39] In addition to giving the usual meaning of *dispensaire*, *Le nouveau petit Robert* notes the influence of the English word (1775) but also points out the French use of the word (1573) to describe a collection of (medical and drug) formulas. *Le petit Littré* (1863) gives another, older meaning: a laboratory for the preparation of substances that enter into the preparation of compound drugs – "the apothecary's shop" is signaled in *The Concise Oxford Dictionary.*

construction, as was often the case in charitable institutions, thus wasting "the money of the poor."[40] The establishment consisted of five rooms: waiting, consultation and dressings, minor surgery, and recovery or rest, with the fifth reserved for lodging the nurse. Nurse Hutter, the key figure in the functioning of the dispensary, soon became the director, with another nurse and woman helper added. Dr Baillet became an adjunct and the busy Calot came in to do surgery. The availability of Rothschild hospital doctors was vital to the functioning of the dispensary. In 1894 Dr Pierre came on board to take charge of eye, ear, nose, and throat cases. Expansion continued slowly, with even two (male and female) small dormitories added. With the coming of the automobile, handling the victims of road accidents became part of the dispensary's activity, no doubt encouraged by Henri, who was keenly interested in everything about the automobile, including its potential for medical disaster as well as medical progress. In 18 months doctors did over 200 operations, including a few laparotomies or abdominal incisions. Common procedures included operations for abscesses and whitlows and uterine curettages. There were 44 cases of syphilis. Henri mentions one circumcision, for a moral rather than a religious reason. After picking up a bad habit from his lubricious nurse, according to observant parents, a child of eighteen months was cut and cured within a week. This is the only mention of the practice of surgery with a moral purpose, which was usually practiced on women.[41] With the founding of *Le Dispensaire Henri de Rothschild* medical care for the poor of Berck became a social model much talked about but less frequently imitated.

Business was soon booming, much encouraged by the popularity of free care. Patients came from all areas of France. Soon the rich, demanding the same privileges as the poor, started exploiting the system. It is easier for the rich to act poor than the other way round. Eighteen months after opening, the dispensary got new regulations limiting totally free care to residents of Berck but still giving others free medical and surgical care; anyone in extreme distress could also get everything free. New abuses by lying patients led to even more regulation of non-medical charity and of house calls.

With Thérèse's support, Henri expanded the dispensary. The purchase of Perrochaud's chalet permitted the construction of a two-story building, with six rooms on the ground floor. The laboratory was transferred into a big room in a neighboring chalet. There were fourteen cages for "experimental animals, which could be injected with pathological products taken from the sick for diagnosis." Henri said that his first scientific work (1896) was research on the

---

40 Calot and de Rothschild, *Essai sur l'assistance médicale et chirurgicale*, 11–13.

41 See Ann Dally, *Women under the Knife. A History of Surgery* (London, 1991), 159–64, on the clitoridectomy, a subject on which there is an enormous literature. See John Duffy, "Clitoridectomy: A Nineteenth-Century Answer to Masturbation," under the rubric of *The Female Genital Cutting Education and Networking Project* online at http://www.fgmnetwork.org/articles/duffy.htm.

toxicity of camphorated naphthol (a concoction of one part naphthol and two parts camphor), which was used to prevent suppuration in acute tonsillitis and to treat tubercular ulcerations of the tongue. The Rothschild hospital in Berck had experienced an alarming number of fatalities in using this product. Henri gave some dogs intra-articular injections, resulting in their dying in convulsive agony. *Voilà*: the explanation of the fatal results in children.[42] Photography and moulage immortalized the "interesting cases." By 1903 the dispensary had become a real little hospital with seven beds for surgical patients. A surgeon and a doctor directed the establishment, which was supervised by a woman manager. The dispensary required the services of one male and four female nurses. Daily consultations continued with free medications, orthopedic apparatuses and prostheses always available for the "deserving poor," who could also get free goods such as sterilized milk, and tickets for bread, meat, charcoal, and other essential items. Commentators have indulged the reader with many statistics. Between 1892 and 1894, the dispensary received 2437 sick (922 men, 844 women, and 671 children); patients stayed for a total of 1732 days. And the optimistic report on healing noted that there were 878 cures and 329 notable improvements. In the year 1908 there were 830 days of hospitalization for patients, 3570 various consultations, 4609 cases of minor surgery with dressings, and 29 cases of major surgery. And in 1908 babies were given 8558 bottles of milk (500 gr).[43] Looking back from the year 1929, Henri was able to provide an impressive summing up of the record of his dispensary over a quarter century.[44]

> Figures for 1903–28
> Days of hospitalization – 19,776
> Consultation of different sorts – 54,888
> Minor surgery and dressings – 92,794
> Major surgery – 498
> Casts for fractures, etc. – 1474
> Bottles (500 gr) of milk distributed – 263,062
> Baths given – 4831
> Bandages and house calls – 1026

Henri does not seem to have been particularly interested in the conventional notion of immortality, but Thérèse probably thought of the dispensary in the same way she thought of her activities at the hospital: "Faire le bien conduit à l'immortalité."

In 1931, the year his mother died and the dispensary closed, Henri also sold the hospital to the Fondation Franco-Américaine de Berck for 2,225,000 francs.

42 HR, *La Lignée française de la famille Rothschild 1792–1942. Etude historique et biographique* (Oporto, 1942), 116.

43 Docteurs Calot and Henri de Rothschild, *Le docteur Henri de Rothschild à Berck-sur-Mer, and Le dispensaire Henri de Rothschild* (Paris, 1895), 44–6.

44 *Exposé des titres et travaux scientifiques du Docteur Henri de Rothschild*, 49–50.

The German invasion in World War II destroyed the hospital, which had been renamed for the surgeon Adolphe Jalaguier (1853–1924). Jalaguier, known for his pioneering surgery, was recognized for his long history of operating on children suffering from harelip, clubfoot, and coxalgia.[45] A resurrected institution was named the Centre Calvé, named after Jacques Calvé (1875–1954), a well-known Berckois name in the history of orthopedics.[46] As is often the case in post-Vichy France, history connived with crime to make it easy for people to forget the origin and history of some institutions.

A Patient's Voice

After hearing doctors praise themselves so much for their work at Berck, one would certainly like to hear from a patient or two. And we can, indirectly through the novel. In 1923 Jeanne Galzy's novel *Les Allongés* received the highly desirable Femina prize.[47] The novel, by a former patient of the Maritime Hospital, gave a nasty shock to the Berckian medical industry, which was used to ingesting a rich diet of friendly official discourse and praise, much of it no doubt deserved. Galzy suffered from Pott's disease, and one of her sharpest memories was the odor of "dissolving flesh," the sweet stink of dressings and of iodoform. "Am I in the house of the dead," she wondered. Death lurked behind every bed; one out of every ten patients died, said the morose Italian patient. (Galzy peopled the novel with many nationalities: Spanish, Italian, Greek, Argentine, Polish, Russian, and American.) Corpses were carted off secretly at dawn in order to protect the curative reputation of "this town without a cemetery." She might have dealt with some more mundane but serious hospital problems such as rampant ringworm. Or the hospital as a terrible environmental polluter producing a nauseating stench and dangerous sanitary conditions, enjoyed by squadrons of delighted flies and mosquitoes at Berck-Plage. Perhaps most irritating for doctors was the shocking originality of the novel in dealing with patients, their feelings, fears, and hopes, rather than with the medical experience per se. "La Maison des Sables" had never been the subject of such scrutiny, even in a novel.

A serious reply was not long in coming, in a novel with an uplifting title (*Prisoners in Body, Free Spirits*) meant to offer hope to the sick of Berck, who also

---

45 Jalaguier practiced at the *hospice des Enfants-Assistés* between 1898 and 1918.

46 On Jacques Calvé (and his Calvary) see www.chirpédiatric.org, site of the Société Française de chirurgie pédiatrique, "mon Profil," (mardi 12 avril 2005).

47 Jeanne Galzy (1883–1977) was a prolific and popular author, whose works included books on saints (Theresa of Avila), the private life of André Chénier and George Sand, as well as novels with seductive titles, such as *Jeunes filles en serre chaude* and *La femme chez les garçons*. Republished by Gallimard in 1975, *Les Allongés* (Paris, 1923) was a bestseller of yesteryear with at least sixty-seven printings.

had the novel dedicated to them.[48] The authors clearly attempted to counteract the negative impression of Berck being spread far and wide by Galzy's sizzler. The beach of tortures was really the beach of hope. Doctors were busy in the novel, but not too busy to cultivate a good bedside manner, especially when meeting patients for the first time, a situation described by the authors as a sort of dueling match. An operation of thirty-nine minutes on a knee is described in some detail. "On devient savante à Berck, hein!??" The danger of a doctor's relying on an x-ray poorly done is counterbalanced by the all-important clinical examination. A couple of German and Swiss doctors are found incompetent in the diagnosis of their patients, now happily in the care of superb French doctors. Patients' rights are given an airing in a description of the filing of "official" complaints and in patients putting pressure on the prefect to permit them to stay in establishments not approved by the ministry of health. Unlike in Galzy's novel, in Remys' novel organized religion has an important role: there are a bishop, a priest, saints, Christ, and Masses. All that is needed for comfort, if not salvation. Of course the "miracle" is medicalized – no ambiguity here. "Is Berck perfect? No, for one must tell the truth, even to one's benefactors. Criticism is easy but proves nothing. Berck is envied by the rest of Europe." A fairer treatment of the sadness and hope in Berck, perhaps, but not so good a read as the somber *Les Allongés*, which gave so many thousands of readers a frisson of pleasure on their vicarious visit to "the house of the dead."

---

[48] Jean-Robert and Gabriel Remy, *A Corps prisonniers, âmes libres. Berck.* (Lille, 1928; 2nd edn, Bresle, 1928).

Chapter 3
An Education at the Paris Faculty of Medicine

I am in favor of reducing the death rate.[1]

Why and how Henri de Rothschild became a physician was duly recorded by the doctor himself in his later years.[2] Since his father (James Edouard) had ended up in the bank in spite of beginning a brilliant legal career, Henri was able to claim that he was the first in his family to break with the family's occupational tradition. The origin of his interest in medicine was a family affair. James Edouard associated with the great doctors of the day who came to see his sick father, Nathaniel: Charles Richet, Apollinaire Bouchard, Alfred Fournier, and Charcot, a doctor detested by Fournier. In 1867 his father's interest in the increasing interaction between the law and medicine led him to participate in the founding of the *Société française de médecine légale*. Since Henri was only nine years old when his father died in 1881, much of the influence probably came from the stories told to him by family and friends.

The influence of Henri's mother on his decision to become a doctor was not inconsiderable. For about ten years (approximately 1884–1895) she was ill and stayed in her bedroom or on a chaise longue in her boudoir for weeks at a time, though she seemed able to supervise care of her children and to undertake her favorite works of charity in hospitals, schools, and nurseries.[3] Henri remembered vividly the hospital atmosphere of the family residence invaded by the famous doctors. After she told the doctors about her hopes for Henri's becoming a doctor, they indulged him by talking up the profession, especially as a source of great intellectual and moral satisfaction. Medical studies were, Henri said, a sort of continuation of his home life for ten years. Even before marrying James Edouard, Thérèse had a history of service in the healing arts. In her native Frankfurt am Main during the Franco-Prussian war she helped look after wounded prisoners,

---

1 Knock in Jules Romains, *Knock* (Paris, 1924), 36.

2 Henri de Rothschild [HR], *Croisière autour de mes souvenirs*. II: *Mes maîtres et mes amis à la faculté et dans les hôpitaux* (Paris, 1936).

3 Dates and details differ slightly, depending on the condition of Henri's memory. HR (André Pascal), *Une dame d'autrefois. La Baronne Mathilde-Henri de Rothschild 1872–1926* (Lausanne, 1946), 64 ff.

and she cared for wounded German prisoners in World War I.[4] After her marriage to James Edouard she took a great interest in the establishment at Berck-sur-Mer; after he died she became devoted to it. Writing towards the end of his life, Henri leaned to the idea that the doctors who visited his mother had a greater influence on him than his compulsory visits to the children's hospital in the Pas-de-Calais. He was not always of this opinion.

The Road to the Faculty

When Henri was about six years old his mother decided that he, like his English cousin Walter, should be encouraged to become a zoologist.[5] Since Henri's good work was rewarded with gifts, he soon had a sizeable collection of insects and stuffed animals and birds, specimens bought from Emile Deyrolles, a specialist in these memories of life, whose shop was in the rue du Bac. On his tenth birthday he received a stuffed chimpanzee sitting on a tree branch. This fellow primate kept him company for two years. Then the arrival of Gustave Hariet as a French tutor ended Henri's budding career as a natural scientist. Hariet was unable to stand the stink of science (odors of carbolic acid, camphor, and naphthalene); nor did he appreciate the higher entomological aesthetic embodied in the insect collection. Hariet managed to get the menagerie shipped off to storage in Thérèse's residence in Gouvieux. Later in life, Henri did not record any distress over this early change of direction in his life. Thérèse agreed reluctantly to Hariet's scheme because he proposed a new hobby for Henri, collecting autographs, letters, and manuscripts of famous people. So began the famous collections that eventually ended up in the Bibliothèque nationale.

Although Henri's zoological career was short-circuited, his relations with the worlds of zoology and entomology were not completely severed, and as a later patron of the sciences he had several significant research connections with these sciences. He supported the work and publication of the research in the third volume of the entomological encyclopedia, published by the Presses Universitaires de France, which dealt with the voracious xylophagous (wood-eating) beetles in French tropical Africa.[6] Pierre Lesne took six years to research and write this scientific monograph, of use to both researchers and loggers, he hoped. In this arena Henri was known as a man who supported "the scientific development and the industrial exploitation of our [French] colonial domain."[7] The carcinologist

[4] Thérèse-James de Rothschild, *Pages détachées du cahier d'une jeune fille* (privately printed, 1920).

[5] Walter de Rothschild (1868–1937), son of Nathaniel Mayer and Emma, Thérèse's sister.

[6] Pierre Lesne, *Les coléoptères bostrychides de l'Afrique tropicale française* (Paris, 1924); series: *Encyclopédie entomologique*, 3.

[7] Lesne, *Les coléoptères bostrychides de l'Afrique tropicale française*.

Louis-Eugène Bouvier gratefully noted in his preface to the work that it had been conceived and executed in as close to scientifically ideal conditions as possible, thanks in large part to Henri's support. Bouvier's approval of this scientific and potentially practical work flattered the author and his patron both by his praise and his status: he was a member of the academy of sciences and a professor at the national museum of natural history. A destructive pest threatening French colonial economic interests had been identified, thus showing the common interest of science, motherland, and capitalism, essential ingredients of the Weltanschauung of not a few Rothschilds.

Between 1881 and 1894 Henri's mother condemned him to spend his summer vacations at Berck-sur-Mer. James Edouard liked to rough it up in his chalet built in a wild area of the dunes. Thérèse enjoyed the area too, especially with a Rothschild hospital to patronize. After the death of her husband she continued her visits, accompanied by her two children, their English maids, and the female German teacher. Issuing directives and orders, she played an authoritative Florence Nightingale part at the hospital, while Henri played with "hunchbacks, cripples, and disabled children."[8] Looking back much later, Henri sighed that his mother was unaware of the danger of infections from these gibbous and coxalgic children; she thought that they were weak, perhaps undernourished, rather than sick with tuberculosis. It seems that Thérèse wanted her children to become familiar with human misery and pain in the hope that they would follow in a Rothschild tradition of doing something to alleviate human suffering.

According to Henri, Thérèse believed that the practice of medicine is an apostolate rather than a profession. In July 1886 Thérèse told the astonished director of the hospital in Berck-sur-Mer to have a doctor introduce the fourteen-year-old Henri to the different medical departments, including viewing the dressing of wounds and observing surgery in the operating room with "its torture equipment." Both German tutor and the director tried unsuccessfully to get her to postpone her plan. Henri later said that he was too young to have been aroused by feelings of pity and charity in seeing the treatment of patients.

Like his visits to the pharmacy and kitchen, the hospital experience was more or less entertaining for him as a child. Whether he was left indifferent to the experience, as he claimed, is open to doubt, for he also recognized that it did develop a sensitive side of his personality. It may be that his mother wanted him to become a doctor in order to take over the hospital. Even if Henri's reactions were not exactly those hoped for by Thérèse, medical routines became more familiar to him than those of banking and business. So his mother's medical cult – he says that after she reached the age of sixty, living among the sick and the people who cared for them became a mystical experience for her – though it did not convert him to medicine, was probably not without its conditioning effect.[9]

---

8 HR, *Croisière*, II, 41–2.

9 HR, *Croisière*, II, 43–4.

Writing his memoirs in the 1930s, Henri remembered that when he reached the age of eighteen he was still thinking of the sick and handicapped children he had played with on the beach in Berck. In fact, he said that the whole Berckian medical experience came back to him. He admitted that in spite of deep disappointment and disenchantment with his odd childhood, he had become aware of the deep gulf separating rich and poor. So it was possible for him to conclude that the whole experience was in large part responsible for his choosing a medical career and advantageously preparing him for a life of medical charity. Like most people Henri was not exactly sure why he ended up in his chosen career. Certainly it is clear that he later derived a certain satisfaction from having been present if not at the creation then at the eventual transformation of Berck into a genuine medical-surgical city. Even more satisfying was the knowledge that his family had played an important medical and social role in the development of Berck.

There were a few obstacles on the road to the faculty of medicine but none that a bright young Rothschild could not overcome, especially if he were a prodigious worker like Henri. After finishing his *année de seconde* at the Lycée Janson-de-Sailly, Henri switched to the Lycée Louis-le-Grand. In this elite Lycée establishment top teachers assured that students were offered a superb education, according to elite definition. His year in *rhétorique* was one of academic slavery because he had to prepare for two different university-given examinations, the first part of the *baccalauréat ès lettres* and the *baccalauréat ès sciences restreint*. Earning the second diploma was necessary to make up for a year lost when his mother unwisely made him repeat his *classe de quatrième* in order to keep him firmly under the maternal yoke for one more year.

With his "limited" science diploma he could enter the program for the *officiat de santé* – *officiers* were no longer so innocent of scientific knowledge as Charles Bovary. This was a real piece of luck, for the rank of health officer was abolished in 1892. (Doctors were happy to lose competitors, even if rural areas would lose medical care while waiting for more doctors to be churned out by the faculties.) Once in the program for the *officiat de santé*, Henri was permitted to transfer to the program for the doctorate after obtaining the *baccalauréat ès lettres complet*, which he received on successfully completing the lycée year in philosophy. Once again he had to undertake two tasks: this time, to enter the lycée class in philosophy and register in the university program. Since he had done so much natural history, physics, and chemistry, along with Latin and French courses, Paul Brouardel, then dean of the faculty of medicine, one of his mother's doctors, was able to let him skip the scientific program of physics, chemistry, and natural sciences (PCN) required of students with little scientific baggage. In order to change his matriculation from one program to another, Henri needed a high-level recommendation, especially since he had not been able to take the PCN courses with their laboratory work. It was not necessary to go higher than Brouardel, who asked Dr Pupin, secretary of the faculty, to arrange the matter. Pupin, Brouardel's chief of staff, his *éminence grise*, notorious for his "cuisine bureaucratique," appreciated the cigars and game sent by Henri on later appropriate occasions.

Henri thus gained a year, compensating for the time that his mother had caused him to lose in lycée and winning the right to enter the faculty of medicine as a second-year student. He thus escaped the cruel dilemma facing him because the rules of the *Assistance publique* established an age limit of twenty-five years for taking the *internat* examinations while the military regulation required him to be an *interne* at twenty-four or a graduated physician at twenty-five if he wished to do his military *voluntariat*, a special engagement of a year, or military service as an officer rather than a simple soldier.

On entering the faculty of medicine in November 1891, Henri partially escaped the family compound of the avenue de Friedland. He still had to spend October with his mother in Gouvieux, where he enjoyed his leisure time in firing at rabbits in the park of the residence. Thérèse was distressed at the possibility of his falling into moral turpitude in the Latin Quarter. She was, according to the diagnosis of her son, the "slave of an eternally tortured conscience";[10] so she sometimes peppered her victims with absurd demands, which had to be taken seriously nevertheless. The first victim in this case was Brouardel, who had been treating her for ten years. He pointed out in vain that Henri was nineteen years old and that it was not a serious matter if he led the normal life of a young person. Exactly what Thérèse did not want. Not that a serious student in medicine had much time for fun after courses, laboratory, and hospital. But Brouardel could only satisfy the demanding mother by assigning two faculty doctors for some sort of surveillance of the potential roué. The dean still hoped that on Saturday night at least Henri would be allowed to relax with young friends in order to prepare for the next arduous week. A frightful business, Thérèse murmured bitterly, just before the dean escaped with his "eternal cigarette dangling from his lips."[11]

Thérèse next summoned another of her doctors, Charles Périer, an old friend who was then head doctor of the *Chemin de fer du Nord* and a surgeon at the Lariboisière hospital after 1881.[12] The patients in his department were chiefly workers ("mécaniciens, chauffeurs, ouvriers des ateliers et des dépôts de la Chapelle, de Saint-Denis et de la grande banlieue") and passengers injured in railway accidents.[13] Henri was already a voluntary student worker in Périer's department at Lariboisière. In his last lycée year Henri had visited the Lariboisière, Hôtel-Dieu, and Salpêtrière hospitals in the company of the eminent doctors whom Thérèse regarded as her friends; and on Thursday afternoons he visited the laboratories of

---

10 HR, *Croisière*, II, 43–4.

11 Lucien Nass, *Pauvres docteurs! Moeurs médicales* (Paris, 1906), 6.

12 Henri writes Perrier, but I assume he meant Périer. Charles Périer (1836–1914) became a *chirurgien des hôpitaux* in 1872, when he was named a *professeur agrégé* at the military hospital Val-de-Grâce; he resigned from the army about four years later.

13 Périer wrote several short works in occupational medicine, some of which were notices distributed to the workers at the *Chemin de fer du Nord* on hygiene, alcoholism – a liter of wine at 8–10 percent alcohol was the daily limit –- tuberculosis, syphilis, and work accidents.

the faculty of medicine and of the Pasteur Institute. Périer was expected to be a friendly spy reporting back to the matriarch on Henri's work habits and conduct; in another sense, he was a substitute father. Henri later identified Périer as his first teacher in the practice of medicine and as a sympathetic person of good will towards him in these student days. Lucien Picqué, assistant to Périer at Lariboisière, initiated Henri into the rituals of the surgical art. Henri assumed at one point that his mother worried about student drinking, gambling, seducing and being seduced by young women, and carousing in cafés. Thérèse, seeing that Périer assumed that she was thinking of the dangers of "contagious diseases," emphasized that it was not disease but rather the moral danger of "immoral behavior and vice" that worried her. Périer solved the problem by turning Henri over to Marie Nageotte-Wilbouchevitch, a hospital *interne*. Shocked at first, then reassured by the idea that a serious woman preparing her medical thesis would be completely absorbed in her work, Thérèse was finally satisfied on the issue of her son's moral safety in the Latin Quarter. Once she was convinced that the doctors and surgeons who came to the avenue de Friedland would keep her totally informed about Henri's new life, a valet summoned Henri to the "maternal boudoir" to hear judgment.

This exercise of maternal power more or less coincided with Henri's own plans. Like his father, he chose an unusual occupation for a nineteenth-century Rothschild, though his devotion to the work ethic was pure family ideology. A timid, reserved young man, little interested in "distractions à la mode," he hardly justified his mother's fears about his possible life of decadence. And of course, as Henri admitted, he was already leading a life of Aristotelian virtue, with moderation guaranteed by fidelity to his "bonne amie," an older mistress acquired from the household of a relative's mistress. An arrangement with a woman twice his age worked out well and became in memory, as is often the case in such affairs, an Eden for the troubled mind. The setup also conformed to contemporary male bourgeois wisdom on ideal outlets for the young male libido.[14] Henri regretted more than once that his own sons did not follow his own bad example when they were eighteen years old.

The Hospital Scene

On the day after Périer's visit to the avenue de Friedland, Henri, accompanied by his sister's governess, was taken in his mother's brougham to the Lariboisière hospital. In the Saint-Côme ward, which reeked of iodoform and carbolic acid – the use of "chemical antiseptics" was common by this time – Charles Périer met students and young "medical scientists" to begin the rounds of patients. Nageotte-Wilbouchevitch supervised Henri's activities and kept him busy. Of Polish origin,

[14] Nicely explained to Thérèse by Brouardel: "une maîtresse d'un âge mûr, fidèle et pot-au-feu, est la sécurité pour un jeune homme de bonne famille comme pour ses parents." She was not amused. HR, *Croisière*, II, 46.

the petite, thin, short-haired woman, who was addressed as *Monsieur l'interne*, had no interest in the frivolities of female fashions, as Henri quickly noted. Her authority and clarity of speech were matched by her mastery of her duties. Just what one might expect of a woman who was the second female to pass the examinations for the *internat*. Augusta Klumpke, another foreigner, had been the first. Both women, necessarily fully Frenchified, married well-known French medical men. Klumpke married Jules Dejerine and followed him in his speciality of nervous diseases. Dejerine replaced Peter at the Necker hospital, where Henri came into contact with him for the study of internal pathology and basic medical diagnosis. Wilbouchevitch married Jean Nageotte, a big name in neurology who rose to a chair at the Collège de France; she too followed her husband in devoting her professional life to studying nervous diseases and psychiatry. During World War I she was the chief assistant of the surgeon Adolphe Jalaguier at the military hospital Val-de-Grâce; so she became "la vaillante doctoresse." Some of this experience provided material for Henri's plays.

Périer's department at Lariboisière gave Henri an introduction to emergency medicine, though the term was not yet in use. The daily stream of railway accident victims, whether employees or passengers, often suffered from large traumatic lesions such as fractures of the skull, the pelvis, arms, and legs as well as facial mutilation. A doctor could look back on this marvelous opportunity for observation and even for supervised action with gratitude and enthusiasm. Henri called it an "admirable school of emergency medicine."[15] Before x-rays (discovered by Röntgen in 1895) came into use it may be that doctors needed to be more skillful or at least more careful in setting broken bones. But of course all this exposure as a student volunteer was only a prelude to the real business of becoming a doctor, namely years of study and work in the faculty of medicine.

Germ Theory

Henri came into medicine at the time when germ theory had conquered surgery, with the non-believers either dead or in the position of fighting a losing battle against antiseptic and aseptic measures. He was also one of the last students of Michel Peter, a serious critic of Pasteur's microbial imperialism; he mentions only the high-level practical instruction given by this "eminent clinician."[16] When news of Listerian methods reached France some surgeons were immediately interested enough to cross the channel to see exactly what Lister had done to reduce his surgical mortality rate in Glasgow. The protean concept of Listerism is, in Lawrence's words, "a catchall for a heterogeneous collection of practices,

[15] HR, *Croisière*, II, 228.

[16] For a brief defense of Peter, see Bruno Latour, *The Pasteurization of France* (Cambridge, Mass., 1988), 29–30. Translated by Alan Sheridan and John Law.

statistics, and theories that were gradually perceived (created even) by the end of the nineteenth century as a single historical entity." In Britain "roughly between 1867 and 1880 some surgeons invoked Lister's name to justify all or some of their practices, statistics, and theories, and others did not." But then Listerism "became successfully identified with a germ theory of the type promoted by Robert Koch and the surgical practices said to be based upon it." But no matter how skeptical one is of the historical myth of Listerism, one principle survives: "carefully applied chemical dressings were superior to other means in reducing surgical mortality in the late nineteenth century."[17] Not to be forgotten: the steam spray apparatus that put out a spray of carbolic acid, sterilizing and poisoning the atmosphere of operating rooms and sick rooms; the spray was soon recognized as a danger to surgeons and patients. In 1868 Charles Périer, along with his friends and future famous surgeons Edouard Nicaise (1838–96) and Félix Terrier (1837–1908), went to see Lister's setup in Glasgow and Spencer Wells's in London. Just Lucas-Championnière (1843–1913) and the gynecologist Samuel Pozzi ("le charmeur," 1846–1918) had preceded them and returned enthusiastic missionaries of Listerism. Périer and friends became equally fervent disciples of "Lister's method."[18] Périer (1836–1914) along with Lucas-Championnière, a big name at the Tenon hospital (20th arrondissement) from 1881 to 1887, was a key figure in introducing antiseptic surgery at the Lariboisière hospital; he introduced an antiseptic room in 1887, one of the first installed in France – his colleagues soon asked for the same. With a reputation for being an old-fashioned family doctor, Périer was a popular practitioner. In the hospital, where he became head of surgery, he was known as brilliant and impetuous, one of the first to do abdominal surgery successfully.[19] *Le Progrès médical* played an important role in the spread of Listerism by publishing some of the works of these pioneers. As long as the older surgeons skeptical of germ theory survived, some younger believers in the theory tricked them by

---

[17] Christopher Lawrence, "'A Time to Heal': The Diffusion of Listerism in Victorian Britain," *Bulletin of the History of Medicine* 74 (2000): 618–19; see also his book *Medical Theory, Surgical Practice: Studies in the History of Surgery* (London, 1992). Indispensable in the consideration of Listerism is the article by T. H. Pennington, "Listerism, its Decline and its Persistence: The Introduction of Aseptic Surgical Techniques in Three British Teaching Hospitals, 1890–99," *Medical History* 39 (1995): 35–60.

[18] Samuel Pozzi, *Quelques observations à propos du pansement de Lister appliqué aux plaies d'amputation et d'ablation de tumeurs* (Paris, 1876); Edouard Nicaise, *L'antisepsie dans la pratique de la chirurgie journalière* (Paris, 1896). Félix Terrier, the editor of the *Revue de chirurgie* from 1881 to 1907, author-reviser (with Maurice Péraire) of a *Manuel de petite chirurgie* (original work by A. Jamain (1816–62); 8th edn, Paris, 1901), published a *Petit manuel d'antisepsie et d'asepsie chirurgicales* (Paris, 1893) – also coauthored with Péraire; the opening lecture in his course in his *Cours de médecine opératoire* (Paris, 1893; 8th edn, 1901) was on antisepsis and asepsis.

[19] *Bulletin de l'Académie de médecine* 41 (1914): 418; *La Presse médicale* 81 (1914): 743; and Michel Dupont, *Dictionnaire historique des Médecins dans et hors de la Médecine* (Paris, 1999).

hiding sterile dressings under dirty ones. At least this happened at the Hôtel-Dieu in the late 1870s, when the good results obtained by using the sterile cotton wool dressings concocted by Alphonse Guérin became known.[20]

Henri noted that the second group to go to Britain was among the first in Paris to do successful – meaning that the patient survived – ovariotomies. In a statistical survey of the operations he did at the Saint-Louis Hospital during two years in the 1880s, Lucas-Championnière boasted of having done 237 successful major operations (amputations, hernias, excisions of the scrotum); in his 128 operations on the female abdomen, he was less successful – 8 deaths (6.62 percent mortality) – with ovariotomies for cysts being more dangerous (2 deaths out of 28 operations, that is 7.14 percent mortality). In another total of 321 operations on males and 142 on women, he boasted of a low mortality of 0.43 percent. It was striking to Lucas-Championnière that these excellent results were obtained in the most miserable of circumstances: the patient was placed on a mattress resting on a wooden table in flimsy structures previously occupied by victims of smallpox; the material should have been burned according to hygienists. The important thing, apart from the experience of the surgeon and his faith in the antiseptic method, was the total absence of suppuration (the formation and discharge of pus). A mini-revolution had taken place in Paris surgery. The glory of Lister was to have freed surgery from its empirical prison to bring it into a scientific state. Lucas-Championnière dedicated his book on antiseptic surgery to Lister.[21] When Philip Hair spent four months in Paris hospitals after graduating from Edinburgh in 1866, he found that there was nothing approaching Lister's treatment of wounds; instead, too weak solutions of carbolic acid were being used in a very slovenly, indiscriminate way. The three cases of ovariotomy he observed were fatal. The application of Lister's treatment in the Edinburgh clinical wards produced the best results.[22] A generation later Hair would probably have found some difference because of the influence of the French Listerians.

---

20 Victor Veau, "L'Oeuvre chirurgicale de M. Jalaguier," in *Adolphe Jalaguier (1853–1924)* (Paris, 1925), 35–48, from the *Journal de chirurgie* (décembre 1924). William Tod Helmuth, *A System of Surgery* (4th edn, New York, 1879), 237–8, 239–45, noted that Guérin's generally successful "occlusive and compressive dressing with wadding" was based on the principle of "the complete exclusion of atmospheric germs." Given the advantages of "Lister's antiseptic method," Helmuth recommends it to surgeons for a trial, especially in hospital practice.

21 Just Lucas-Championnière, *Chirurgie antiseptique. Principes, modes d'application et résultats du pansement de Lister* (2nd edn, Paris, 1880); *Statistique des opérations faites ... mai 1887 à mai 1889* (Paris, 1889); and *Le passé et le présent de la méthode antiseptique* (Paris, 1899). He wrote a classic monograph on the treatment of hernias: *Cure radicale des hernies* (1887; new edn, Paris, 1909). Pennington notes that John Tyndall described Lister's achievement as a revolution in surgery, changing art into science.

22 Letter by Philip Hair, M.B., *Lancet* (19 Oct. 1867), 502.

Henri's entry into the Parisian medical world of the 1890s coincided with this triumph of antiseptic surgery in hospitals. The basic elements of dressings were carbolic acid, corrosive sublimate (mercuric chloride), permanganate of potassium, iodoform, ether-iodoform, and some concoctions developed by ingenious doctors like Just Lucas-Championnière, whose powder achieved some popularity. Lucas-Championnière considered sublimate to be a dangerous and mediocre antiseptic in surgery and obstetrics and iodoform to be a bit better but far inferior to carbolic acid. After Koch showed in 1881 that sublimate was a superior killer of bacteria, its use spread in Germany. In 1884 Lister approved of the dangerous if effective mercurial disinfectants, though sublimate could not be used in a spray because of its toxicity and lack of volatility.[23] The new surgeons, operating in a new conceptual world, amused their students with horror stories about the great scalpels of the past, some of whom were still in action when Henri appeared on the medical scene. The great trinity of famous surgeons who were unbelievers in Listerism was still around in the 1890s: Armand Desprès (1834–96), Jules-Emile Péan (1830–98), and Aristide Verneuil (1823–95). One of Velpeau's favorite students, Desprès, after interning and enjoying the honor of being laureate of the faculty and of the *Assistance publique*, became an *agrégé* and a hospital surgeon before the age of thirty. His studies of erysipelas and muscle tumors did not make him so well known as his articles in the *Gazette des Hôpitaux*, of which he was editor for a while. He was the very model of the witty, sarcastic, even mocking Parisian, too gifted for his own good: a gymnast and a singer like Wurtz (who also sang while working), a skater like Maisonneuve, and even an engraver. The independent and liberal Verneuil was a popular professor whose *Eloge de Robert* attacked the system of medical education for its wasting of students' time and its killing of scientific initiative and independence. Péan is immortalized in a portrait of him teaching at the Saint-Louis hospital by his friend Henri Gervex, better known for his painting *Rolla*. In the early 1890s the French medical world was treated to a spectacular quarrel between Péan and Verneuil over priority in inventing and applying a hemostat.[24] Non-Pasteurians but great doctors.[25]

Henri condemned the entire crew of germ-doubters for refusing to admit obvious truths and reacting to principles of the experimental method with ill-considered contradictions and absurd acts resulting from excessive pride, professional jealousy, and often barely concealed bad faith. Péan, who had a reputation as the most skillful surgeon of his time, was not unusual in arriving in top hat, black dress with white tie, protected by a serviette around his neck, to operate at Saint-Louis. Even some believers in germ theory dressed similarly in the early days of Listerism. Operating coats came into use in the 1880s, at least

---

23 Pennington, *Medical History* 39 (1995): 38.

24 "Le débat Verneuil–Péan," *L'Illustration – Années 1892–1898* 106 (Paris, 1895): 72.

25 For biographical titbits, see Paul Labarthe, *Nos médecins contemporains* (Paris, 1868), and Pierre-Nicolas Sainte Fare Garnot, *L'Hôpital Saint-Louis* (Paris, 1986).

in Germany and America, to protect surgeons from sprays, blood, and infected patients. Verneuil, who concocted a theory of the "traumatic virus or poison," perhaps had doubts about his scorn of germ theory when he finally agreed to plunge his hands into a solution of carbolic acid before operating, though this concession had little effect on the grim statistics of his department. A faculty professor and member of the Academy of Medicine could afford to be a bit more philosophical about the risks of serious surgery. Desprès went too far in ignoring filth and germs when, as his daughter's obstetrician, he allowed her to come close to death with an infection, perhaps puerperal fever; called in at the last minute, Adolphe Pinard barely managed to save her. This empirical event did not change his mind about germ theory. Henri called it an "incident invraisemblable" and classified him as one of the last dirty surgeons of the past.[26]

Rejection of or lack of interest in germ theory did not necessarily signal a surgeon's lack of interest in sanitary conditions in the operating theater. After a successful operation to remove a blood cyst from a patient's left ovary, Péan once commented favorably on the use of alcohol dressings even though the operation had to be carried out in unsatisfactory sanitary conditions. He made similar observations after doing an emergency operation on a female patient to drain thirty liters of liquid and then remove a tumor weighing thirteen kilos. Henri might have been surprised to learn that the operation was a success.[27] After operating on hemorrhoids, Péan would insert a tampon of cotton wool treated with iodoform into the anus.[28] Whether or not germs existed, they had to be killed. In reality, sanitation and hygiene were becoming as important as the surgeon's skill.

In his canonical work on daily surgery, Desprès noted that in his early student days at the Hôtel-Dieu, of the three surgeons in action there, Philippe Boyer lost fewer patients than other surgeons because he did the dressings himself. Desprès listed two alcohol dressings among those to be used at the end of the treatments of wounds. He found Lister's use of phenol (carbolic acid) so complicated that it should not be recommended. It lacked only the rites of exorcism. Though there were some wounds and operations in which Lister's dressing was as good as the alcohol dressing, its disadvantage was that it provoked a cauterization effect and prevented suppuration – Desprès apparently accepted a revised version of the doctrine of "laudable pus," whose formation assumed drainage from the affected

---

26 HR, *Croisière*, II, 53. Pinard wrote an article on Semmelweis for the *Annales de gynécologie et d'obstétrique*, 2nd series, 3 (1906): 641–54; see Robert Delavault, *L'Asepsie un demi-siècle avant Pasteur: Ignace Semmelweis 1818–1865* (Paris, 2007), in the collection *Médecine à travers les siècles*.

27 Jules-Emile Péan, *Ovariotomie; l'ovariotomie, peut-elle être faite à Paris avec des chances favorables de succès?* (2nd edn, Paris, 1869), 30, 33, 45.

28 Péan, *Leçons de clinique chirurgicale professées à l'hôpital Saint Louis pendant les années 1887 et 1888* (Paris, 1892), 692. Péan noted that expertise on cysts of the uterine parenchyma was a French specialty, particularly at Saint-Louis.

area. Camphorated alcohol possessed virtues that could not be lightly discarded. As Peter J. Kernahan has shown, some surgeons like George Callender got excellent results from "a pre-Listerian program of cleanliness," while refraining from criticizing the new germ gospel. One of the major problems with germ theory was "Lister's collapse of causation into a single etiologic agent … difficult for surgeons to accept."[29]

In his discussions Desprès did not mention germs. Not even in his discussion of hemorrhoids, though they were as common as varicose veins; the pathological changes torturing the rectal-anal and leg areas are similar in both afflictions. Hemorrhoids gave Desprès an opportunity to indulge in a Cheyne-like commentary on the vices of civilization. Piles were often caused by the good life. Binges, tiredness, and constipation were not excluded in his catholic etiology, but he emphasized that they were one of the punishments men suffered as a result of having enjoyed "an excess of women." Sexual excess could also produce orchitis, which might be matched by metritis in the co-enjoying wife. Desprès did not entertain the notion of other possible relations. Such were the joys and medical sorrows of the newly married before facing pregnancy and death.[30]

Puerperal fever – Tarnier's discovery

Puerperal fever was the major single cause of maternal mortality in the pre-Pasteurian age. By the 1880s it was becoming rare even in hospitals; of course it was still safer to have a child at home attended by a midwife rather than a doctor.[31] But even long after the antiseptic age arrived, deaths from this fever accounted for forty percent of British maternal mortality. Of equal medical importance was the fact that the fever was a professional cross borne by the accoucheur. The Parisian obstetrician Stéphane Tarnier illustrates nicely the dilemma faced by the hospital doctor who accepted the statistical knowledge available by the 1860s on puerperal fever mortality. When Tarnier was an intern in the Maternité hospital in 1856 1 in 17 deliveries ended in the tragedy of a dead mother (2237 deliveries and 132 deaths). Tarnier classified the disease as an epidemic, which was as common outside the hospital as inside it – or so it was commonly believed until Tarnier put his keen observational powers at the service of an embryonic epidemiology. Since the facts he observed "en ville" did not agree with common opinion, Tarnier

[29] Peter J. Kernahan, "Causation and Cleanliness: George Callender, Wounds, and the Debates over Listerism," *Journal of the History of Medicine and Allied Sciences* 64 (Jan. 2009): 1.

[30] Armand Desprès, *La chirurgie journalière* (1877; 4th edn, 1894). The prolific Desprès also wrote on depopulation, syphilis, La Fontaine's fables, and the nursing sisters (*Les soeurs hôspitalières … la laïcisation des hôpitaux* (Paris, 1886)).

[31] W. F. Bynum, *Science and the Practice of Medicine in the Nineteenth Century* (Cambridge, 1994), 205–6.

did a comparative statistical study of the puerperal fever mortality in the old 12th arrondissement and in the Maternité. The work gave him a medical thesis, a memoir, and a shocking argument.[32]

Discussion of the subject at the Academy of Medicine revealed the alarm caused in the ranks of doctors by a maternal mortality seventeen times greater at the hospital than in Paris generally. Alfred Velpeau, who had a considerable reputation with the scalpel, convinced that Tarnier's figures were wrong, asked Adolphe Trébuchet to check them. Trébuchet came to roughly the same depressing conclusion as Tarnier, but in a piece of fine tuning he found that city maternal mortality was 1 death out of 250 live births rather than 1 death out of 322 births. (Comparable mortality in London was 1 death for every 309 births.) Returning to the fray in 1862, Tarnier restated his figure of 1 out of 322 and increased the mortality at the Maternité to the deplorable level of 1 maternal death out of 14 births. Other hospitals being no better, the best thing for an expectant woman to do was to give birth at home. Although varying figures were served up by different experts, who had their own agendas, the most complete and perhaps the best statistics were, Tarnier argued, those provided by J.-F. Malgaigne and published in the official bulletin of the ministry of the interior.[33]

Years	**1861**	**1862**
Hospitals	1/10.42	1/14.64
Bureaux de bienfaisance	1/194.12	1/164.66
City, excluding the above	1/169.80	1/160.88

It was cold comfort that the provincial hospitals had about the same maternal mortality. Hospitals in cities such as Vienna, Munich, Leipzig, and St. Petersburg were little better than those in Paris. A bleak maternal mortality landscape dominated Europe.

The etiology of disease in pre-Pasteurian medicine was dominated by miasmas, which could be divided into further enlightening categories like "puerperal miasmas." Tarnier showed his ingenuity by finding that puerperal miasmas impregnated the walls, objects, bedclothes (and so on) of the rooms occupied by women lying in; the women's life in common in an area containing women already sick was disastrous. The only solution Tarnier could think of was to have the hospitalized women put in a separate area for a period of up to eight days

[32] S. Tarnier, *Recherches sur l'état puerpéral et sur les maladies des femmes en couches* (thesis, Paris Faculty of Medicine, 1857); *De la fièvre puerpéral observée à l'hospice de la Maternité* (Paris, 1858). For the apotheosis, mostly deserved, of Tarnier (researcher, educator, popularizer, and a revolutionary in obstetrics, surgery, and medicine,) see the fine work by Scarlett Beauvalet-Boutouyrie, *Naître à l'hôpital au XIXe siècle* (Paris, 1999).

[33] Tarnier, *Mémoire sur l'hygiène des hôpitaux de femmes en couches* (Paris, 1864), 6.

immediately after they gave birth.[34] Why not abolish the maternity hospitals? First, abolition would deprive pregnant women of the professional skill available only in the hospital and the free service provided for the "poor and pregnant in Paris."[35] And maintaining the doctors' skills was dependent on a supply of pregnant women. True, Tarnier confessed, it was a secondary consideration, but maternity hospitals were "a resource for clinical teaching, and for doctors, and for midwives, and the suppression of this resource would leave the pregnant woman a victim of all the enterprises of ignorance and empiricism." The advance of medical science was dependent on the sacrifice of a number of new mothers. This cruel dilemma must have weighed heavily on the conscience of the few doctors who thought about the subject. After Tarnier's work it was difficult to ignore the issue.[36]

In 1875 Pierre Budin, Tarnier's *interne* at the Maternité, went to Edinburgh to observe Lister's practices. In 1878 Budin also did the rounds of maternity institutions in Holland, Germany, Austria, Russia, and Denmark. Armed with foreign knowledge, Budin was able to convince Tarnier to use carbolic acid systematically in the fight against puerperal fever. Paul Bar, another of Tarnier's *internes*, had experimented with sublimate as an antiseptic, which was regarded as an improvement on Tarnier's techniques of isolation and ventilation. The older generation was not paradigmatically immune to innovations recommended by younger doctors, at least if the doctors were under firm patriarchal control.

Obstetrics: the labor of Adolphe Pinard

In the late nineteenth century, obstetrics was still connected to surgery; it was a part of the surgical empire, though this had little meaning for pregnant women, most of whom were fortunate enough not to have to come into contact with a surgeon. The pregnant poor went to the Maternité, where professional midwives supervised deliveries. Surgeons took over only in difficult or abnormal deliveries, though in some hospitals the *Assistance publique* added a few delivery beds to the general medicine rooms. The curse of the system was infection, a problem caused by the way medicine was practiced and which, doctors concluded, could only be cured by more medicine. The battle against bacteria was accompanied by a reform of institutional and professional structures. Budin requested the setting up of special services for delivery of babies along with the creation of a corps of physician-accoucheurs. In 1882 Paris municipal councilors, Lanessan

---

34 Beauvalet-Boutouyrie, *Naître à l'hôpital*, 319, refers to Tarnier's system, involving separation of mothers, doctors, nurses, interns, and midwives with a drop in mortality from 12.4 percent in 1871 to 2.8 in 1879.

35 Rachel Ginnis Fuchs, *Poor and Pregnant in Paris: Strategies for Survival in the Nineteenth Century* (New Brunswick, NJ, 1992).

36 See S. Tarnier, *De l'asepsie et de l'antisepsie en obstétrique ... leçons professées à la clinique d'accouchements*, collected and edited by Dr J. Potocki (Paris, 1894).

and Bourneville supported the idea. The result was that the *Direction générale de l'Assistance publique* created a class of hospital accoucheurs, recruited by competitive examinations much like the system for recruiting doctors and surgeons in the departments of Paris hospitals. The first competition, in 1882, admitted four doctors, including Budin, to the new positions. This new hierarchic (and hieratic) status for obstetrics also marked the moment when, according to Henri, "obstetrical technique took on a new importance in the domain of the medical sciences, thus gaining a privilege denied it until then."[37] A scientific-bureaucratic change of considerable magnitude complemented the antiseptic "revolution" evident in obstetrical practice after 1875.[38]

By the 1890s the "theory of antisepsis" had fully penetrated obstetrics, but as Adolphe Pinard regretted, puerperal fever still killed too many women. *Professeur agrégé* at the faculty of medicine in Paris and accoucheur of the Lariboisière hospital, Pinard took the usual keen interest of the intelligent doctor in the history of his profession and churned out several useful surveys of the history of obstetrics in Paris hospitals. Lariboisière had opened in 1854 with the maternity section becoming a separate department in November 1882. Pinard calculated that the 12,580 women who delivered up to 1 January 1889 experienced a total mortality of 0.74 percent with 0.39 percent being due to "puerperal infection." The antiseptic liquid that Pinard used initially (1882–84) for vaginal irrigations and for wet compresses applied to the vulva was a 1 percent phenyl solution aromatized with essence of thyme. On the advice of Bouchard, Pinard changed the solution to one containing mercury iodide and potassium mercury iodide, among other things. A petroleum jelly containing phenyl made examinations safe. In 1885 there were 757 deliveries in house with 15 maternal deaths (6 from puerperal fever) and 1312 external deliveries with 5 deaths. Pinard emphasized the importance of all hospital personnel being skilled in the antiseptic method; "all must have faith."[39] It is still difficult to convince medical personnel to follow sanitary practices without fail; washing hands seems especially difficult.[40]

In a study published in 1896 on the treatment of puerperal fever, Pinard and Victor Wallich found that during 1894 in the *Clinique Baudelocque* out of 2137 women who delivered or had miscarriages, 7 died. Four women died from puerperal fever and 3 from eclampsia, which is a complication of preeclampsia, a condition formerly called toxemia.[41] These figures indicate a remarkable drop in deaths from septicemia during the decade 1883–94, from 2.78 to 0,18 percent.

---

37 HR, *Croisière* , II, 228.

38 HR, *Croisière*, II, 219–315.

39 The Conclusion in Adolphe Pinard, *Du fonctionnement de la maternité de Lariboisière et des résultats obtenus depuis 1882 jusqu'en 1889* (Paris, 1889).

40 "Handwashing and Use of Examination Gloves," *Lancet* 351 (1998): 571.

41 A. Pinard and V. Wallich, *Traitement de l'infection puerpérale* (Paris, 1896). Deaths from preeclampsia are rare in the USA, but there is an increase in cases of the disease, which produces high blood pressure, albuminaria, and oedema. Linda Carroll, "Dangerous

Pinard and Wallich attributed the change to the methodical institution of continuous irrigation. In 1894 out of the 123 women who were infected, or considered as such, only 29 had stayed in the room for women awaiting delivery; all the others were in labor and dilated when they arrived, with 6 having had examinations or operations outside the clinic. So it was difficult to know where this latter group had become infected. And since a change of personnel could considerably affect results, Pinard and Wallich emphasized the importance of training the personnel in the latest theory and practice. Out of the approximately 60,000 births in Paris in 1896, about 27,000 took place in the establishments of the *Assistance publique*; the rest were presumably home deliveries handled by the city's 3700 doctors, midwives, and health officers.[42]

The training of personnel changed to accommodate discoveries being made about infection-producing bacteria. Pasteur's work on "puerperal septicemia" appeared in 1879–80. The articles he published in the bulletin of the Academy of Medicine eventually reached a large medical audience. In 1889 Fernand Widal's thesis showed that the microbe responsible (*streptococcus pyogenes*), which entered the system through the uterus, could give rise to different forms of puerperal fever. In 1888 J.-A. Doléris, a hospital accoucheur, found that the old procedure of curettage advocated by Récamier about the mid-nineteenth century but abandoned, could still be an effective means of treatment.[43] After 1895 the fight against puerperal fever entered a new phase with the introduction of serum derived from animals that had been vaccinated against the germ. When it became known that a serum would be effective against only a specific bacterium, doctors like Pinard and Widal emphasized the importance of first getting a pre-treatment diagnosis identifying the specific germ causing the disease. Widal's work showed the different forms of streptococci. And after Marmorek's research was published in the *Annales de l'Institut Pasteur* in 1895 it became clear that treatment of certain diseases needed to be preceded by a "bacteriological diagnosis" – the germ had to be identified.

Medical students had only a short time to learn about delivering babies and the bacteriology relevant to childbirth. True, by the 1890s the newly trained students knew the theoretical basis of antisepsis, but Pinard received them during only a month for their *stage* or practical experience at the *Clinique Baudelocque*. Every two weeks a group was phased in for a month. The obstetrical education of students had improved slowly over the century. A "cours d'accouchement" had been introduced at the Hôtel-Dieu in 1794. When Siebold visited Paris in 1831 students had no place to learn the practical side of delivery. The same was true in many other towns. In Bordeaux midwives with faculty diplomas were found in the

Complication of Pregnancy Becomes More Common," *The New York Times* (10 July 2001), D7, D10.

42 Paul Brouardel, *La profession médicale au commencement du XXe siècle* (Paris, 1903), 39.

43 Pinard and Wallich, *Traitement de l'infection puerpérale*.

1840s to be as ignorant as medical students.[44] Assisting at a delivery was one of the few things considered immoral for an early nineteenth-century student. Then in 1834 the first chair of clinical obstetrics was created in Paris. Paul Dubois, Pajot, and Tarnier were among its distinguished holders. By 1880 a single department was clearly inadequate for handling 600 doctors. Even in 1890, according to Pinard, some students were becoming doctors without ever having examined a woman or having been present at a birth. When Pinard was the head of the birth clinic connected with the Paris Faculty of Medicine, he found that out of 135 students the number of times a student received delivery training ranged from 2 to 5, with 43 students assisting at only two events. So when students took the relevant fifth medical examination, the results could be disastrous if they had not been assiduous in the area. (Work experience outside official courses might have helped.) Pinard added that the results for the women delivering might be even more disastrous. He was convinced that obstetrics could not be taught according to the existing medical-surgical model of pedagogy.

As we have seen, Henri de Rothschild entered medical school at a time when the theory and practice of medicine had changed as a result of Pasteur's germ theory and also as a result of a growing medical consciousness and even guilt over the high mortality accompanying medical intervention. And the acceptable level of mortality was constantly being revised downward as scientific discoveries identified more and more of the causative agents of disease and etiology fed into actual doctor–patient relations. This growing concern over the success of medicine in treating the patient manifested itself in an increased attention to detailed statistical analyses of results obtained in surgery.

Mortality figures at the end of the nineteenth century indicate that an operation was still a dangerous business. Consider the statistical reports done at the Bichat hospital in the *Service des consultations spéciales et service hospitalier* during the 1890s.[45] In 1892 the number of sick treated was 10,528, with most patients showing up in August, vacation time. Forty-nine deaths occurred among the 593 patients operated on: 15 deaths among those having abdominal surgery and 19 deaths among the 238 women whose genital organs required surgery. No one died among the 32 males whose genital organs were cut. Mortality was still at about the same high level in 1899, when 206 operations on female genital organs resulted in 20 deaths compared with no deaths for the 28 operations on the male apparatuses. Gender equality appears in a conflation of figures for 197 abdominal operations on males and females with 39 deaths. Grim as these figures appear to us, they should be placed in the context of the 12,105 sick who were treated

---

44 M. Barnetche (professeur d'accouchements, etc.), "Considérations sur l'hospice de la maternité de Bordeaux," *Journal de médecine de Bordeaux* (1843): 200–1.

45 Félix Terrier, *Statistique des opération pratiquées à l'Hôpital Bichat (service des consultations et service hospitalier) pendant l'année 1892 [–93, 1898–99]* (Paris, 1893–1900).

in the external surgical *consultation*; 385 of this number also had operations not requiring hospitalization.

Doctors made a serious effort to implement the latest chemical-killer strategies in the warfare against germs. The report of 1893 noted that solutions of phenyl were no longer used to wash wounds, hands, instruments, or operating surfaces, though this Listerian panacea was still used as a spray in waiting rooms to keep down dust and make them easier to clean. There was a limited use of a solution of calomel (mercurous chloride) and a concentrated solution of boric acid. Asepsis was displacing antisepsis, especially in the operating area, which was scrubbed down with soap and filtered, boiled water. Further cleaning was carried out in the space where the patient was operated on. For dressings there was sterilized talcum powder, ordinary cotton wool, and sterilized lint. Instruments required different sterilization procedures. The "German procedure," employing caustic soda, was unpopular because it took the nickel off instruments. By the 1890s the latest technology for sterilizing instruments was the Mally sterilizer that used glycerine at 125 to 130 degrees centigrade, followed by a bath in a corrosion inhibitor, sodium nitrite (made with filtered water) at 111 to 116 degrees. In order to survive, most germs required the cooperation of careless personnel. As Pinard never tired of warning, it is easy to make a mistake in the struggle to keep the patient free from a life-threatening infection.

Henri's Medical Heroes[46]

Henri believed that his lost lycée year might have prevented him from ascending to the status of *interne*, a sort of medical or surgical resident in the hospital. The so-called but aptly named *externe* could observe patients, perform certain tasks, generally "unskilled," and keep records, but he (rarely she) never enjoyed the privileges of the "marshal's baton"-wielding *interne*. Most candidates failed the examinations for the *internat*. Among famous failures we find Léon Daudet and even Charcot, though the latter did well enough to get classified as a provisional intern; Daudet had probably lost interest in becoming a doctor, and he was certainly more interested in pursuing Jeanne Hugo than studying for the *internat*.[47] The casualty rate is not surprising, given the fact that only enough doctors were passed to fill the few positions available. Henri failed in 1896, when 564 candidates competed for 60 internships. Anatomy was his weak spot, with a score of 7 out of a possible

46 In the Han period (206 B.C. – A.D. 220), Chinese biographers would indulge in an account of the people their heroes had read; not a bad idea. Gilles Manceron, *Segalen* (Paris, 1991), 7.

47 Christopher G. Goetz, Michel Bonduelle, and Toby Gelfand, *Charcot. Constructing Neurology* (New York, 1995), 292–5; for a different spin on Daudet's experience, see Marie-Christine Pouchelle, *L'hôpital corps et âme. Essais d'anthropologie hospitalière* (Paris, 2003), 167.

15 points in the written examination. He did well in pathology, with 12 out of 15 points. The range of anatomy examination scores in his group of 12 (11 present) candidates ranged from 14 to 7 points and in his pathology group of 10 examinees from 13 to 9 points. He was not admitted to the oral examination. Uninterested in repeating the grim ritual, Henri went on to an astonishingly productive medical career, as perhaps only a Rothschild *externe* could do.[48]

After being named "externe des hôpitaux," Henri spent a year with Paul-Jules Tillaux (1834–1904), whose expertise in anatomy was rewarded by having a fracture named for him, and the experience familiarized the student with dislocations, fractures, and minor surgery. But Tillaux was simply "a great surgeon of the old school." Henri was particularly fond of Pierre Budin, his "très vénéré maître," whose "excellent advice" guided his early career. The initial encounter, in 1893, was not promising. Being rewarded with a bronze medal on becoming an *externe* in 1892 did not guarantee a friendly welcome by the professors. Henri the student supplicant went to see Budin to ask for a place as an *externe* in his department at the Charité hospital. The name Rothschild produced a rather cold welcome. "… I am very strict with my students and tolerate no irregularity," the professor warned. Henri replied that there would never be an occasion to reproach him. Even when he got married, Henri took just a short leave in order never to miss a single tour of duty, which in these particular circumstances, Budin noted, in a moment of rare levity perhaps, was an act of great merit. Budin soon came to have a different reaction to the name Rothschild; praising his former student in 1902, he noted that Henri learned about duty in the family, which also taught him to do good. In time the "kind and patient teacher" became a friend whose presence in times of happiness and sadness gave encouragement and consolation. Budin took the place of a father for Henri, who emphasized this relationship by saying that Budin considered him as a son.[49]

Georges Dieulafoy (1839–1911) makes an appearance in Proust's *Le Côté de Guermantes* to consult with Dr Proust, Marcel's father, at the deathbed of Marcel's grandmother.[50] Another of Henri's faculty fathers, Dieulafoy was

---

[48] AP-HP, 761 Foss. 20 (761 Foss. 1–72 covers "Personnel médical: concours et prix.") See Thomas Neville Bonner, *Becoming a Physician. Medical Education in Britain, France, Germany, and the United States, 1750–1945* (New York, 1955), 107, 129–30, and Guy-Marie Lucien, *Cent cinquantenaire de l'internat des hôpitaux de Paris* (thesis, Paris Faculty of Medicine, 1952).

[49] Speeches by HR and Pierre Budin, in *Discours prononcés à l'inauguration de la Polyclinique Henri de Rothschild, le 19 décembre 1902* (Mâcon, 1902).

[50] *Le Côté de Guermantes* (1920–21) is the third part of Marcel Proust, *A la recherche du temps perdu*. Zola delved into Dieulafoy's *Manuel de pathologie interne* for a touch of realism when he wanted to describe the agony of Dr Pascal in *Le docteur Pascal* (Paris, 1893). See "Biographie de médecins célèbres de l'antiquité à nos jours," www.medarus.org/Médecins/MédecinsTextes/dieulafoy, and Anne-Marie Bernard, *Le Monde de Proust vu par Paul Nadar* (Paris, 1999), 42.

always a conspicuous figure at any of the medical gatherings centering on Henri's medical activities. A habitué of the Rothschilds, a collector of paintings of the romantic school, he was also one of the flock of well-known doctors who looked after Henri's mother. So Henri's initial meeting with Dieulafoy was less formal and more friendly than the one with Budin. Like Budin, Dieulafoy had a story about the beginning of their relationship, which began at the Necker hospital. The dialogue developed in the professor's catechismal form. Dieulafoy: "My dear Rothschild, I would be delighted to have you as a student, but in my department we begin work early." Henri: "I know." Dieulafoy: "We finish late." Henri: "I know." Dieulafoy (perhaps surprised at this lack of frivolity): "You will have to arrive early and leave late; you will do autopsies, make observations – you will be the low man on the totem pole." Henri: "Quite!"[51] Henri was a model student, the first to arrive at and the last to leave the hospital. And he volunteered to do the boring tasks shirked by many others. Dieulafoy was surprised (again) to find that Henri kept up this impressive performance throughout his stint in the department. In his memoirs, Henri would later dub Dieulafoy his "grand patron." During two years as an *externe* in Dieulafoy's department Henri continued studying internal pathology and during the "eloquent professor's" Thursday teaching at Necker, he first learned to examine a patient and give a diagnosis. So he had much to thank the "master clinician" for. The third year of his *externat* was spent in Fournier's department at the Saint-Louis hospital. Although known as a leading medical researcher, Fournier had a reputation for being good to students. Fournier allowed Henri to develop the clinical skills acquired under Dieulafoy and to diagnose venereal and skin diseases, sometimes difficult to do.

Many doctors like to trace their intellectual heritage back to Hippocrates, but Dieulafoy settled for Sydenham, "the English Hippocrates," who had also been recommended by Bretonneau and Trousseau. As indicated by the holdings of Sydenham's works, including translations, in French libraries, the apostle of the bedside tradition was popular in the land of the clinic. In 1896 Dieulafoy proudly climbed into the faculty's *chaire de clinique*; ten years before he had become faculty professor of internal pathology. He considered himself lucky to have been a student in the brilliant clinical period at the Hôtel-Dieu during the reign of Trousseau, a man of Tours, like Dr Rabelais. Dieulafoy spoke so well that many people thought that his clinical lectures were delivered extemporaneously; faculty gossips attributed this rhetorical skill to his roots in the Midi. He was from Toulouse. Henri admired Dieulafoy for having been able to leave the old "non-Pasteurian" school and, though over fifty years old, accept germ theory. This switch was not a bad idea for someone who was a believer in the redemptive power of surgery and whose great successes in treating diseases in the body cavities justified the audacity and temerity of its practitioners. And medical studies were soon modified to give surgery its place in the sun. Having done a surgical internship for two years with Velpeau and Denonvilliers, Dieulafoy was an enthusiastic promoter of the

---

[51] HR, *Croisière*, II, 131–3.

new partnership between medicine and surgery. Fernand Widal credited Dieulafoy with having "created the medical-surgical movement; he drew doctors out of their timidity, transforming their medical temperament."[52]

Perhaps. But Dieulafoy deplored the conservatism of official medicine, at least in his conversations with Henri once the latter had entered the medical profession and begun a career of hospital building. French medicine needed more experimentation and the development of a new diagnostic. And, Dieulafoy urged, this was the direction in which Henri should push the medicine practiced in his hospital. In Parisian hospitals the heads of departments rarely got the opportunity to treat the sick by calling on the most recent advances in physics, chemistry, and biology. Hoary rules, sacred routines, and the ideology of the administrators of the *Assistance publique* all militated against any attempt to adopt the latest medical-surgical idea or practice and still less to move ahead of the leaders in their fields. Hence the importance of Henri's new Polyclinique in the rue Marcadet, where Dieulafoy hoped to see one of the signs of the rebirth of French medical leadership. The death of Dieulafoy in 1911, a few years after the deaths of Pierre Budin and Paul Poirier, represented, Henri later lamented, the disappearance of the last of his "grand patrons." Of course the *grand patron* did not really disappear: as Vergez-Chaignon points out, he evolved from a polyvalent physician dividing his time among hospital, faculty, and private clients to the hospital doctor, a researcher, administrator, and man of the latest medical science.[53]

One of the mentors chosen by the dean (Brouardel) to keep an eye on Henri was a surprising choice. Périer recommended the director of the *Ecole pratique* of the faculty, Paul Poirier (1853–1907), who was interviewed by Thérèse to make sure that her son would be in Poirier's own laboratory and under his wing even at lunchtime. Poirier was not keen on this odd arrangement but accepted it since he kept an open table for students and friends anyway. Thérèse did as much as she could to control Henri and, above all, prevent him from wasting time. So every day Henri would go lunch chez Poirier in the lodging provided for him at the faculty *Ecole pratique*, next to the Dupuytren museum. Sometimes Poirier lunched chez Charcot on the boulevard Saint-Germain.[54] Poirier was a fantastic character, the talk of the town, a dandy, a fashion horse, who zipped from faculty to hospital driving his own Panhard. He had a reputation as a great surgeon, which he believed was justly deserved. Many people, including lots of women and some powerful friends, agreed. In 1870 he met and became a close friend of the top lawyer and politician Waldeck-Rousseau, who was married to one of Charcot's daughters. So

---

[52] HR, *Croisière*, II, 151–2. On the successes of the new "surgical therapeutics," see Georges Dieulafoy, *Clinique médicale de l'Hôtel-Dieu de Paris 1896–1897* (Paris, 1898), 17–21. Dieulafoy was at Tenon from 1879 to 1881.

[53] HR, *Croisière*, II, 216–17, and Bénédicte Vergez-Chaignon, "Le Médecin," in Jean-Pierrre Roux and Jean-François Sirinelli (eds), *La France d'un siècle à l'autre. Dictionnaire critique* (Paris, 2000), 511–12.

[54] HR, *Croisière*, I, 221 ff.

thanks to his unusual mentor, Henri met literary men, lawyers, journalists, young surgeons, and also some of the "dangerous creatures" his mother wanted to keep him away from; he did not seem to suffer any ill effects from any of the encounters chez Poirier, who was flattered by singers as "le premier gigolo de Paris." Poirier enjoyed the publicity.[55]

In 1887 Poirier had been nearly ruined by the Pranzini scandal, which was the subject of a successful book by Henri years later.[56] Pranzini was a famous criminal who murdered a friend of Poirier's, the high-class tart Régine de Montille, along with the chambermaid and her daughter. Following an established custom, students in Poirier's laboratory, who were doing a dissection of the executed murderer Pranzini, made wallets from the cadaver's skin. Anthropodermic bookbindings were more common. *La Lanterne* used news of the practice (and the fact that the police also received a wallet) to stir up politicians and to sell papers. It is probable that Gaston Variot was behind the articles. Variot had lost to Poirier in the competition for the single available *agrégation d'anatomie*, an event that led him to hate the faculty and Poirier; Variot later recognized that there was no basis for the accusation against Poirier.[57] The politically well-connected Brouardel was able to ride out this affair of a few days and save Poirier's skin. He was not able to save him from the sharp pens of Léon Daudet and Paul Bourget.[58]

In the preface to his medical thesis, Henri referred to the four years during which he did dissection in Poirier's laboratory, temple of anatomical science and surgery. Contrary to much gossip about Poirier's absences, Henri refers to the master's constant and vigilant supervision. Not just a ritual formula in this case. It seems that Poirier was not initially happy to see Henri show up to learn anatomy at the *Ecole pratique* because the professor suspected some frivolous intentions on the part of the young Rothschild. One of Henri's favorite professors and friends,

---

55 In 1904 Poirier moved from Tenon, where he had been from 1889 to 1903, to the Lariboisière hospital. Léon Daudet put him in his novel *Les Morticoles* (Paris, 1894) as the handsome surgeon Tismet de l'Ancre, understanding and obliging surgeon of "femmes du monde." On the novel, see Toby Gelfand, "Medical Nemesis, Paris 1894: Léon Daudet's *Les Morticoles*," *Bulletin of the History of Medicine* 60 (1986): 155–76, and chapter 8 of Mary Donaldson-Evans, *Medical Examinations. Dissecting the Doctor in French Narrative Prose 1857–1894* (Lincoln, Nebraska, 2000). In the second volume of his *Souvenirs et polémiques*, entitled *Devant la douleur* (1914), "édition établie par Bernard Oudin" in the collection "Bouquins" (Paris, 1992), Daudet handed out kudos to a few doctors while castigating others. Paul Bourget gave Poirier a fictional dramatic role in his novel *Le Sens de la mort* (1915). See Jacques Mialaret, *Paul Poirier, 1853–1907* (Paris, 1965), 1, 9.

56 André Pascal (HR), *Pranzini. Le Crime de la rue Montaigne. Avec reproduction de documents authentiques* (Paris, 1933), 466. This work was translated into English.

57 A.-B. Marfan, "Nécrologie – Variot (1855–1930)," *Le Nourrisson* 18 (1930): 206–8. Though supported by some big guns, Variot was also a sore loser to Marfan in the competition for a faculty chair in 1914.

58 Léon Daudet's comments on the medical profession are easily found by using Oudin's excellent index to Daudet's *Souvenirs et polémiques*.

Poirier was a skillful dissector of the mind and emotions as well as a master of the scalpel in the dissecting theater. Henri appreciated both theaters, profiting from Poirier's moral judgments and his prudent, enlightened advice as well as his teaching of anatomy.

Poirier had succeeded the eccentric and brilliant Farabeuf (1841–1910), whose bizarre appearance, odd clothes, and curious delivery were offset by skillful teaching, blackboard virtuosity, and good dissecting skills. An excellent organizer, he "renewed and codified anatomy teaching and surgical medicine," and "inspired and supervised the construction of the buildings of the *Ecole de Dissection*."[59] The author of a canonical manual on surgery, he trained many anatomists and probably most of the surgeons in Paris hospitals. Nearly blind, he retired in 1902 confident that the faculty would pick his choice for succession, not his notorious rival, Poirier; the professors cooperated, but the higher powers did not: the *Conseil supérieur de l'instruction publique* refused to ratify the faculty choice and thereby gave the minister the opportunity to pick Poirier.

Farabeuf was a hard act to follow. Poirier's hagiography assures us that he did it without any serious problems because he possessed a surplus of the pedagogical qualities esteemed in the medical faculty. Poirier was a startling change from Farabeuf, who fascinated by his oddness. The dapper professor's pleasing if small physique, his ease in speaking combined with a mastery of the audience, his keen intelligence, his productive industriousness, his power to inspire, and his choice of top-quality collaborators "ensured his enormous and deserved success." His research on lymphatic vessels and the publication (with Charpy and an army of associates) of an encyclopedic treatise on anatomy gained him a modest international reputation.[60] Henri said that he and associates spent some time over a period of about four years collecting items to serve as illustrations in this *Traité d'anatomie*.[61] Poirier's activities give us a glimpse into the surgeon's life as well as of the role he played in the development of surgery in Paris hospitals. An important part of Poirier's influence is visible in his communications and above all in his criticisms, often acerbic, of the communications of his fellow surgeons at the *Société de Chirurgie*. Meetings were not tepid affairs, especially when Poirier aroused passions by bruising big egos. Not that Poirier was the only one to indulge in a "virulent and icy courtesy," though he excelled at it, and his skill encouraged the others, especially wounded colleagues. Poirier spoke nearly as often as the garrulous Tuffier, who in 1904 spoke fifty-eight times on many subjects. Reynier, Guinard, and Michaux, and even Terrier and the icon Tuffier, were Poirier's frequent targets.[62]

Poirier and Henri both had a passionate interest in three subjects: asepsis, appendicitis, and cancer.

---

59 G. Cordier, *Paris et les anatomistes au cours de l'histoire* (Paris, 1955), 78.

60 Cordier, *Paris et les anatomistes au cours de l'histoire*, 78–9.

61 HR, *Une dame d'autrefois*, 79.

62 Mialaret, *Paul Poirier, 1853–1907*, 3.

Once asepsis came to be regarded as indispensable, discussion turned to the modalities of aseptic procedures (including the preparation of the patient's skin and the surgeon's hands), the usefulness of gloves, and techniques of sterilizing instruments and the different kinds of equipment.[63] Doctors had enough latitude of decision for things to go seriously wrong as well as right in the operating theater. At the Tenon hospital there was still careless behavior as personnel passed, without taking the proper aseptic measures, from the autopsy to the operating room. The subjects of aseptic discussion have changed but the difficulty of maintaining eternal vigilance in surgical cases keeps discussion (and infection) a permanent reality in the hospital.

Anesthesia and aseptic procedures made modern surgery possible, allowing the surgeon to create a quasi-autonomous empire in medicine for nearly a century until it became "integrated into wider therapeutic strategies."[64] The path of progress was not a smooth one as surgeons squabbled over issues and techniques. The appendectomy, first performed in the 1880s, illustrates how difficult it was for the great men to agree on a single approach to medical conditions. The word appendicitis seems to have been used first by R. H. Fitz at the inaugural meeting of the Association of American Physicians in 1886.[65] Discussion of the acute condition was driven by a mortality of eighteen percent in Paris, and even up to thirty-five percent in Henri Chaput's department, though it is difficult not to accept Chaput's argument that he could not be held responsible for patients showing up with general peritonitis, which caused the death of seventeen out of forty-eight patients, compared with no mortality for the thirty-one ordinary cases. Chaput, along with Dieulafoy and Poirier, was in the pro-operating camp.[66] Dieulafoy insisted that the medical treatment of appendicitis did not exist. Poirier's dogma maintained that as soon as the diagnosis is certain or even a simple suspicion exists, the surgeon must take out the appendix. Some doctors still prescribed the application of leeches and believed that only the formation of an abscess was a clear indication of the

63 Pennington, *Medical History* (1995), 39 (1): 39, notes aseptic procedures like boiling instruments, sterilizing dressings, use of steam at atmospheric pressure, and the autoclave.

64 On the evolution of surgery, see Roy Porter, *The Greatest Benefit to Mankind. A Medical History of Humanity* (New York, 1998), 597–627.

65 The appendix has recently been found to be of immense importance to the fetus in immune system functions and excellent for reconstructive surgery of the bladder and ureter. See Loren G. Martin, "What is the Function of the Human Appendix?" ScientificAmerican.com, article posted 21 October 21 1999, and Carl Zimmer, "The Riddle of the Appendix," *The New York Times* (9 August 2005), science section.

66 On the importance of Chaput in the history of surgery, see Jacques Poilleux, "Portrait de Henri Chaput (1857–1919), www.bium.univ – Paris 5.fr/acad -chirurgie/séances … 2006. He wrote the chapter on "Les anus contre nature et les fistules stercorales" in the multivolume *Traité de Chirurgie* (Paris, 1892), edited by Simon Duplay and Paul Reclus. Chaput headed surgical departments at the hospitals La Pitié (1900–01), Broussais (1901–06), and then Lariboisière.

need for an operation, which was generally a simple incision and drainage. In Poirier's surgical philosophy, Frederick Treves's successful drainage of Edward VII's appendix in 1902 was classified as "a temporization that nearly killed the king."[67] Henri Diriart noted that in the Béarn in the early twentieth century, well-informed patients refused operations in the clinic; on one occasion his father had to use the kitchen table to perform an emergency appendectomy (successful) on a woman patient.[68] The prudence of these patients was not unjustified.

The unclear etiology of appendicitis has not prevented doctors from having strong opinions on the subject. Henri followed one group's medical opinion in rejecting "the old theory" that the affliction is caused by cherry stones, grape seeds, birdshot, and other small bodies that become lodged in the organ. We pretty much dismiss this theory too, though there has been at least one cherry pip found in an inflamed appendix, and it has been argued that hundreds of cases of appendicitis can reasonably be blamed on seeds.[69] Henri subscribed to the idea put forward by Dieulafoy in his faculty lectures of 1895 that the problem occurred when the opening between the appendix and the intestine became blocked, causing inflammation. So the research task was to search for the causes of this occlusion rather than investigating the foundations of the popular medical theory on the inflammation-provoking migration of gravel into the appendix. Blockage and putrefaction were the processes at the center of the new etiology; microbes produced acute inflammation leading most often to a perforated appendix. The danger was that a gangrenous mass would drop into the abdominal cavity, thus ensuring peritoneal disaster. For Henri here was a satisfying coherent theory drawing upon extensive clinical experience and pointing the way to an effective treatment. And he could praise one of his teachers for making a first rate contribution to the literature on a modern medical scourge. Of course he did not give a detailed discussion of theories of obliteration such as that of Charles Talamon. Doctors knew where to find such discussions, and the public should not be overburdened with surgical minutiae.[70]

Believing that medical advances should be made known through popular propaganda, Henri showed in 1897, with a long article on appendicitis, that he could compete with the best of facile pens in the game of "vulgarisation populaire."[71] A dramatic opening: "In the past few years a new illness has become known ... appendicitis." And while the doctor might deplore the number of its victims, he could applaud the numerous works written on the subject by doctors and surgeons.

67 Mialaret, *Paul Poirier, 1853–1907*, 14.

68 *Réception du docteur Henri Diriart*, Académie de Béarn, séance publique du 8 mai 1976 au parlement de Navarre (Pau, 1976), 26.

69 Roger W. Byard, and others, "Acute Appendicitis in Childhood: Did Mother Know Best? A Pathological Analysis of 1409 cases," *eMJA*, 169 (1998): 647–8.

70 Charles Talamon, *Appendicite et pérityphlite* (Paris, 1892).

71 HR, *L'appendicite. Notes de vulgarisation populaire* (Paris, 1897), extract from the *Revue générale internationale scientifique, littéraire et artistique* (7 janvier 1897).

The dramatic nature of the affliction ensured that it got its share of publicity, but Henri noted that its causes and especially knowledge about its serious consequences if untreated were not known widely enough. Even doctors did not always take the necessary precautions with their patients to avoid the fatal complications that could arise from inflammation of the vermiform appendix. Doctors were good at taking a patient's history and in doing a physical examination – still the best way of diagnosing appendicitis – but they did not know much about the best treatment for it. Henri claimed that there were lots of deaths attributed to violent shock, the cold, or the absorption of some harmless small foreign body, when in reality death resulted from an undetected attack of appendicitis allowed to degenerate into peritonitis. Following Dieulafoy's description of this "terrible illness," an experienced doctor could diagnose appendicitis in its early stage by observing symptoms such as vomiting and constipation and by noting the localization of the pain at McBurney's point.[72]

Henri may have been suffering from an overdose of optimism, for it turns out that even in our advanced age about nine percent of the cases of appendicitis in men and a startling twenty-three percent in women are misdiagnosed. The difficulty with women seems to be a "more complex anatomy [than men] in the right side of their abdomen," and the difficulty with surgeons is that "nearly one in four appendix removals in women of childbearing age" are unnecessary. Technological advances do not necessarily increase the physician's clinical acumen.[73] But this situation results directly from the surgical philosophy developed in the late nineteenth century after anesthesia and antisepsis/asepsis allowed for the surgical empire to dominate medicine. Dieulafoy's dogma warned that "one will never regret having operated too soon; one will always regret having operated too late."[74] Progress made by modern surgery – a vague but irrefutable formula – made appendicitis much less serious. Opening up the abdomen had become a safe operation if, Henri added, it were done by a skillful surgeon. The professional result of this development was a shift in the turf arrangement: surgeons captured appendicitis from physicians. Dieulafoy tried to save something for medicine by declaring that there are certain illnesses that are medico-surgical, meaning that the turf has to be divided between the doctor who diagnoses and the surgeon who operates. Henri concluded his analysis by proclaiming the authority of the surgeon, the savior who intervenes to save patients before their death from peritonitis. "One owes one's salvation to the surgeon alone, on condition of abandoning oneself to him

---

[72] Charles McBurney (1845–1913), American surgeon. "The point on the surface of the abdomen which lies on a line from the tip of the hip-bone to the navel and one-third of the way along it, which is the point of maximum tenderness in appendicitis" (*The New Shorter Oxford English Dictionary*).

[73] "Many Appendix Ops 'Unnecessary'," BBC News, 9 October 2001.

[74] HR, *L'Appendicite*, 18.

completely, that is to say without discussion of the timeliness of the operation and especially without wanting to delay an operation he judges urgent."[75]

Henri subscribed wholeheartedly to the surgical imperative for cancer as well as for appendicitis.

The long history of breast cancer operations, which seem to have been by far the most common type of cancer surgery until well into the nineteenth century, reaches back into late antiquity. By the late nineteenth century the radical mastectomy along with the prostatectomy had entered the repertoire of the adventurous surgeon. By the time Henri left medical school there were few parts of the body that had not been brought into the scalpel's domain. Poirier can be regarded as a modest pioneer in cancer surgery and an advocate of the school of radical extirpation. Whether the afflicted organ was the tongue, breast, or uterus, among others, Poirier insisted on early intervention and a radical excision of the lymphatic glands, the villains of propagation of the disease, according to the latest medical theory. This approach assumed that the lymphatic system and the bloodstream were separate; the eventual discovery of their complete integration showed the theoretical bankruptcy of the radical surgical approach, at least in the treatment of breast cancer, by the 1970s.[76] Paul Segond, perhaps willing to accept the position of his fellow great surgeons, worried about the "surgical aberrations" of which others might be guilty. Poirier exuded confidence. Surgery had made great progress, and so he and colleagues operated better than their teachers, and their students would operate better than they did. Though his general belief may be true, his example is hardly convincing. Some old surgeons were still using their fingers to pluck a few ganglions from armpits, and naturally their cases had a poor prognostication. Others, like Poirier, taking the radical approach to the afflicted organ and the lymph glands got "incomparably better results."[77] Fellow members of the Society of Surgery kept discussing the issues for weeks. Poirier's surgical treatment of cancer of the tongue was approved by Henri Hartmannn, J.-L. Faure, Pierre Sébileau, and Edouard Quénu. It was not easy to doubt a man who accepted patients judged inoperable by colleagues and presented their cases to the Society as cures two years later. Defining cure was not a priority. Younger colleagues and those, like Henri, training under Poirier were convinced that Poirier's path was the road to progress. With Pierre Delbet and G.-S. Roussy, Poirier was one of the founders of the *Association française pour l'étude du cancer*. Henri also joined the group.

Sometimes Poirier's surgery worked, sometimes it did not. In the absence of a scorecard of the sort we have nowadays, we have to judge anecdotally, which

[75] HR, *L'appendicite*, 17. Henri does not mention Adolphe Jalaguier's classic chapter on appendicitis in the second edition (1895) of the *Traité de chirurgie*; Victor Veau, in his obituary article on Jalaguier (*Journal de chirurgie*, Dec. 1924) says that the chapter was still valuable in 1924; in 1901 Jules Ferron dealt with the "technique de Jalaguier" in his thesis.

[76] Porter, *The Greatest Benefit*, 604.

[77] Mialeret, *Paul Poirer, 1853–1907*, 14.

necessarily means considering the results of operations on famous people. In 1905 Poirier operated on Maurice Bunau-Varilla, flamboyant scoundrel and editor of the famous paper *Le Matin*, for appendicitis with peritonitis.[78] The price for recovery was a temporary stercoral fistula. When Poirier found that Waldeck-Rousseau was suffering from cancer of the pancreas, he called on the hero of the cholecystectomy, Hans Kehr, to operate; but the patient died during exploratory surgery. Not that much could have been done anyway in this case. The next year Poirier got the grim news that he had the same disease, took leave and ended up dying in a *Maison de santé* in Auteuil. He died in 1907 after a massive self-administered injection of morphine. After funeral rites were celebrated in the church of Saint-Germain-des-Prés, he was buried in his native Normandy. Henri was among those speaking at the graveside.[79] Poirier left half a million francs to Henri with instructions that he should establish a hospital in Granville for the study of all matters relating to maternity and infant care. Henri carried out his duty, and Jules Pams, then minister of agriculture, officially opened the hospital in 1911.[80]

A view from the top: Brouardel looks at the profession in 1900

Henri de Rothschild entered medical school at the time of its greatest hopes, strains, and political pressures between the Revolution and our own day. At the end of his career, Paul Brouardel surveyed the French medical scene. Medicine begins with disease.[81] Here Brouardel could count many victories and hold out hope for more. The efficacy of "new methods" had been demonstrated against the child killer diphtheria and the frightening if rare disease rabies. More serious general killers such as tuberculosis, typhoid fever, and cholera were better understood, and though they were by no means eliminated, the way in which they became epidemic was better understood. Knowledge was seen as the beginning of prevention. Brouardel, who was president of the *Société de médecine publique et d'hygiène professionnelle de Paris*, admitted that there was a lot of disease in

[78] See the coruscating sketch of this "flamboyant, mad-dictator type of press magnate" in Theodore Zeldin, *France 1848–1945* (2 vols, Oxford, 1977), paperback volume *Taste and Corruption* (Oxford, 1980), 182–4.

[79] Mialaret, *Paul Poirier, 1853–1907*. Dominique Meyniel, *Tenon, l'hôpital de Ménilmontant* (Paris, 2008), 55, praises Poirier as "one of the creators of modern cancerology, ... a great anatomist," and a contributor "to the founding of the nursing school of the *Assistance publique*."

[80] François Huguet, *Les professeurs de la faculté de médecine. Dictionnaire biographique* (Paris, 1991).

[81] Brouardel, *La profession médicale*, 5–8. At the beginning of the autumn term in 1899, speaking as dean, Brouardel told students of the medical profession's new social role as a public figure. See chapter 5 of Pierre Guillaume, *Le rôle social du médecin depuis deux siècles 1800–1945* (Paris, 1996).

working-class families, though he did not refer directly to social conditions of disease, probably because that would have introduced politics, specifically the role of politicians in public health. The clinician and pathologist Charles Bouchard did not hesitate to recognize the impossibility of ignoring "the influence of social conditions upon the individual's propensity for disease."[82]

Brouardel did identify an interest of the political class in the health of the working class, an interest coinciding with the scientific revolution in medicine. "Thanks to the work of Pasteur [no mention of Koch], we can declare that there are avoidable diseases; their agents are known ..." He might have mentioned the growing presence of the medical profession in elected political offices. So not only were people looking to the new medicine for protection from diseases, they were reminding the new doctors that "promises had been made in the name of science." Brouardel noted too the political anxiety about the "depopulation" of France. This being a difficult matter of regulating reproductive sexual behavior in favor of a larger population – one attempt was to make abortion illegal – politicians turned to doctors for advice about prevailing diseases and often got answers to more questions than they asked. A reduced mortality could compensate for a declining birth rate. As Brouardel put it, "Since France cannot be forced to procreate, at least we can prevent those who are born from dying." In addition to curing disease on an individual basis, the doctor now had to show officials at all levels of government how to avoid disease.[83]

The new doctors knew more than their predecessors, and there were more of them to put the new scientific medicine into practice. In 1893 there were 1963 doctors in Paris; by 1900 there were 2846, a one third increase in 7 years. Brouardel argued that the result was a serious decrease in salaries because each doctor's number of patients dropped from 280 to 146. Older doctors complained about the faculty's turning out all these new doctors without a warning on "the extremely grave crisis in the profession."[84] An influx of foreign students aggravated the situation: in 1894 a quarter of the medical students were non-French. This foreign invasion was dealt with by a law of 1897 requiring any individual who wished to practice in France to possess the *baccalauréat* degree in order to get a state medical degree (*doctorat d'Etat*); otherwise, the degree granted was a purely university degree (*doctorat d'université*), which did not allow the holder to practice in France. The number of foreign students dropped rapidly to about 100 seeking the purely university degree. Another problem was not so easily solved. In 1894 there were about 5000 medical students in facilities that could serve a maximum of 3000. At the request of Brouardel, the minister of education sent out to the educational bureaucracy a circular putting the brakes on expansion; for a number of years a

82 Andrew Aisenberg, *Contagion, Disease, Government, and the "Social Question" in Nineteenth-Century France* (Stanford, 1999), 84, 87. Aisenberg notes anti-Pastorian Michael Peter's supporting view on the social conditions of disease.

83 Brouardel, *La profession médicale*; see chapter 4, 59–208, esp. 59–60.

84 Brouardel, *La profession médicale*, 38–48.

policy discouraging students from pursuing a medical career kept the number of students at about 4000. The system was still churning out annually a good number of doctors, rising from 595 in 1890 to 1211 in 1898. Brouardel calculated that between 1859 and 1901 French faculties graduated 8440 doctors. In 1902 there were more than 16,000 doctors practicing in France. The foundations of the later vast medical machine were solidly in place. French doctors were probably correct in believing that they were too thick on the ground. By the end of the twentieth century, the number of doctors was approximately 190,000, about 1 doctor for every 300 people, instead of 1 doctor for every 2500 people in about the year 1900. Over the course of the century, doctors classified as specialists rose from 5 to about 50 percent of the profession.[85]

What good resulted from this efficient production of doctors? Given the roles of public health measures and better nutrition in improving the longevity and wellbeing of populations, this is an unanswerable question. Nevertheless, we have an answer. Brouardel argued that there was a correlation between falling mortality rates and the increasing number of doctors. In 1891–93 the French death rate was 23.7 per 1000 and in 1896–1900 it was 22.0 per 1000. And in the mutual associations formed to fight disease through better medical care and mutual help, the death rate was 16.0 per 1000. Having three million members, the *Mutualités* had a considerable positive influence in promoting good health. In Paris, with the greatest concentration of doctors, the death rate per 1000 was 24.3 in 1886 and 20.6 in 1900. The wealth and health of the Ile-de-France are not of recent vintage. Brouardel's weakness for statistical speculation led him to calculate that there were 100,000 fewer sick people in Paris in 1900 than in 1886. Whatever the validity of the statistical arguments, few people cared to argue against the case that more and better medical care resulted in a healthier population.

In his plays Henri de Rothschild successfully exploited to good dramatic effect the problems and ethical dilemmas of the new doctor, including the arrival of the woman doctor. Brouardel noted that the state of malaise in the medical profession so evident in 1900 was reflected in the move to "fix" the rules of medical deontology (a fancy word for ethics) and in the discussions about the rights and duties of doctors both in their relations with one another and with their patients. For Brouardel medical ethics dealt with only one side of the issue of the so-called "extremely grave crisis" of the profession. Its deep causes lay in the progress of science, especially the discoveries of Pasteur, and the notoriety given by the non-scientific press to all of the conquests, true or hypothetical, in the medical domain. Had not a large number of parents pushed their offspring into "a career where they will find, they believe, honor and profit?" Brouardel was inclined to place most

---

[85] Vergez-Chaignon, "Le Médecin," in Roux and Sirinelli (eds), *La France d'un siècle à l'autre*, 511; see also her book *Le Monde des médecins au XXe siècle* (Bruxelles, 1996). See George Weisz, *Divide and Conquer. A Comparative History of Medical Specialization* (New York, 2006), xv–xvi, for a distinction between the nature of specialization in the nineteenth century and in the twentieth (1890s to 1940s).

blame for doctors' troubles on the politicians, who, following the lure of social change, passed laws making the practice of medicine more difficult.[86] Not that it stopped students from flocking to the profession, whether in the hope of saving humanity or of making money, and the two aims are not mutually exclusive. But of course they had a different social outlook from Brouardel's, whose career (and life) was about to end.

The new century seemed to Brouardel to be much more medicalized, in a general sense, than the preceding one, though he did not say so explicitly. He noted how the press in 1900, compared with that of thirty years before, dealt with all the issues of medicine and public health. No newspaper was without its daily dose. There were articles on the great discoveries, newly discovered germs, new surgical operations in the antiseptic-aseptic age, the quality of drinking water, and the adulteration of food and wine; and there were all sorts of advertisements for medicaments to treat nearly every disease. The press has never turned back from this direction. Like us, Brouardel was the victim of his own Whiggish epistemology. "In the sciences, truth is absolute ... In the arts [humanities], the absolute does not exist, for all is relative ...Now in the practice of medicine all is relative."[87] So the nearer that practice moved towards science, the more certain it became. Medicine was condemned to worship Isis if it wanted to keep those promises about curing diseases. But doctors found that patients increasingly demanded much more than the cold comfort of science.

Looking back from the early 1930s over his career in medicine Henri was no less Whiggish than most historically minded doctors are in boasting about the tremendous medical progress western man enjoyed in the nineteenth century, especially in the post-Pasteurian era. Henri was particularly impressed by the results achieved in his own area in medicine, pediatrics.[88] True, in the period 1874–90, a time of squabbles, there were hardly any results in "the fight against infant mortality." But about 1892, "the art of curing underwent a profound evolution" because of Pasteur's discoveries – Koch was again ignored – which not only gave doctors an explanation of the etiology of diseases and infections but also "certain means of preventing and fighting them." The inauguration of the Pasteur Institute in November of 1888 by the president of the Republic gave official approval to germ theory. Pasteur's methods being adopted, "our *maîtres* in the art of healing were not slow in accomplishing miracles." One of these miracles, Henri believed, was Tarnier's getting rid of puerperal fever in his hospital department. Antisepsis brought gangrene and septicemia under control in the hospital. The development of an anti-diphtheria serum seemed also to bring about a mini-miracle. We now see things differently, with the mortality curve in steep descent before the introduction of the serum, as seems to be the case in other diseases with their serums and vaccines. The medical memory and statistics are two different historical categories

86 Brouardel, *La profession médicale*, 11, 29–30.

87 Brouardel, *La profession médicale*, 23.

88 HR, *L'oeuvre philanthropique du lait* (Paris, 1902), 6–8.

of understanding. But few historians would not agree with Henri's assertion that "With the discoveries of Pasteur and Lister surgery entered a new era," with an ever-expanding empire because of the boldness of surgeons, no longer held back by fear of infecting their patients.[89]

Germ theory led to a reorganization of medical turf. Henri put this in dramatic terms. "As a result of being able to open the abdominal cavity without infecting it, gynecology passed nearly completely from the control of the doctor to that of the surgeon."[90] There was not a turf war in a classic sense because medicine, animated by the higher cause of obtaining the maximum of cures possible, evolved in a more peaceful and unifying way. Or so he believed. The barriers between medicine and surgery along with those between obstetrics and puericulture broke down. The new theory of the origin of disease required the close collaboration of doctors, laboratory workers, surgeons, accoucheurs, and pediatricians to defeat the recently identified enemy. But basing the progress of scientific medicine on germ theory imposed a new program with innovations in the methods of diagnosis and the rise of an elite group for the treatment of diseases. Henri identified two members of this elite in Parisian medicine, "two *grands maîtres* of French science to whom we owe this second evolution in the art of healing": Budin and Dieulafoy.[91] Budin's harnessing of science, medicine, and politics to produce a shakeup if not a revolution in the care of infants, along with his promotion of Henri's medical career, can be seen as a reasonable pretext for this grand claim. But Dieulafoy? Henri's argument was that this great clinician definitively established the pathology, symptomatology, and treatment for appendicitis. As we have seen, Dieulafoy, championing the surgical approach, brought in the surgeon (inevitably one of his friends) to operate in his presence, thus co-opting a potential rival and establishing a medico-surgical partnership for the benefit of the patient. Not that the French escaped "the cult of the surgeon" or the advent of "the fashionable surgical disease," both topics of Henri's plays.[92]

What this analysis ignores, or at least treats as a sub-text, in its deification of Pasteur is what Alain Contrepois describes as "the integration of medical bacteriology into the diagnosis and treatment of patients." Contrepois draws attention to the "interaction of clinical and bacteriological approaches," in late nineteenth-century medicine, with the "bacteriological diagnosis in the laboratory" being the "true extension of clinical medicine." Dieulafoy and Bouchard were two of the major figures in the harnessing of the new medical speciality of "infectious pathology" to the established anatomical-clinical approach to medicine.[93] So

---

[89] HR, *Notes ... Budapest* (Paris, 1897), v–viii.

[90] HR, *Croisière*, II, 228.

[91] HR, *Puériculture et centres d'élevage* ((Paris, 1931), 8.

[92] Bynum, *Science and the Practice of Medicine in the Nineteenth Century*, 137; see the chapter on surgery in Porter, *The Greatest Benefit to Mankind*, 597–627.

[93] On this topic, including a reduction of the significance of the broader concept of the so-called Pasteurization of France, see Alain Contrepois, "The Clinician, Germs and

soon after the Great War it would not have been possible for Henri to talk about the spread of the influential German bacteriological model, even though it was integrated into hospital medicine, and Henri was always proud of the latest medical practice in his establishments. Perhaps one should not exaggerate the integration of clinic and laboratory, for as late as the 1950s the pediatrician Robert Debré deplored the typical designation of lab work as examinations complementary to the primary clinical examinations. Debré aimed for an integrative approach in his new pediatric hospital.[94] Henri, curiously ignored in the pediatrician's forays into medical history, would have had no trouble in agreeing with him.

Infectious Diseases: The Example of Charles Bouchard [1837–1915] in Paris," *Medical History* 46 (April 2002): 197–220.

94 Robert Debré, *L'honneur de vivre. Témoignage* (Paris, 1974), 412.

Chapter 4
Henri de Rothschild's Medical Empire in Paris

He who gives dominates.[1]

When he was eighteen, Henri de Rothschild wrote a short Whiggish essay (dedicated to his mother) intended for all the ladies engaged in charity who enjoyed being members of patriotic and national organizations such as the *Œuvres de l'Union des Femmes de France* and the Red Cross.[2] In stating a number of truisms on charity and in exhuming some historical (more or less) facts about medical care, Henri gave us some insight into the genesis of his own career in medical charity. His explanation of the charitable impulse assumed that the divine hand had encoded the golden rule in the human heart. What would happen to humanity if there were not people who would help the unfortunate and the sick? With all the poverty, suffering, unhappiness, illness, and moral corruption in the world, high-minded people like his mother would always be able to satisfy their desire to do good.

Henri vaguely recognized the existence of ancient medicine and even that of the Arab world before he leapt into the late nineteenth century. Christianity improved on ancient customs, but scientific progress and the development of the modern state transformed the concept of charity by bringing new resources to public morality. Neatly avoiding any reference to the seizure of church resources during the French Revolution, Henri merely noted the contemporary growth of hospitals, orphanages, asylums for the aged, and various kinds of schools – all of the vast welfare structure inspired by public charity. And private charity continued; indeed with the fantastic growth of capitalism, it increased or at least seemed more spectacular than it had been for some centuries. Henri believed that medicine had been the most valuable auxiliary of *la bienfaisance*, a concept similar to *la charité* but perhaps without any theological baggage.

Claiming that no science had experienced so many revolutions as medicine, Henri nevertheless believed that post-Hippocratic medicine took giant steps on the road to certainty only to be derailed for centuries by an excess of imagination. So much for the history of medieval medicine. Still, history helps us understand the

---

[1] Fernand Braudel, *The Mediterranean and the Mediterranean World in the Age of Phillip II* (Berkeley, 1996), II, 826.

[2] Henri de Rothschild [HR], *Etablissements hospitaliers et secours médicaux dans l'antiquité* (second edn, Mâcon, 1890).

nature of modern medical science. Medicine deals with many objects, but thinking about the different means that took the art to its perfection shows that one must go back to the sources from which the different parts had their origin and growth. The degree of certainty achieved in medical science has not been achieved by combining facts but by the multitude of discoveries and observational precision. Only a return to the history of medicine can reveal the path of progress taken by the art as well as the insight of the great men into the cure of diseases. Henri's history was shaky but his ideology was progressive.

The Hospital that Henri Built

When in late 1895 he established a *Consultation de nourrissons* in an empty shed on the old Rothschild hospital property in the east of Paris, Henri had no idea of how the popularity of the establishment would lead him into the hospital business. The beginning aim of Henri's Picpus institution was to guide nursing mothers through a program of "medical supervision" and to distribute free sterilized milk. Two new areas, general medicine and surgery, were added later, with a dozen beds to hospitalize sick nursing mothers and their babies. Expansion included two annexes for a laboratory with an atelier for photography and a department of orthopedics and radiography. Among the young patients were a large number with rickets, scrofula, and tuberculosis. The *consultation*/polyclinic took on the proportions of a small hospital. It soon had three to six daily hospitalizations chosen from among the most seriously ill. In eight years, the records showed 69,282 consultations and 76,000 hospitalizations. The hospital's emphasis was on pediatric service. At the *Exposition universelle internationale* of 1900 in Paris the jury report on Henri's Picpus exhibit called his establishment a dispensary and a small hospital. The exhibit received honorable mention.[3] Fortunately for the booming patient population, the polyclinic moved to its new premises in the rue Marcadet (18th arrondissement) in 1902.[4]

One problem with the Picpus address was that he had to waste an hour to travel there from his rented residence in the Avenue d'Iéna. And two Rothschild hospitals on the same property might have been excessive for the area, at least compared to the medically shortchanged northern area of the city. He finally found an old milk shop of 600 square meters in the rue Marcadet. After six months of remodeling, the building could be called a hospital and inaugurated as such after he defended his thesis and became free of his duties to the *Assistance publique* (1898). By 1901 the need for expansion showed the wisdom of moving the polyclinic to the rue

---

3 Report online at http://cnum.cnam.fr/CGI/fpage.cgi?8XAE580.4/334/100/758/0/0. The jury report on the *Exposition* of 1900 gives 40,000 as the number of people treated annually – no details are given; medicaments given were over 100 daily, reaching perhaps 45,000 annually.

4 The Rothschild Archive, London [RAL], 000/930: 58-1, 168–71.

Marcadet, where he found lots of land with easy access, permitting the building of a much bigger establishment with better organization. The experience gained in five years allowed Henri to organize on the basis of information better than that he started out with in the rue de Picpus. In a great number of cases hospitalization of children now seemed indispensable; his building on the rue de Picpus was not satisfactory for that scale of operation. Henri boasted that his Marcadet system provided a model for others during the next quarter century.[5]

The new hospital, planned by Henri-Paul Nénot, the architect of the new Sorbonne (University of Paris), measured 1400 square meters, with the medical facilities on the first floor and four dormitories for 25 adults or children on the second floor. Care was first limited to pediatrics, babies being brought in by their mothers; but then adults needing care started showing up and were not turned away. In the new hospital Henri decided to accept the sick whose state required care in the areas of general medicine, surgery, dermatology, women's diseases (including those specific to pregnant women), pediatrics, orthopedics, eye, ear, nose and throat, dentistry, and even nervous and mental problems. To assure a "rational treatment" he needed the latest therapeutic resources. So the new polyclinic was endowed from the beginning with well-equipped laboratories for histological, bacteriological, and chemical research, as well as for photography, radiography, sterilization and galactology (research on milk). Three *internes* and a pharmacist complemented 15 medical personnel, who were under a female director and a midwife. As well as being the titular head of the *consultation de nourrissons* and of surgery, Henri put himself at the top of the establishment in all medical and administrative matters. But this apparent *Übermensch* knew how to delegate power to competent colleagues.

The glittering ceremony marking the inauguration of the Polyclinic H. de Rothschild on the rue Marcadet in 1902 gives us an idea of the importance of the hospital and the prominent socio-political position occupied by Henri in Third Republican Paris. The minister of public education (J. Chaumié) presided over the affair. Henri, Mathilde, and his sister Jeanne received the guests, who were comforted by an entrance quivering with live plants and a courtyard "artistically decorated."[6] Among the more than 300 guests were the president of the municipal council, the prefect of the Seine, the prefect of police, the mayor of the 18th arrondissement, senators and deputies, municipal councilors, a covey of professors and doctors, including Zadoc-Kahn, and another Rothschild famous for her medical charity, Henri's mother. Henri led a large contingent, including the minister, on a tour of the impressive premises, and as an enthusiast of automobile racing, he made sure that they did not miss the ambulance. The short speech by the minister expressed admiration for the intelligent organization and practical layout

[5] HR (André Pascal), *Une dame d'autrefois. La Baronne Mathilde-Henri de Rothschild 1872–1926* (Lausanne, 1946), 83–4.

[6] HR, *Une dame d'autrefois*, 83–4.

of the hospital, at once a polyclinic, a dispensary, and a center of education. And a politician could especially appreciate the fact that it was in a populous area of Paris. The Republic was grateful and the government congratulated the founder. On no day in his life could Henri have indulged his appetite for adoration more than on 19 December 1902.

Opened to the public on 1 January 1903, the new establishment had the advantages of profiting from the lessons learned from the old hospital and the fact that there was no general hospital in the quarter of the *Grandes Carrières* – a reference to the area's old gypsum quarries. The clientele increased so rapidly that alongside the services for treating babies, the administration had to organize a hospitalization service for adults of both sexes. So after a while the polyclinic was transformed into a true hospital with regularly organized departments under the direction of competent specialists.[7] Looking back, nearly thirty years after the opening, Henri said that it was really in 1908 that the Marcadet establishment was transformed into a true hospital. This is a few years later than the date one might deduce from some other sources, which seem tweaked to speed the institution along the road to greatness. The *Consultation de lait* with its distribution of sterilized milk was ended when similar organizations appeared in the quarter. During May 1904 out of 1304 patients, 332 were newborns and 538 were children. The number of male adult patients reached 185 and female patients 249. Moving to a higher level of medical prestige, the hospital provided medical and surgical care for children and adults of the 18th arrondissement; its surgical service developed considerably, with its 35 beds reserved preferably for patients who had been operated on and for the increasing number of victims of accidents on public streets. Within a couple of years about 4000 patients were being seen annually with about 15,000 consultations a year. There were so many people at certain times that departments were overwhelmed, and rules had to be established to ensure the rejection of cheats pretending to be poor in order to get free medical care, which could include chemical analyses, bacteriological cultures, and inoculations, in addition to medical attention and medicaments. In 1909 alone 28,000 dressings were done, 11,000 free prescriptions given out, 18,000 liters of milk given away, and 281 orthopedic devices applied. In over 20 years, from June 1903 to December 1924, 2667 sick people were hospitalized, including 1681 cases of major surgery. There were 221,371 consultations with free distribution of medicaments, 195,254

[7] The medical personnel included L. Brunier (assistant to Henri), *Consultation de nourrissons*; Baillet, general medicine; A. Péchin, ophthalmology; Pierre Bonnier, ear, nose and throat; Léopold Lévi, neuropathology and psychiatry; P. Ehrhardt, surgery; C. Ducroquet, orthopedics; L. Netter, laboratory research; Valensi, pharmacy. Source: HR, "Polyclinique H. de Rothschild," in *Actualités Médico-chirurgicales* (Paris, 1911). Henri later noted Abel Desjardins under "services annexes" for surgery.

liters of milk, and more than 1500 layettes.[8] A mini-medical industry was booming in the 18th arrondissement.

It is not easy to estimate from surviving documents what it cost Henri to run his medical establishments. In 1899 he made a payment of 80,000 francs to Hélios (*Société de produits hygiéniques et alimentaires*). The jury report of the *Exposition* of 1900 gave the annual cost of running the Picpus clinic at 60,000 to 80,000 francs. As early as 1904 (January–July) there is a record of one expense of 62,025 francs for his Marcadet polyclinic; later institution building greatly increased spending. The first round of installation of scientific equipment cost about 200,000 francs.[9] Many minor and some major bills have survived. The plumbing bill in 1899 came to 2186 francs. One expense listed for Marcadet in May 1901 is about 3030 francs but another bill for a month (without a date) is just over 8890 francs. Other bills for that year total 7151 francs. For October 1903 there are two separate lists, one running to just over 4774 francs and the other to just over 5489 francs. Then for November 1903 the salaries for personnel are given as 4437 francs. Other bills due for March 1904 add up to 1815 francs. An extraordinary bill in November 1903 came from the city for washing down the building, amounting to 3793 francs. We can get a better idea of the cost from the survival of a "Relevé des dépenses" for July 1904 showing the cost of the Polyclinic for that month as 8930 francs, and for the period 1 January to 30 July of 1904 as 62,024 francs. In July 1905 the list of expenses for the polyclinic included 6609 francs for general service and 3293 francs for patients. His support of medical publishing entailed all sorts of heavy expenses. Two bills for photography, presumably illustrating some disease or other, in July and December 1905 totaled 3572 francs. Collaboration by the physicians Brunier and Netter on his *Revue d'hygiène et de médecine infantiles* did not come cheap, if the amount of 4040 francs paid to them in the same year is any indication. Payments to G. Kadar for printing and engraving and to Protat for printing ran between 2342 and 6376 monthly for both in 1905, though the payment in March was for 18,419 francs. Publication of the third volume of his *Traité d'hygiène et de pathologie du nourrisson et des enfants du premier âge* and number 6 of the *Revue* in 1905 cost 19,613 francs.[10] Printing bills, which could be considerable for journals he supported, are not included in these figures; nor is the cost of medical books and journals, including many German publications, for the excellent library at Marcadet. In January 1920 Henri bought 30 shares of the publishing company Félix Alcan for 22,500 francs. Perhaps his printing bills

---

[8] HR, "Polyclinique H. de Rothschild," in *Actualités Médico-chirurgicales*, and RAL 000/930: 58-1, 168–71, 200.

[9] Though many of Henri's papers have survived their Franco-German–Russian voyage to the RAL, much appears to be missing, making it impossible at present to give total expense figures.

[10] "Henri de Rothschild 1899–1911," Archives nationales: Centre des archives du monde (CAMT), Roubaix, 132 AQ 5914 and RAL 000/930: 58-1, 210.

convinced him that publishing was a good investment, and Alcan looked like a good bet.[11]

Militarized as auxiliary hospital 78 during World War I, with its nursing personnel attached to the *Société de secours aux blessés militaires*, the Marcadet establishment was designated as a treatment center for the seriously wounded. Henri paid for the entire functioning of the center during the war, which saw 821 wounded soldiers admitted for a total of 54,359 days of hospitalization. Seventy surgical beds were set up for the severely wounded. Pierre Delbet was the head surgeon and Pierre Ehrhardt the head doctor. Between 1916 and 1918 Henri supplied to the appropriate organizations the materials necessary for treating burn and blister victims by the wax method. In a post-war reorganization at Marcadet, surgery was given renewed importance with the appointment of Gaston Picot, who, unfortunately for historians, was more expert with the scalpel than the pen.

The Great War had a considerable impact on medicine both technically and institutionally. There was greatly increased state intervention. The medical corps was mobilized, meaning an astounding if temporary growth of medicine controlled by the state. It also became obvious during and after the war that French medicine and public health were inferior to practices in a few other countries, notably the United States. The Rockefeller mission to France (Commission for the prevention of tuberculosis, 1917–22) "aimed at hygiene education and the modernization of health-care services," initially at least to protect American soldiers from TB and venereal diseases.[12] In France no one was more aware than Henri of the peculiarly French health problems and the need to emulate the best medical practices of other advanced countries.

The Marcadet polyclinic, a totally philanthropic work, had a double goal in Henri's opinion: first, to serve the sick poor and, secondly, to constitute a center of study, research, and scientific teaching. This dual mission distinguished Henri's from James's hospital. With all departments functioning regularly, it was not difficult to attain this goal and even go beyond it. Specialization demanded new consultations for diseases of the digestive tube and of the nervous system, as well as for arthritic affections. In 1908 an independent department of major abdominal surgery and gynecology came into existence. In 1909 modernity arrived with a big splash in the creation of a department of radium therapy to treat cancer patients. Henri proudly announced that there then existed no better-equipped hospital for the treatment of the poor of Paris in the best possible way. The polyclinic rapidly became a vast and varied field of medical science studies. Scientific documents from different departments soon accumulated in large numbers. Such potential

---

[11] RAL 000/930: 58-1, 168–71, 172–82, 197, 199, 200, 202, 203.

[12] [11] See Pierre Guillaume, *Le rôle social du médecin depuis deux siècles 1800–1945* (Paris, 1996), chapter 7 ("Les Répercussions de la première guerre mondiale"), and *Research Reports from the Rockefeller Center* (Spring 1996), 5: http://archive.rockefeller.edu/publications/resrep/rr1996.pdf. See also Jean-François Picard, "American Patronage and French Medicine", http://picardp1.ivry.cnrs.fr/.

medical enlightenment did not remain hidden. In 1904–05 Henri and collaborators published a work of three hefty volumes on the hygiene and pathology of infants and young children.[13] At about the same time he was publishing articles, based on clinical research on subjects such as infant dyspepsia and whooping cough, in the journal he had founded in 1902.[14] Pediatrics was now a fast expanding field.

The journal (*Revue d'hygiène et de médecine infantiles*, with its annex the *Annales de la Polyclinique H. de Rothschild*), appearing every two months, carried articles by the hospital's medical personnel and also gave statistical information on the departments' activities.[15] In order to give the personnel the information needed for research, writing, and practice, Henri put at their disposal a library of 70 French and foreign periodicals and eventually more than 15,000 books and theses in pediatrics, obstetrics, and gynecology. French hospitals did have libraries, though they were allowed to fall into decay.[16] Robert Debré noted that he was innovating in establishing a library in his post-World War II pediatric hospital when he insisted on the importance of a library, whose books and journals were disposed of by his successor.[17] The laboratories were available for both research and learning. Teaching was furnished with the latest technology. The laboratory of photo-radiography put together a collection of interesting documents frequently used by lecturers in the courses they taught. The 300-seat room reserved for teaching and lectures contained the latest projection equipment. The top specialists and scientists in Paris were invited to give lectures and courses. And they happily responded to the Rothschild invitation.

In 1903 Pierre Budin taught a course in puericulture and infant feeding for the "society ladies" who provided the lay assistance necessary in programs to help women in delivery and their infants. These charitable bourgeois women followed Budin's lectures with the greatest interest. In 1904 Louis Netter, laboratory head at the Marcadet hospital, gave a course in bacteriology, which was well attended by a large number of doctors and foreign medical students. Then there was a more or less fallow period in the program, though different single lectures continued, given by fairly well-known people on standard medical topics. In 1909, in response to

---

13 *Traité d'hygiène et de pathologie du nourrisson et des enfants du premier âge* (3 vols, Paris, 1904–5). "Collected and published by Dr H. de Rothschild."

14 *Revue d'hygiène et de médecine infantiles et Annales de la Polyclinique H. de Rothschild.* Another well-known journal in the same field was the *Journal de clinique et de thérapeutique infantiles*, absorbed by the *Gazette des maladies infantiles et obstétriques*, 1893–. Gaston Variot, "Editeur scientifique."

15 Bourneville, "Visite aux œuvres du Dr H. de Rothschild," *La revue philanthropique*, 20 (1906–07): 487, praised the *Annales*, similar to the reports put out by English hospitals, as a model that all hospitals, especially those in Paris, should imitate.

16 Gérard Tilles and Daniel Wallach, "December 23rd, 1886: The Foundation of the Medical Library of Saint-Louis Hospital (Paris)," at www.bium.univ-paris5.fr/sfhd/ecrits/fonda_eng.htm.

17 Robert Debré, *L'honneur de vivre. Témoignage* (Paris, 1974), 413.

requests by a large number of people, Henri organized a series of lectures covering contemporary issues in pathology and therapy. Henri moved on many levels in Parisian society, which showed perhaps an excessive interest in medicine, or so he sometimes said in moments when he was fed up with bourgeois babbling about medicine. But on the professional level he recognized a genuine public interest that should be satisfied. Some of the biggest names in French medicine, some of the most famous professors in the faculty of medicine, and some of the most distinguished specialists in the hospitals welcomed the opportunity to spread the pathological and therapeutic gospels. The series was a great success with the large mixed medical and lay audience, who warmly applauded the lecturers. Dieulafoy spoke on the value of doing blood cultures in diagnosing infectious diseases; Delbet and others spoke on cancer, including radium therapy, obviously two topics that interested the doctors as much as their patients – cancer mortality had doubled within ten years. Desjardins spoke on contemporary surgical methods. Thoinot, a member of the Academy of Medicine, enlightened his audience on the notorious "secret médical."[18]

After the transformation of 1908 and the experience of the war years, the next big change in the Marcadet hospital came after the death of Mathilde de Rothschild in August 1926. In light of her work in the medical field, lay and social though much of it might have been, Henri decided that the best way to perpetuate his wife's memory was to reconstruct and enlarge the hospital, whose new name became *La Fondation Mathilde-Henri de Rothschild*. Henri bought the contiguous property of a garage and ateliers for the expansion. Much of the old construction was demolished and a new wing built on a surface of about 900 square meters. In order not to interrupt medical services, the work was done in two stages, though the hospital did close during the second half of 1928. In line with the medical dream of the day, the new Marcadet establishment was "a true surgical hospital," with thirty-five beds for indigent patients, including dormitories and isolation rooms, and eleven comfortably fitted and furnished rooms for patients of a higher social class – this novelty (a sort of boutique medicine) was testimony to the success of the hospital and the reputation of its doctors. One part of the premises contained the consulting rooms and the rooms for general medicine, operations, orthopedic surgery, ear–nose–throat practice, stomatology, diseases of the heart and blood vessels, and so on. Radiology, apparatuses for the administration of medical electricity, laboratories, and other essentials of medical practice were found in another part of the premises. The number of monthly consultations by the end of the 1920s exceeded 3000, averaging 1200 days of hospitalization and 35 cases of major surgery. The nursing staff included a director, a head nurse, and 15 certificated nurses, all of whom were female. There were also a laboratory head with an assistant, a radiologist, and a pharmacist – a complete hospital. There was no religious requirement for admission as a patient. The hospital founded in

[18] The lectures, published under the aegis of Polyclinique H. de Rothschild, were given in May and June of 1909; see reference to *Traité d'hygiène*, in note 13 above.

1852 by James-Mayer (*Hôpital-Fondation de Rothschild*, 11th arrondissement) still maintained its old policy of free medical care for Parisian Jews and indigent patients from the neighborhood.[19] In the 1930s the Marcadet hospital had to start charging fees, though 20 percent less than those of the *Assistance publique* hospitals. Interesting sick cases were still treated without charge, which cost Henri over 100,000 francs annually. Hospital maintenance, new materials, instruments, apparatuses, and so on added further personal expenses.

Rothschild family connections with the Marcadet hospital continued for some years after Henri died in 1947. During the four years of the German occupation in World War II, the hospital was pillaged and transformed into an army barracks. Medical materiel had been transferred in 1939 to Compiègne (Oise) for the organization of a military ambulance group, headed by Henri's daughter-in-law, the baroness James-Henri, and general evacuation of the hospital took place in the spring of 1940. The German soldiers amused themselves by destroying or burning relics, photographs, and records. Henri particularly regretted the loss of Mathilde's memorabilia, including her wartime decorations, which had been kept in a glass case in his office at the hospital. At the end of 1944, with the departure of the Germans, the hospital was restored to a working condition with the old department heads returning to work.[20] Henri had made the Association Hôpital Mathilde-Henri de Rothschild responsible for the running of the hospital; the arrangement was continued by his daughter Nadine (Madame Adrien Thierry) and then by their children. Life at the hospital continued, at least for a while, much as it had before. Some patients were happy; a few were not and sued, which was then a hopelessly optimistic action in France. In 1957 Jane Nemre, aged eighty-two, enjoyed a successful operation to remove cataracts. The hospital's *Livre d'Or* records her joy in a poem celebrating the existence of a place that was "nearly a paradise on earth," with special praise for its unbeatable director, Juliette Thibault.[21] The death of baroness James-Henri in 1959 was a blow to the organization, for she had been a strong supporter of the hospital. But Henri's sons Philippe and James continued their support, at least financially. Membership in the Association cost 1000 francs annually. A one-time payment of 10,000 francs could be substituted. Philippe and his wife did that in 1959; so did Philippe's brother, James, as well

[19] HR, *Exposé des titres et travaux scientifiques du Docteur Henri de Rothschild* (Saint-Ouen, 1929). The guide *Paris charitable, bienfaisant et social* (new edn, put out by the Office central des oeuvres de bienfaisance, 1936) has entries for both Rothschild hospitals. "La Fondation Mathilde-Henri de Rothschild, 199 rue Marcadet, XVIIIe arrondissement. Hôpital-dispensaire. 40 lits. Gratuité pour les indigents. Consultations médicales tous les jours, à 9^{h}." The hospital in the twelfth still held a *Consultation de nourrissons* on Thursdays. On the architecture of the building on the rue Marcadet, see Henri Defrance, *Nouveaux hôpitaux, maisons de santé, maternités, etc.* (Paris, 1930).

[20] HR (André Pascal), *Une dame d'autrefois. La Baronne Mathilde-Henri de Rothschild 1872–1926*, 295–6.

[21] Archives de Paris, Perotin 8/Roth/77/1 11 and 12.

as Adrien Thierry, and Jacques Thierry and his wife. In 1970 the total assets of the Association amounted to 1,793,208 francs 30 centimes. The Association was dissolved on 3 October 1975, with the establishment becoming a private clinic.

Clinical Research and Treatment of Patients

Henri often used the word experiment. He took a reasonable view of himself as a force in French medical research. After the founding of the Marcadet hospital, Henri never refused to accept a professional who wanted to experiment with a new therapeutic method, provided that it did not present any serious danger to the patients. Medical reaction to this program was sometimes hostile. Colleagues whose theories and methods were tested and found medically unsound or ineffective responded with attacks, sometimes violent, against the bearer of bad tidings. Unlike some more vulnerable researchers, Henri was able to disdain what he called offensives of questionable impartiality and courtesy, while continuing to apply the treatment in question if he found his patients reacting favorably to it. Often he was confirming therapeutic results already obtained in other countries, though perhaps introducing foreign novelties was not necessarily the best way to win support from the French medical community.

Not every therapeutic trial had a happy ending. About 1913 Alexander Marmorek (Pasteur Institute) tried out his controversial anti-tubercular serum at the hospital. Marmorek's unshakeable faith in his serum seems to have equaled Koch's in glycerin extracts of the tubercle bacillus; both concoctions turned out to be equally inefficacious. After a few months of experimenting had elapsed, Henri regretfully recognized that the serum did not, as he delicately put it, have the high curative properties attributed to it by its creator. After the Great War he was pleased by the "conclusive results" obtained by the trials he supported to test the anti-tubercular vaccine of a more famous researcher at the Pasteur Institute, Albert Vaudremer. In addition to the Marcadet hospital in Paris, Henri could introduce new medical and scientific skills at the Nathaniel de Rothschild hospital in Berck-sur-Mer. One of the first *internes* of the Berck hospital, Robert Ducroquet, was given free rein to practice orthopedics. Ducroquet's great skill and classic technique, along with the use of apparatuses that not all doctors approved of, justified Henri's confidence and permitted him to claim that many of nature's unfortunates were thus enabled to taste a little physical wellbeing and the joys of life. But it is clear the Marcadet hospital was more important for Henri.

What exactly was the nature of the work carried out in the Marcadet hospital by Henri and by other researchers, either on their own or in collaboration with him?

Endocrinology

Given Henri's desire to be associated with leaders in medical research, including its application to the care of patients, it is not surprising to find him passionate about the thyroid gland. Though the thyroid gland had been known since antiquity, endocrinology, which deals with the structure and especially the function of the organs of internal secretion, did not become a hot research area before the late nineteenth–early twentieth century. As it became known that the endocrine or ductless glands secrete chemicals into the blood (and lymph) – Frederik Ruysch (1638–1731) had assumed that the thyroid did something similar – research became interested in how metabolism works, that is, how these glands regulate body functions. Pharmaceutical companies were not far behind researchers – indeed, often worked with them – in pursuing "the therapeutic use of organ extracts."[22] In 1835 Robert Graves described exophthalmic goiter and is now honored by having hyperthyroidism called Graves–Basedow disease. Long connected to goiter and cretinism, which came to be related, the diseased organ became the victim of surgical enthusiasm, though, as the Medawars point out, "the classic way ... of demonstrating endocrine function is to extirpate the gland, observe the consequences, and then demonstrate that normality can be restored by replacement of the gland or by injection of an extract made from it."[23] Research on the thyroid gland brought under the medical gaze another disease, myxoedema, referring to adult hypothyroidism or under-activity of the thyroid, which dulls both body and mind. In the 1890s treatments with thyroid extract and then the addition of iodine to the diet entered into therapy.[24] Looking at the big picture, Joseph Fruton argues that in "the 1890s a pattern was set for the interplay of physiological and chemical investigation that characterizes present-day research in endocrinology ... in which academic scientists collaborate (and compete) with their colleagues in commercial enterprises."[25]

In 1908, responding to the request of colleagues, Henri and Léopold Lévi brought out a collection of their publications and communications on the thyroid and pituitary glands over the preceding eighteen months. The collection was medically significant enough to have appeared in the publications of the *Société de biologie*, the *Société de neurologie*, and the *Société médicale des hôpitaux*, among others. It was assumed that doctors would be happy to have in a convenient book form these articles dealing with the normal and pathological functioning of the organs. Charles Achard, professor at the Paris Faculty of Medicine, gave

---

22 Joseph S. Fruton, *Proteins, Enzymes, Genes. The Interplay of Chemistry and Biology* (New Haven, 1999), 475; see also the section on endocrinology in Roy Porter, *The Greatest Benefit to Mankind. A Medical History of Humanity* (New York, 1998), 562–70.

23 P. B. and J. S. Medawar, *Aristotle to Zoos. A Philosophical Dictionary of Biology* (Cambridge, Mass., 1983), 77.

24 Iodine is "required for the synthesis of the thyroid hormones thyrosine and tri-iodothyronine"; iodine deficiency in the human diet leads to goiter or enlargement of the thyroid. Sir William Gull first described myxoedema in 1873. John Walton and others (eds), *The Oxford Medical Companion* [OMC] (Oxford, 1994), 342, 435.

25 Fruton, *Proteins, Enzymes, Genes*, 476.

the collection an academic benediction in a four-page preface.[26] Achard noted the oddity that the endocrine glands occupied an important place in contemporary medicine though "the quasi-fabulous period of their history just ended." The mystery surrounding these organs had just been lifted with the revelation of their physiological functions and the diseases, particularly myxoedema, resulting from their malfunctioning. Achard emphasized their importance in a great number of events of both "normal and pathological life." The pathology of the thyroid revealed a great variety of causes and effects of diseases, many of which were dealt with in this hefty volume. The two doctors were certainly interested in treating a variety of ailments assumed to result from various glandular problems: dry extracts derived from internal secretion glands were administered to patients suffering from chronic rheumatism, asthma, and hypo- and hyperthyroidism, and migraines. The migraine headache was a common condition treated by doctors. In addition to the common migraine, there were sexual, menopausal [*hysteria cephalia*], and ovarian migraines.[27]

Walther's grafting of a sheep's thyroid – an intriguing experimental fling in medicine – inspired A. Mignon to write his thesis (1895) on a case of exophthalmic goiter following typhoid fever. Doctors took note. But Henri confessed that the real starting point for his and Lévi's work on the thyroid was encountering a case of chronic progressive rheumatism in a sixty-year-old patient who, in a fall from a bicycle about twelve years earlier, had damaged his right knee with the affection spreading to tissues and joints to such a degree that by 1904 the patient was in a wheelchair. The patient was "cured" after taking a series of doses of thyroid extract as tablets. Doubt existed about the cure because it had not started early enough. A similar case, reported in the *Presse médicale* in 1905, established the fact that giving similar treatment to a rheumatic patient aged forty-seven, who had been suffering since he was twenty-four years old, did not eliminate deformation of limbs and ankylosis (immobility and fixation of a joint). Still, there was improvement, which led Henri to conclude that there was reason to treat incurable chronic cases as well as the less serious cases, assuming that the doctor recognized the signs of malfunctioning of the thyroid.

The favorable outcome of the treatment of one patient led the doctors to try it on other rheumatic sufferers. A thirty-four-year-old patient provided a challenge: she had been afflicted after the age of seven, the crises becoming severe after the age of seventeen. Treatment had included aspirin, pyramidon, and sodium salicylate along with stimulation from the application of a pointed cautery. Progressive improvement was noted after fifteen doses (0.10 ctg each) of thyroid extract had been taken at the rate of two to three per day. After two years of treatment the patient

---

[26] HR and Léopold Lévi, *Etudes sur la physico-pathologie du corps thyroïde et de l'hypophyse*, (Paris, 1908). Preface by Charles Achard, "professeur agrégé à la faculté de médecine, médecin à l'hôpital Necker."

[27] For Lévi's communication to the neurological society of Paris, see "La migraine commune," *Revue neurologique* 13 (1905): 166–72.

was completely cured, with even the deformations disappearing. On one occasion the patient was the victim of medical error when she was overdosed with more than twice the prescribed dose as a result of being given the wrong tablets. The doctors regarded it as an enlightening incident showing the necessity of detailed medical supervision of treatment and providing a sort of unintended experiment showing the influence of thyroid extract on a patient. The diarrhea, nervousness, insomnia, hot flashes, and "thermophobia" – some of the "phenomena of the Basedownian series" – suffered by the patient served the cause of science.[28] It was not unusual for doses of medication to be administered to the limit of producing intoxication to observe its maximum effect: potassium bromide for epilepsy and arsenic for chorea were two well-known examples. (Bromides, which depress the central nervous system, were formerly used as sedatives and tranquilizers.) Eighteen months after treatment was stopped, the thirty-four-year-old patient was well, too well, perhaps, for she was able to wear pointed shoes and get married without consulting her doctors.

Working with Lévi, Henri claimed to be among the first to study the endocrine glands. The claim needs clarification. In 1911, when this new branch of medicine was in the course of becoming a special area, they declared themselves to have been participants in that evolution.[29] This seems to be a nice safe statement. It could be backed up with a fair amount of evidence. Their work was included in the complementary teaching program of two hospitals (Laennec and Hôtel-Dieu) and it got attention at medical congresses such as that of the mad-doctors and neurologists meeting in 1908 at Dijon. Speculation abounded about the relations between the thyroid and nervous and mental diseases. Maxime Laignel-Lavastine flattered the researchers by borrowing considerably from their work on the thyroid. So did Joseph Grasset in his three-volume classic *Traité élémentaire de physico-pathologique et clinique* (1910–12). In his work *Neurasthénies et psychonévroses*, Hippolyte Bernheim recognized that, according to the endocrine gospel of Lévi and Rothschild, neurasthenic states are often the result of autointoxication stemming from thyroid malfunctioning.[30] Not without a touch of irony, Henri and his collaborator noted that some of the facts they had discovered were verified so quickly and established so solidly in medical literature that Lévi and he no longer needed to be mentioned as having discovered them.

[28] Karl Adolph von Basedow (1799–1854) described thyrotoxicosis (hyperthyroidism) and treated it with iodine. OMC, 78.

[29] HR and Léopold Lévi, *Nouvelles études sur la physico-pathologie du corps thyroïde et des autres glandes endocrines* (2nd series, Paris, 1911).

[30] Hippolyte Bernheim, *Neurasthénies et psychonévroses* (Paris, 1908), 39.

Syphilis

Brieux's play about syphilitics (*Les Avariés*) was a piece of fiction too real for the censors to allow it on the Paris stage in 1901.[31] So one of France's most famous playwrights had to play in Liège and Brussels. When the censors came to their senses after three years of waiting and lifted the interdiction, the play opened at the Antoine theater in February 1905. *Les Avariés* was dedicated to Alfred Fournier, whose ideas were vigorously articulated by the doctor in the play. Syphilis, like alcoholism and tuberculosis, was a great killer; it was also a great killer of children. Perhaps one out of seven Parisian males was infected, and the infected males were blamed for spreading the disease to nineteen out of twenty infected women. "Men – the bastards – give you the disease and then put you in prison for it," observed one poor prostitute. Brieux's doctor gave impassioned speeches on the need for public enlightenment on a disease that needed to be treated like any other disease, that is, without shame or punishment. In Paris infected women were relegated to a separate part of the Saint-Lazare prison. "Syphilis is like certain women; it gets angry only when neglected." The doctor emphasized the importance of beginning an early and mostly successful treatment, but he forbade marriage and reproduction during three or four years in order to protect women, who would pass on the disease to their babies, which is exactly what happened in *Les Avariés*. The treatment of syphilis was then in its mercurial period, and that was where Henri de Rothschild appeared on the clinical stage.

Henri was proud of the role he played in introducing new therapies, especially the administration of arsphenamine or "606" (trade name: Salvarsan), the highly touted new German treatment for syphilis, a rather prevalent disease in Paris, and not only among its 85,000 or so prostitutes. He became a Parisian apostle of Paul Ehrlich (1854–1915), the immunologist whose name has been immortalized largely because of his treatment for the *morbus gallicus*.[32] Although he did not express much interest in Ehrlich's antibody formation theory or *Seitenkettentheorie*, Henri, as a practicing physician running a hospital, showed great interest in Ehrlich's concept of chemotherapy with its dream of a magic bullet, allowing the doctor to become a medical *Freischütz*.[33] Henri's promotion of the new treatment for syphilis made up an important part of his medical career. He spent six months of the last year of his *externat* in the *service* of Alfred Fournier (1832–1914), whose chair of dermatology and syphilology, established in 1879, made the Saint-Louis

---

[31] Brieux, *Les Avariés* (Paris, 1909); a work in its 31st edition did not need to give the author's first name (Eugène; 1858–1932).

[32] "606" was the 606th arsenical compound concocted by Ehrlich's shop. Henri never mentioned the role of Sachahiro Hata, Ehrlich's assistant, in testing the compounds.

[33] See Anne Marie Moulin, *Le dernier language de la médecine. Histoire de l'immunologie de Pasteur au Sida* (Paris, 1991), especially 90 ff and 231 ff; W. F. Bynum, *Science and the Practice of Medicine in the Nineteenth Century* (Cambridge, 1994), 162–8; and Porter, *The Greatest Benefit to Mankind*, 450–4.

hospital into a leading center of syphilology in the city that was in the running for the title of world capital of syphilis.[34] Fournier had come on the medical scene with considerable éclat: after interning in the *Hôpital des Vénériens*, he published the much-admired lectures on syphilis by his *maître*, the great syphilologist, Philippe Ricord (1800–89). As a professor at the Hôtel-Dieu, Fournier's learning did not alienate students, while his bedside manner gave comfort to patients; he moved to Saint-Louis in 1876.

Henri refers to his friendship with Fournier's son Edmond, and one could find this relationship slightly at odds with Henri's previous accounts of his being kept a prisoner by his mother. Perhaps his shyness had led him to exaggerate the rigors of a cloistered childhood. After Dieulafoy advised him to spend a few months in Fournier's department, Henri was able to take advantage of being at dinner at the Fourniers to ask the professor to let him spend some time at Saint-Louis. Fournier couldn't stand Charcot, his powerful competitor at the Salpêtrière; Fournier's modification, in 1876 and in 1879, of Charcot's dogmas on the separation of syphilis and the nervous signs of *tabes dorsalis* (locomotor ataxia) and general paralysis was elevated to the status of a medical controversy between the school of one hospital and the other.[35] People who were invited chez Fournier were treated to a dog show in Charcot's honor. Fournier's Great Dane, Dacia, snoozed under the dining room table during dinner, coming out only when a servant served coffee. Putting a lump of sugar on its nose, Fournier would ask the dog what it thought of Brouardel. "What do you want to do with him?" The dog would not budge. Other well-known names would be mentioned. The dog would keep still. Then Fournier would cry out "what would you do with Charcot?" With a jerk of its head the dog would send the lump of sugar flying into the air, catch it, and swallow it. Fournier was rich and his rich patients made him richer. Charcot, who had what used to be called a "belle clientèle," also basked in the brilliant culture of the haute bourgeoisie: his salons were adorned with paintings by Corot, Goya, Franz Hals, and Jan Steen, along with other cultural status symbols, which were kept in the company of a sculpture of Ganymede (Catamitus) by Madame Charcot. Henri would have been equally at home with either great doctor.[36]

---

34 Claude Quétel, *History of Syphilis* (Baltimore, 1990), 137. Translated by Judith Braddock and Brian Pike.

35 Charcot died in 1893; Noguchi and Moore did not "discover the trepona in the cerebral cortex of general paralytics, thus verifying Fournier's theory," before 1913. Quétel, *History of Syphilis*, 324.

36 Charcot (1825–93) married the rich widow Augustine Durvis in 1864; in 1884, for over a million francs, he bought the eighteenth-century *Hôtel de Varangeville* at 217 boulevard St.-Germain, today the *Maison de l'Amérique latine*. See Professor Charcot, *Leçons du mardi à la Salpêtrière* (Paris, 2002), Avant-propos, and Christopher G. Goetz, Michel Bonduelle, and Toby Gelfand, *Charcot. Constructing Neurology* (New York, 1995), 268–304.

It is hard to know how many people were afflicted with syphilis, in spite of the various guesstimates we have. Fournier's records indicate that over a long career he saw 20,000 patients. In 1925 one governmental estimate put the number at about four million, one tenth of the French population; in 1929 the estimate for the number of infected had risen to an astounding eight million, which seems excessive even in a period as mythically lustful as the 1920s. Quétel calls the figures "inflationary statistics."[37] One estimate put the annual number of deaths from syphilis in the late 1920s at 140,000.[38] Young doctors, or even old ones, were not generally familiar with diagnosing the disease. It was learning the diagnostic gaze necessary to recognize syphilis that Henri appreciated chez Fournier. Keenly appreciative of the theater, Henri also appreciated Fournier's "dazzling" pedagogical style, especially when the professor, taking his students on rounds of patients, found an impressive chancre and told them to study it: "Mettez-vous ça dans l'oeil, Messieurs les externes"; he would then sweep on to another patient. Even more satisfying for Henri was the knowledge that some of the most eminent doctors misdiagnosed the disease as tuberculosis or cancer. Though Fournier certainly advanced understanding of the disease, congenital syphilis in particular, he did not come up with a new and more effective therapy. Medical lore honors Fournier by attaching his name to gangrene resulting from a fulminating infection of the scrotum and to a couple of other disagreeable conditions.

Henri cites the case of a woman who had gone for three or four visits to hospitals of the *Assistance publique*, even getting hospitalized in the department of Paul Poirier, where she was diagnosed as suffering from cancer of tubercular or syphilitic origin. The doctors offered her a cure by amputation, which she refused. Henri ordered the mercury treatment. In about a month and a half, the extensive ulceration had completely scarified. In addition to showing the superiority of Fournier's shop, Henri got a scientific presentation out of the case. He had photographed the whole process of treatment and presented the case with the healed patient to the *Société de Dermatologie*, presided over by Fournier himself. The end of the story showed the legal danger of dealing with this disease, especially in wives. On going back to Poirier's department to complain about the incompetence shown in her case, the woman treated by Henri found out for the first time that she had syphilis, which she, chaste wife, could have caught only from her husband. The subject of a divorce by his wife-victim, the husband sued the *Assistance publique* for violation of the professional (medical) secrets law and won the case along with an indemnity award.

In the pharmacopeia for the treatment of syphilis there were a couple of dozen mercurial preparations, including ointments, The old exterior treatments

---

37 Quétel, *History of Syphilis*, 199 and 320 (note 1). During the 1930s the number of cases of syphilis recorded in the USA, with a population of about 123 million, was 267,000, compared with 162,000 for gonorrhea. *Encyclopaedia Britannica* (Chicago, 1943), 23: 46.

38 Louis Devraigne, *Vingt-cinq ans de puériculture et d'hygiène sociale* (Paris, 1928), 337. He flattered syphilis as "the great abortionist."

included baths with sublimate, rubbings, fumigations with cinnabar or red sulfide of mercury, and eventually hypodermic injections. One of the most famous internal treatments was the administration of van Swieten's liqueur, a foul-tasting concoction containing one of the salts of mercury, which ruined the digestion but was so efficacious that doctors modified the formula to make it more palatable and less deadly to the stomach.[39] But Henri and collaborators (L. Brunier and Louis Netter) found that van Swieten's liqueur was at least a good substitute for calomel (mercurous chloride) in treating chronic digestive troubles in non-syphilitic infants.[40] Ricord's pills, containing a mercurial dose of five centigrams, enjoyed a good reputation as a cure but had side effects similar to the liqueur. Doctors were not at a loss in handling this dangerous medication. Dupuytren and Ricord added opium to the treatment; other doctors recommended a stimulating diet; and still others followed treatment with a dose of four grams of sodium borate in a glass of water. More convenient administration of counter measures included Dethan's pastilles of potassium chlorate or Vigier's pastilles of sodium borate. If the patient were in the tertiary stage of syphilis, potassium iodide could be effective in eliminating syphilitic ulcers and even syphilitic paralysis; Ricord recommended this medicament. Laroze's sirup, which used bitter oranges to make the stuff quasi-palatable, was recognized as efficacious but with serious side effects that might require suspension of treatment and resumption with smaller doses. Ulceration caused by treatment could be prevented by another medicine, the administration of Gilbert's sirup and alum gargles.[41] Syphilis was a disease ready for a new treatment.

In the issue of *Le Temps* on 26 October 1910 Henri wrote a long account of a visit to Ehrlich's Institute in Frankfurt. Why this visit would be of interest to the bourgeois readers of the newspaper was made clear in his opening sentence: "In just less than three months '606' has been monopolizing conversation in all circles; I will say even in all the salons the only issue is the new remedy."[42] Henri thought that the enormous publicity given in the press to Ehrlich's discovery was the chief reason for public interest in "606". Ever optimistic concerning the scientific enlightenment of the masses, Henri convinced himself that the public

---

39 Léopold Métayer, *Les injections intra-musculaires de sublime à doses rares et élevées dans la syphilis; comparison avec le calomel et l'huile grise* (thesis, Paris Faculty of Medicine, 1899), pointed out that sublimate or mercuric chloride could not be used in all cases.

40 HR, "Valeur thérapeutique de la liqueur de van Swieten chez les nourrissons atteints de troubles digestifs chroniques avec atropie," *Revue d'hygiène et de médecine infantiles* 2 (1906): 109–43. He gave a related paper at the international congress of medicine (Lisbon) in April 1906.

41 Dr Paul Labarthe and others, *Dictionnaire populaire de médecine. Usuelle d'hygiène publique et privée* (2 vols, Paris, n.d.; 3rd edn, 1890), II, 988–96.

42 HR, "Une Visite chez le Professeur Ehrlich," *Le Temps* (20 octobre 1910). Unless otherwise identified, all quotations in this and subsequent paragraphs are from the article.

was eager to learn everything about any "discovery destined to revolutionize a science, especially when this science is medicine." This publicity inspired passionate debates with ignorant and informed partisans in the opposing camps of doubters and believers. Doctors themselves were not reticent to join in the quarrel, even before there was enough scientific evidence available on which to base "a serious and exact opinion." Henri was particularly disturbed by fellow doctors who used their experience and authority to write articles for the popular press claiming that nobody ever died of syphilis, a truism for primary syphilis but a piece of medical bad faith bound to mislead a public mired in a state of medical ignorance. One had to look forward to the final reckoning with the disease, and here Henri enthusiastically provided a list of horrors, some more probable than others: general paralysis, cerebral hemorrhaging, gummas in different organs, aneurysms, and cancers that often develop in syphilitics. Not to mention the death of infants from congenital syphilis. It was simply criminal to say that syphilis does not kill.

Henri recognized that Ehrlich's treatment by "606" or Salvarsan, a toxic arsenic compound – in the literature there are also references to trivalent arsenicals or arseno-benzol compounds – was the subject of a "violent and unjust polemic," partly because many doctors had a vested interest in treating syphilitic patients with mercury in its different combinations. The wave of hostility and skepticism that greeted "606" in France was perhaps a bit of a surprise. Neither Ehrlich's distinguished scientific reputation nor his Nobel Prize (1908) seemed to weigh in favor of a warm welcome for an ostensible venereal panacea. Following the Rothschild tradition, Henri carefully avoided any mention of post-1870 skepticism of and even hostility to anything German. Quite to the contrary, was not France friendly on principle to inventions and discoveries arriving from abroad? Nor did he mention the speculation that "606" was a Jewish cure for a Jewish disease; the Proustian judgment that "syphilis marked the Jewish body" would have been foreign to his scientific discourse.[43]

For a doctor – and Henri was writing as a doctor – the proper course of action would be to delay judgment until one had personally observed the facts and concluded what the advantages and disadvantages would be in prescribing the medication. When people asked him about the new treatment, he therefore replied that he could not say anything about it. This was not a position that a doctor claiming to be one of the leading practitioners of scientific medicine in Paris could maintain for long. So he and his friend E. Emery (the clinical head of Fournier's department) decided to experiment with "606" in the Marcadet polyclinic. Eight seriously ill patients who had not responded to other treatments were injected with "606" over a fortnight. In one particularly touching case, the patient was an eleven-year-old girl who had been immobilized for four years with infectious arthritis in a knee and treated unsuccessfully for a long time in a Paris hospital; she was now

[43] Sander L. Gilman, *Jewish Frontiers. Essays on Bodies, Histories, and Identities* (New York, 2003), 127, 141.

facing an amputation. After receiving an injection she became sufficiently well to get up and start walking after three days. Henri's exultation at results from the use of "606" was expressed in religious language. "Filled with wonder and amazement, I was present at true resurrections, miraculous cures." Not knowing anything about the medication she received or about the debates surrounding it, the child's recovery could not be the result of suggestion or of simulation. Henri noted that he was not alone in his faith, for his medical colleagues had achieved similar remarkable results. The English expert L. W. Harrison summed up with cross-channel sobriety. "The effect of a single dose of this remedy is usually to cause the spirochetes to disappear from the discharge of syphilitic sores in 24 hours and syphilitic lesions [to] heal with a rapidity which was a source of great wonder to those who had toiled in the treatment of syphilis with the help of only mercury and preparations of iodine."[44] Such enthusiasm would not be seen again in medicine until the advent of sulfa drugs and antibiotics.

Henri pioneered in organizing a *Consultation* for the ambulatory treatment of syphilis by using "Ehrlich's method." Convinced of the superiority of Ehrlich's over all other treatments, he established the *Consultation de syphilothérapie* in his polyclinic. Since the polyclinic could not hospitalize patients suffering from syphilis, as was the general rule for patients receiving heavy doses of arsenical compounds by intravenous injection, the doctors created the method of "ambulatory treatment." It was so efficacious that Ehrlich eventually came to Paris to see it in action, and this method of treatment spread rapidly, or as rapidly as a new treatment with a foreign pedigree could be expected to spread among Paris doctors who had invested in another treatment. In 1911 Gaston Lorreyte noted that French doctors did not share the general enthusiasm for the Teutonic treatment. Some doctors argued that intramuscular shots of "606" worked better if given after injections of soluble mercury salts, though both medicaments were needed for a successful treatment.[45]

One of the stories about "606" that bothered Henri was that people surrounding Ehrlich had invented the whole history of a cure for syphilis in order to make a killing on the stock market in buying and selling shares of the company associated with manufacturing the product. According to this version of events, there was no new miracle treatment for one of the most devastating of modern social diseases. Henri thought that this sort of scientific scam was highly unlikely. But the Rothschilds

[44] *Encyclopaedia Britannica* (1943), 23: 44. The film *Dr. Ehrlich's Magic Bullet*, starring Emanuel Goldenberg (Edward G. Robinson) and Ruth Gordon came out in 1940.

[45] Some of the big names in spreading the Salvarsan gospel in publications such as the *Annales des maladies vénériennnes*, the *Bulletin de l'Académie de médecine*, and the *Journal de Médecine de Paris* were: Henri Hallopeau (who had long used arsenic to treat syphilis), Léon Bizard, and Louis Durœux. See also Gaston Lorreyte, *Contribution à l'étude du traitement de l'hérédo-syphilis par l'injection d'arséno-benzol au cours de la grossesse* (thesis, Paris Faculty of Medicine, 1911), and Lévi-Bing and Louis Durœux, *Annales des maladies vénériennes* (mars 1911).

were already the target of numerous attacks based precisely on this sort of financial fantasy and, given their financial prominence in France, Henri could not take the chance of becoming involved, even remotely and unintentionally, in any sort of scandal, especially one Jewish and German. (And the anti-Dreyfusard pot was still simmering.) So in order to set his conscience completely at ease he decided to visit Ehrlich, then director of the Royal Institute of Experimental Therapy in Frankfurt. (Henri later said that he and E. Emery visited Ehrlich's institute in Frankfurt and also went to Berlin, but this seems to be the same trip he wrote up in *Le Temps*.) Presumably Henri's command of German was useful during the visit; he did not mention the fact that Ehrlich was also Jewish and was also affected by the new wave of anti-Semitism infecting Europe. He emphasized that his report would be exclusively scientific, though, given the nature of the accusations against Ehrlich, not without moral relevance. Nor does cigar-connoisseur Henri mention the fact that Ehrlich was a serious addict to this kind of oral satisfaction: Ehrlich was notorious for walking around with a box of cigars, of which he smoked twenty-five a day.

When questioned about the commercial exploitation of "606", Ehrlich told Henri that he got no commercial benefits from sale of the product. Ehrlich observed that he could have made a fortune off the product along with ensuring himself a large annual income like the inventors (Emil Fischer and Joseph von Mering) of Veronal, the brand name of diethyl barbituric acid or barbital, marketed by the Bayer Company. Not that he did not think that a lifetime's labor should not earn material advantages; he just did not care for luxury and needed very little to get along, except to fund his scientific work, which was supported by "friends of science and humanity." The cost of development of "606" had been the equivalent of 300,000 French francs, part of which had come from "donors," including the Speyer foundation (Georg-Speyer-Haus) and part from his 1908 Nobel Prize award, shared with Ilya Mechnikov, for work on immunity. Höchst produced the first large amount of "606", about 65,000 doses, paid for by the Georg-Speyer-Haus, which had been founded by Frau Franziska Speyer in 1906 to provide a research laboratory (Research Institute for Chemotherapy) for Ehrlich next to his institute. The close connection developing between pharmaceutical companies and medical science was not discussed; it was a subject that would interest Henri greatly after World War I, when he would engage in some activities more akin perhaps to those of Ehrlich than those of Fischer and Mering, at least in the sense that he put enormously more money into medical research and patient care than he ever got out of the drug business.[46] Henri reported that any royalties Ehrlich received from "606" went into the foundation and maintenance of an institute of biological chemistry – perhaps he meant chemotherapy.

[46] See Bynum, *Science and the Practice of Medicine in the Nineteenth Century*, 167, for reference to the connection between Ehrlich's institute and drug companies (Farbwerke Cassella and Höchst) in the patenting, production, and marketing of Salvarsan and Neosalvarsan.

Both German and foreign medical practitioners who treated patients with "606" agreed to send Ehrlich detailed observations of the results. Ehrlich's published articles gave the results of the clinical experiments using "606" in the treatment of about 14,000 patients with syphilis. These observations were organized according to regions and accompanied by photographs of patients before and after treatment. A later volume gave a complete bibliography of the articles. Making the new chemotherapy more significant was the fact that a large number of the people treated had failed to respond to mercury treatments. Primary, secondary, and tertiary syphilis cases were treated. And, of great importance, only twelve or thirteen patients had died. Critics of the administration of "606" claimed that injecting the arsenical compound had produced cases of amaurosis and dangerous poisoning. Ehrlich told Henri that no such cases had been reported to him. Neither could the reported deaths be attributed directly to "606". After reading the reports on the deaths, Henri agreed with Ehrlich. The cases found were deaths from other causes: infectious pneumonia, occurring two weeks after the injection; a ruptured aneurism, which had not been detected; and general paralysis with the patients already in a coma. Some patients died from advanced stages of the disease, with the relatives having been told that the treatment would not work in such cases. There were exceptional counter-indications of course, but ninety percent of syphilitics could be treated without any danger. Not that this opinion was generally accepted in Paris, Henri lamented, but he hoped to contribute to a change of opinion. Henri thought it important to emphasize that no treatment works in all cases; for example, in children's hospitals there might still be a death rate of twelve to fourteen percent from diphtheria and croup, but this was great progress compared with the days before the advent of serums, when the death rate was sixty to eighty percent. Doctors accepted the efficacy of Roux's serum. Of course neither the serum nor "606" would produce favorable results in dying patients.

Administering "606" in small, successive doses was soon recognized as ineffective, for the organism became immunized, with the microbes slowly regaining their original virulence as the medicine lost its efficacy. So theory required that one had to administer a devastating first strike against the disease. If the treatment were begun when the chancre first appeared, it was easy to destroy the spirochete (bacterium *Treponema pallidum*). The key therapeutic idea of this great *therapia sterilisans* was to strike early and hard with the new weapon. Henri worried about what was called recidivism in the apparently cured patient, that is, the survival of a number of bacteria too small for the Wassermann test to detect but which could cause a flare up later by more active and more dangerous germs. (The test, dating from 1906, did give some false positive results.) This recidivism was a danger associated with patients receiving only one injection. A new technique prescribed a first intravenous injection followed in three or four weeks by an intramuscular or subcutaneous injection. Ehrlich noted that in certain difficult cases, a third injection might be required. Indulging in the caution typical of the practicing physician, Henri wondered if even then the patients treated by "606" might not suffer from a recurrence of the disease, caused by bacteria that had not been killed by the injections. Only time would tell, he sighed, but the immediate happy results were undeniable, he emphasized. Intramuscular injections with the medication in an aqueous solution turned out to be a defective method of treatment because of poor absorption of the active ingredient; and because of pain, patients often refused a second injection. The injections were usually made deep into the muscles of the buttocks, which were then energetically rubbed to speed up absorption. Any unabsorbed liquid could form very painful cysts. A later procedure of doing repeated smaller injections solved some of the problems associated with the old method of one big ghastly shot. Injections with the medication in an oil emulsion turned out to be better tolerated and could even be used in cases where the intravenous injection could not. It also soon became clear that the treatment needed to be administered by a skilled person.

Henri's organization switched to Neosalvarsan or "914" when it became available. Treatment was free. (Neosalvarsan was easier to use and more patient-friendly but not so active therapeutically as the powerful "606".) In four years (1910–14), his establishment treated 5646 syphilitics. With the coming of war in 1914, rates of venereal disease shot up, with many serious cases needing hospitalization: the army had to hospitalize 456 syphilitics between August 1915 and February 1916. Sick soldiers received intravenous injections of Neosalvarsan or sometimes of mercury cyanide.[47] In 1919 Henri reorganized his *Consultation*, with Emery remaining as the head and Morin coming in as a collaborator. By the 1920s there were numerous dispensaries in Paris devoted to the treatment of syphilis, and Henri took pride in being among the pioneers in introducing "606" into France. Along with Emery, Henri created "a real center of teaching" and published a volume of the first lectures given by doctors on "this new and exciting therapy." Having been told that some women would be present at the lecture he gave on the treatment of syphilis, Emery declared that it would not be exclusively medical.[48]

Radiation

Medicine was full of radiation after the 1890s. Some of Henri's old professors gave him advice on lines of experiment to follow.[49] The diagnostic possibilities of x-rays were soon exploited after Röntgen's discovery in 1895. After the Curies isolated radium from pitchblende in 1898, the destructive-therapeutic potential

---

47 See A. Mignon, *L'évolution du Service de Santé pendant la guerre 1914–1918*, I, 625–7. *Le Service de Santé pendant la guerre ...* runs to 4 vols (Paris, 1926).

48 HR, *Croisière autour de mes souvenirs. II: Mes maîtres et mes amis à la faculté et dans les hôpitaux* (2 vols, Paris, 1933–36), 326, and Dr E. Emery, "La méthode d'Ehrlich," *Actualités Médico-chirurgicales* (2nd series, 1912), 20–52.

49 HR, *La Lignée française de la famille Rothschild 1792–1942. Etude historique et biographique* (Oporto, 1942), 97–105.

of the element was soon recognized.[50] Fournier, an enthusiastic supporter of exploiting the work done by the Curies, was the first person to speak to Henri about the use of radium in the treatment of cancer; indeed, he spoke of miracles being achieved in England and Austria while lamenting the fact that France could not afford this excessively expensive therapy. Henri Dominici, Fournier's student, later known for his therapeutic "tube de Dominici," wanted to offer radium therapy to patients but could not find any radium; here is where Henri came in, though it was not easy even for him to find any. Radium then cost 1,500,000 francs a gram. After a few months he had acquired 25 centigrams, which was divided between Dominici (20 cg) and Pierre Delbet (5 cg). Along with Paul Poirier and the neuropathologist Gustave Roussy, Delbet was a key figure in the founding in 1906 of the *Association française pour l'étude du Cancer*, which occupied the scientific turf, leaving political and social action to the *Ligue contre le cancer*. [51] (Rector of the academy of Paris after 1937, Roussy was removed from office in 1940 as a result of the application of the statute on Jews.) At the same time Poirier called for the creation of an *Institut de Cancer* "to stimulate and sustain initiatives while also centralizing research results." Germany and England had already moved in this direction, while France had established a league only in 1892, which had disappeared for lack of funding. The project for establishing the institute was more successful. A committee of Roux, Bouchard, and Debove attracted 300,000 francs in a few weeks; Henri contributed 10,000 francs.[52]

Dominici's work converted Henri to radium therapy. "Dominici (1907) showed that equal efficacy is obtained through a greater thickness of tissue if the beta-rays and the less penetrative part of the gamma-rays are stopped by suitable filtration. This most important discovery led to the use of radium or radon foci enclosed in heavy metal cases, which filter all but the gamma-rays."[53] Radium-226, the most stable isotope of radium, decays to radon, a colorless, radioactive element, first isolated by Ramsey and Gray in 1908. "For decades it was used as a source of beta particles and gamma rays in radiotherapy."[54] In 1912 Dominici became the head of a center for the free treatment of cancer (*Centre de Radiumthérapie*) that Henri set

[50] Bettyann Holtzmann Kevles, *Naked to the Bone. Medical Imaging in the Twentieth Century* (New Brunswick, NJ, 1997), Part I ("The X-ray Years"), 9–141.

[51] On the *Ligue contre le cancer*, founded during World War I, see Patrice Pinell, *The Fight Against Cancer: France 1890–1940* (London, 2002). Translated by David Madell. See also Pinell, "La Ligue contre le cancer," in Annette Wieviorka (ed.), *Justin Godart. Un homme dans son siècle 1871–1956* (Paris, 2004, 2005), 163–8. Mathilde de Rothschild was prominent in the league.

[52] Elisabeth Hausser, *Paris au jour de jour. Les événements vus par la presse* (Paris, 1968), 245.

[53] Claudius-François Regaud, "Radiumtherapy," *Encyclopaedia Britannica* (1943), 18: 908. After 1913 the word Curietherapy was used to describe the use of radioactive material in therapy.

[54] OMC, 843.

up in the rue Pergolèse (16th arrondissement), where it had laboratories of physics, chemistry, histology, and photography in "a modest pavilion." The building also housed a waiting room for patients, a room for applying dressings, a room where the treatment was given, and an office-library where Dominici could talk to his colleagues about the treatment. With the discovery of medical applications of radium, enthusiastic and sometimes chauvinistic experts were soon touting another panacea. An advertisement for the *Laboratoire pharmacologique du radium* (27 rue de Miromesnil) promised that radium products given by injection, ingestion, or ionization could be an energetic modifier of nutrition, an analgesic, as well as a treatment for tumors, cancers, infections, run-down condition, and a means of increasing the therapeutic effectiveness of medications. G. B. Shaw squawked "at present [1911] the world has run raving mad on the subject of radium."[55]

As soon as the results of initial experiments were known, Henri was told of the therapeutic advantages of the treatments, as in the case of using radium to treat cancer patients. At least half a gram of radium was needed to treat a serious number of cancer patients. Because of the difficulties of production and the competition of American and English laboratories, only a small quantity of radium was available. So in 1910 Henri set up a factory at St. Denis ("le laboratoire de Saint-Denis") for the production of radium from radioactive materials imported from Portugal. In the first year of operation a gram and a half of radium was extracted from 800 tons of Portuguese mineral. More than half a gram went to Dominici; the rest went to surgeons in Paris hospitals to use in experimental treatments. Mathilde suggested that the first gram of radium produced in the second year of operation at St. Denis be given to Marie Curie for the *Institut du Radium*, and the gift was given in Mathilde's name. The "factory" was later devoted to the production of luminous equipment for use in the trenches and in submarines. Henri then gave a gram of radium to the *Service de Santé militaire* to be used in the *Service de la Doctoresse Laborde au Grand Palais*, in the new setup he later called the Hospital of the *Grand Palais*, a special facility for treating soldiers suffering from painful scars or traumatic neuritis.[56]

The factory at St. Denis produced between two and a half and three grams of radium annually over a fifteen-year period; seventy-five percent was given to the medical community and twenty-five percent was sold to cover a small part of the expense of running the factory. Once the Belgian company *Union minière du Haut-Katanga* started producing fifty milligrams of radium from a ton of Congolese uranium oxide (a variety of uraninite, a mineral form of uranium oxide containing tiny amounts of uranium, radium, etc.), there was no point in continuing

[55] *Le Radium*, a monthly publication, promising to publish everything about radioactivity, began in 1904 and continued until it was absorbed after World War I by the *Journal de physique théorique et appliquée*. Shaw's remark is in the "Preface on doctors" (31) of the Penguin edition (1946) of his play *The Doctor's Dilemma* (1911), first produced in London in 1906.

[56] HR, *Une dame d'autrefois*, 311.

the Portuguese-dependent factory of St. Denis. Two technicians handled radium operations because it was not advisable, according to conventional ignorance of the period, for a young man to be exposed to the dangers of radium for more than six hours a day. After 1919, on the initiative of Roux, the *Institut du Radium* of the University of Paris joined forces with a special department of radium therapy at the hospital of the Pasteur Institute. (In 1909 the University of Paris and the Pasteur Institute had decided to construct the *Institut du Radium* to house a research laboratory for Marie Curie along with a Pasteur Institute laboratory for Claudius Regaud's study of the biological and medical effects of radioactivity. The *Institut du Radium* was finished in 1914.) Henri's operation in St.Denis supplied it with part of the radium it used. Cancer treatment was becoming important in Paris. Dominici died too young, but the therapy was already being presented as valuable in treating cancer patients. A bit later Claudius Regaud identified "some general diseases, of which rheumatism is the most favourable type," for treatment by the use of radon "with the highest degree of success."[57] Henri continued to be a major figure in the support of radium therapy and radiotherapy, which refers to treating diseases by the application of various kinds of radiation, particularly x-rays. Marie Curie's promotion of x-rays during the Great War gave a considerable boost to this new diagnostic technique: with 200 fixed posts and 20 vehicles ("petites Curies"), it was possible to take over 1 million x-rays in the period 1917–18 alone.[58] The medical discourse on the use of the new technologies was positive and full of hope; no iatrogenic cloud yet darkened the patient's horizon, though, as we now know, there were many martyrs to therapeutic radiation.[59]

In 1919, when an organization was set up to administer the radium that Henri had made available for medical purposes, it was only fair that it be named the *Fondation Henri de Rothschild*. Delbet insisted that its scientific aim was closely tied to its humanitarian object. The foundation was non-profit, though it planned to sell at cost some of its production for the benefit of people who could afford to pay for radium therapy; most of the production went to the poor patients in the hospitals of the *Assistance publique*, which could not afford to give them radium therapy. The text of the first year's report, by an old surgical hand, indicates that medical science had become crudely clinical: "progress can only be achieved by treating the sick."[60] The Radium Institute of London, with its use of tubes of bromide of radium and tubes of emanation, provided a model for the Paris

---

57 Regaud, "Radiumtherapy," *Encyclopaedia Britannica* (1943), 18: 908; the date of this article is probably 1929! Note the ambitious title of the book by Jean Regaud: *Claudius Regaud (1870–1940). Pionnier de la cancérologie, Créateur de la Fondation Curie. Chronique de sa vie et son oeuvre* (Paris, 1982).

58 Françoise Thébaud, *La femme au temps de la guerre de 14* (Paris, 1986), 92.

59 See "Les martyrs des rayons X," in Jacques Borgé and Nicolas Viasnoff, *Archives des médecins* (Paris, 1995), 171–4.

60 Fondation Henri de Rothschild, *Rapport de M. le professeur Pierre Delbet* (Paris, 1919), 3.

institute. One of the first questions that had to be answered, after money had been found to buy the radium, was how the element would be used to treat patients. Given the difficulties and dangers of using radium, it was fortunate for patient and doctor that the gaseous element radon, a product of disintegration, could be used "safely" if enclosed in tubes; radiation could then be measured and controlled, following tables provided by the manufacturer, and the treatment would have the same therapeutic effects as radium. These tubes could also be used in a doctor's office. Everything seemed under control for the great medical trial to begin. Where was the science in all this?

In a section entitled "scientific research" in his report, Delbet admitted that radium could be used to treat tumors without achieving any scientific progress. This was what happened most of the time. He found some discussions about radium therapy to be "models of incoherence," a serious accusation in the French medical world. In the use of radium to treat cancer of the uterus, some doctors claimed to have achieved cures, while others were proclaiming only the bad effects of the treatment. Delbet explained the paradox by noting that some cancer cells are stimulated by radiation while others are killed; different cancers react differently. In these contradictory situations the deciding histological examinations had not been done, and so the discussions were sterile. Even in reports published by institutes of radium therapy there was no more accurate information. No wonder the use of radium had not spread more. Delbet concluded that ignorance and confusion along with unskillful treatments had aggravated the evil and turned many doctors and surgeons away from radium therapy. He proposed a collective effort to get the profession out of the mess quickly.

In order to establish the effects of radiation on the cells of different types of cancer and the reaction of tissues according to the intensity and duration of radiation, Delbet called for the clinical, radiological, and histological control of the process, with biopsies being done before and after treatment. A person qualified in microscopy would examine tissues from biopsies, operations, and autopsies, all supplied by the "collective work." All documents would be centralized in a real archive of radium therapy. Regaud volunteered to organize the archive. Results stemming from the collective work would be published in the bulletins of the *Association française pour l'étude du cancer* after a public professional discussion. All that remained was to cure the patient – the most difficult task of all.

When the *Association* (later *Société*) *française pour l'Etude du Cancer* was founded in 1906 at the instigation of Poirier, Henri was a founding member and became the treasurer. Bouchard became president when Poirier, the first president, died in 1907, and Pierre Delbet the general secretary, with headquarters at the "Ecole de médecine" of the University of Paris. Henri contributed 40,000 to

60,000 francs annually for the publication of the *Atlas du cancer*, edited by Delbet. When *La Fondation Curie* was created in 1920 to fund activities like those of the *Institut du Radium*, it received a transfer of the annual subvention that was at the disposition of the *Fondation Henri de Rothschild pour les savants*. This fact may explain the figure of two million francs that some sources claim Henri gave to the institute. (The famous *Institut Curie* was born in 1970 from the joining of the *Institut du radium* and the *Fondation Curie*.) Henri took responsibility for the Institute's statutory endowment – meaning making the first legal gift – and budget.[61] He was also a member of its *Conseil d'administration*. Philippe joined his father on this council and later became a vice-president for life. Henri was supposedly among the herd of males in love with Marie Curie, which even if true had nothing to do with his support for radium therapy. Nor is it likely that if Marie Curie were aware of this supposed affection, she would have had any interest in a married Jewish lover, especially after the scandal generated by her pre-war affair with Paul Langevin. (News of the Langevin–Curie affair broke in November 1911.) Nor have I found any mention of Curie joining Colette for a cruise on Henri's yacht, the *Eros*. Henri's membership in the Franco-Anglo-American League against Cancer (founded in 1918 on the initiative of Justin Godart) provided an international symbol of the prominent role he played in anti-cancer efforts. He contributed generously to an organization emphasizing anti-cancer propaganda as well as to charity for poor victims; Mathilde's "fêtes de charité" supplied most of its annual budget. By the 1920s technology was already generating more than its share of medical optimism and an impressive number of institutions. Henri believed that the one was justified and the others necessary. It was all just a normal part of scientific development.

On 26 December 1923, Henri made sure that he played a conspicuous role in the celebration of the twenty-fifth anniversary of the discovery of radium. Discourses by scientists, physicians, and politicians at the *Fondation Curie* and at the Sorbonne filled the day, but the evening was more exciting for the representatives of "l'élite glorieuse et incontestée" of French scientists and other lucky guests, including a cabinet minister: an invitation to a well-lubricated and gastronomic affair at Henri's *Château de la Muette*. Henri gave a speech whose text runs for eleven pages in which he presented himself as a friend of science and of scientists, as one who had been captivated by the multiple applications of radium and its emanations. Henri reminded the guests how difficult the early days had been when the only raw material available was the Portuguese mineral. He evoked the memory of some of the great doctors he had known, especially Fournier. Nor were the guests allowed

---

61 1919 budget for the Oeuvre du radium

Installation............ 5000 francs
Secretary............... 3600
Assistants.............12,000
Histologist............ 8000
Total.....................28,600

to forget the unselfish collaborators of Dr Regaud in the different departments of that mini-empire of radiation, the *Fondation Curie*, to which he had contributed the 4,000,000 francs recovered from his gifts to the *Œuvre philanthropique du vin* when it was transformed into a commercial society. It can be claimed without too much exaggeration that the *Fondation Curie* with its strategic and financial support of the beginning of the war on cancer was not only a model imitated by French cancer treatment centers but was also "the cradle of world radiotherapy" in the 1920s.[62] Henri also undertook to give a subsidy of 200,000 francs annually to the institute; the agreement was for 10 years, and he gave the subsidy for 5 more. Henri did not mention the banker André Lazard, a supporter of radium therapy; like the University of Paris and the Institut Pasteur, Lazard seems to have been eclipsed in the Rothschild celebration by the great doctors of the day. Everyone enjoyed drinking toasts to Marie Curie and to the memory of Pierre Curie as well as to those who worked in the laboratories with only one thought: the mutually interactive process of alleviation of human suffering through scientific progress. Even in the history of celebrations at *La Muette* this one was probably the most memorable, something Henri recognized in saying that the date would remain engraved in the family memory as an event of unique character.[63]

Electromagnetic Radiation

Electricity has been part of medicine since the eighteenth-century experiments of Galvani. In the nineteenth century electricity moved beyond neurophysiology to therapy, with gynecology providing an area of experimentation. During his year as an *externe* at *La Pitié* Albert Pegoud became interested in Théophile Gallard's use of direct current to treat uterine fibroids. He reviewed the literature, especially that published in the United States, where Cuttler, using acupuncture needles inserted into the uterus through the abdomen, claimed to have reduced or stopped the growth of twenty-three out of thirty-six tumors and completely eradicated three out of the thirty-six. Using a battery specially set up to deliver the required current, Pegoud was unable to duplicate Cuttler's results. Pegoud found no change in the volume of tumors receiving the current, and indeed it had a slight tendency to cause them; nor did the current stop or reduce hemorrhaging.[64] The failure of electrotherapy in one

---

62 See http://www.curie.fr/fondation/musee/histoire.cfm/lang/_fr.htm.

63 *XXVe anniversaire de la découverte du Radium. Allocution prononcée par le Dr Henri de Rothschild* (La Muette, 26 décembre 1923). A special printing.

64 Albert Pegoud, *De la valeur des courants continus dans le traitement des tumeurs fibreuses de l'utérus* (thesis, Paris Faculty of Medicine, 1881). Pegoud notes that the procedure was first done in the United States in the 1870s (Cuttler, 1871); he refers to Gallard, *Leçons cliniques des maladies des femmes* (1873); and notes that Friedrich Semeleder gave detailed instructions in the *Wiener Medizinische Presse* in 1876 (numbers 50 and 52). Dr George Apostoli was an apostle of electrical treatment in gynecology in the 1880s: uterine fibroids, metritis, and an aid in birthing. Apostoli wrote the foreword

medical area did not discourage electrical enthusiasts, and with the improvement of equipment and the method of current delivery by the early twentieth century, this type of treatment was not unusual. In 1910 Jules Renard remarked that after finding his blood pressure, heart, and liver to be "normal," his doctor subjected him to high-frequency currents for his unidentified illness. Renard died shortly thereafter.[65] The therapy is still with us, at least in torture, and possibly it helps stroke victims recover motor skills.[66]

Henri was an enthusiastic supporter of the application to general pathology of all available "electrical methods," that is, electromagnetic radiation, which then included diathermy as well as use of infrared and ultraviolet light.[67] Diathermy is medically defined in several similar ways; the following definition is from the *American Heritage Medical Dictionary*: "the therapeutic generation of local heat in body tissues by high-frequency electromagnetic radiation, electric currents, or ultrasonic waves." In London Arthur Waugh had his rheumatism treated with twenty minutes of infrared radiation (so-called heat radiation), directed to his "hinder parts," followed by an erotic massage.[68] Henri's scientific curiosity, along with his desire "to serve science," was encouraged by his son Philippe, whose scientific bent carried him so far as to take a doctorate in physics at the University of Paris.[69] On returning from a jaunt in 1930 to the United States to further his scientific education, Philippe asked his father to experiment with some electrical machines that produced "artificial fever" for therapeutic purposes: short wave radio frequency. He saw the machines in the laboratories of General Electric in Schenectady and found an improved version being used by Dwight Carpenter at the Rockefeller Institute in New York City. Carpenter was improving the condition of patients suffering from general paralysis and even obtaining cures. The results were comparable to those obtained by "malaria therapy."[70] The young Emile

---

to Rudolf Temesváry (Budapest Gynecologist), *Ueber die Anwendung des Elektrizität bei Frauenkrankheiten* (Vienna, 1890).

65 Jules Renard, *Journal 1887–1910* (Paris, 1990), 996. Georges Duhamel, *Les Maîtres* (Paris, 1937), 163, has his character Professor Chalgrin, on the advice of D'Arsonval, consider trying "la haute fréquence" for his pressure and generally poor state.

66 See "Electricity to Brain may Aid Motor Skills," *The New York Times* ("Science Times"), 27 Jan. 2009, D6, reporting on a study published in *The Proceedings of the National Academy of Sciences* on 21 Jan. 2009.

67 "The technique can be used to apply warmth to structures beneath the skin, like muscles or joints, or in surgery to cause heat coagulation and necrosis by localized intense application." OMC, 205.

68 Alexander Waugh, *Fathers and Sons. The Autobiography of a Family* (2004; New York, 2007), 116–17.

69 "Thèses présentées à la Faculté des sciences de l'Université de Paris par Philippe de Rothschild. Première thèse." *Etude de quelques applications de la pulverisation cathodique des métaux...* (Paris, 1931).

70 Edward M. Brown, "Why Wagner-Jauregg Won the Nobel Prize for Discovering Malaria Therapy for General Paresis of the Insane," *History of Psychiatry* 11 (2000): 371–82.

Halphen, an accompanying ophthalmologist, stayed behind, at Philippe's request, in order to become fully acquainted with this new method of treatment and its applications. Henri decided to try out the treatment in his hospital after Halphen returned with precise information and plans. Halphen was given carte blanche to get the machines, which, if possible, Henri wanted made in France. Under the supervision of the engineer Poittevin, the Compagnie Générale in Paris built two different apparatuses. With the collaboration of his friend Jules Auclair, Halphen carried out several months of experiments before reporting results to Henri and about fifteen of his colleagues at a dinner organized for that purpose. A conference of specialists presided over by Arsène d'Arsonval, physicist and a big name in electrophysiology, considered the therapeutic results, which created a stir in medical circles. Using short wave radio frequency for heat therapy became an accepted practice and is still around.

Henri asked the doctors to send their patients for treatment and to supervise it themselves. Interest in the new equipment spread quickly. Some heads of departments in the Paris hospitals got a gadget, with the neurologist Louis Crouzon of the Salpêtrière being on top of the list of favored specialists. In July 1931 the international congress of radiology met in Paris; the clinician, immunologist, and radiologist A.-L.-G. Béclère, one of Henri's old professors, presided over the gathering. Halphen and Auclair gave a paper, and congress goers were invited to visit the Marcadet hospital. Henri was quite keen on keeping French medicine on the mythical cutting edge of science and in showing his hospital's use of any new medical technology to foreigners. After a year of treatment of over 300 patients by *électropyrexie* (inductopyrexia), as it was called, Henri concluded that the most diverse chronic diseases could benefit from an improved diathermic therapy, or at least it seemed, as he carefully put it, that there were a priori grounds for thinking so. A close collaboration of doctors with Poittevin over a two-year period slowly improved the machines. Henri was proud to be the patron of young doctors eager to join him on the moving frontier of medical technology harnessed for the better treatment of disease.

Burns

One of the medical areas in which Henri eventually acquired a certain amount of fame was the treatment of burns. Certain occupations in the new industrial civilization of the nineteenth century resulted in a large number of serious burns victims and demanded a new speciality in occupational medicine, itself a new growth medical sector. The *grands brûlés* were conspicuous among the patients rushed to the Lariboisière hospital for treatment: they included locomotive drivers, mechanics, forge workers, and rolling mill operators. Henri referred particularly to the *brûlés* of "the family railroad" (the *Compagnie du chemin de fer du Nord*). The treatment of burns is a dramatic and difficult business, especially in the case of extensive damage with deep lesions. Périer's department treated burns victims in the traditional nineteenth-century way, though the antiseptic movement had improved things slightly. Henri noted that burns remained very painful for treated patients and even if they did not die, they required many months to recover. Since Périer's unit had so many suffering burns patients Nageotte-Wilbouchevitch looked for a way to dress their wounds more efficiently and less painfully. As a young aide, Henri followed her work closely. Her technique was to use a brush to clean out the wounds with warm water and soap, then brush on a thiol or mercaptan as an antiseptic, and finally apply a layer of cotton held in place by a wide bandage. When the dressing was removed after ten days to a fortnight, the wound had usually partially scarred. This antiseptic treatment of burns gave Nageotte-Wilbouchevitch a doctoral thesis and a bit of fleeting fame before the "technique" disappeared into the limbo of abandoned medical practices.[71] Henri wryly noted that he was perhaps the only one who remembered this "technique opératoire," which he whiggishly classified under the rubric of mistaken ideas. At this time there was little or no discussion of the psychological trauma suffered by burns victims.[72] The next significant advance in the treatment of burns took place after 1914, when the war provided an abundance of burns victims. During the war Henri was lured into trying a new, better burns therapy. (See Chapter 7, "Rothschild Medical Service in World War I".)

Medical and Drug Business

Physicians increase their incomes by entering into all sorts of lucrative arrangements with pharmaceutical companies. Always interested in dispensing the latest scientifically based medicine and in supporting private enterprise, Henri promoted several drugs with the hope of profit for both patient and promoter. Perhaps his model product here was Veronal rather than Salvarsan. In May 1930 he visited the headquarters of the chemical company Riedel-de Haën Aktiengesellschaft in Berlin to negotiate the distribution in France of two of the company's products, Noctal and Dormalgin (*Nocténal* and *Alpagine* in French); he also hoped to get the German company to distribute the product Orga-mine (Orgamine) or lactoserum, which he had produced and successfully sold in France.[73] So we have here German tranquilizers and sleeping pills and a French ferment promoting good digestion, with an attempt to create consumers across the frontiers for products promising to

---

[71] Marie Nageotte-Wilbouchevitch, *Traitement antiseptique des brûlures* (thesis, Paris Faculty of Medicine, 1893). She did later work in orthopedics. See her *Atlas manuel de gymnastique orthopédique, Traitement des déviations de la taille* (Paris, 1903), and *Traitement des déviations de la colonne vertébrale et de l'insuffisance respiratoire* (2nd edn, Paris, 1937). She also did work on Pott's disease. She became president of the *Société de pédiatrie* de Paris in 1931.

[72] See Elisabeth Bursaux, "La grande brûlure est un drame physiologique et psychique," *Le Monde* (23–24 juillet 2000), 16.

[73] In addition to their active chemical ingredients, Noctal and Dormalgin contained starch and talc as excipients. Noctal also contained lactine or sugar of milk.

benefit consumer and seller, or so Henri thought. The plan was expensive. Then there were the issues of assessing competition from similar products on the French market and of determining how the German drugs would be marketed in France. Having his own hospital was a big advantage: in July 1930 Riedel sent 400 tablets of the two drugs for use in his hospital. A contract over several years specified millions of tablets. Henri's papers contain a page of calculations on the cost of launching a pharmaceutical product in France.[74] Among the major expenses were advertising in medical journals, 100,000 francs; samples for 15,000 physicians, 150,000 francs; visits to physicians, 130,000 francs; and more samples, 270,000 francs. Estimations ran from 900,000 to 1,700,000 francs. In the end not even Henri was willing to proceed with this gamble.

Spending this amount would no doubt have been justified if the profits could be assured and competition was not difficult to overcome. But more important was the project of getting Riedel involved in a sort of business exchange in which they would sell the French product lactoserum or Orgamine. An expert on patents, A. Monteilhet, thought that the brand "Orgamine" could be sold in Germany without any legal problems with patents. The company called Laboratoire Orga-Mine (Etablissements Saint-Benoist, 6bis rue Monsieur, 7th arrondissement), made and sold the lactoserum; it would import and oversee the distribution of the German drugs, a task that would be facilitated by its existing commercial relations with some French pharmacies. The first letter (31 May 1930) from Riedel after Henri's visit said that it was in German because the writer supposed that Henri knew German very well; this appears to be true, though, for business purposes, Henri got it professionally translated.[75] There are only a few words he (presumably) looked up and then noted in French on the letter. (To translate the business correspondence from Riedel Henri used the services of a translation bureau in Paris.) Riedel graciously conceded that if there were need to correspond with the Laboratoire St.-Benoist, it would do so in French, "naturally not very elegant."

Riedel was interested in introducing into Germany the surgical version of lactoserum, but first they had to test it and then give it a trial by German doctors. This product was patented in France under the name "Orgamine" but in Germany as "Cytosteryl"; it was used to disinfect wounds, put into dressings, used in lavage, and applied in other surgical procedures. The producer claimed that in addition to its disinfecting power, Orgamine had nutritive properties that nourished cells while healing scars were forming. P. Mazé of the Pasteur Institute, who was Henri's collaborator in developing the product, would oversee the manufacturing process. Henri said that the study and preparation of lactoserum was first suggested to him by the veterinarian Vallé, who knew that chemists and biologists had analyzed and published articles on this product, essentially the liquid remaining from cow's milk after the coagulation of proteins and albuminoids, which in other circumstances is called cheese making. Henri set up a small laboratory at Vaux de

[74] RAL 000/930: 58-1.

[75] RAL 000/930: 58-1.

Cernay, where, with the help of Mazé, the product was scrutinized. After a year a product was ready for industrial preparation in a bigger laboratory and for large-scale distribution to hospitals. Later production shifted to an industrial laboratory for pharmaceutical specialities.[76] Scientific and social certainty was assured by the status of institutions and individuals: research scientist-professor at the Pasteur Institute and baron-physician of a great banking family. (The information about Mazé's role was noted as confidential.)

One problem Riedel noted right away was that sometimes a vial of Orgamine turned cloudy, meaning it was contaminated. The Germans wanted a detailed explanation. It was a problem in quality control, perhaps, but not easy to explain, given its sporadic nature. Easier for the French than the Germans to accept this doubt. As it turned out, it did not matter, for Riedel could not do anything with Orgamine in Germany until the product was recognized in the same reliable category of effective medicines as Noctal and Dormalgin, introduced in 1924 and 1926 respectively, after years of testing. If studies of the products in schools of pharmacy and university clinics produced good results, the number of collaborators was doubled or tripled in order to get good results from the largest possible number of patients. After the publication of research results, a date was chosen to launch the product in commerce. Sixty-two articles on Noctal and forty-five articles on Dormalgin had appeared in professional publications. They were accepted as first-rate medicines. Pernocton, a barbiturate used after 1927 to induce anesthesia, had garnered thirty publications on the road to acceptance. Orgamine was not in the same category at all: there were no comparable reports on it in French medical publications or even unpublished reports by reputable French doctors. Riedel assumed that the product was undergoing testing and that the results would eventually be available.[77] This blow came in early January 1931. Then some time after, Henri decided that he could not pursue a commercial interest in Noctal and Dormalgin; his letter in late July 1931 told Riedel that it was a pity because doctors and his friends had observed good results from use of the drugs. Though there are no readily available figures, lactoserum, under separate medical and surgical labels, sold well to pharmacies and to doctors; veterinarians had their own special internal brand. Doctors got a discount of twenty percent. (Bills in Henri's papers indicate that some lots used in his medical practice came from the Richer Pharmacy on Avenue Marceau.) Orga-mine (*Laboratoires de biochémie médicales*), a limited liability company, on the rue Van-Loo in the 16th arrondissement, capitalized at ten million francs, advertised itself as supplier to civil and military hospitals. In time a variety of this medicine has migrated to the health food store category with

[76] HR, *La Lignée*, 111–12.

[77] RAL 000/930: 58-1, 158 has a dossier on lactoserum with a chemical analysis of the composition of an ampoule in terms of dry extract per liter (62.13 gr), sugars (53.475 gr), ashes (4.265 gr), and nitrogenized matter (3.190 gr). Impressive precision but perhaps medically useless in terms of what the active ingredient is; an undetermined matter (1.2 gr) is not encouraging. RAL 000/930: 58-1, 167 has letters from Armand Vagne, Firma J. D. Riedel.

a less impressive therapeutic name, whey. So Henri was continuing in the great tradition established by Metchnikov (1845–1916; Pasteur Institute, 1888–1916), who in the last decade of his life took a slight detour from his work on immunity to preach the lactic acid gospel of longevity: pure cultures of lactic acid bacteria added to skim milk (yogurt, kefir, kumiss, etc.) prevent intestinal putrefaction, thus avoiding dire consequences for the gastrointestinal system and the kidneys.[78] Henri's success with the feeding of infants and in reducing their mortality is a story with a more scientific and more successful ending.

[78] Elie Metchnikoff, *Quelques remarques sur le lait aigri* (1904), from the *Essais optimistes* (Paris, 1907).

Chapter 5
The Science of Infant Feeding

> The heart and milk of a mother can never be replaced.[1]

> One can judge the level of a civilization by looking at the curves showing the [historical] drop of morbidity and mortality in early age.[2]

In February 1901 *les Remplaçantes*, a play about wet-nurses by Eugène Brieux, began a successful run at the Antoine theater in Paris; in eight editions by 1907, the play also enjoyed a considerable success with the reading public.[3] The hero of the play is Dr Richon, an old country doctor, who receives Dr Tirelle, a Parisian physician visiting the sticks in order to examine a wet-nurse before she is hired to suckle the baby of a Parisienne. Richon does not allow his patient-mothers to give their babies the bottle. In that at least, he and the bourgeoises of Paris are in agreement. Breastfeeding is in fashion. (The medical view was that well-off society women in France were not in the habit of breastfeeding.[4]) Of course it is not possible for a Parisian woman to be shut up for a year because "an unfortunate accident made her a mother." So wet-nurses are in demand, preferably unmarried mothers, for they are cheaper and unencumbered. Nearly all the women from Richon's village go to Paris as wet-nurses: the area is "maintained by the misery and vice of Paris." The nursing activity brings in money and venereal disease. When Richon gets invited to a Paris salon to entertain the natives, the tables get turned as he denounces the system that draws wet-nurses from the countryside, thus leaving the rural cemeteries full of babies who had to be given the bottle because their mothers were suckling *les petits parisiens*. (The death of the wet-nurse's baby is a key event in the fine film *La Ravisseuse*, 2005.) A bureaucracy was responsible for running the system: a *bureau de placement* required wet-nurses to bring their babies to Paris for scrutiny and then sent the babies back to ignorant relatives. The country doctor gives the Parisian women something other than the social scene to think about.

---

1 Adolphe Pinard, cited in Edmond Lévy-Solal, *La Puériculture* (Paris, 1919), 32.

2 Robert Debré, *L'honneur de vivre. Témoignage* (Paris, 1974), 669.

3 Eugène Brieux, *Les Remplaçantes* (8th edn, Paris, 1907). Two of his other plays are of related interest: *Le Berceau* (1898) and *Maternité* (1903).

4 Madame Bronislas Dluski, *Contribution à l'étude de l'allaitement maternel* (thesis, Paris Faculty of Medicine, 1894), 10.

Over the centuries it has been recognized that nothing is better for babies than mother's milk. Back in 1894 Bronislas Dluski argued that research showed that breastfeeding is the only rational way to feed infants, benefiting both mother and baby; reasons for not breastfeeding being social, it was up to society to suppress any obstacles to it. Breastfeeding has been promoted recently with both reasonable and extravagant claims: it boosts an infant's immunity as the mother's antibodies help fight infection; it gives more protection against gastroenteritis, childhood diabetes, ear infections, and allergies like eczema; it also reduces the child's risk of falling victim to modern plagues such as obesity and depression.[5] Some of the latest titbits of research claim that breastfeeding may boost social mobility and even intelligence. Quite a preventive medicine; or so it was until our science-based civilization poisoned the milk with tiny amounts of nearly every contaminant known to woman, including levels of DDT residues and PCBs exceeding U.S. federal food-safety levels.[6] Until well into the nineteenth century, wet-nurses and mothers breastfed most live-born babies until they were weaned or died of one of numerous infant diseases. The medical profession was in general agreement that the breast of the baby's mother was the safest and most nutritious method of infant feeding.[7] Henri de Rothschild sang its praises in a short work published in 1902. "Its chemical constitution and its biological qualities are such that unlike all other milks, it is well assimilated and only in exceptional cases gives rise to serious gastrointestinal problems."[8]

Yet as an industrial–commercial civilization metastasized, with more and more women entering the urban workforce, fewer and fewer mothers breastfed their babies. As Catherine Rollet has emphasized, the wet-nursing business developed along with industrialization.[9] In 1902 Henri was concerned with another aspect of the issue: it is "not always possible for poor women to breastfeed their infants when they have to work to support a household."[10] "The nursing industry" grew enormously in nineteenth-century cities because of the expansion of a population of fertile workingwomen. Whereas the rich could afford to keep wet-nurses at home and the middle class could send their infants to officially approved and supposedly

---

5 For a recent paean see John Walton and others (eds), *The Oxford Medical Companion* (Oxford, 1994), "infant feeding," 409. Recent research does not find breastfeeding to give much defense against asthma or allergies. Lion Murard and Patrick Zylberman, *L'Hygiène dans la République. La santé publique en France ou l'utopie contrariée 1870–1918* (Paris, 1996), 349, 354, insist that there is no simple correlation between breastfeeding and gastroenteritis; rather, infant mortality is a "total" social fact depending on the level of public health.

6 Florence Williams, "Toxic Breast Milk?," *The New York Times Magazine* (9 Jan. 2005), 21–4.

7 Fanny Fäy-Sallois, *Les nourrices à Paris au XIXe siècle* (Paris, 1980), 134, 161.

8 Henri de Rothschild [HR], *L'oeuvre philanthropique du lait* (Paris, 1902), 3–4.

9 Catherine Rollet, *Les enfants au XIX*[e] *siècle* (Paris, 2001), 27.

10 HR, *L'oeuvre philanthropique du lait*, 13.

safe wet-nurses, the poor, especially single mothers, could only afford the worst of wet-nurses, many of whom just fed the infant artificially, which was fraudulent and usually dangerous. Near the end of the nineteenth century about one tenth of the infants (an annual figure of about 100,000) in France had wet-nurses at home. But we have to keep in mind, as Charles Maygrier discovered at the Charité hospital in this period, that over seventy percent of mothers at least started their babies on the breast rather than the bottle.[11] Brieux's Dr Richon also wanted to see breastfeeding made easy for working mothers; this would possibly have meant the establishment of facilities in the workplace: the Mulhouse (Mülhausen, 1871–1918) model of a nursery in the factory showed that the idea was workable. Giving women six weeks of post-partum paid leave reduced infant mortality from forty to twenty-five percent, a piece of knowledge leading to the German law of 17 July 1878. In Switzerland women got eight weeks of leave after delivery. At the international congress of public health and demography (1900) held in Paris, Adolphe Pinard had to be satisfied with a resolution passed stating that every salaried woman was entitled to rest during the last three months of gestation.

By 1900 the *Assistance publique* was distributing 800,000 francs annually in monthly amounts of 10 to 20 francs to each needy woman in Paris who breastfed in whole or in part. It was estimated that 65 percent of infants in 1910 were fed artificially; over three quarters of these babies suffered from working mothers. In 1910 the potentially lethal *biberon à tube* (nipple with a tube to the milk supply) was outlawed; many nipples were not made of pure rubber and could not sustain the temperature needed for sterilization. The complex *biberon Robert* had two tubes with bottle, valve, and nipple; the tubes and nipples of even cleaned *biberons* retained numerous colonies of microbes, as well as pus and blood from lesions in babies' mouths.[12] In 1896 it was estimated that 17,355 Parisian babies out of the 58,516 born –about one tenth of whom were born outside wedlock; now it is over 50 percent – were sent to generally unsupervised country wet-nurses: 4561 were breastfed and 12,794 were bottle-fed. Henri noted that out of 60,000 live births in Paris, 18–20,000 babies (or about one third of the infant population) were put out to nurse, 3000 on the breast and the rest on the bottle; 30 percent died during the first year, 25 percent during the second year, and of the survivors (about

---

11 See Catherine Rollet and Marie-France Morel, *Des bébés et des hommes. Tradition et modernité des soins aux tout-petits* (Paris, 2000), 147–8, and Rollet, *Les enfants au XIXe siècle*, 27. Charles Maygrier, *La Consultation des nourrissons à la Charité de 1898 à 1901, "Extrait de L'Obstétrique (15 mai 1901)"* (Paris, n. p., 1901), out of 2080 infants leaving the *Consultation* after 11 to 15 days, 71.58 percent were breastfed, 23.22 percent were given both breast and bottle, and 5.19 percent were exclusively bottle-fed sterilized milk.

12 Jack D. Ellis, *The Physician-Legislators of France. Medicine and Politics in the Early Third Republic, 1870–1914* (Cambridge, 1990), 219; Pierre Budin, *Femmes en couches et nouveaux-nés – Recherches cliniques et expérimentales* (Paris, 1897), 264–5; and Rollet and Morel, *Des bébés et des hommes*, 160.

10,000) 20 percent had TB or rickets.[13] Cow's milk has been the usual liquid of replacement for mother's (or wet-nurse's) milk. But substituting the udder for the breast in an urban environment was a capitalist enterprise full of danger for the health of the suckling.

In the nineteenth century doctors developed a model of the perfect wet-nurse, including requirements for her breasts; they had been working on the model since antiquity. The second-century (AD) classic work *On Gynecology* by Soranus established many of the dogmas that would guide the medical profession for centuries.[14] By the time that Henri became a doctor it was accepted (by doctors at least) that only a doctor could certify that a woman was a good wet-nurse. (Mario Bellocchio's superb film *La Balia* [*The Wet Nurse*, 1999] is not entirely bereft of historical verisimilitude in its presentation of the profession.) She should be between the ages of twenty and thirty-five in order to produce milk with the right balance of butterfat, casein, water, and sugar. Brunettes are generally preferable to blondes and redheads, the last having a dangerous libido and watery milk, which tends to produce infant diarrhea. Big breasts are not important; perhaps they should even be avoided. The breast should be pear-shaped with blue veins visible and have enough holes in the nipples to permit easy feeding. The best milk is from a nurse who had a baby from two weeks to two months before she begins wet-nursing. The nurse's baby as well as her milk should be examined. The careful doctor may also look at the milk through a microscope, then the new tool of the modern doctor. Diet and hygiene demand attention. If the wet-nurse starts menstruating again, it is not a reason to change nurses, though the baby may experience minor digestive upsets from the changes produced in the milk by menstruation.[15] Pierre Budin had shown that menstruation, though much discussed, usually had little effect on the quality of mother's milk; nor did pregnancy usually have any effect, at least in over seventy percent of the cases he studied.[16] The sexual relations of wet-nurses

13 "Les Rothschilds – Gouvieux-Chantilly 1880–1930," in *Bulletin de la Société historique de Gouvieux* (Oise), no. 4, 1992: 149; HR, *Dépopulation et protection de la première enfance* (Paris, 1900); Rollet and Morel, *Des bébés et des hommes*, 147–60; and Rollet, *Les enfants au XIXe siècle*, 27. Jules Renard, *Journal 1887–1910* (Paris, 1990), 395, noticed in Château-Chinon, "Des petits Parisiens en nourrice, tout nus sur les seuils."

14 Soranus' *Gynecology*, translated by Owsei Temkin (Baltimore, 1956), 90–103; Yvonne Knibiehler, "Allaitement," in *Dictionnaire de la pensée médicale,* ed. Dominique Lecourt (Paris, 2004), 30; and Danielle Gourevitch, *Le mal d'être femme: La femme et la médecine dans la Rome antique* (Paris, 1984), 233–59.

15 Henri cites A. Lesage, *Traité des maladies des enfants* [sic], II: 596 ff.: HR, *Les troubles gastro-intestinaux chez les enfants du premier âge* (Paris, 1898), 5, and *L'allaitement mixte et l'allaitement artificiel* (Paris, 1898), 18. The reference to Adolphe Lesage (1862–1952) may be to his *Traité des maladies de l'enfance*; Lesage's classic work is *Les maladies du nourrisson* (Paris, 1911).

16 Budin, *Femmes en couches et nouveaux-nés – Recherches cliniques et expérimentales*, 374–9. Much of the work in this volume was done with his intern (Dr Chavane) after 1892 and published in journals such as the *Annales d'hygiène publique et*

pose a delicate problem. They should be rare and not result in pregnancy. But relations should not be prohibited, for a frustrated wet-nurse produces bad milk. (Research had not yet established the relation between breastfeeding and sexual arousal, both in the mother and, as a result of odors produced by the mothers and the babies, also in nearby women.) The pregnant wet-nurse may have to be dropped if the baby shows signs of serious digestive problems, and she is also advised to abstain from sexual activity, if possible.[17] Obviously the wet-nurse has to be free of communicable diseases; the problem is that once they can be observed, it may be too late. The medical examination of wet-nurses included scrutiny of mouth, anus, and genitalia, all sites where syphilis might be detected.[18]

Towards the end of the nineteenth century the business of "selling mother's milk" underwent a transformation before being largely replaced by bottle-feeding.[19] As the death rate of delivering mothers from puerperal fever was reduced from 15–20 percent to near 1 percent, the serious problem of infant mortality began to occupy political and medical attention. Lévy-Solal remarked that in 1900, with about 26,000 more deaths than births, France needed more coffins than cradles.[20] Alarming mortality figures were thrown around: in working-class neighborhoods, between 33 and 86 percent of newborns died, with the most shameful mortality record occurring in the Nord. A study of 681 cities and towns for the period 1892–97 showed that in the largest cities 18.4 percent of all newborns died before their first birthday; for the Nord, the percentage was 28.3.[21] General infant mortality in Germany about 1900 was high, about 23.6 percent, compared with 15.6 percent

---

de médecine légale. The book is dedicated to Lawson Tait (1845–99), the superb English surgeon who, in Christopher Lawrence's words, "helped gynaecology mean surgery." Dluski, *Contribution à l'étude de l'allaitement maternel*, 97, also concluded that a new pregnancy had little effect on the health of the baby being nursed by the mother.

[17] HR, *Soins à donner aux femmes en couches et aux nouveaux-nés* (2d edn, Paris, 1909). Lectures given in the *Hospice de la Salpêtrière* for the municipal school for male and female nurses of the city of Paris. On "Mating Signals," see online BBC News, 24 April 2002.

[18] Paul Labarthe and others, *Dictionnaire populaire de médecine. Usuelle d'hygiène publique et privée* (3d edn, 2 vols, Paris, 1890), article on "Nourrice," II, 548–50, and Fäy-Sallois, *Les nourrices à Paris au XIXe siècle*, 174–92.

[19] See chapter 7 ("The End of the Wet-Nursing Business") in George D. Sussman, *Selling Mother's Milk – The Wet-Nursing Business in France, 1715–1914* (Urbana, 1982), and Béatrice Fontanel and Claire d'Harcourt, *L'épopée des bébés, une histoire des petits d'hommes* (Paris, 1996), section on "nourrir."

[20] Lévy-Solal, *La Puériculture*, 8.

[21] Ellis, *The Physician-Legislators of France*, 219. Different sources give different figures for infant mortality, with doctors compiling their own figures in mini-studies, such as that by Dluski, who in her *Contribution à l'étude de l'allaitement maternel* did a study (1894) of 420 infants at the *Clinique Baudelocque* to find that breastfed babies had a mortality of 10.8 percent and bottle-fed babies a mortality of 45.7 percent.

in France.[22] Babies often died from "infant cholera," a label for different forms of gastroenteritis afflicting those less than a year old; it is estimated that more than one third of the deaths resulted from diarrhea.[23] Jules Simon affected the military metaphor in 1891 in declaring that a battalion of 180,000 infants perished annually. Henri noted more prosaically that out of 1000 live births between 200 and 250 died in their first year and that this mortality was due in most cases to bad or poorly regulated feeding.[24] These figures were more optimistic than the ones he had given two years earlier (1900). In Paris and the better-off departments about 35 per cent of bottle-fed babies under a year of age died from gastrointestinal troubles. Doctors, always generous with the transfer of responsibility, blamed wet-nurses for spreading diseases. Théophile Roussel, a long practicing and locally popular doctor from the Lozère who turned politician, with interests ranging from pellagra to the protection of abused and abandoned children, tried to change things. He managed to get a law ("la loi Roussel") passed in December 1874 establishing national responsibility for the administrative supervision of the guarding of pauper children up to two years of age, of paid wet-nursing, and weaning. Each of the country's departments would have a medical inspection service, whose reports on babies would be transmitted by departmental committees to a higher commission in the ministry of the interior, the coordinating agency.

The Roussel law and its amendments looked good on paper but produced poor results. It is not surprising that Brieux's Dr Richon condemned the Roussel law as useless; he also denounced the *Préfecture de police* for not enforcing the law because of the danger of disturbing the habits of the Parisian population. Then at the *Congrès international d'hygiène* (Paris) in 1875 Bertillon and Monot made the sensational claim that the departmental mortality for nurslings was ninety percent though only seventy-five percent in more favored departments.[25] It is not surprising that in this shocking situation a dangerous organization such as the Office of Wet-

---

22 Petre Trisca, *La protection du nourrisson et de la maternité en Allemagne* (Paris, 1926), 20: the lowest in Europe was in Sweden–Norway: 9.6 percent; the highest was in Russia: 27.2 percent. By 1914, according to Trisca, Germany had lowered the rate to 16.4 percent. See L. Emmett Holt's historical sketch (1905) of infant mortality online at www.neonatology.org.classics/holt.html.

23 Charles Maygrier, *Les Consultations de nourrissons* (Paris, 1903), 2. "Gastroenteritis is a nonspecific term for various pathologic states of the gastrointestinal tract. The primary manifestation is diarrhea, but it may be accompanied by nausea, vomiting, and abdominal pain." There was no mention of the viral origin of gastroenteritis. See www.emedicine.com/EMERG/topic213.htm.

24 See Rachel Ginnis Fuchs, *Poor and Pregnant in Paris: Strategies for Survival in the Nineteenth Century* (New Brunswick, NJ, 1992), 60, and HR, *L'oeuvre philanthropique du lait*, 13.

25 Séverin Icard, *L'alimentation des nouveaux-nés. Hygiène de l'allaitement artificiel* (Paris, 1894), xvii, quotes Bertillon as giving a mortality of 710/1000 in Paris and 240/1000 in the department of the Seine for babies not fed by their mothers. Icard was a doctor at the *Grande-Miséricorde (Service des enfants)*; his book was honored by the Academy of

Nurses in Paris would have to close shop, though it was soon realized that not all infant mortality could be blamed on "the cupidity and negligence of wet-nurses."[26] Some observers noted that there was a higher mortality among illegitimate children, whether fed at home or put out to wet-nurse.[27] In Paris, between 1885 and 1907 infant mortalities ranging from sixty-two percent to seventy-one percent were common in poor areas like the fourth and eighteenth arrondissements; the percentages for rich arrondissements like the eighth and sixteenth ranged from three to eight per cent.[28] Bergeron, later a permanent secretary of the Academy of Medicine, found the figures humiliating for France.[29] Optimists, in an anti-German mood, called Roussel's law "la loi de la sécurité nationale."[30]

The municipal council of Paris became increasingly worried over the growing mortality of bottle-fed babies. In the period 1871–1914 twenty-eight doctors served on the council, though after 1900, as the council moved to the right, the number elected dropped to two or three as lawyers and journalists became more successful in incarnating the modern political type. Since the doctors, mostly well-known medical personalities who preached the latest scientific gospel, were often of high social status, they were able to influence legislation aimed at promoting

Medicine – "prix de l'hygiène de l'enfance, 1891" – and by the *Société protectrice de l'enfance de Paris*, "Médaille de vermeil, 1892."

26 HR, *L'allaitement mixte et l'allaitement artificiel*, vi–vii and 272–7. Henri gives the infant mortality (1893–97) for the *Maternité* hospital *consultation* as 5.69/100 (20 deaths out of 351 children followed regularly), none of which were due to gastroenteritis; for his Picpus Polyclinique (1896–97): out of the 1067 children who were brought to his *consultation*, only 350 came regularly, and of the 83 of the regulars who received free sterilized milk, only 1 died of diarrhea – 2 others, who never came back, also died. For the *consultation de nourrissons* of Dr Chavane in the rue du Chemin-Vert (1895–97) there was a total mortality of 9.09/100, including 1 death from diarrhea for the 99 children who came regularly for more than a month. Henri also points out that Dr Drapier in Rethel (head doctor of the *Crèche Hippolyte-Noiret*) published an article in *Obstétrique* (Sept. 1896) showing a drop in deaths in 1893 from 13/100 to 2.80/100 when the milk was changed from boiled to sterilized milk.

27 Lévy-Solal, *La Puériculture*, 8.

28 Nancy L. Green, *The Pletzl of Paris. Jewish Immigrant Workers in the Belle Epoque* (New York, 1986), fits Jewish infant mortality into the category of poor arrondissements.

29 Budin used the figures in his *Femmes en couches et nouveaux-nés – Recherches cliniques et expérimentales*, 260–1, cited by HR, *Puériculture et centres d'élevages* (Paris, 1931), 2.

30 Icard, *L'Alimentation des nouveaux-nés*, xviii. For a defense of the Roussel law, see Joseph Grancher, J. Comby et A.-B. Marfan (eds), *Traité des maladies de l'enfance* (5 vols, Paris, 1897; 2d edn 1904–05); 5: 70–1; Comby points out that the effectiveness of the law depended on the amount of money departments spent to implement its provisions, with serious application resulting in a considerable reduction in mortality.

public health.[31] Looking at the 358 physician-legislators of the Third Republic between 1870 and 1914, Jack Ellis found that most were moderate republicans, with the more conservative doctors sitting in the senate rather than the Chamber of Deputies.[32] In spite of the interest of national and municipal physician-legislators (sometimes overlapping categories) in promoting public health, reform on a national scale was tardy. The health code drafted in 1932 under the Cartel des Gauches on the initiative of Justin Godart was not finished until after World War II. (Health regulations had been codified in the U.K. by 1875.) Herds of infected dairy cows were not uncommon in a country lacking legally enforced inspection. In the land of Pasteur, the process of pasteurization was finally legally defined in 1955 as a procedure for the preservation of milk.[33]

In 1897 Paul Strauss, municipal councilor and powerful advocate for reform, proposed the establishment of a commission to study the sanitary measures needed to fight infant diarrhea and to regulate the sale of milk in Paris. Roussel dubbed Strauss "le nouveau Saint Vincent de Paul" because of his support of the care of abandoned children.[34] Budin became the secretary of this milk study commission (*Commission pour l'étude du lait*). A report published in the municipal bulletin in 1898 caused quite a stir. A sub-commission recommended that raw and insufficiently sterilized milk be replaced by properly sterilized milk and that free and low-priced milk be distributed to needy nursing babies, as well as to the poor sick and old people; only nurseries using sterilized milk would be given municipal financial help. In order to spread the new sanitary gospel, French doctors came up with the idea of combining medical and feeding facilities in hospital baby clinics – *Consultations de nourrissons/gouttes de lait*. In 1892 the director (Ernest Peyron) of the *Assistance publique* authorized Budin, then accoucheur at *La Charité*, along with his *interne* Chavanne, to open a *consultation* with the purpose of continuing to see women with the babies he had delivered; milk could be given only to the needy.[35] The *gouttes de lait* for the distribution of milk were usually attached to

---

31 Nobuhito Nagai, *Les conseillers municipaux de Paris sous la Troisième République 1871–1914* (Paris, 2002), 145–65.

32 Ellis, *The Physician-Legislators of France*, 93–5, 118–21.

33 Murard and Zylberman, *L'Hygiène dans la République*, 364–6.

34 Strauss was also a *conseiller général*, a senator, and the *ministre de l'hygiène, de l'assistance et de la prévoyance sociales* for twenty-six months in the 1920s. Initiator of projects to build hospitals, asylums for pregnant and delivering women (*Asile Michelet* and *Asile Léo-Delibes*), he also got the Paris municipal council to subsidize Roux's research at the Pasteur Institute in 1895 after Roux had communicated at Budapest the results of his work on an anti-diphtheria serum. See *Célébration à l'Hôtel de Ville des cinquante années de mandates publics de M. Paul Strauss* (Paris, n.d.); the Pasteur Institute and the association of the mayors of the Seine also honored his career with celebrations and interminable discourses. He was a great pillar of the Third Republic.

35 Maygrier, *Les Consultations de nourrissons*, 6. The *Conseil de surveillance* added the restriction on the distribution of milk.

the medically oriented *consultation*, which was not an expensive development, for only a balance, a milk sterilizer, and a doctor's devotion were needed, according to Charles Maygrier, a later accoucheur at *La Charité*. (The term *goutte de lait* was fluid, its meaning changing over time; after the first international congress of the *gouttes de lait* in 1905, the coverage was extended from infancy to include early childhood of poor children, no matter how they were fed. When the term *gouttes* came to imply that at least in some *gouttes* a doctor might be available for the children who could not afford a private physician, the term *consultation* became more important and, Paul Strauss argued, should be indicated in the name of the organization.[36]) Some private *consultations* were created in dispensaries and nurseries. Dr Boissard had one at the Tenon hospital (20th arrondissement). After the *Conseil général de la Seine* got in on the act, five more *consultations* were created. But these nine organizations oversaw only a small part of the 650,000 liters of milk consumed daily in Paris. The working class and the poor (two overlapping categories) were still badly served, if at all.[37]

The purpose of these distribution centers and other institutions was to provide working-class quarters with cheap milk containing the nutritionally correct amount of butterfat, about forty grams per liter. Twenty-five centimes a liter gave a small profit for the establishment of other centers. Prodded by Budin, Henri documented the functioning of the milk business in France, where, unlike in Germany and Denmark, producers and retailers were *not* inspected, nor the milk controlled by technicians chosen by the police. Henri had earlier used the analyses of samples done by the municipal laboratory of the city of Paris, which found that the fat content of milk sold in the city contained twenty-five to thirty grams of fat per liter instead of the thirty-five grams that the producers had agreed on as a minimum. At one point it was found that so-called whole milk really had over thirty percent of the fat skimmed off, though in the 20th arrondissement of Paris only about twelve percent of the milk was watered down. Henri found it strange that producers, sellers, and, for a long time, the public were uninterested in the issue of good quality milk demanded by public health officials and pediatricians.[38] If the water were from the Seine, the baby was exposed to typhoid fever germs. Later municipal laboratory testing of the milk supplied to the arrondissements of Paris found that the fat content of milk was found to be too low (about twenty

---

36 Paul Strauss, "Bulletin," *La revue philanthropique* 17 (1907–08): 127–8. Budin always emphasized the importance of the breast: "La meilleure goutte de lait est celle que l'enfant trouve dans le sein de sa mère," cited in Louis Devraigne, *Vingt-cinq ans de puériculture et d'hygiène sociale* (Paris, 1928), 5.

37 HR, *L'oeuvre philanthropique du lait*, 5–6. By about 1903 there were twenty-five *consultations* in Paris: thirteen under the *Assistance publique* and twelve dependent on private charity. The sixth, fourteenth, eighteenth, nineteenth, and twentieth arrondissements each had three *consultations*. See Maygrier, *Les Consultations de nourrissons*, 8–9.

38 HR, *La Lignée française de la famille Rothschild 1792–1942. Etude historique et biographique* (Oporto, 1942), 111.

grams) only in the 10th arrondissement (rue Lafayette), a surprise in a rich quarter. In the rest of Paris, it became more usual to find too much fat (fifty to fifty-eight grams, instead of the usual Parisian thirty-seven to thirty-eight grams) because milk suppliers added the fat in order to avoid being accused of skimming the milk or worse. The discovery of quantitative fraud and its public exposure and legal danger presumably led to the change.

The national government promoted the establishment of *consultations/gouttes* in the provinces. Not that we should forget the work of individual doctors such as Dr Dufour, who is credited with having established in 1894 at Fécamp the first *goutte de lait* in the provinces; his company sold sterilized milk to the rich and used the profit to give milk to the poor. He recorded a drop from 40 to 16 percent in infant mortality. By 1907 in the Yonne, land of chablis, the consumption of milk by infants was promoted by the prefecture, even to the extent of making the establishment of *consultations* obligatory. There were soon 129 *consultations* in operation. Some doctors, including the medical syndicate, were opposed to possible competition; even some medical inspectors were hostile to free services provided by governmental organizations. The striking fall in annual infant mortality – from 205/1000 to 60/1000 in Auxerre from 1898 to 1904 – after the establishment of *consultations*, supported by the *Société protectrice d'enfance*, made long-term opposition difficult. The position of the national government was made clear when the ministry of the interior sent copies of the book *Les consultations de nourrisons*, by Drs Marois and Mocquot, to all of the prefects in France. The prefect of the Yonne took pleasure in quoting from the preface by Budin: "No more children should die from gastroenteritis."[39]

There was little discussion of what may be a specifically Norman problem, namely the contribution of alcoholism to infant mortality. Towards the end of the nineteenth century the annual infant mortality rate in Rouen was given as 33/100 (live births). Poor children were victims of the vicious practice of being served black coffee laced with eau-de-vie, presumably Calvados, which, added to the milk, was also a well-known Norman soporific for cranky babies. According to the Rouen doctor Raoul Brunon, it was the spread of alcoholism in women that caused them to replace milk and soup with the new caffeine-loaded alcoholic drink. Rich children suffered from alcoholism for a different reason: they were given alcoholic medicinal wines to control their dyspepsia. Rich children also ate too much meat, though Brunon does not specify what diseases resulted from this excessive consumption.[40]

As a result of encouragement from Budin and of his own interest in a great problem in public health, Henri soon played a major role in the baby-feeding

39 *La revue philanthropique* 21 (1907): 705–11.

40 Raoul Brunon, "Alcoolisme des enfants en Normandie," *XIIIe Congrès international de Médecine. Paris 1900. Comptes rendus. Section de Médecine de l'Enfance* (Paris, n.d.) 5: 640–1. The proceedings were published by A.-B. Marfan, who was the secretary of the section.

revolution. Public and private organizations sprouted up to help pregnant women and to save babies; *refuges de convalesence*, like that at Fontenay-aux-Roses, took women in for two to four weeks to help their postpartum recovery and to give instruction on how to bring up baby. When he was an *externe des hôpitaux* (and later a *moniteur*) in Budin's department at La Charité, Henri was surprised by the excellent results obtained in baby feeding by the *consultation/goutte*. Henri speaks of all this in terms one might expect of a religious experience – and he was finding one of his callings: "from then on [1894] I became attached to the study of this exciting issue of infant hygiene."[41] Six months after entering Budin's department, Henri rose to the lowly if useful rank of tutor (*répétiteur).* Henri showed the same keen attention to Budin's ideas and teaching when the latter moved his *consultation* to La Maternité in 1895. After two years of experience chez Budin, in October 1895 Henri, encouraged and guided by the professor, opened an establishment "to succor babies." Quarters were made available for him by the board of directors of the Rothschild hospital in the rue de Picpus. Henri's uncle Alphonse was president of the board. The big isolated pavilion in a garden housed the first privately founded *consultation de nourrissons/goutte de lait* in Paris. There were six beds in two dormitories, a room to prepare sterilized milk, a pharmacy, and a laundry. Though he did not yet have his degree, Henri, supported by distinguished collaborators – to use a classic phrase – from chemistry, bacteriology, and hygiene, founded a work that would serve as a model to numerous similar *consultations* and *gouttes* in France and abroad. Budin recommended some experienced "pediatricians." Originally organized along the lines of Budin's model, Henri's *consultation*, which eventually took on the impressive name of *Polyclinique H. de Rothschild*, began with personnel supervising maternal breastfeeding and distributing sterilized milk for poor children.[42]

Emile Duclaux, director of the Pasteur Institute, recognized the high scientific level of Henri's work on milk when (1901) he invited Henri to give some lectures at the Institute on "Pasteurian theories applied to the dairy industry."[43] Speaking

---

[41] HR, *L'oeuvre philanthropique du lait,* 5–6 and HR, *Bibliographia lactaria. Bibliographie générale des travaux sur le lait et sur l'allaitement jusqu'en 1899* (Paris, 1901), introduction.

[42] Dates differ slightly in different sources. Henri listed the founding of these organizations in the section "assistance" of his *Exposé des titres et travaux scientifiques du Docteur Henri de Rothschild* (Saint-Ouen, 1929). 1896 – Fondateur de la Polyclinique H. de Rothschild, 82, rue de Picpus, Paris; 1899 – Fondateur de "l'Œuvre philanthropique du lait," à Paris. According to Marie-Claude Delahaye's superbly illustrated *Tétons et tétines – histoire de l'allaitement* (Paris, 1990), 151–2, the Picpus *consultation* provided free milk for twenty-five mothers for up to twelve months; others while waiting to get into the free milk group paid half price (thirty centimes a liter) for the milk, which was distributed by the pharmacist Lamouroux, attached to the *consultation*. Four irregularities on a mother's card led to exclusion from the program.

[43] HR, "Les théories pasteuriennes appliquées à l'industrie laitière," lectures given at the Pasteur Institute and published in 1901 by the *Revue générale de chimie pure et*

in the "maison de Pasteur" was an anxiety-creating honor; so Henri was proud of and reassured by Budin's presence at these lectures showing how pasteurization had brought progress to the French milk industry, which had fallen behind other countries in applying science to production. In the United States, Canada, Germany, Switzerland, Holland, Sweden, Norway, and Denmark, the milk industry was "guided by science."[44] Two sciences that were relatively new, at least in name, had transformed the processing and sale of milk. Biochemistry provided the tools to study the elements of which milk is composed along with the laws governing their formation and interactions; its theories provided solutions to a large number of problems and enigmas. In his exhaustive *Bibliographia lactaria* (1901), Henri added another relevant activity: "new theories on yeasts and the perfecting of methods of investigation and analysis." A second science, microbiology, shed new light on the agents present during the decomposition and fermentation of milk. Pasteur's work on microbes was the foundation of this branch of scientific scrutiny, or so everyone who spoke at the Institute felt obliged to say.[45]

The subject of infant feeding became a near obsession of hygienists, the public health professionals.[46] Milk even seemed to be the product most interesting to the general population. Henri wondered what natural product could really be of more concern than milk: the only food of babies, an effective therapeutic agent, and a food of choice for every type of weak or sick person. At the turn of the twentieth century, experts believed that milk contains all the elements necessary for good infant nutrition. "Milk, a complete food," is still a nutritionally accurate slogan.[47] Within the structure of scientific knowledge of the time, before vitamins had been discovered and used to construct a new nutritional paradigm, this was a reasonable dogma on feeding. It still is, at least up to the age of five months.[48] Milk also served as an efficacious medicament in a certain number of infections in some of the body's main organs (kidneys, heart, stomach); this function has since largely

appliqué and also separately as a fascicule.

44 HR, *Contribution à l'Etude de l'industrie laitière en France et dans les principaux laitiers d'Europe et d'Amérique,* (Paris, 1902), 5, extract of the *Revue d'hygiène et de médecine infantiles*, I (1902), no. 1.

45 On the "Pasteurian revolution" in pediatrics, see Patrice Pinell, "Pédiatrie," in Dominique Lecourt (ed.), *Dictionnaire de la pensée médicale* (Paris, 2004), 853–7.

46 HR, *Bibliographia lactaria.* "8,400 indications bibliographiques soigneusement vérifiées. ... 2 suppléments pour 1900 et 1901" (Paris, 1901), ix.

47 For a recent eulogy of milk, see *NutriNews* (Jan. 2002) on "le lait, un aliment complet."

48 Jean-Philippe Girardet (Trousseau hospital, Paris), argues that up to the age of five months milk alone is the perfect food for babies, who also risk developing allergies and hypertension among other problems if other food is introduced too early. Reported in *Yahoo actualités–santé*, 19 Nov. 2001, based on an article in *Panorama du Médecin*, 8 Nov. 2001. In January 2002 the journal *NutriNews* repeated the good news on milk, the complete food.

disappeared except for whey therapy, yogurt indulgence, and other fermentation-based hopes and follies.[49] Henri noted that the milk industry had been completely transformed within a few years by a large increase in consumption and the closely connected application of changing scientific ideas. Like brewing, milling, and sugar production, the milk industry had become a true science – a rather vague label it is true but meaning that top scientists worked for the industry, especially in Switzerland, Denmark, and Germany.[50]

What sort of science did the dairy researchers do? Of course the composition of milk was an important subject, including comparisons between the mammary secretions of women, cows, asses, and other mammals. Asses and goats had the reputation of being free from some diseases, including syphilis.[51] Henri carefully made reference to Duclaux's work as basic for investigations into the activities of microorganisms in the transformation of milk. (Pasteur's classic paper on lactic acid dealt with a subject that eventually proved important for the explanation of malolactic fermentation in wine, though he did not know of the positive role of lactic acid-producing bacteria in transforming the tart malic acid into the softer lactic acid.) Henri was passionate about the transformation of lactose into lactic acid accompanied by the release of carbon dioxide, a transformation showing the action of the non-pathogenic microorganisms, the ferments. One of the key ferments that researchers worked on was casein (a phosphoprotein of milk containing combined phosphoric acid), which we associate with cheese and plastics; Henri thought about it as a key component of mother's milk. As with wine, so with milk: pathogenic organisms infected the liquid; the difference was that in milk the pathogens could transmit infectious diseases. Some people worried about tuberculosis and hoof and mouth disease. Milk was also recognized as an excellent medium for the growth of bacteria that could be transferred to babies through careless hands. (Plates magnifying microscopic pictures of the actor bacteria were prepared in the polyclinique.) But the transmission of TB and other infectious diseases through the consumption of raw or insufficiently heated milk was considered to be rare. What worried doctors like Henri was the so-called "infant cholera" or gastroenteritis of the newborn caused in 95 percent of cases by

---

49 Whey (*le petit lait, lactosérum*) is still among the highly recommended food supplements – e.g., "Whey to go" from Solgar. The Whey Protein Institute recommends it for helping to meet a variety of "medical challenges" running the gamut from breast tumors to cholesterol reduction. HR and P. Mazé gave a long communication on the subject to the Academy of Medicine in Paris on 4 June 1929: "Le lactosérum en thérapeutique chirurgicale et en thérapeutique vétérinaire."

50 HR, *Bibliographia lactaria*, ix.

51 Delahaye, *Tétons et tétines*, notes that the *Assistance publique*, following a request by Professor Parrot, *Hospice des Enfants-Assistés*, set up a stable of asses to feed syphilitic children; one ass fed two babies daily. Delahaye has also published *Bébés au biberon – petite histoire de l'allaitement* (Paris, 2003), and with Didier Lett, *Une histoire de l'allaitement* (Paris, 2006).

the omnipresent *Bacterium coli*. (The bug was renamed *Escherichia coli* in 1919 to honor Theodor Escherich, discoverer of the bug and a pioneer in pediatrics in Vienna.[52]) This disease was blamed for most infant mortality in Paris and the provinces.[53] Even politicians were alarmed enough to call on science for cheap help.

Henri pointed out that consumers were the first to benefit from safe milk and willingly paid for the increased cost when they knew what they were paying for. The rich man is perhaps a little optimistic about the food values of the poor. Behind the general concern about the hygienic and economic conditions of production, there lurked a double problem: how to get cheap good quality milk while protecting the consumer from fraud. The consumer, being in the unfortunate position of not knowing that the price of milk increased, or even doubled, for good reason, became a likely victim of fraud and likely to expose her family to danger from cheaper but adulterated milk, a tricky liquid to identify by taste. Milk seemed to present problems in tasting similar to those presented by wine, another product often adulterated in the post-phylloxera era. Only "a true expert [could] determine the quality of milk by tasting it."[54] And only a chemist could recognize its chemical properties and nutritive value. The general public continued to judge milk as its ancestors had: "milk is good if it doesn't turn on boiling."

Consumers were finally protected by the same factor that counteracted the lack of scientific enlightenment on the part of dairy farmers and peasants. The industrialists preparing milk products for sale pasteurized or sterilized the milk. Pasteurization meant heating the milk to seventy-five degrees centigrade for five minutes immediately after milking and then cooling it quickly. This process was used for urban areas, where milk was consumed within twenty-four hours of milking. If the milk were cooled down a second time to two or three degrees above zero, it could be stored in cellars until shipping time. Basically, the destruction of microorganisms by heating made it possible to transport and conserve milk without the addition of more or less toxic chemical products.[55] The spread of refrigeration was helped considerably by laws prohibiting the addition of chemical preservatives to milk, among other liquids. Still the consumer could be misled into wrongly assuming that pasteurized milk was safe for a long time after purchase.

Sterilization provided a better guarantee of safe milk. Franz Soxhlet's method of sterilization meant heating the milk in a sealed container up to a temperature of 98 degrees centigrade for 40 minutes. The milk would then keep without refrigeration for 36 to 48 hours. (Few people had an icebox.) Soxhlet's original double boiler or bain-marie, dating back to 1889, underwent inevitable technical modifications over the years. Henri believed that an "absolute sterilization of milk at a humid

52 "Theodor Escherich," in www.whonamedit.com.

53 HR, *Les troubles gastro-intestinaux chez les enfants du premier âge*, 15.

54 HR, *Les troubles gastro-intestinaux chez les enfants du premier âge*, 15, and *Bibliographia lactaria*, introduction.

55 HR, *Bibliographia lactaria*, introduction.

temperature of 115 degrees C for fifteen minutes kills all micro-organisms and spores."[56] The happy result of these technical advances in providing safe milk for babies was clear in Budin's department at the *Clinique d'Assas*, where the use of sterilized milk and careful supervision ensured that there were only rare cases of gastroenteritis, even during Parisian heat waves, when infant mortality could rise above 75 percent of infants less than a year old. So that politicians would appreciate the contribution of the medical profession to public health, Budin did not fail to note the drop in infant (0–1 year of age) mortality from 134/1000 to 115/1000 in the decade up to 1903, even in hot summers like that of 1898. One can also mention July 1900, when the temperature hit 40 degrees centigrade. Authors, picking different years and ages, get different rates of mortality. A.-B. Marfan, in a lecture given in 1915, advanced the following mortality figures for 1000 infants between one month and one year: 1892–95 – 258; 1896–1906 – 220; 1901–05 –164; 1906 – 145; 1909 – 143.[57] An added advantage of the sterilization of milk was that it could even help Europeans in their tropical colonies by controlling their gastrointestinal diseases, or at least those that came from milk, both as a safe food and, modified, as an effective medicine.[58]

The basic science on which the safety of milk depended was identical in different countries, but the modalities of scientific application and regulation differed according to national and cultural values. In spite of his praise of the Pasteur Institute and of Budin's department, Henri found France to be behind much of the western world in the milk industry and in assuring the safety of its product. Always keen on studying medical progress outside France and introducing therapeutic advances into Paris, often through his own institution, he undertook a study tour of European countries leading in the milk industry.[59] In Denmark, Switzerland, and Germany, the dairy industry had understood the need to put competent people in charge, meaning people who kept up to date in industrial chemistry and bacteriology. University professors and distinguished chemists did not hesitate to serve as technical advisers in model establishments. This was pretty

56 HR, *Les troubles gastro-intestinaux chez les enfants du premier âge*, 15, and *Bibliographia lactaria*, introduction.

57 Pierre Budin, "La ville de Paris et la mortalité infantile" (lecture given on 4 December 1903 in the *mairie* of the 4th arrondissement…), *La revue philanthropique* XIV (1903–04): 381–416; on Antonin Marfan, see Maurice Genty, *Les Biographies médicales*, 2d series, "Les Maîtres d'aujourd'hui" (Paris, 1930–36).

58 HR, *Bibliographia lactaria*, introduction. Henri also recommended the treatment of gastroenteritis with skim milk to which a lactic acid culture was added, pasteurized and then sweetened. The treatment was tested at his Polyclinic. HR, "Traitement de la *gastro-enterite* par le lait écrémé acidifié," *Revue d'hygiène et de médecine infantiles* 2 (1903): 484.

59 HR, *Notes sur l'hygiène et la protection de l'enfance d'après des études faites à Berlin, Saint-Petersbourg, Moscou, Vienne et Budapest* (Paris, 1897).

much what happened in the wine industry in the twentieth century.[60] The higher agricultural institute of Copenhagen had a special chair for the dairy industry.[61] There were twelve scientific establishments (large experimental stations) doing studies for the German milk industry. Some German universities had agricultural institutes where the theory and practice of dairy farming were intellectually respectable, scientifically important, and therefore productive in publication. Henri visited model dairies in Berlin and Frankfurt am Main where the administrative council was composed of doctors and veterinarians responsible for the application of the rules of modern hygiene to the functioning of the stables and dairies. Thirty-two dairy schools covered the Reich: nine only accepted female students, ten accepted both male and female, and the rest fell into the male domain. Organized into big federations, the industry supported five weekly newspapers. The scientific and commercial sectors interacted in a way similar to that of the scientific and productive sectors of the industry. In most large towns a laboratory for analysis and research supervised the regulation of the sale of milk. In many towns there were *Kindermilchanstalten*, which distributed milk guaranteed to be fresh and pure from healthy cows. (A more rigorous version of the *gouttes de lait*, which were, in their simplest form, milk distribution centers for poor babies and children.) Science could also produce profits in ordinary ways. Switzerland supplied most condensed milk to the European market. Henri thought that France could learn much from its competitors about modernizing its dairy industry.

France had a large dairy industry with big problems. At the beginning of the twentieth century there were about 6,700,000 French dairy cows producing annually 800,000,000 hl of milk, one fifteenth of which was consumed in Paris as milk, butter, and cheese.[62] About 5900 cows lived in the city of Paris. Less than a half dozen big wholesale milk-processing firms did the filtering, pasteurizing, and conditioning that allowed the milk to survive safely for 16 to 24 hours, even in Paris. The presence of adulteration was matched by – some would say caused by – an absence of science.[63] In 1897 the municipal council of Paris turned down a proposal to create a municipal school of dairy science, though the recommendation came from its own commission for the study of milk, made up of hygienists and scientists. This failure was not so serious as it might have been if a course in dairy science had not existed at the Pasteur Institute. The department of analysis

---

60 See Leo A. Loubère, *The Wine Revolution in France – The Twentieth Century* (Princeton, 1990), and Harry W. Paul, *Science, Vine and Wine in Modern France* (Cambridge, 1996).

61 HR, L'industrie *laitière au Danemark. Rapport adressé à Monsieur le Ministre de l'Agriculture* (Paris, 1902), reprinted in *La Industria Lechera* (Buenos Aires, 1922).

62 On French and Parisian diets, see Harry W. Paul, *Bacchic Medicine. Wine and Alcohol Therapies from Napoleon to the French Paradox* (Amsterdam, 2001), 225–7.

63 For information of the early years of the Paris municipal laboratory and controversy surrounding its test results, see Harry W. Paul, *From Knowledge to Power. The Rise of the Science Empire in France 1860–1939* (Cambridge, 1985), 214–20.

and applied chemistry offered a course in theoretical dairy science with practical analyses. The course was given in the annex of biochemistry, under the guidance of Auguste Trillat, known for his work on alcohols and milk. And in 1902 Henri offered a ray of hope to those who despaired of French backwardness. Although the milk industry did not offer big advantages to businesses wanting to follow scientific methods rigorously, things were improving. Schools of dairy science were few and poorly attended; the industry, wallowing in a routine that triumphed over the application of scientific principles, nearly ignored new developments. Henri provided cogent arguments for a shakeup in the French dairy industry.

In 1902 perhaps the situation was not quite so bad as it was being painted. Henri scrupulously noted the favorable signs of change in France. There was an *Ecole nationale d'industrie laitière* in Mamirolle (Doubs), a subsidized *Station laitière* in Olmet (Cantal), eight *Ecoles pratiques de laiterie*, and some *Ecoles de fromageries*. In some departments the organization of the milk industry into cooperative societies had developed considerably. In Paris a *Société d'encouragement à l'industrie laitière* published the journal *L'industrie laitière*. The economic importance of the dairy industry was increased by the fact that France was a debtor country in cheese and butter. In 1899 imports of cheese were worth 29,000,000 and exports 11,000,000 francs, imports of butter were worth about 17,000,000 and exports about 7,000,000 francs. A surplus was produced by exports of salted butter worth 58,000,000 francs with little of this product imported. A powerful sub-text of Henri's analysis of the dairy industry was that science could make France a more competitive dairy power.[64]

In the movement to supply safe milk to babies and children, scientific medicine happily cohabited with pediatric practice. Budin and Henri were especially aware of the progress made in Germany, Denmark, and Sweden. Soxhlet in Munich seemed to tower above most others in the relevant area of research. His publication in 1891 of the first results obtained in the study of the effects of the consumption of sterilized milk earned him a role of founding father. In France Budin was the first to apply the "new method." As in the "pasteurization" of wine, so in the sterilization of milk, technique was of the highest importance. And what seemed a German patina on Pasteurian science was really a successful German technique. Budin obtained excellent results in feeding milk sterilized in a bain-marie. (Budin was against premature weaning and "artificial feeding," but when "natural feeding" was not possible, he advised the use of sterilized milk.) Henri's tour of the facilities of the countries advanced in the production of safe milk and the publication of his observations were an impetus to reform in Paris (and France).

In Paris Henri made a considerable contribution to the effort of getting milk distributed to the needy: his *Œuvre philanthropique du lait* (established in 1899) rented special places in densely inhabited working-class quarters (e.g., Belleville

64 HR, *Contribution à l'Etude de l'industrie laitière en France et dans les principaux laitiers d'Europe et d'Amérique* (Paris, 1902); reprinted from the *Revue d'hygiène et de médecine infantiles*, 1 (1902).

and Charonne) and hired trustworthy personnel to handle distribution and accompanying paperwork. A milk supply company in Paris furnished the milk at the same price and in the same conditions as the milk it sold to the *Assistance publique*. The managers of the depots had lists of those qualified to buy the milk at a low price or to receive it free. Numbered coupons were also sold at headquarters in the rue Cambacérès (8th arrondissement) to philanthropic societies, dispensaries, nurseries, and people who dispensed charity: they then gave the coupons to their objects of charity. In areas where there were few depots, milk could even be delivered to where the consumers lived.

By June 1901 the *Œuvre philanthropique du lait* was distributing over 15,000 liters of milk monthly. In the first semester of 1901 the *Œuvre* distributed 357,868 liters of fresh milk and 83,279 liters (201,875 bottles) of sterilized milk. By 1902 the *Œuvre* had 14 depots operating in Paris, with Henri's old friend and colleague Dr Achille Hauser (1867–1956) directing the operation. Over a 30-year period the *Œuvre* distributed a daily average of 100,000 liters of safe milk. The *Œuvre* soon began paying its own way and started buying milk to give away, all without need of subventions. Over the next 30-odd years the *Œuvre* expanded until by 1933 it had 834 depots for the sale of milk. One report gives the astounding number of 1500 depots of distribution. The money spent annually for milk aid amounted to 187,457 francs, and the value of the coupons sold was 2,095,173 francs. By then Henri had long turned everything over to Hauser, who added new items to the depots, including food products such as charcuterie. Henri's medical interests were concentrated on *La Fondation Henri et Mathilde Rothschild* in the rue Marcadet.

Although head of the *Œuvre philanthropique du lait*, Hauser acted as director without taking a salary. Science and charity seemed compatible bedfellows. Hauser enjoyed an intimate, profitable relationship with Henri and his family, beginning with James-Edouard when Achille was a child.[65] Madame Katz, director of the Rothschild hospital in Berck-sur-Mer, had a fertile sister married to a grocer near Mulhouse. In 1875 Achille left his nine siblings to pass the summer with his aunt at the seashore. James, taking a liking to the lad as well as recognizing his potential, provided for his education. In 1904 Achille named his son James after his benefactor. During their stay at Berck-sur-Mer in 1883 Henri and Achille became friends. Promoted by Henri's mother, the friendship continued in Paris and during their studies in the faculty of medicine. After surviving the ordeal of the examinations for the *externat*, Achille became Arthur's personal physician and remained on call until the patient refused to follow medical advice to give up a serious addiction to Havanas. Achille and Arthur used to meet frequently at the Rothschild property in Vaux de Cernay. The social relationship with Henri flourished, turning into a medical-commercial affair.

When in 1898 Henri established the organization to distribute milk to needy babies, Achille seemed like a natural choice for director. In 1911 Achille also became the director of an organization for the distribution of a more famous French

[65] *Bulletin de la Société historique de Gouvieux* (Oise) 4 (1992): 86.

food, wine – good, unadulterated, cheap wine, a rare commodity in working-class establishments. (Henri got out of the distribution of wine from the Midi when the *Œuvre philanthropique du vin* became the *Société des Vins Hauser*.) Achille showed superb entrepreneurial skills in helping the poor, which did not exclude helping himself.[66] The Hauser milk-shops he created in 1899 flourished, joining up in 1913 with the *Société des Fermiers Réunis*, a big milk distributor in Paris. These milk-shops also distributed groceries in agreement with the Vilgrain stores. In 1940 the name changed to the *Laiteries parisiennes*, which distributed butter and *fromage blanc* (made in their own milk collection centers in departments outside Paris) along with standard food items.

The main problem in the production and distribution of milk, apart from sanitation, was quality control. Henri had several battles with big milk suppliers and even with dairy farmers in the Sarthe before he was able to get his own milk empire established. Hauser was able to put the Rothschild name to good use in overcoming some obstacles. Then Henri's *Œuvre* was able to establish a milk collection center and a model dairy on one of the biggest farms near Paris, at La Ferté-Bernard in the Sarthe, and thus control its own milk supply. The superior quality of the milk, which was filtered and generally pasteurized, was evident in a content of 38–40 grams of fat per liter. Henri had to spend close to a million francs (over 800,000 in any case) to establish this model plant, which processed 6000 liters daily, and he became unhappy with the cost of the operation after a year. After Hauser came into the operation, the expensive home delivery of fresh or sterilized milk was stopped and the milk then sold in special boutiques. Legally, Henri gave the plant to the *Œuvre philanthropique du lait*, which built 14 such enterprises over the next 40 years. Over a generation the *Œuvre* opened 134 depots and distributed milk in 80,557 needy cases, a work of charity that Henri calculated as worth 2,095,173 gold francs. In a commercial reorganization after 1907 the organization became an industrial company, a non-philanthropic competitor in the milk business. The good news by 1925 was that it was hardly possible to find adulterated or contaminated milk in Paris.[67]

The *Œuvre* did not please milk dealers. In 1908 the commercial milk business enjoyed a legal victory over the *Œuvre* when the *Syndicat des Crémiers de Paris et des départements* (milk dealers' union) took the philanthropic organization to court, which was, in this case, the *Tribunal de Commerce de la Seine*. The union claimed that the *Œuvre*, by posing as a charitable organization, was making large profits from selling milk without having to get trade licenses and pay taxes. In

---

66 Terminology differs in different sources. In The Rothschild Archive [RAL] 000/930: 58-1, 162 there is the following precise and apparently legal description of Hauser's business. "Laiteries A. Hauser, fondées en 1899 par le docteur Henri de Rothschild. Hauser Frères et cie. … Capital 3.400.000 francs. Siège, 39 rue de Surène, 8th arrondissement [in 1905 the address was given as 59 rue Vandamme, 14th]. Service de livraisons 178 et 178bis rue de Vaugirard ,15th."

67 HR, *La lignée*, 90–1.

spite of the *Daily Mail*'s proclaiming that the Paris milk dealers' union had won a suit against Henri de Rothschild, his counsel was able to convince the commercial court that having turned over all his interest in the philanthropic milk business to Hauser, he was not personally involved. But the union did win its case. The tribunal pointed out in its decision that though there was charity involved, the *Œuvre* was still a commercial enterprise and therefore designations such as *Œuvre humanitaire* and *Œuvre de bienfaisance* had to disappear within a week of the date of the decision. The *Daily Mail* noted that the tribunal ordered the words "Rothschild Foundation" and "The Philanthropic Pure Milk Foundation" removed from all Rothschild shop fronts. Every day's delay would have brought a fine of the equivalent of two pounds instead of the forty pounds asked by the plaintiff.[68]

The dairy industry probably had little love for Henri after the harsh report he did in 1908 on its practices. This report, done for the commission on milk of the *Ligue contre la mortalité infantile*, dealt only with the processing of milk in big industrial establishments, where pasteurization and sterilization were standard practices.[69] Milk collected from different farms underwent treatment that could include filtering, pasteurization or sterilization, homogenization, and skimming before transport of the finished product to points of distribution and sale. Filtering was essential because ignorant and careless workers usually milked the cows; machines had the potential of improving sanitation in this sector. The aim of the report was to encourage the dairy industry to furnish consumers with good quality milk. One would think that the industry itself would be eager to do this, but the serious shortcomings specified in the report indicate that this was not the case.

The modern milk-processing plant was, at the time of this report, a technical marvel designed to assure the perfect integrity or pureness of milk: its apparatuses made it into a real laboratory. In most foreign dairies, which Henri knew well, there existed "absolute scientific rigor, ensuring that the prescriptions of modern science are scrupulously followed." (He made good use of German literature.) Such was not the situation in France, where old routines continued in spite of the beneficial influence of graduates of the *Ecoles de laiterie*; on farms there simply were not enough trained personnel to ensure that "a cheap product like milk was treated with the same scruples as an expensive product." Henri made it clear that the industrial dairies supplying Paris were generally run according to the correct scientific methods. Since the problem was on farms where the high price of equipment made it impossible for them to modernize their processes, it was useless to try to force them to buy the apparatuses needed to collect and keep the milk in an aseptic way. Inspectors and veterinarians visited these farms but, given the remoteness of the farms, this supervision worked better on paper than in reality. Legal action against some culprits for illegal skimming and watering down

---

68 *Gazette des tribunaux*, 47 (18 February 1908) and *Daily Mail* (21 January 1908), in RAL 000/930: 58-1, 220.

69 *Ligue contre la mortalité infantile – Commission du lait. Rapport présenté par le Dr Henri de Rothschild. Traitement du lait récolté* (Mâcon, 1908).

seemed to promote virtuous behavior by others, at least temporarily. Only the big establishments could be trusted to deliver a pure product.[70]

Not all modern developments in the processing of milk were completely beneficial without modification to ensure preservation of some of the product's desirable qualities. Pasteurization (e.g., 80 degrees centigrade for 5 minutes) destroyed pathogenic microorganisms causing measles, German measles, scarlet fever, typhoid fever, diphtheria, and TB, but it was only a partial sterilization because the destruction of lactic acid bacteria requires a temperature of 105 degrees C for 10 minutes. Some doctors argued that these processes diminished the nutritive value of milk, though they did not have the conceptual basis to make a strong case, except for the possibility that heat destroyed the diastases (amylases), thereby altering the biological state of milk. Henri was able to use an article by Hippius in the *Jahrbuch für Kinderheilkunde* (1905) to argue that heating milk to 85 degrees C for 2–3 minutes does not essentially change the biological state of milk. These debates are reminiscent of the debates over the pasteurization of wine. With an ideal method of pasteurization, milk keeps its chemical and biological properties. More important from the viewpoint of infant mortality, the milk is aseptic without being sterile. In any case, Soxhlet, Budin, Marfan, Variot, and others had shown that in a great number of cases sterilized cow's milk was often better tolerated than mother's milk. Henri hastened to add that much remained unknown in infant therapy and pathology.

In 1924 Henri noted that sterilized milk was not much used any more to feed babies. A new feeding paradigm had come into existence based on "modern principles according to which children must be fed living milk, pasteurized for only a few minutes."[71] Scientific progress can be a personally depressing business. Henri could afford to be quite objective and even enthusiastic about the obsolescence of his own work.

One thing about the application of science to consumption is that the modification of products never stops. Usually for the benefit of industry, it sometimes benefits the consumer. One of the novelties in 1908 was the homogenization of milk, though it was a new process not much used. Since the etiology of many diseases was unknown, any new food process ran the danger of being blamed for causing a disease. In this case it was scurvy; knowledge of vitamins, ascorbic acid (C) in particular, was years away. The advantage of homogenization was that the milk could not be skimmed illegally. Henri noted that crooks would need to switch to watering, which was worse for the consumer. Showing how unwise it is for an expert to make predictions in his area, Henri declared that homogenization would not become an industrial process. (Some self-proclaimed experts on heart disease believe that would have been a good thing.) One thing was certain, Henri concluded, when the modern dairy applied scientific methods in good conditions,

---

70 *Ligue contre la mortalité infantile – Commission du lait. Rapport présenté par le Dr Henri de Rothschild.* Quotations from the report cited in note 69 above.

71 RAL 000/930: 58-1, 218.

it could supply a germ-free, non-adulterated product. Science could not guarantee quality, of course, but the old technical skill of tasting could. Milk samples had to be tasted when the milk was brought in to the factory from different sources. Differences in quality, freshness, and wholeness made it essential for a highly competent person to determine which batches of milk should be mixed and if any batch should be rejected because it would alter a large quantity when integrated into it. Like the production of good wine, the production of good milk was a total work of art dependent on science.

Violent social change creates circumstances extremely favorable to the sale of adulterated food. Milk was one of the leading products capable of being reinvented with profitable opportunities for fraud. Condensed or concentrated milk provided a classic case of adulteration, especially during World War I. In 1917 Henri and the Lyonnais veterinarian Charles Porcher did a scientific exposé of the problem.[72] A large number of foreign brands of condensed milk invaded the French market because of wartime shortages of regular milk. These products varied considerably in nutritional value, though in the non-informative commercial culture of the day customers were kept ignorant of such information. Ignorance and marketing, often commercial twins, confused condensed milk with different varieties of preserved milk and did not distinguish between whole and skim or sugared and non-sugared milk. The authors bluntly accused businesses of exploiting consumer ignorance to increase profits. This work with Porcher earned an official accolade in the *Bulletin municipal officiel de la ville de Paris* in 1918, when the *Conseil d'hygiène et de salubrité* of the department of the Seine noted the authors' "remarkable work."[73]

Unlike the United States, France had no legislation regulating the composition and labeling of condensed milk. This type of milk was notorious for its low fat content: the milk was heavily skimmed to make butter, which sold at a high profitable price. Condensed milk, being a manufactured product, should have a constant composition, with a minimum fat content of 33–35 gr per liter. Henri and Porcher also wanted the degree of concentration to be fixed at 66 percent water and 34 percent dry extract, or 5 percent higher in water and 5 percent lower in dry extract should legislators desire to legislate a weaker concentration. Most fraud occurred in non-sugared condensed whole milk, as a result of the insufficient degree of concentration rather than in any bad chemical quality of the original milk. Labeling requirements could go a long way in checking fraud. The label, in the language of the consumer, should give net weight, in grams for France, and the variety, whole or skim, and not vague words like rich and pure.[74] The authors

---

[72] *L'Industrie des laits concentrés et la fraude*, by Dr Henri de Rothschild, *Médecin aide-major de 2e classe, et Professor Charles Porcher, de l'Ecole vétérinaire de Lyon* (Paris, 1917). "Communication faite à la Société des Experts-chimistes de France le 14 février 1917."

[73] *Bulletin municipal officiel* (14 January 1918) in RAL 000/930: 58-1, 220.

[74] Weight stated in ounces provided an excellent opportunity for fraud because the old French *once* equaled 30.6 gr and the English ounce, 28.35 gr. The *Service du Ravitaillement*

noted that the word *condensé* was not so good as the word *concentré*, which was in increasingly frequent usage. The degree of concentration with instructions for use had to be stated in liters and not in parts, which differ according to parts by weight or by volume. Adding antiseptics should be forbidden. A last point made by Henri and Porcher dealt with the feeding of children. The label should carry the advice "For feeding children, consult a doctor." (This good advice would, if followed, extend control by the medical profession over mother and baby.) One of the feeding problems, especially for infants, arose from the fact that sweetened milks were not sterilized; with a high content of flora, these products needed to be made in hygienic conditions.

The authors ended on a note of commercial patriotism. The condensed milk market was large, and France had the high-quality milk along with the technical and mechanical resources to enter this market, monopolized in 1917 by Swiss, Dutch, American, and Italian products. During the war and after, Henri produced his share of patriotic encouragement for the French economy. In his *Exposé des titres* (1929) Henri noted with satisfaction that as a result of the work done by Porcher and himself, the government required that condensed milk sold in France carry a label in French giving essential information about the product.

By the end of the nineteenth century the milk industry and the medicalization of baby-feeding practices had spawned a research empire whose subjects spewed out an enormous number of publications. The special commission of scientists created in 1897 by the Paris municipal council included in its proceedings the most recent results in research on milk. What was lacking in 1900 was a general bibliography on milk and baby feeding. And Henri provided this in 1901 with the publication of an exhaustive *Bibliographia lactaria*; his work on baby feeding had led directly to organizing this enormous work, which listed 8400 medico-scientific works. Henri and Duclaux, who wrote a preface, saw the book as evidence of the triumph of science. Milk, an essential food and prime necessity, now belonged to science. Duclaux, at his Whiggish best, declared that errors are always corrected in science, thus ensuring the triumph of truth. Science ensures its triumph through patience and hard work. The adherence of scientists to the experimental method produced this miracle. And led to Henri's superb *Bibliographia lactaria*.

The bibliography was divided into three parts. First, works categorized under the heading of the general study of milk, including as subjects the milk of women and cows and other mammals, milk products such as kefir and whey, sterilization and pasteurization, condensation and preservation, and industry. The general category also included physiology, pathology, analysis, bacteriology, hygiene and legislation, fraud and adulteration, diet and therapeutics, and the transmission of diseases. The second part of the work dealt with baby feeding, and the third part listed patents. The periodicals in which articles appeared were listed along with the authors cited in the entire work. Publications in the major scientific languages were covered. Researchers seemed to have left no teat untouched: cat's milk,

wanted labels to indicate whether the milk was whole or skimmed and sugared or not.

sow's milk, the fat in porpoise's milk, and, in a comparative vein, the antagonism between the milks of human females and of bitches. This bibliography was a great tool of science that could have only been done by an individual with Henri's resources, energy, and medical knowledge.

Chapter 6
A New Medical Speciality: Pediatrics

> The medicine of children and especially babies is not simply 'scaled down' adult medicine. It is a totally different game.[1]

We have seen that in 1892 Pierre Budin, then accoucheur at *La Charité*, succeeded in creating a *consultation spéciale de nourrissons* to tackle the problem of reducing infant mortality. Henri praised Budin for launching a real crusade to save babies, done with the material support of some of his patients and the approval of the *Assistance publique* – diplomatically, he did not note its institutional inertia. A basic problem, as Budin and his colleagues saw it, was the issue of power: the accoucheur had control of the baby for only nine days after its birth. This was the "short period" – short for Budin, Henri, and their allies – corresponding to the time specified by regulations of the *Assistance publique* for stays of new mothers in its maternity establishments. The department head determined exceptions. Budin succeeded in his fight against this system when he opened his model *consultation* at *La Charité*. Rachel Fuchs calls his institution "the first well-baby clinic," the beginning of "schools of motherhood."[2] His radical innovation gave the accoucheur control over the baby's feeding and medication for twelve months. Though some doctors in pediatrics opposed this turf grab, the *Directeur général* of the *Assistance publique*, Ernest Peyron, supported Budin. Paul Strauss was able to influence Peyron in favor of Budin's plan. One would hesitate to say that the scientific evidence in the case did not convince the *Assistance publique*, but political pressure also counted.[3]

In 1894 Henri's training in puericulture took a new turn when Pierre Budin introduced him to Mademoiselle Hénault, the head midwife at *La Maternité*. Henri later seemed satisfied to have been present at the birth of what he later called the new medical science of puericulture, a word that was laughed at when introduced

---

[1] Patrick Keating, *The Bluffer's Guide to Doctoring* (London, 2000), 23. See note 4 below for definitions. In 1921 Pierre Nobécourt, in *La Presse médicale* (19 février 1921), noted that "the great English pediatrician" Charles West (1816–98), a founder of the Hospital for Sick Children in Great Ormond Street (1852), compared doctors who enter a children's hospital for thc first time to travelers to a country whose language and customs they do not know.

[2] Rachel Ginnis Fuchs, *Poor and Pregnant in Paris: Strategies for Survival in the Nineteenth Century* (New Brunswick, NJ, 1992), 146.

[3] Charles Maygrier, *Les Consultations de nourrissons* (Paris, 1903), 6, and Louis Devraigne, *Vingt-cinq ans de puériculture et d'hygiène sociale* (Paris, 1928), 15.

in the 1860s but caught on after the 1890s, when big doctors started using it, and it was no longer merely a matter of "pipi, caca, lolo, dodo."[4] Henri found himself in the midst of a changing and expanding system for raising babies. The *consultation* led to an *Ecole pratique d'élevage* for mothers and wet-nurses along with a sort of information service. The *consultation* also became a laboratory for "rational experimentation" on infant feeding. Hundreds of physiological and pathological observations led to the development of rules for different types of feeding and, more difficult, to the treatment of many of the inherited and contagious infant diseases.[5] The model organization at *La Charité* required mothers of the babies delivered by Budin to stay in the hospital for ten to fifteen days. This stay was not regarded as dangerous or excessive or as pampering the patient but rather as an ideal measure of the control essential for the healthy development of the baby and probably for the successful future pregnancies of the mother. Some mothers who needed further convalescence went from the hospital to the municipal asylum in Fontenay-aux-Roses. Budin recommended breastfeeding by the mother or, when needed, by wet-nurse.

Budin's system reached a small number of mothers, for well into the twentieth century over ninety percent of babies were born at home, two thirds of them with a midwife assisting.[6] So they had to be reached in other ways, one of which was through "popular meetings" bringing together mothers of different quarters of Paris in order to teach them how to feed their infants properly and what mistakes

---

[4] "Pissing, shitting, eating, sleeping." According to the *New Shorter Oxford Dictionary*, this old word puericulture (E. 20, from French) now refers to the rearing of children as a skill or a branch of sociology. The word p(a)ediatrics (L. 19) is defined as "that branch of medical science that deals with childhood and the diseases of children." *Le nouveau petit Robert* (1993) shows the difference in usage of the French words. La puériculture (1865, from Latin puer + culture): "Ensemble des méthodes propres à assurer la croissance et le plein épanouissement organique et psychique de l'enfant (jusqu'à l'âge de 3 ou 4 ans)." La pédiatrie (1872): "branche de médecine qui traite des maladies des enfants." *Le Journal de Pédiatrie et de Puériculture* presently advertises itself as dealing with, among other topics, general pediatrics, fetal and neonatal medicine, and practical puericulture. Fanny Fäy-Sallois, *Les nourrices à Paris au XIXe siècle* (Paris, 1980), 128, elevates Alfred Caron to the rank of founder of puericulture; Caron wrote *La puériculture ou la science d'élever hygiéniquement et physiologiquement les enfants* (Rouen, 1866). Pinard's book on the subject, *La puériculture du premier âge*, came out in 1904. Cottet-Dumoulin says that in 1999 the *Institut de Puériculture de Paris* was the only establishment in France to use the word. See note 8 below.

[5] Henri de Rothschild [HR], *Puériculture et centres d'élevage* (2d edn, Paris, 1931), 1–5, and Budin's account in the *Journal de clinique et thérapeutique infantiles*, 21 (1897): 413–15.

[6] Catherine Rollet, *Les enfants au XIX*[e] *siècle* (Paris, 2001). According to Maygrier, *Les Consultations de nourrissons*, 42, in 1899 the number of babies delivered under the aegis of the *Assistance publique* was 34,181, of which 16,294 were born in *maternités*, 11,927 were delivered by the *bureaux de bienfaisance*, and 5960 by qualified midwives.

to avoid. A series of talks, the brainchild of the municipal council, inaugurated by Budin in the presence of colleagues, assumed high political importance with the attendance of the prefect of the Seine. Henri was certainly pleased to hear Budin mention approvingly the *consultation* started by "one of our students." In praising Henri's free distribution of free milk at his *Laiteries philanthropiques*, Budin promoted him to his "excellent student," who funded the centers in memory of his grandmother, la baronne Nathaniel [Charlotte]."

Budin died of pneumonia in 1907 at the age of 56. By then there were nearly 500 *consultations/gouttes* in France. A large committee, including Henri and Madame Pasteur, set to work to perpetuate the memory of the great doctor who did so much good. In 1909 the *Fondation Pierre Budin* was inaugurated to promote breastfeeding and puericulture. Henri, Budin's loyal medical son, played a large role in all this. Budin's wife, carrying on her husband's work, was able to open up a serious *Ecole de puériculture et d'allaitement*, including a "model dispensary," in the rue Falguière, in the 15th arrondissement, with an 18-year lease costing 20 francs annually for a site provided by the municipal council. Louis Devrainge, accoucheur at the Lariboisière hospital, became the director of the school. Henri supported the Budin foundation for over 30 years. The school was a modest monument to a leading figure in the birth of pediatrics.[7]

The famous accoucheur Adolphe Pinard (1844–1934), the "apostle of puericulture," including *puériculture intra-utérine*, was the first professor appointed (1890) to the chair of clinical obstetrics at Baudelocque, his fiefdom until he retired in 1914. After the war he went into politics, becoming deputy during the period 1919–27. (The Paris Faculty of Medicine created the Baudelocque clinic (second Paris chair of obstetrics) in 1890 in the gardens of the *Maternité* hospital. The clinic is named for the obstetrician Jean-Louis Baudelocque (1746–1810), for whom Napoleon created the first chair of obstetrics.) Pinard, a well-known medical personality of the Belle Epoque, viewed puericulture as medical eugenics, whose aim was the improvement of the human race by providing medical scrutiny of couples before they reproduced along with paying attention to the development of the fetus and caring for mother and baby. Known for his mellifluous advocacy of breastfeeding, Pinard organized a branch of the charitable society *Allaitement maternel*, which was supported by an elite bevy of bourgeoises.[8] Advocate of a

---

[7] *La revue philanthropique* (1907), 21: 814; Henri de Rothschild [HR], *La Lignée française de la famille Rothschild 1792–1942. Etude historique et biographique* (Oporto, 1942), 92.

[8] Fuchs, *Poor and Pregnant in Paris*, 146. According to Marianne Cottet-Dumoulin (*épouse* Robinot), *Une grande œuvre médico-sociale: l'Ecole de puériculture de la Faculté de Médecine de Paris 1919–1970* (Mémoire, Faculté des science humaines et sociales – Université René Descartes-Paris V, 1999), in 1908 Mme de Rothschild (not further identified) gave 1,500,000 francs to the *Société d'allaitement maternel*, founded in 1876 by Marie Béquet de Vienne. See also online: http://www.whonamedit.com/doctor.cfm/3199.html.

similar gospel, A.-B. Marfan (1858–1942), pediatrician and professor, argued that puericulture must base itself on the principles of Galton and Pinard, meaning the application of eugenics to the function of reproduction. A delicate matter, to be sure, Marfan admitted, but if the issue were put in terms of advice to couples not to procreate while under the influence of alcohol, morphine, or cocaine, or suffering from syphilis, what rational person could possibly object?[9]

Looking at developments in infant feeding and care in a general historical context, one is tempted to see the emergence of a new branch of medicine. George Weisz distinguishes the medical specialization of the nineteenth century from that of the twentieth century (1890s to 1950): the former period was one of small groups straddling medical faculties and of teaching hospitals with specialist private practice being of minor importance; in the latter period specialization became "the dominant form of medical practice."[10] Pediatrics was one of the "new life-stage" specialties that developed in nineteenth-century medicine, though enthusiastic historical sleuths find its embryonic roots in much earlier times, with al-Razi's work on the diseases of children establishing his claim to pediatric paternity. Al-Razi (865–925) also owed something to his teacher al-Tabari, but, like most pedagogical debts, the influence seems obscurely limited to something in child development. In the European Renaissance pediatric efforts are better known than the medical glories of Baghdad during the Abbasid Caliphate: on the historian's list we find Pietro Bagellardo's work published in 1472, Bartholomaeus Metlinger's *Regiment der jungen Kinder* (1473), and Thomas Phaer's book on children (1530). The Enlightenment of the eighteenth century was particularly fertile in pediatric advances, even institutionally, with the establishment in 1787 of the Viennese private *Kinderkrankeninstitut*, which became a small children's hospital in 1837; distinguished names are easy to cite: Nicolas Andry de Boisregard in France, Nils Rosen von Rosenstein in Sweden, Michael Underwood in England.[11] Doctors had definitively discovered children's diseases; what to do with them was another matter. Andry, a controversial figure, professor, finally got round in 1741 to writing a famous book at the age of eighty-three: *L'Orthopédie, ou l'art de prévenir et de corriger dans les enfants, les difformités du corps*. He was possibly another

---

9 See Cottet-Dumoulin (*épouse* Robinot), *Une grande œuvre médico-sociale: l'Ecole de puériculture de la Faculté de Médecine de Paris (1919–1970*), and Edmond Lévy-Solal, *La Puériculture* (Paris, 1919), a report presented to the 5th section of the Congress on mother and child, presided over by Pinard, at the *Congrès Interallié d'Hygiène Sociale pour la Reconstitution des Régions dévastées par la Guerre*, Paris, 22–26 April 1919. On Marfan, see Maurice Genty, *Les Biographies médicales*, 2nd series, "Les Maîtres d'aujourd'hui" (Paris, 1930–36), 225–55.

10 George Weisz, *Divide and Conquer. A Comparative History of Medical Specialization* (New York, 2006), xvi.

11 For some key events in the development of the "new life-stage speciality" of pediatrics see Roy Porter, *The Greatest Benefit to Mankind. A Medical History of Humanity* (New York, 1998), 382–3.

medical father – of orthopedics this time, or at least he invented the word; and using the principle of straightening the sapling (the "tree of Andry") he imposed the same treatment on children's limbs. Pioneering specialists like Percivall Pott, Jacques Delpech, Georg Strohmeyer, and William John Little made orthopedics an important nineteenth-century specialty that became an integral part of pediatrics. (See chapter 2 on the children's hospital at Berck-sur-Mer.)

Writing a classic text established the reputation of a doctor and sometimes ensured that he would be labeled as at least one of the founders of a speciality. So Rosen von Rosenstein's book on *The Diseases of Children and their Remedies* (1764) established his reputation as the author of a textbook serving as a model for pediatric texts for several generations and even as "a founder of modern paediatrics as a medical specialty."[12] Works by Michael Underwood (1737–1820), John Cheyne (1777–1836), and Charles-Michel Billard (1800–32) also fall into the category of key texts in the history of pediatrics. In the history of institutions, the establishment in 1802 of the Paris public *Hôpital des Enfants Malades* (at first for boys only) has generated high historical praise, especially on its own website: "premier établissement pédiatrique au monde" and even "inventeur de la pédiatrie," though the *Oxford Medical Companion* uses the event as proof that the French were leading the way – and this judgment could be easily extended to clinical medicine. During most of hospital history children and adults shared the same facilities.[13] In 1828 Billard published a pioneering systematic text in clinical pathology based on his work at the *Enfants Malades*, and the three volumes on children's diseases by Frédéric Rilliet and Ernest Barthez became "the bible for doctors for the next 25 years."[14] But there was a serious component missing in French pediatrics. As Pierre Nobécourt pointed out in his opening lecture when he took over the Paris faculty *chaire de clinique médicale des enfants* in 1921, until 1863 the faculty of medicine did not teach pediatrics: "triste constatation!"[15] This deficiency is part of the story of the growing pediatric ascendancy of Germany, symbolized by the

---

12 See the entry by A. White Franklin and R. D. H. Boyd on "Paediatrics (pediatrics)," in John Walton and others (eds), *The Oxford Medical Companion* (Oxford, 1994) [OMC], 714–15.

13 In 1926 the *Hôpital Necker* and the *Hôpital des Enfants Malades* were put under the same administration. See http://www.hopital-necker.aphp.fr/Deux-siecles-et-demi-d-histoire.html. "Newborns went to the Foundlings Hospice, while the Pitié and St. Antoine orphanages admitted young children." Guenter B. Risse, *Mending Bodies, Saving Souls. A History of Hospitals* (New York and Oxford, 1999), 294.

14 OMC, 714. Frédéric Rilliet and Ernest Barthez, *Traité clinique et pratique des maladies des enfants* (3 vols, Paris, 1843); 2d revised and expanded edn, 1861; 3d edn, 1891, and expanded by Barthez and A. Sanné, 1891.

15 Pierre Nobécourt, "Leçon d'ouverture – chaire de clinique médicale des enfants" (6 Jan. 1921), in *La Presse médicale* (19 février 1921).

publication (beginning in 1868) of the *Jahrbuch für Kinderheilkunde*, and then of the United States.[16]

Henri Roger (1809–91), a doctor at the *Enfants maladies* who had published on children's diseases, started teaching a supplementary course, but he retired in 1874 without any chair established for the subject.[17] Then in 1878 the faculty got a professorship in the subject for Parrot, a doctor at *Enfants malades* whose identity is now difficult to trace, though he is said to have come from a family of artists. He died in 1883. In 1885 Joseph Grancher (1843–1907), a really serious appointment, took the chair as "professeur de clinique infantile." A medical expert on tuberculosis, he was connected with big names in Parisian medicine and was a collaborator with Pasteur on the rabies vaccine. But Grancher had less of an impact in pediatrics than might have been expected because he was often sick.[18] Victor Hutinel replaced Grancher between 1889 and 1892, when Marfan took over; Hutinel finally got the chair when Grancher died in 1907. An important figure in French clinical medicine, honored by having his name attached to several diseases, including a liver disease ("Hutinel's cirrhosis"), Hutinel had been teaching internal pathology for eleven years before becoming "professeur de clinique des maladies de l'enfance" at *Enfants Malades*. He was the logical choice for president of the first congress of the international association of pediatrics, which met in Paris in October 1912.[19] Since pediatrics had become much too complex a subject for one man to handle, Pierre Nobécourt was given responsibility for hygiene and infant medicine. Hutinel pushed for another professor to take care of the teaching concerning babies. And in 1914 Marfan became professor of the baby business, that is, "professeur d'hygiène et de clinique de la première enfance"; he moved to the *Hospice des Enfants Assistés* after World War I. Marfan was clearly the big name in French pediatrics by then.[20] (One of Marfan's students, Robert Debré

[16] Abraham Jacobi (1830–1919), a German pediatrician, emigrated to New York in 1853, established the chair in pediatrics at New York Medical College in 1861 and went on to organize societies, begin journals, and promote the opening of children's departments in New York hospitals. See C. Becket Mahnke, "The Growth and Development of a Specialty: The History of Pediatrics," *Clinical Pediatrics* 39 (2000): 705–14. Jacobi is another "father" of the specialty.

[17] Henri Roger, *Seméiotique des maladies de l'enfance ... leçons* (Paris, 1864); see also his *Recherches cliniques sur les maladies de l'enfance* (Paris, 1872–83).

[18] Toby Gelfand, "11 January 1887, the Day Medicine Changed: Joseph Grancher's Defense of Pasteur's Treatment for Rabies," *Bulletin of the History of Medicine* 76 (2002 Winter): 698–718. With J. Comby and A.-B. Marfan, Grancher was editor of and a major contributor to the *Traité des maladies de l'enfance* (5 vols, Paris, 1897; 2d edn, 1904–05).

[19] Victor Hutinel, *L'enseignement de la pédiatrie à la Faculté de Paris. Leçon d'ouverture faite le 21 décembre 1907 à la clinique des maladies des enfants* (Paris, 1907; reprinted from the *Bulletin médical*, 25 Dec. 1907). Hutinel was the key author of the collaborative effort *Les maladies des enfants* (5 vols, Paris, 1909).

[20] Nobécourt, "Leçon d'ouverture – chaire de clinique médicale des enfants"; see also his classic *Précis de médecine des enfants* (7th edn, Paris, 1942); with the super-prolific

(1882–1978), was in charge of the Rothschild hospital (Picpus) during the German occupation in World War II.)

Ignoring earlier pioneering efforts in this "new life-stage specialty," Henri argued that in the late 1890s "a new branch of medicine ... [was] transforming itself," with its practitioners staking out an important piece of medical turf. Pediatrics, "the art of raising babies, or caring for children," previously connected to general pathology, was fast becoming autonomous. A new era had dawned, according to the promoters of scientific medicine. Much of the revolutionary impetus came outside the embryonic specialty. After the 1870s the hygiene of babies (less than a year old) had been completely transformed by input from bacteriology and chemistry. The use of sterilized milk had significantly cut infant mortality. Weak and sick babies were surviving in greater numbers thanks to the success of chemists in transforming cow's milk. The incubator created by Stéphane Tarnier in 1883 saved the life of many prematurely born babies. This technology's founding myth reveals that when Tarnier saw a chicken incubator at the *Jardin d'acclimatation*, he thought of replacing the egg with a baby. Nearly all preemies of seven to eight months used to die; the excellent results with the incubator led the *Assistance publique* to purchase forty by 1900. In any case, infant mortality dropped and continued to drop, whether because of scientific medicine or food. This is a false dichotomy, as it turns out, because better milk was the work of scientific medicine.[21]

By the 1880s it was difficult for a doctor serious about scientific medicine to ignore germ theory. In 1889 Budin enrolled in the course in bacteriology at the Pasteur Institute. A short time after, Georges Dieulafoy did the same thing. Henri said that Emile Roux took control of Budin's education as a biologist; the teacher found the eminent physician to be an excellent student. Budin thought that bacteriological information was so important that he gave the people in his own department a clinical lecture every Saturday morning. The acquisition and transmission of new knowledge was a minor problem compared with that of overcoming institutional inertia. Budin was fortunate in being able to profit from the technical expertise of the heads of his laboratories of biology and chemistry (Charles Michel and Maurice Nicloux) in carrying out analyses of milk, blood, and feces.[22]

Léon Babonneix, he edited the five volumes of the *Traité de médecine des enfants* (Paris, 1934); among his more interesting works is *Eléments de puériculture à l'usage des jeunes filles du Maroc* (Paris, 1922).

21 HR, *Notes sur l'hygiène et la protection de l'enfance d'après les études faites à Berlin, Saint-Pétersbourg, Moscou, Vienne et Budapest* (Paris, 1897), introduction, v–viii. Adolphe Pinard, *Stéphane Tarnier, 1828–1897* (Paris, 1898); Pinard also gave the *Eloge* for Tarnier at the Academy of Medicine in December 1908. On the history of the incubator, see Scarlett Beauvalet-Boutouyrie, *Naître à l'hôpital au XIX*[e] *siècle* (Paris, 1999), 324–31.

22 HR, *Puériculture et centres d'élevages*, 9–10. Niclaux (1873–1945), who had both medical and science doctorates, became the head of the laboratory at the medical

One unintended consequence of establishing the Picpus *consultation*/polyclinic had been that Henri's field of scientific scrutiny became much richer, permitting him to fulfill Budin's wishes by recording extensive personal observations and providing the data for his hefty books on feeding babies – over one thousand observations of babies whose feeding was mixed (breast and artificial) or only artificial, that is, cow's milk.[23] *L'allaitement mixte et l'allaitement artificiel* (1898) was dedicated to Budin, who had provided the inspiration for the work and read the manuscript. Henri never ceased to express his gratitude for Budin's decisive influence on the orientation of his scientific career.

At this point in time Henri was preparing his doctoral thesis. He proposed to do chemical and biological research on milk and to apply the new methods of pasteurization and sterilization to infant feeding. He did the work but followed the advice of his mentors in not defending his thesis at that moment because of potential disturbances by demonstrators from the rabid right at a defense of a thesis by a prominent Jew during a hot moment in the Dreyfus affair. So he decided to publish the research as *L'allaitement mixte et l'allaitement artificiel* and, in the same year (1898), prepared a partially new thesis (on the gastrointestinal problems of infants) to defend at a more appropriate moment.[24] Later in life Henri said that his *consultation* accepted only sick babies, thus differing from Budin's *consultation*. Both babies and science benefited: most babies were cured and Henri collected a great number of observations, information for graphs, and photographs to use in his two substantial works on infant feeding.[25]

Henri organized his thesis on infant gastrointestinal disorders according to medical principles of the day, giving them a slight twist to accommodate the specifically pediatric subject. The work dealt with etiology, bacteriology, clinical symptoms, dietary prevention of infection, curing specific infections, and a regimen for sick babies. In all of the gastrointestinal disorders, the predominant syndrome is diarrhea. Why write a new work on this old topic? It could be argued that infant therapy had taken a new direction since the mid-1880s. First, it had

---

faculty's *Clinique Tarnier* (old name was the *clinique d'accouchement, rue d'Assas*); he did interesting work on the passage of alcohol and other poisons from the mother to the fetus as well as studies on the nutritive value of milk. He was the founder of the *Société de chimie biologique*.

23 HR, *L'allaitement mixte et l'allaitement artificiel* (Paris, 1898).

24 HR, *Les troubles gastro-intestinaux chez les enfants du premier âge. Etiologie, pathogénie, symptomatologie et traitement. Alimentation des nourrissons dyspeptiques.* Paris Faculty of Médicine. "Thèse pour le doctorat en médecine présentée et soutenue le mercredi 29 juin 1898, à 1 heure par Henri de Rothschild. Né à Paris le 26 juillet 1872, ancien externe des hôpitaux de Paris, ancien moniteur d'accouchement à la charité, médaille d'argent de l'académie de médecine (Paris, 1898). Président: M. A. Fournier, professeur. Juges: MM. P. Budin, professeur, Poirier et Gilles de la Tourette, agrégés." The thesis has an enormous bibliography of French, English–American, and German works and an index of authors cited.

25 HR, *Une dame d'autrefoi*, 82.

been shown that the number of gastrointestinal sicknesses could be reduced by a rationally administered program of safe feeding. Second, bacteriology had established the cause of the infections. Once the toxin of the pathogenic organism was discovered, an antitoxic serum could be administered. After seven years of research, Adolphe Lesage of the Pasteur Institute, an expert on gastrointestinal diseases, including green diarrhea, managed to come up with a serum to treat "infectious gastroenteritis."[26] Of course Henri argued that it is better to prevent than treat a disease, and here the major weapon was sterilized milk.

The major difficulty in dealing with these infant disorders was the ignorance of many doctors in the area of infant hygiene, especially concerning feeding. Only a small number had taken advantage of the programs set up at the two hospitals *Maternité* and *Charité*. Budin had set up a special *consultation* at the Tarnier clinic for doctors and students. (The *Clinique Tarnier* received this name in 1897. An extension of the medical faculty led to the demolition in 1878 of the old *Hôpital des cliniques*, with its delivery clinic being transferred in 1881 to a new building in the rue d'Assas in the 6th arrondissement. In the 1980s it became part of the Cochin hospital empire.[27]) The subject slowly expanded on the fringes of the medical curriculum. Not that one can blame the doctors for their reluctance to jump on the latest scientific bandwagon: the question was which wagon? Even the introduction of sterilized milk did not end controversies about infant feeding and digestive disorders. Henri pointed out that experts, basing their advice on a selection of facts and observations, proposed very different methods of preparing and composing infant formulas. Many but not all of the differences could be explained by differences in the composition of milk from different cows. There was, for example, less fat in the milk of Dutch cows than in that of Norman cows. Many factors had to be brought under control before the science of infant hygiene could convince doctors to speak with one voice. Proof of effective diagnosis and treatment could only be provided by clinical medicine, which is exactly what Henri did in a series of "clinical observations," carried out in his Picpus establishment and published partially in his thesis and fully later. To achieve scientific clarity, Henri classified his observations into three groups. First, the infants who, contrary to what doctors generally believed, perfectly tolerated pure sterilized cow's milk; this milk was tolerated even by very young infants (fifteen days to three months), including those of normal weight and those underweight. (A low-weight baby can be defined as one weighing 2.5 kg.) Second, a certain number of infants who suffered from acute or chronic digestive disorders caused by overfeeding or by milk of bad quality for periods from eight days to three months. This second group lost weight for an average of eight days and did not seem to tolerate sterilized

[26] Among his works, see Adolphe Lesage, *Le Traitement des gastro-entérites des nourrissons et du choléra infantile* (Paris, 1906). He was an important figure in the history of pediatrics. See www.pasteur.fr/infosci/archives/les0.html.

[27] Emmeline Deroin, *La Maternité de Paris de 1850 à 1900*, "Université de Paris V. Ecole de sages-femmes Baudelocque. Mémoire de fin d'études de sage-femme" (Paris, 2005).

milk. But little by little they were brought round to tolerating it and generally after about a week started to gain weight. The third group referred to two unusual cases where success was due to a special diet, either cold milk or kefir.

Henri's thesis presented many of the arguments and conclusions present in *L'allaitement mixte et l'allaitement artificiel*. Infant digestive disorders are most often the result of a defective diet, whether the baby is breastfed or bottle-fed. The illness of the breastfed baby could be just as serious as the acute or chronic gastroenteritis of the bottle-fed baby. Though Henri gave credit to Escherich for his description in 1886 of the pathogenic microorganism *E. coli*, he used the term *bacterium coli* and noted that Lesage had completed the work. The chronic form of gastroenteritis could usually be cured; the acute form often developed too quickly for any effective therapeutic action. Intestinal antiseptics produced some successful results; stomach flushing and enemas using various chemical concoctions also helped. In treating the disease the doctor had to monitor the general state of the infant. This meant controlling fevers, fighting dehydration, and treating skin problems. There was no point in curing an infant's diarrhea only to have it die from some other illness.

A doctor in 1908 was far better able to handle infant gastrointestinal disorders than his medical ancestor could in 1878. He understood the etiology of gastroenteritis. "General pathology" had furnished the medical profession with agents and means to treat the problem, ranging from flushing out of the digestive plumbing to giving hypodermic injections of serums. In grave cases where there was an urgent need to calm the stomach because of gastric intolerance of food, the doctor could use a potion with bromide or cocaine, or just water with chloroform – Henri got the best results from this last calmative. Calomel enjoyed favor as an antiseptic and a purgative. Among the intestinal antiseptics, benzoate of naphthol enjoyed a certain success. Fevers were treated with a wide variety of pharmaceuticals, including hypodermic injections of a solution of benzoate of soda with citrate of caffeine and, of course, sulfate of quinine. To "fight dehydration and stimulate nutrition" required subcutaneous or intravenous injections of a serum, preferably Hayem's, a concoction including salt, sodium sulfate, and distilled or sterilized water. Some skin abnormalities were treated with powders containing, among other things, talc and zinc oxide but only after the infant had been washed in a boric acid solution. More serious skin problems required repeated baths in a sublimate solution and the application of pomade. Heroic medicine for "les petits malades."

The treatment for a dyspeptic baby followed a precise program designed to ensure the infant's survival. (The term dyspepsia covered all digestive disorders.) The sick infant was first given only water for three days in order to clean out its system and rehydrate it. If the baby were breastfed, the program would likely be simple, with twenty to thirty grams of milk being given in three feedings over three hours. The mother required some basic mathematical skills as well as the ability to squeeze the milk out of her breasts during the non-feeding period. A baby with an easily irritated stomach might need a little chloroformed water. If the infant were not breastfed, treatment was more complex. Germans were better at this treatment. Ingenious German pediatricians – Henri used the expression "pediatric doctors" – had concocted mixtures to replace mother's milk and cow's milk. Gaertner's *Fettmilch* (concentrated) gave good results in the feeding of sick babies who needed to regain lost weight. The closer the milk was to mother's milk, the better it was for the dyspeptic infant's inflamed digestive system. Pure milk often got good results. In some cases the individual baby's idiosyncrasy had to be taken into account: there were cases in which some babies could not tolerate some products. An optimistic Henri noted that in the future French methods would replace German methods. At least the French doctors had gotten to the point where they recognized that many of the infant's problems came from the bad quality of poorly sterilized milk.

After the definitive organization of the Picpus establishment, the free distribution of sterilized milk with the attendant ritual of weighing of babies, considerable numbers of infants were brought in. Between 25 March and 1 December 1896, over 400 infants passed through the doors of the *consultation* and provided Henri with statistical data. They were, for the most part, sick, weak children, often suffering from digestive troubles. Henri took a personal interest in the more rare, interesting cases. The field of study was vast enough to provide material for his extensive work on hygiene and infant feeding. He was able to start the study of problems such as an infant's temporary intolerance of new food; since "temporary" could mean up to 48 hours, and even without diarrhea up to 10 days, it was necessary for the doctor to keep the infant on the new food and use various treatments to achieve tolerance. Like Budin, Henri showed that, contrary to some medical opinion, dyspeptic infants, including preemies, could be cured by feeding them only pure sterilized milk. In the follow-up (weekly or fortnightly) of these babies, he noted that they did not get rickets or impetigo. The rare ones who could not tolerate the milk could be fed either peptonized or maternalized milk, the latter being a concoction processed to be the approximate chemical equivalent of mother's milk. And cold milk worked just as well as warm in certain cases. So high-quality sterilized milk and better feeding habits lowered infant mortality considerably. Therapeutic action, even with Lesage's antitoxin serum, was less certain in its results, for in some serious cases, the baby could not be saved.

Henri thought that his work on infant feeding presented a theoretical as well as practical interest, though of course the practical lessons dominated. The rules of daily medical practice are derived from the careful and repeated examination of facts. It is assumed that the axiomatic fact, the bedrock of science, is certain and incontrovertible. A number of rules formulated by Budin after 1894 had been confirmed by this scientific procedure. The time had come by 1898 for a systematic presentation of these rules while informing the reader of recent advances. Henri declared that *L'allaitement mixte et l'allaitement artificiel* gave convincing proofs, buttressed by graphs and statistics. It was a modern work of medical science, even in its admission of further puzzles for future researchers to solve. "The digestive tube of nursing babies still presents oddities that are difficult to explain" (p. 177).

Henri's medical career "advanced" with the specialty, as he became a "moniteur d'accouchements" and adjunct to the two doctors in charge of Budin's *consultation*. Keeping this connection and duty after entering Dieulafoy's department, as he passed through the grind of a medical training, showed how seriously Henri was attached to the infant-feeding business, which was indeed a matter of national concern.

Henri's personal research contribution to the theory and practice of baby feeding appeared in a substantial number of publications.[28] Like most of his colleagues doing serious research, he did not discover anything startlingly new but worked within an accepted pediatric paradigm to provide solid scientific support for what the medico-scientific community generally accepted. The basic fact with which medical and public authorities had to wrestle was the high death rate from "gastroenteritis" among bottle-fed babies less than one year old; breastfed babies had only about one sixth of that death rate. Henri attributed the high mortality of these babies to the bad quality of milk sold in the poor quarters of Paris and ignorance of the rules of proper feeding on the part of inexperienced mothers; even if the milk were unadulterated, too frequent or excessive feeding could cause problems. An examination of the "non-digested" stools made this diagnosis possible. He later added another factor: hot weather provokes alteration of the milk and the development of microorganisms normally found in milk but not necessarily at a high enough load level to cause problems. The milk could contain chemicals such as formaldehyde and salicylic acid (a derivative of phenol, added to preserve the liquid) as well as possibly contaminated water, added to increase profits. Such additions were illegal.[29] Improperly or carelessly processed milk might contain pathogenic microorganisms or yeasts capable of infecting babies. Dirty feeding equipment also had been identified as a common problem in causing infant diseases.

---

[28] Among these works, the most substantial are *Quelques observations sur l'alimentation des nouveaux-nés et de l'emploi raisonné du lait sterilisé* (Paris, 1897); *Hygiène de l'allaitement. Allaitement au sein, allaitement mixte, allaitement artificiel, sevrage* (Paris, 1898), translated into Italian in 1902 by Dr Gino Gelli; and *L'allaitement mixte et l'allaitement artificiel*. In the last work Henri notes that his personal contribution to the subject was to provide the figures for 1067 children cared for at his Polyclinic from 25 March 1896 to 15 December 1897. For more publications, see "Principaux travaux sur le lait et l'allaitement," *Exposé des titres et travaux scientifiques du Docteur Henri de Rothschild* (Saint-Ouen, 1929), 20.

[29] Henri and Dr L. Netter wrote a report on "L'aldéhyde formique comme agent de conservation du lait" for the *Société scientifique d'hygiène alimentaire rationelle de l'homme* following the discussion over the communication by Emil Behring at the congress in Kassel on 27 September 1903; see their article "Recherches sur la conservation du lait par le formel," *Revue d'hygiène et de médecine infantiles* 4 (1905): 334–52.

In *L'allaitement mixte et l'allaitement artificiel* Henri noted how two of the major problems of feeding had been solved.[30] First, the breastfed baby who seemed to have gastroenteritis was found in reality to be suffering from repeated indigestion that became chronic. The cause of the problem was too frequent sucking for too long, and once the hours and duration of the feeding sessions were regulated, the problems that threatened to become serious usually disappeared. The milk of clean mothers rarely contained pathogenic organisms, often a danger to babies who were bottle-fed or were fed both by breast and by bottle. This infected milk often produced sick babies, whose diseases were explained in pre-Pasteurian times by learned complaints about the nature of the cow's milk – too much fat, too much casein, too rich. When switching to milk from goats or asses did not cure the victim, the mixed feeding itself was incriminated as the cause of any problems. Only with the coming of "the era of modern bacteriology" was the mystery solved, when the microorganisms that were the agents of diseases such as tuberculosis, scarlet fever, diphtheria, and, above all, infant diarrhea, were shown to be present in cow's milk. Once sterilized, the cow's milk was nearly as good as the mother's, or so Henri and nearly everyone else thought at the end of the great bacteriological century. Only recently have we learned that mother's milk contains important unsaturated fatty acids important for the physiological development of human babies and that cow's milk should be cut with boiled water before being fed to a baby. Instinct and experience have historically favored the superiority of mother's milk; now the not entirely concordant voices of science support that view.

Henri prescribed that a breastfed baby who did not gain weight should be put on a mixed regime, which could include maternalized milk, peptonized milk, or simply sterilized cow's milk, as determined by the pediatrician. Gaertner and Backhaus had introduced maternalized milk for babies who had problems with more traditional feeding. Although human milk has about the same fat content as cow's milk, it has only half as much protein and twice as much carbohydrate.[31] At the end of the nineteenth century, doctors used a comparative analysis of the two milks that assigned slightly more water, much more lactose, and much less casein and salts to human milk than to cow's milk. The fat content was found to be about the same.[32] The "lait maternisé" was cow's milk processed to have the qualities of human milk, or at least the same level of casein, fat, and sugar.

---

30 HR, *L'allaitement mixte et l'allaitement artificiel*, ix–xi; on bacteriology, Henri cites E. Duclaux, *Le lait, études chimiques et microbiologiques* (Paris, 1887; 1894) but he gets the title a bit mixed up.

31 Mother's milk contains forty percent casein and sixty percent soluble proteins; cow's milk contains eighty percent casein and twenty percent soluble proteins. Calves gain weight three times as fast as babies. See Michaëla Bobasch, "Choisir un lait approprié pour remplir le biberon des nourrissons," www.lemonde.fr/web/imprimer_article/0,1-0@2-3238,36-352457,0.html.

32 HR, *L'allaitement mixte et l'allaitement artificiel*, i. See HR, *Notes sur l'hygiène et la protection de l'enfance d'après les études faites à Berlin, Saint-Pétersbourg, Moscou,*

Some babies, particularly those who had the misfortune to be born prematurely or sick, including those with an incompletely formed digestive tube, could not even tolerate their mothers' milk or that of a good wet-nurse. For them the proper milk might be "peptonized" milk, a concoction invented by Budin and Charles Michel to make the protein soluble by a process of "predigestion." (Pepsin is an important digestive enzyme, secreted by the stomach, which breaks down proteins into polypeptides. Obtained from the dried mucous lining of the stomach of a pig, sheep, or calf, it was used medicinally.)[33]

Knowledge of the sterilization of milk spread in rich families because of the effort of accoucheurs and doctors. The poor were helped by the *consultations de nourrisson/gouttes de lait*, an agency useful not only for the distribution of sterilized milk but also for instructions on its consumption in order to prevent it from being mixed with water. In the *consultation*, teaching mothers the proper procedures was as important as caring for the babies. Henri sighed that the struggle against disease was nothing compared with the fight against the ignorance of parents, which is why he believed that the *consultations* were, above all, educational centers to teach mothers about feeding babies. At his *consultation* in *La Maternité*, Budin saw the babies once a week in order to control and record developments; so the *consultation* was a true school for mothers. Recording a baby's development was also a way of detecting problems at an early stage, when they were more likely to be treated successfully. The establishment was "not only a hospital but … a center for the teaching of pediatric medicine."[34]

Henri could proudly complain, in the great Rothschild tradition, of bearing up under "a crushing task" from June 1894 to December 1898. And the whole thing was a family affair in one striking way. Henri married at the age of twenty-three, and he always remained grateful for his wife's strong support of his medical career. Mathilde's reputation for leading a frivolous social life, a valuable safety valve for the under-employed rich female, is not fully deserved. Budin was the accoucheur for the couple's nicely spaced births of two sons (James and Philippe) and daughter (Nadine) in 1896, 1899, and 1902. All survived into adulthood.

By the time that Henri published his pamphlet *L'Œuvre philanthropique du lait* (1902), he had become a leading figure in the movement to keep babies alive and well by providing good nutrition and basic medical care. By then he had also founded the *Œuvre philanthropique du lait* (1898) to organize the distribution of milk and had begun collaboration with the *Revue philanthropique*. The *Revue*,

Vienne et Budapest, 8–14, for a discussion of the production of "maternalized" milk by the Gaertner and Backhaus processes.

33 HR, *L'allaitement mixte et l'allaitement artificiel*, conclusion. The *New Shorter Oxford Dictionary* banishes the word peptone to the region of "now rare": a protein made soluble by partial digestion; *Le Nouveau Petit Robert* is more encouraging for this word dating back to 1857: "mélange obtenu par la dégradation des viandes sous l'effet d'enzymes (pepsine, pancréatine, papaïne)."

34 RAL 000/930: 58-1, 168–71.

founded in 1897 by Paul Strauss (editor) and others as the official organ of "the fight against infant mortality," published the first French studies in puericulture and infant hygiene. Henri aided the publication. Budin introduced Henri to Strauss. Henri became one of the first members as well as the longtime treasurer of the *Ligue contre la mortalité infantile* (later called the *Comité national de l'enfance*), an organization established in 1902 by Budin with the collaboration of friends like Strauss and Théophile Roussel, the first president of the league. Alphonse de Rothschild was also among its first members. Budin generously declared that Strauss was the real founder and soul of the league.[35] The league created schools of puericulture, *consultations*, *gouttes*, and trained society ladies to visit poor families. Strauss, then senator of the department of the Seine, prefaced the book *L'Œuvre philanthropique du lait* with a plea ("Against infant diarrhea") coupled with a paean to Henri's efforts to reduce the incidence of this serious disease. Strauss summed up Henri's energetic activities in opening *consultations de nourrissons/gouttes de lait* as total devotion to post-partum puericulture: "he is one of the most zealous propagandists for the protection of children, a man whose words are followed by action."[36]

The fight against infant diarrhea, inseparable from the birth of pediatrics, was linked to a more general cause, a political obsession of the day, "the fight against the depopulation of France," which Charles Maygrier called one of the most preoccupying social issues of the day – "a national peril." The number of live births per 1000 French women (15–50 years old) was only 102, comparing poorly with Prussia's 150 and Bavaria's 156. France needed 900,000 additional births each year to match German fertility.[37] Strauss the politician was enthusiastic about the action being taken to protect young children by cooperative or at least complementary municipal organizations. And no better private model existed than Henri's *Œuvre philanthropique du lait* for the organization of the *gouttes de lait* for distributing good fresh milk to poverty-stricken mothers as well as selling milk cheaply to low-income families. An effort was made not to compete with small

[35] Budin, "Ligue contre la mortalité infantile," *La revue philanthropique* 15 (1904): 231–6, notes that the league had some success in Algeria, with Arab mothers as well as colonials, and in Madagascar – "nothing is more curious than to see the photographs from there: mothers bring their small black babies to be weighed and all listen carefully to the advice they are given" (234).

[36] HR, *L'Œuvre philanthropique du lait* (Paris, 1902), 3–4: "Contre la diarrhée infantile," preface by Paul Strauss.

[37] HR, *Dépopulation et protection de la première enfance* (Paris, 1900), a lecture given at the *Union scolaire* on 14 November 1900. Henri notes that depopulation is a relative term measuring population growth, though there were more deaths than births in France during 1890–95, with a turnaround in 1896–97. Henri followed the crowd in blaming the low birth rate on disease, particularly TB, alcoholism, and occupational poisoning. See also Maygrier, *Les Consultations des nourrissons*, 1, and Séverin Icard, *L'alimentation des nouveaux-nés. Hygiène de l'allaitement artificiel* (Paris, 1894), ix.

retailers by checking the financial status of recipients. Rothschild charity could not appear to be threatening "le petit commerce."

By 1902 Henri considered himself sufficiently expert in the baby business to set forth the basic rules for organizing and running a *Consultation de nourrissons/goutte de lait*, both organizations that were becoming part of the Parisian maternal landscape.[38] By encouraging the formation of numerous local committees, Strauss and Budin had carried out a "philanthropic crusade" for the spread of these institutions throughout France. Those functioning so well in Paris, like the Rothschild organization, provided the model to be copied. A good *consultation* became a bit more complex than in its embryonic days, requiring at least four rooms, comprising waiting and consulting rooms, a room for the preparation of sterilized milk, a room for the distribution of milk, and the office of the directress responsible for the business part of the operation, which included essential detailed record keeping. Keeping records required the subjection of mothers to a strict discipline: delinquents were denied service after two infractions of the rules. Normal babies required a fortnightly visit; babies with problems had to be seen every week. Success of the *consultation* depended on the firmness of the doctor and directress. Rewards were given for obedience. And the budget for rewards and "assistance en nature" (goods and food) to mothers had to be large.

Unlike back in 1897, when he did not view breastfeeding as far superior to all other types of feeding, Henri now (1902) declared that the doctor's role was to encourage breastfeeding by all possible means. More breastfeeding meant that less sterilized milk would have to be distributed – a view to economy, acceptable if the measures resulted in the maintenance of safety and good nutrition for the babies. Encouragement to mothers to adopt breastfeeding included the distribution of layettes, medications, meat, money, and other goodies. The use of sterilized milk would be a measure of last resort in cases where the mother did not have enough of her own milk to feed the baby. Mixed feeding and especially artificial feeding had to be exceptional. Given the interesting contrast of this view with his view of 1897, we must assume that Henri was putting forward policy guidelines for a successful *consultation de nourrissons/goutte de lait* and not necessarily an argument based on the statistics provided by experimental science. Infant mortality was not an issue. When artificial feeding began to spread, sinister English and American influences could be detected. According to Henri, snobbery was one factor in explaining why French mothers adopted this foreign fashion.[39]

The distribution of sterilized milk was perhaps the most delicate matter to handle in the organization. In Henri's frank analysis, the *gouttes de lait* were

---

[38] HR, *Les Gouttes de lait – Organisation d'une "Goutte de lait" et d'une "Consultation de nourrissons*" (Paris, 1902), extract of the *Revue d'hygiène et de médecine infantiles* 1/5 (1905).

[39] HR, *Puériculture et Centres d'élevage*, cited in Cottet-Dumoulin (*épouse* Robinot), *Une grande œuvre médico-sociale: l'Ecole de puériculture de la Faculté de Médecine de Paris (1919–1970)*, 12.

eminently philanthropic organizations allowing mothers to feed their babies in a certain rational manner with the lowest possible expense and risk. Their potential for reducing scandalously high French infant mortality rates in the provinces made it imperative in the view of their Parisian advocates that every commune establish a model philanthropic organization to save thousands of bottle-fed French infants from a certain death. Doctors had a major responsibility in promoting the establishment of *consultations*. Local, private, and state personnel could collaborate in the effort as in the establishment of another Paris model, the *Dispensaire de Belleville*, founded by Gaston Variot in 1892 with private gifts and municipal and state grants in order to serve the working poor in that northeast part of the city. Variot, a prickly and prolific pediatric doctor in Paris, was convinced that reducing infant mortality depended on eliminating the ignorance of mothers, and few did more than he by writing and by preaching the lactic gospel to "women of the people" to achieve that aim. His *goutte de lait* distributed industrially sterilized (108 degrees C) milk to help the effort "to preserve and multiply our brave *race gauloise*, whose genius will continue to shine on the world." This was written in 1916.[40]

There seems to be a remarkable consistency in the medical advice given to mothers over the years. In the absence of evidence of a patriarchal plot to keep women domesticated through having them breastfeed their offspring, it is reasonable to assume that medical experience found mother's milk best for the health and development of children. It was also cheap. In 1930 *Le Progrès médical* carried a substantial review of the three main baby-feeding methods.[41] The author began with the basic dogma that diet is the core of pediatrics. His first dietetic point was that breastfeeding by the mother is best for the baby; second best is breastfeeding by a paid wet-nurse. The third best choice is artificial feeding, a term that pointedly contrasts this method with that of breastfeeding, which is natural. In contrast with the first two methods, the third nearly always causes feeding problems, no matter how carefully the process is controlled. According to an advertisement for *Lactagol* in the same publication, many of the mother's mammary problems could be alleviated by use of this miraculous powder, which promised to stimulate the mammary gland into high production as well as maintain the quality of the milk. There is no place like a medical journal to see the fruitful cooperation of pharmaceutical capitalism and medicine. Like in gerontology, pediatrics provided a remarkable opportunity for doctors to promote pharmaceutical products.

---

40 See G. Variot, *La mortalité infantile et l'ignorance des mères* ("Conférence … réouverture des cours de l'Institut de Puériculture, le 16 novembre 1916"). Variot was one of the pioneers in understanding and using radiology to deal with childhood diseases, including installing a laboratory of radiology at the Trousseau hospital; the facility moved with him to the *Enfants-Malades* in 1900. A.-B. Marfan, "Nécrology – Variot (1855–1930)," *Le Nourrisson* 18 (1930): 206–8. He also wrote a standard medical text, *Traité d'hygiène infantile* (Paris, 1910).

41 A. Lemaire, "Les régimes de nourrissons," *Le Progrès médical* 27 (5 juillet 1930): 1190–6.

Revue d'hygiène et de médecine infantiles

Henri's great interest in infant hygiene and pathology eventually took on an unexpected development because of the different specialists who were attracted to his establishments. To a considerable extent, they came because of Henri's appreciation of their collaboration. The Picpus polyclinic's initial function as a *consultation de nourrissons*, involving regular weighing of infants and distribution of sterilized milk, was soon supplemented by a range of medical activity, which expanded with the opening of the Marcadet hospital and included the medical treatment of deformities (with fitting of prostheses), of nervous pathology, and of diseases of eye, ear, nose, and throat. X-rays and photography were also provided. Before long there had been accumulated a considerable archive of pediatric material, much of it dealing with what doctors considered to be "interesting cases" that provided the fodder for articles in journals and even for books.

Henri finally succumbed to the pressures of friends to fund a journal for exactly that purpose: the *Revue d'hygiène et de médecine infantiles* began appearing in 1902.[42] The chief collaborators were from the universities of Berlin, Paris, Rome, Geneva, Nancy, and Vienna, along with doctors attached to the Rothschild polyclinic. In the first issue of the journal Paul Strauss praised Henri for devoting a good part of his fortune and the best part of his time to pediatrics. And the journal appeared at the right time in the growth of this new area of medicine. It was also the right time for Henri: the new journal became the official organ of the new Marcadet establishment, a "real study center of the pathology of childhood."[43] Young authors were particularly welcome. The journal also provided an outlet for much of the work done by Henri on milk, the milk industry, baby feeding, and syphilis, as well as work by him and his collaborators on subjects such as the thyroid. It provided an analysis of relevant articles in different medical journals, of medical theses, and of medical books. Much of the material later appeared in book form.

Science is succored by journal publication and prizes, the twin pinnacles being respectively the journal *Nature* and the Nobel Prize. Believing that prizes promote research, Henri funded several prizes in order to encourage bright people to do research on baby feeding, not a topic that ordinarily attracted great or at least ambitious minds. The prizes were awarded by the *Société scientifique d'hygiène alimentaire*, whose president was senator Henri Ricard, with Henri as secretary of the society. Two doctors (Michel and Perret) won the substantial first prize of 5000 francs for their memoir on the feeding of babies up to the age of 2 years. The topic of provisioning large cities with milk inspired a number of memoirs so good that even Budin, the head of the evaluating committee, was impressed. Provisioning

---

42 See HR, "Avis aux lecteurs," *Revue d'hygiène et de médecine infantiles et Annales de la polyclinique H. de Rothschild* 1 (1902): 1–2. "Directeur: Dr H. de Rothschild." The review appeared every two months. The administrator and publisher was Octave Doin.

43 HR, "Avis aux lecteurs," 1–2.

included hygiene, technology, transport, legislation and regulation, sale, and social economy. Henri also funded a special prize of 1000 francs for the worthy authors who worked in institutions in Poligny, Toulouse, and the Lozère. The winner of the special prize, Porcher, then at the veterinary school in Toulouse, later collaborated with Henri in an article on milk fraud. Milk research had become a minor medical industry.[44] Henri was the logical choice for secretary of the International Congress on Milk (Supply, Industry, and Depots) that met in Paris in 1905.

Pediatrics – An Academic Growth Industry

By 1904 pediatric medicine had undergone conceptual and institutional changes that pioneers like Strauss and Henri recognized, welcomed, and hailed as evidence of what could be done for mother and baby if politicians and doctors followed the scientific route indicated by the Pasteurian revolution. Strauss recognized the new challenges. In pathological heredity, degeneration was the enemy to conquer. Prenatal care, of prime importance, had hardly begun, as one could see from the discussions over the labor law to help pregnant women. And the Roussel law needed revision to bring it in line with "scientific principles and the data of experience."[45] Henri attributed part of "the great progress of recent years in children's medicine"[46] to the reorganization of Parisian hospital departments that had been brought about by leading accoucheurs and pediatricians, especially Budin, Variot, Josias, and Marfan, and the heads of the *Assistance publique* (Ernest Peyron, Louis Mourier, and Gustave Mesureur). The new scientific gospel had to be spread throughout the system by the lower echelons of the medical establishment. Henri himself played an important role here: over the years he gave a course at the municipal school for nurses (*Hospice de la Salpêtrière*) on the care to be given to women in delivery and to the newborn. The course dealt with recent progress in obstetrics and pediatrics, gave the nurses a practical education in these subjects, and, when published, provided a reliable guide for mothers.[47] The distinction enjoyed by pediatrics in France could be seen in the roles played by French doctors in different

---

44 "Les prix Henri de Rothschild," *La revue philanthropique* 19 (1906–07): 648.

45 HR (ed.), *Traité d'hygiène et de pathologie du nourrisson et des enfants du premier âge* (Paris, 1904). Preface by Senator Paul Strauss. The work is dedicated to Budin and Albert Josias. Henri contributed to the sections on infectious and on nutritional diseases.

46 HR, "Avis aux lecteurs," 1–2.

47 HR, *Soins à donner aux femmes en couches et aux nouveaux-nés*. The six lectures at the *Ecole municipale des infirmiers et infirmières de la ville de Paris* dealt with female physiology, reproduction, hygiene for pregnant women, the role of the nurse in caring for the woman in labor and in delivery, post-delivery physiology, the conduct of the nurse, the physiology, hygiene, and feeding of the newborn, problems of weak and premature babies, and so on.

societies and congresses as well as in the foreign consultations they gave to help in the establishment of real schools of pediatrics on the French model.[48]

New disciplines produce new research that often leads to the founding of new journals. In 1913–14 the first volume of the journal *Le Nourrisson* appeared, announcing in a long title its concern with the hygiene and pathology of the nursling (one month to two years). Up to the age of one month a baby was categorized as the newborn (*le nouveau né*).[49] The age divisions also included second or middle childhood, from two to six or seven years, and third or *grande enfance*, from six or seven to puberty, a state of flux in which the child enjoys the anxieties of adolescence before passing on to the pleasures and tragedies of adult freedom. Although childhood includes the first twelve to sixteen years of life, from a pathological point of view the last category (adolescents) resembles adults; so the treatment of their diseases is more the province of adult medicine than of pediatrics. The other categories provided enough customers for pediatricians.

The editor of *Le Nourrisson*, A.-B. Marfan, was one of that group of doctors whose names are immortalized by diseases.[50] Marfan gave a classic description of the progressive spasmodic paralysis of children with hereditary syphilis. In the hospitals where he did his observations, 25/100 of infant (less than one year old) deaths were due to syphilis. Another of his claims to scientific status was his demonstration that ultraviolet radiation could be used to prevent and to treat rickets. In 1914 Marfan occupied the new chair of hygiene and diseases of children up to two years of age (*la première enfance*) at the *Hôpital des Enfants-Malades*, where he headed the diphtheria pavilion. The chair was transferred in 1920 to the *Hospice des Enfants assistés*, an organization resulting from fusion in 1838 of the efforts of several hospitals to take care of abandoned children and orphans (*Hospice des enfants trouvés et orphelins*). In the middle of the nineteenth century the *Hospice* came under the *Assistance publique* under the rubric of *Service des enfants assistés*.[51] The *Assistance publique* agreed to the transfer of Marfan's

---

48 HR (ed.), *Traité d'hygiène*, introduction.

49 *Le Nourrisson. Revue d'hygiène et de pathologie de la première enfance* 1 (1913–14). A.-B. Marfan, general editor. There were eight other editors from the Paris hospitals.

50 OMC includes Marfan's syndrome under arachnodactyly. See Genty, *Les Biographies médicales*, 2d series, "Les Maîtres d'aujourd'hui," 225–55.

51 After 1961 the migration of responsibility continued to the prefecture of the Seine and then in 1985 to the department of Paris; the reality indicated by the old terminology is now dignified as the *Aide Sociale à l'Enfance*. See the website of the Archives de Paris under "Enfants trouvés – Enfants assistés." About 1896 there were 11,000 to 12,000 children being cared for, according to Hutinel, "L'enseignement de la pédiatrie à la faculté de Paris." Hutinel noted that the children came from "la population la plus misérable de Paris," afflicted with numerous skin diseases. On the bright side: diphtheria disappeared in the early 1890s. In 1920 the death rate of infants with wet-nurses at the *Enfants-Assistés* was 50 percent, brought down to 14 percent by 1927, and 7 percent by 1931. See Rachel Fuchs, *Abandoned Children. Foundlings and Child Welfare in Nineteenth-Century France* (Albany, N.Y., 1984).

chair provided that Marfan become head of the *Institut de puériculture* created at *Enfants-Malades* by the city of Paris and the department of the Seine, thus making the chair (*Chaire d'hygiène de clinique de la première enfance*) a sort of annex of the *Clinique de la première enfance*.

Marfan argued that if pediatrics is a special branch of medicine, it owes its status to the pathology of its earlier periods, particularly early childhood. The distinctive characteristic of the first two years is indicated by the fact that languages have a special word for the child in that stage: infant, *Sauling*, *poppante*, *niño de pecho*, *nourrisson*. The different characteristics of infants require special study, especially for childhood diseases and their effects. The stage of development of *la première enfance* is very special physiologically and no less so pathologically. Nothing defines a person better than a disease. Marfan found that early childhood is distinguished by the great frequency of its unique affections: certain types of digestive problems, athrepsia or insufficient assimilation of nutrients, tuberculosis of the visceral ganglions, and skin diseases, for example. Marfan seemed tempted to say that the infant's nervous system is unique but narrowly avoided this claim. The number of diseases often leading to death still deserved enumeration: convulsive seizures, malformations, and congenital abnormalities. Marfan found hereditary syphilis to be most virulent, with specific manifestations, in this period of childhood.

Of course *Le Nourrisson* did not neglect the newborn baby. Like Budin and Henri de Rothschild earlier, Marfan and his pediatric colleagues considered the first month of a baby's life to be the most special of all. The "obstetrical diseases" proved it: asphyxia, hemorrhages of the nervous centers, infections of the umbilical cord, and purulent ophthalmia, for example. Still the infant was the focus of the journal, and in his introduction Marfan concentrated on justifying the invention of this medical category of young patient. Medicine had among its distinguishing characteristics two of particular importance. First, it gave much attention to food hygiene; since the integration of germ theory into medicine, the safety of milk had been a key concern of pediatrics. Second, the medicine of nurslings necessarily paid attention to the morbidity caused by violation of the rules of infant hygiene. Doctors were rightly obsessed with these factors because of high infant mortality; Marfan used a table to show the morbid anatomy of childhood at the beginning of the twentieth century.[52] It showed deaths per 1000 live births: 1st year – 150 (47 in 1st month and 17 in 1st 5 days); 2nd year – 40; 3rd year – 20; 4th year – 15; 5th year – 12; 5–10 years – 50; 10–15 years – 30. Louis Py came up with a grimmer estimate of an annual mortality of 202/1000 for babies less than 1 year old; over 150,000 infants out of less than 1,000,000 live births died annually.[53] All

52 A.-B. Marfan, *Traité de l'allaitement et de l'alimentation des enfants du premier âge* (1899; 1903; 1906; 4th edn, revised and expanded, Paris, 1930), vii. The book is dedicated to the memory of his father, Dr. Antoine Marfan.

53 In the edition of 1930, Marfan gives infant mortality figures of 200/1000 for the 1st year, 80/1000 for the 2nd year, 40/1000 for the 3rd year, and 25/1000 for the 4th year.

doctors condemned this high child mortality as an important factor in the so-called depopulation of France – the classic trope of the day – and a "threat to the future of civilized nations," a phrase indicating that the white man had heavy burdens at home. The startling contrast of these figures with the low infant mortality achieved in the *consultations* indicates that the pediatricians were reaching a small part of the reproducing population.

Henri wrote a play in 1920 dealing with depopulation and the future of the French people, but it does not seem to have played anywhere. Under the soap-operatic title of *Le plus grand amour* we find references to a speech, articulating the medical wisdom on saving babies, by a professor at the *Congrès de la protection de l'enfance*. The editor of a newspaper with the wakeup title of *Le Chantecler* advertises his intention to give space to the burning social questions of the day, especially the disquieting problems posed by depopulation and the necessary regeneration of "our race." In a eugenics-inspired discussion, an analogy between human reproduction and animal breeding seems perfectly sensible. All of this heavy discussion takes place in the context of a real human drama in which a love-marriage is called off because the father of the bride was thought to have been mentally ill. Fortunately, it turned out after some investigation that the mentally ill person was not the father of the bride at all. All's well that ends well, even in a failed play.[54]

After decades of medical research on baby feeding, the issues remained debatable and many basic questions unanswered, including the ancient ones about alimentation, digestive upsets, and nutrition. Nearly everything was the subject of wavering or of disagreement. Marfan declared that *Le Nourrisson* would try to cut through the debates, identify errors, and establish a solid basis of agreement on basics. Marfan argued for the superiority of breastfeeding (natural) over artificial feeding: was not infant mortality lowest in countries where breastfeeding was most prevalent (Norway and Iceland) and highest where breastfeeding was most abandoned (Germany and Austria)? While accepting the argument that the discoveries of Pasteur and Duclaux had completely modified the practice of artificial feeding, Marfan argued that bacteriology could not explain everything and, he implied, given the continuing high mortality figure, the new science was not the panacea many thought it to be. (Like Budin, Henri, and Variot, Marfan had done his Pasteurian duty in joining in campaigns such as the one against the feeding bottle armed with a germ-laden rubber tube.) Medicine (meaning doctors) had forgotten an old clinical lesson: the laboratory was causing neglect of the techniques of clinical observation. Marfan pointed out that when one tries to deal with subjects that have not been well established clinically, the results are not very useful in medical practice. Oxalemia (an excess of oxalates in the blood) still did

See Louis Py, *La puériculture en France à l'heure actuelle* (thesis, Faculty of Medicine, Toulouse, 1913).

54 HR (André Pascales), *Le plus grand amour* (Paris, 1920); only fifty copies were printed exclusively for rehearsals and staging.

not have a clinical existence; whereas tuberculosis and diphtheria provided models of diseases with a clinically defined existence and were therefore, Marfan implied, better managed medically. The clinical picture followed by enlightenment from the laboratory would produce a more effective medicine. And also establish the priority of the doctor in dealing with diseases and patients. Debré's similar views probably came from Marfan.

Marfan saw the problems of pediatrics basically as an issue of wrong method: medical emphasis on the laboratory had caused clinical observation to be neglected. After thirty years of study, the child's digestive upsets and nutritional needs remained disturbingly obscure. So the study of these problems had to begin again, starting not at the top but at the base; after methodical, rigorous clinical observation had been carried out, the laboratory could enter on the scene to try to cast light on the problems with all the means that physics, chemistry, bacteriology, and experiment put at the doctor's disposal. This new method would perhaps give slower results but they would be more stable, thus avoiding the necessity of changing doctrines and even nomenclature every ten or fifteen years. Marfan's dream of ending the struggle between the clinic and the laboratory was never achieved; indeed, it is probably undesirable to follow Marfan's route. The permanent truce seems to work as well as any scheme. Two separate empires in the medical school: research science (not a pleonasm) and clinical science – the clinic can hardly deny the means of its greatest advances in understanding and treating disease. And, if managed care allows it, in the best of all possible Panglossian worlds, the conscientious doctor can still practice clinical medicine – the bedside diagnostic tradition writ large.[55]

One of Marfan's protégés argued that pediatrics had long emphasized physiological research at the expense of the anatomo-pathological approach, at least in dealing with gastro-intestinal dyspepsia.[56] In dealing with infant diseases, no doubt this is a good thing for the doctor to keep in mind, but for most babies hardly relevant since the non-physiological approach would depend finally on an autopsy. Of course it was useful for the researcher and the *maître* to learn, as a result of thirty autopsies carried out at the *Crèche des Enfants-Malades*, that digestive–intestinal difficulties could be linked to defective feeding, summed up in Marfan's lingo as infants' chronic gastro-intestinal dyspepsia. Even more important was the conclusion that the cure was maternal breastfeeding or, in the impossibility of attaining that ideal, feeding with sterilized milk.

Marfan belonged to the Parisian hospital-university elite. One of the great medico-social works of this group was the creation by the Faculty of Medicine and

[55] On the "four cardinal arts of the good bedside diagnostician ... inspection, palpation, percussion, and auscultation," see W. F. Bynum, *Science and the Practice of Medicine in the Nineteenth Century* (Cambridge, 1994), 33–42.

[56] Marie Hooper-Blackler-Kalopothakès, *Troubles et lésions gastriques dans la dyspepsie gastro-intestinale chronique des nourrissions* (thesis, Paris Faculty of Medicine, 1894). The author, born in Athens, won the "Médaille de l'externat des hôpitaux."

the American Red Cross of the *Ecole de puériculture de la Faculté de Medécine de Paris – Fondation Franco-Américaine* (1 July 1919), located first on the rue Desnouettes (15th arrondissement) and then permanently on the boulevard Brune (14th arrondissement).[57] Members of the administrative council of the school included professors Marfan, Pinard, Victor Hutinel, and Henri Roger. And the baron Dr Henri de Rothschild.[58] The school functioned as a pedagogical center, dispensing technical and practical education to the doctors, nurses, and students who were going to have anything to do with infant feeding. The school eventually came to exercise a useful intellectual function in dispensing the correct scientific teaching on infant feeding, which in the course of a few years had gone from dogmatic certainty to squabbling doubt; scientific advances in nutrition provided a new certainty.

Practices based on science are liable to change as scientists put forward new ideas, possibly even resulting in the agony of paradigm switch, or something of that nature. The practicing doctor is likely to be confused when his scientifically based practice is shown to be inefficacious or, worse, dangerous. The patient is puzzled too and wonders, as Emily Yoffe did concerning hormones, "how could so many doctors get it wrong for so long?"[59] Experts on infant feeding found themselves in a particular doctor's dilemma in the early twentieth century. The medical context of this confusion lay in "the creation of a new category and model of diseases: deficiency diseases."[60] In 1904 Henri had not been entirely convinced by Netter's argument that normal milk is anti-scorbutic because it contains citric acid, though heat destroys it and thus contributes to the appearance of infant scurvy. Henri concocted the ingenious argument that heat might produce peptones in the milk, which cause hematuria symptoms that are similar to scurvy. This illness was easily cured by modifying the infant's diet to include pure milk (from healthy cows), lactose, beef juice, and some raw fruit juice. A cure took place within one to three weeks. According to Henri, the disease was most prevalent in the United States, where the feeding of processed products was farther advanced and fed to the babies of the rich. In any case, he noted, this debate was more an issue for milk production than for biology and would be cleared up when production was put on a scientific basis, as in Denmark and Germany. He gave a paper at the International Congress on the Milk Industry in 1905 arguing that pasteurization could not cause

---

57 See Cottet-Dumoulin (*épouse* Robinot), *Une grande œuvre médico-sociale: l'Ecole de puériculture de la Faculté de Médecine de Paris (1919–1970)*.

58 With fellow professors Grancher and Marfan, Hutinel ("Professeur titulaire de clinique des maladies de l'enfance") is often saluted as a founder of pediatrics in France. Roger (1860–1946), known for his useful contacts with businessmen and philanthropists (sometimes the categories overlap) was president of the council; Pinard and Marfan were vice-presidents.

59 Emily Yoffe, "Hormonal Imbalances" (11 July 2002), http://slate.msn.com.

60 Porter, *The Greatest Benefit to Mankind*, 551; see 551–60, section "Biochemistry and Nutrition."

scurvy, for, after all, in a ten-year period he studied there were only twenty-three cases of scurvy in France.[61]

Casimir Funk invented the misleading word "vitamines" in 1912, but he was on the right etiological track in attributing diseases such as rickets to vitamin deficiencies. By 1922 Edward Mellanby had separated vitamins A and D (the anti-rachitic factor). By 1933 the essential work had been done on ascorbic acid (vitamin C), including the discovery that heat easily destroys it. Experts were not long in warning that heating the milk fed to infants is a good way of causing one disease while preventing another. In recalling this period of debate and confusion, at a crisis stage by 1922, Henri had to protest that Budin's disciples, including himself, were not killing infants! With the discovery that a few teaspoons of citrus juice four or so times a week would prevent scurvy, the crisis evaporated, and sterilized milk regained some of its old popularity. A tempest in a teapot, anyway, for milk, rich in vitamins A and D, does not contain any vitamin C to speak of. The *Ecole de puériculture* quickly spread the new rules to the various organizations involved in infant feeding and in supplying information to mothers and wet-nurses. (By 1933 there were over 5000 *gouttes de lait* in France.)[62]

The World War I slaughter, especially of young males, intensified French discussion of "depopulation," a cause of some medical anxiety during the Third Republic. The French figures still shock us: 1,300,000 deaths – of which the demographic subtext was a missing 1,400,000 births, 1,100,000 wounded, and nearly 400,000 disabled. France suffered 10.5 deaths for every 100 active soldiers, compared with 9.8 for Germany, and 5.1 for the U.K. In addition to dealing with its deplorable state of public health and the new *socially* significant diseases (notably cancer), France needed to produce and save as many babies as possible.[63] The politically promoted idea that the existence of sixty million Germans threatened forty million French also provided an ideological stimulus to coitus and pediatrics. It helped puericulture tremendously that Paul Strauss became minister of public health in 1922. Diffusion of puericultural ideas was in large part due to the enthusiasm of people such as Pinard, Léon Bernard, and Henri de Rothschild. American stimulus was vital. Americans had a low opinion of French public health, and the American Red Cross and the Rockefeller Mission in France after 1917 were vital forces in encouraging the Gallic libido and in reducing French infant mortality.

It is possible to conclude that Jews were prominent in the movement supporting the *Ecole de puériculture*. Apart from members of the Rothschild tribe, one finds

---

61 HR, "Scorbut infantile (maladie be Barlow)," *Traité d'hygiène et de pathologie du nourrisson et des enfants du premier âge*, 736–7.

62 HR, *Puériculture et centres d'élevages*, 17–19. Henri seems to get vitamins C and D mixed up. It has not been known until recently that mother's milk does not have enough vitamin D for the suckling.

63 Patrice Pinell, *The Fight Against Cancer: France 1890–1940* (London and New York, 2002), 66. Translated by David Madell.

among the founding members the Lazard brothers, Willy Blumenthal, and the Kohn couple. Marie Kohn was president of the school's propaganda committee. Rich women were prominent supporters of the school: the baronesses Léonino (Jeanne, Henri's sister) and Edmond de Rothschild and the duchess d'Uzès. The Jewish financial contribution was exceeded only by that of American organizations. Contributions up to the end of 1927 included 1,000,000 francs from the American Red Cross, 550,000 from the League of American Children, 275,000 from the *Comité du Secours national*, and then 100,000 from Edmond, 50,000 from Henri, 50,000 from the *Banque de France*, and a total of 37,000 from Robert and James de Rothschild and Madame Adrienne Thierry (Henri's daughter). In addition to hefty contributions, Edmond and Henri brought an important long-standing social capital that was helpful to the new organization. (Edmond would continue his support of scientific causes with contributions in 1927 to the *Institut de biologie physico-chimique* and in 1928 to the *Institut Henri-Poincaré*.) From the time of its foundation Henri was a prominent active member and officer of the *Association française pour l'étude du cancer*. Looking at these developments with a jaundiced Bourdieuesque eye we might wonder why families like Michelin, Rothschild, Deutsch de la Meurthe, and Dietrich became attracted to the idea of the "useful gift." There may be something in the argument that they saw the need to support the republican cause by engaging in useful social action. Were they collaborating in an unarticulated project of keeping public order through pacifying the poor? This is hard to prove, of course, and throwing a puericultural sop to Cerberus was done officially to save the baby.[64]

One of the explanations of continuing high infant mortality, according to many people, Henri included, was the notorious administrative centralization of decision-making in public health, thus making it difficult to modify programs that did not work. So after the Great War the central government adopted a decentralized approach to saving babies by establishing centers for infant care. During the war mothers had been given moral guidance and material support, which produced a drop in infant mortality. To improve on that welcome trend, organizations known as *centres d'élevage* or *centres de nourrissons* were created in order to place one or two infants with "well-brought up" peasants (farmers), who were paid generously to raise the children. Wet-nurses were also trained for their jobs. What impressed Henri about this scheme was the disappearance of "the old corrupt system" with its fictional administrative supervision of farmed out babies by a doctor appointed by the administration in Paris. In the new system specialist nurses did the rounds, in small cars or on bicycles, visiting forty to fifty children a week. The *Assistance publique* claimed that infant mortality among pauper or abandoned children in the department of the Seine dropped from twenty-seven to about five percent at the end of the 1920s. Whatever the number of babies saved, the new system, based

---

64 Cottet-Dumoulin (*épouse* Robinot), *Une grande œuvre médico-sociale: l'Ecole de puériculture de la Faculté de Médecine de Paris (1919–1970)*, 31.

on elementary training of people in infant feeding and care and on supervision by specialist nurses on the local scene, worked much better than what existed before.

High-minded philanthropic women made a modest contribution to the drop in infant mortality and performed a valuable service in establishing model centers of infant care. Madame A. Weil-Picard organized the first center as a dispensary where a visiting nurse could stay, allowing children to be brought in once or twice a week for a visit to a medical specialist, perhaps a pediatrician. Her good results encouraged emulation: Madame Gonze Boas founded a center at Montmorency. Then Madame Boas de Jouvenal founded a new charitable work (*Association de Travail et d'Assistance*), which proceeded to create several centers. The *Assistance publique* encouraged and supported these private initiatives. A training center for wards came into existence at Orgeval-Maule. Other "dames charitables," as Henri dubbed them, flattered by membership on the governing committee of the *Association de Travail et d'Assistance*, supported new centers. Henri particularly admired the *Fondation Marie Kohn*. She established a well-known dispensary and *centre de nourrissons* at St-Rémy-les-Chevreuse (Seine-et-Oise). The results of Kohn's center for 1929–31 were good, even superb for that time in France. Only three deaths were reported in this period for a total of ninety-three wards passing through the establishment; forty-four wards were in residence on 1 January 1931. The Kohn establishment used the lacto-serum peddled by the company of Pierre Mazé and Henri, who did not draw any tempting conclusions from this fact.[65]

There is an irony in the fact that French mothers have recently been remarkably immune to pro-breastfeeding propaganda. Among ten "industrial nations" France has the lowest percentage of mothers who breastfeed their newborns, 56 percent, compared with nearly 100 percent in Scandinavia and about 70 percent in the U.K. and the United States. Some corrections may be in order, according to research for the year 2000. Japanese women do worse than French women with only 44.8 percent breastfeeding one- to two-month-old infants. For the United States the percentage is 54.7 and for Sweden 80.2. Percentages fall as the infant ages. Paradoxically, good governmental facilities for baby care, keeping mother and baby separated while the mother works, may partially explain this situation. In the United States, the public's prudery makes breastfeeding difficult except in protected areas, though the American Academy of Pediatrics strongly urges breastfeeding.[66] Breastfeeding is strongly related to society's image of the mother. In France, according to one argument, the nursing mother went from being regarded

[65] HR, *Puériculture et centres d'élevage*, 26–36. Henri does not mention the early (circa 1907) Dispensaire de puériculture created by Madame Béquet de Vienne in Paris. For brief comments on nineteenth-century private organizations for the protection of children, including dispensaries and crèches, see Grancher, Comby, and Marfan (eds), *Traité des maladies de l'enfance*, vol. 5, 71–2: mentioned are the works of Dr Gilbert of Le Havre, Madame de Fougeret, Dr Marjolin, and the Parisian *Société pour la propagation de l'allaitement maternal*.

[66] *New York Times* (21 October 2003 and 7 June 2005).

as a milch cow in the nineteenth century to consecration as "a tender mother living an idyllic existence with her infant."[67] But after the Great War doctors ended this idyll by switching mothers to artificial feeding in the interests of scientific medicine, that is, the study of the qualitative and quantitative food requirements and the frequency of feeding children at different ages. At this primitive stage of investigation, scientific observation of breastfeeding was deemed impossible. So the baby became a "digestive tube" and the mother a subject of medical control; the doctor became the "second father," relegating the biological father to the periphery of the child-raising kingdom.[68] This is one explanation of the curious evolution of breastfeeding in France. This explanation of a low French breastfeeding rate would have surprised Henri de Rothschild. He would have considered it a perverse development in medical science, though it can be argued that the health advantages (including lower mortality) of breastfeeding for the baby have been convincingly demonstrated only recently. Henri would strongly disagree. This medicalization of the mother–infant world, enthusiastically promoted by Henri, occurred within the context of the broader, successful social struggle to reduce infant mortality. He would have regretted the loss of the breast but approved the saving of the baby.

---

[67] Yvonne Knibiehler, "Allaitement," in Dominique Lecourt (ed.), *Dictionnaire de la pensée médicale* (Paris, 2004), 33. Not all doctors were convinced of the suitability of breastfeeding for all mothers. Georges Daremberg, *Les grands médecins du XIX*e *siècle* (Paris, 1907), 124–5, in a warning about overenthusiastic philanthropists, says that 50 percent of mothers cannot nurse properly.

[68] For a seductive presentation of this scenario, see Knibiehler, *Dictionnaire de la pensée médicale*, 33–4. Also on the medicalization of society, blamed on Pasteur's doctrines, public health actors, and the Great War, see Pierre Guillaume, *Le rôle social du médecin depuis deux siècles 1800–1945* (Paris, 1996), 95–101, 143.

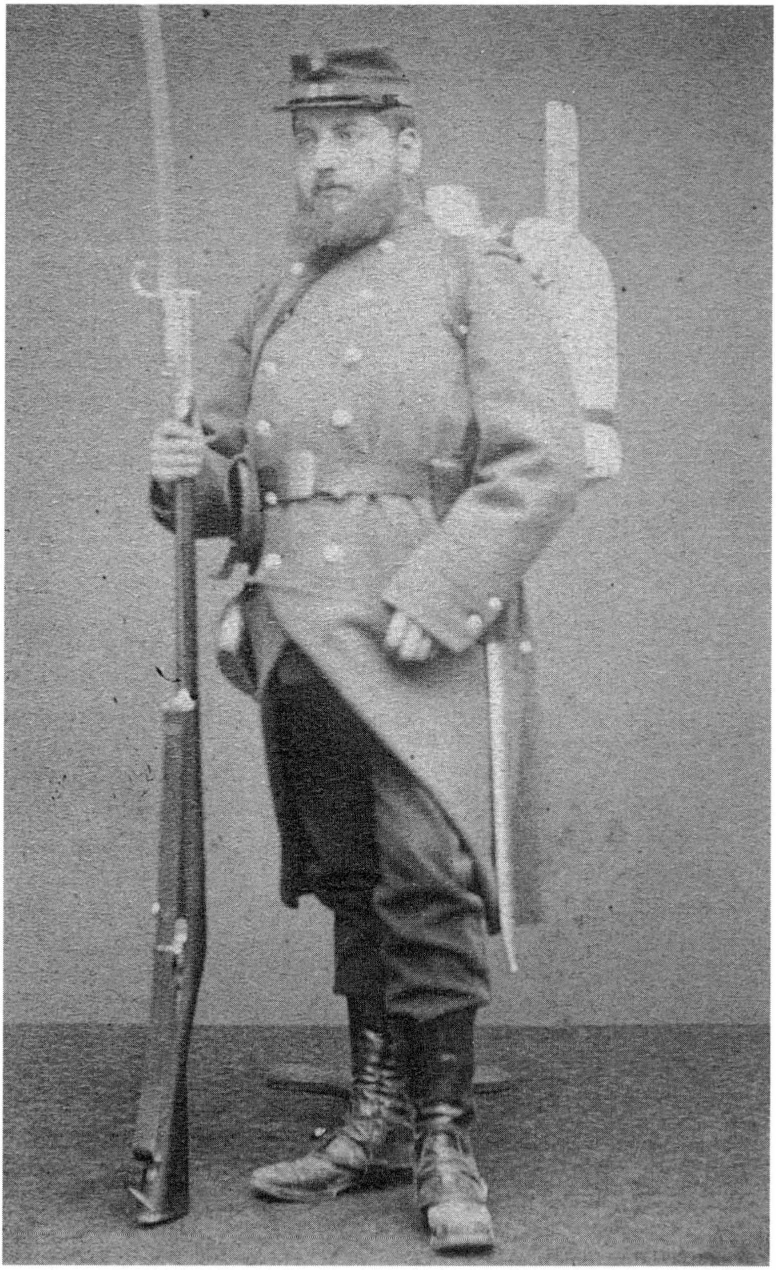

Figure 1 James Edouard de Rothschild (1844–1881, father of Henri) in uniform during the Franco-Prussian war. The Rothschild Archive, London.

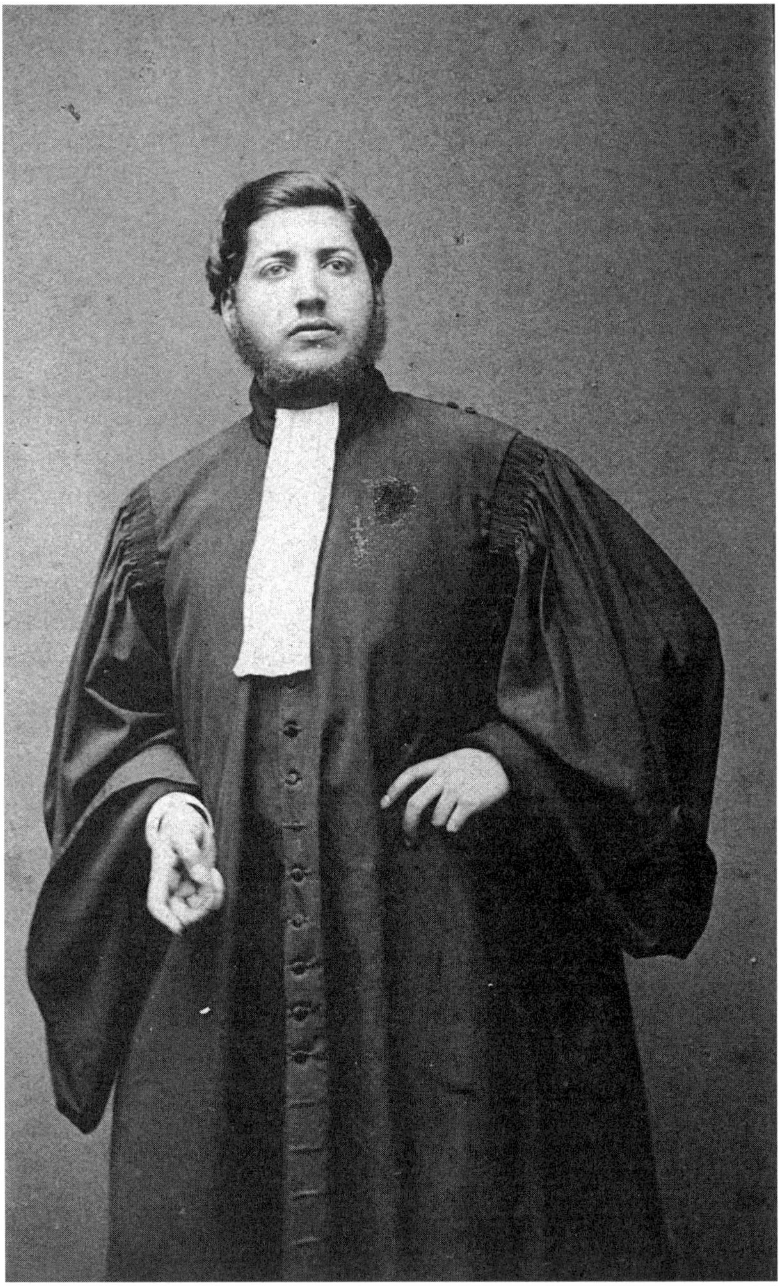

Figure 2 James Edouard de Rothschild in legal dress; he was briefly a practicing lawyer. The Rothschild Archive, London.

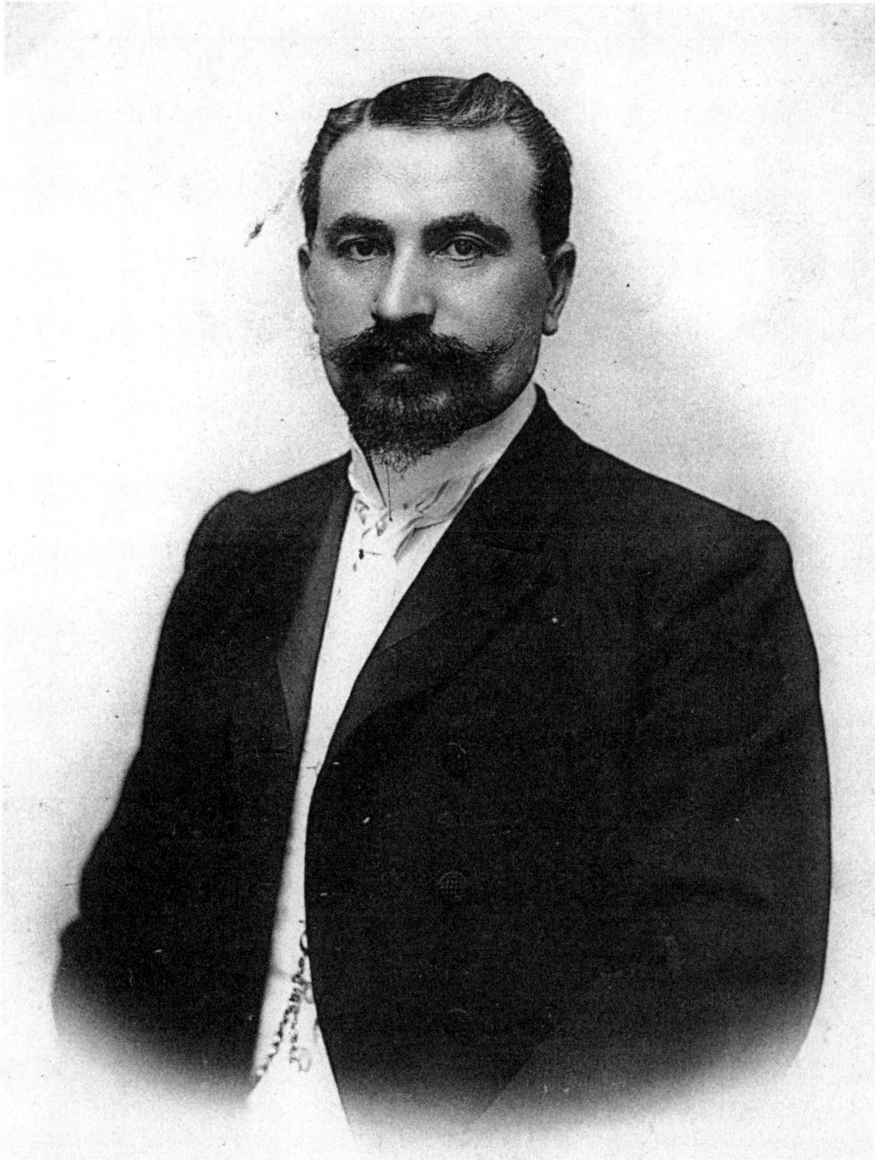

Figure 3 Dr. François Calot, head surgeon at the Rothschild hospital, Berck-Plage. The Rothschild Archive, London.

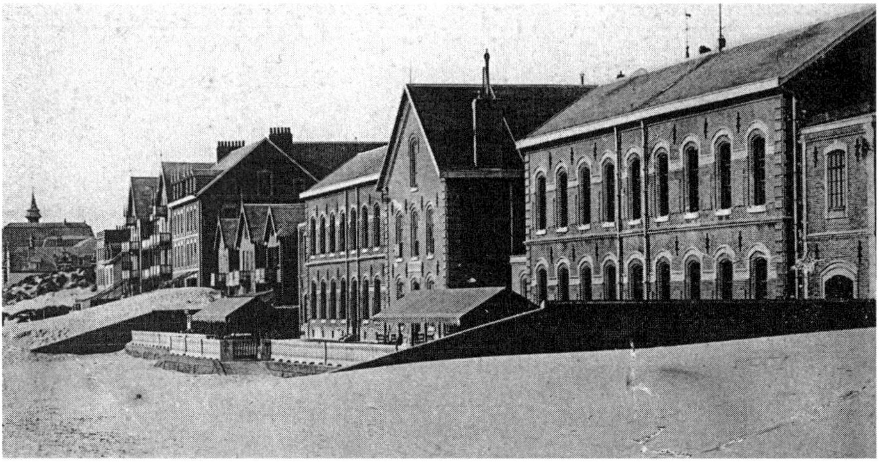

Figure 4 The Rothschild hospital at Berck-Plage, built by James Edouard and named after his father, Nathaniel. The Rothschild Archive, London.

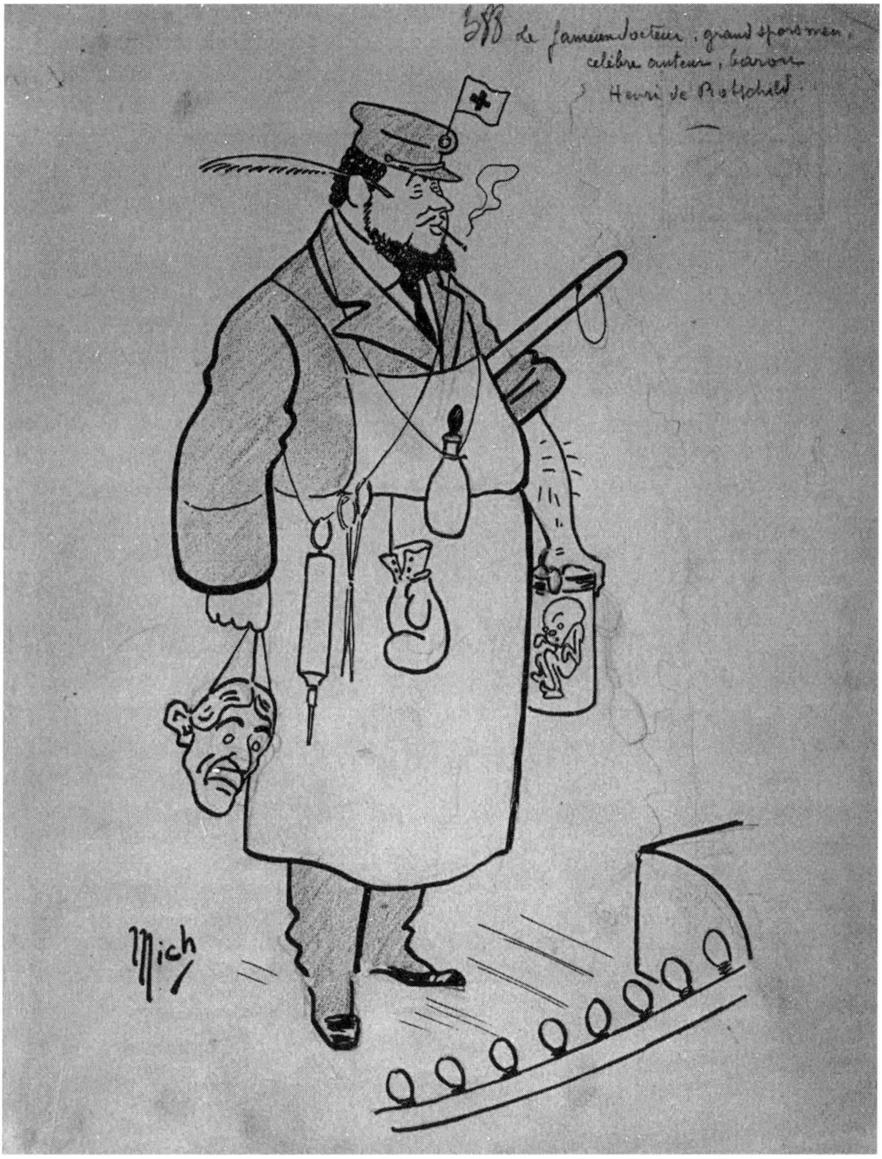
Le fameux docteur, grand sportsman,
célèbre auteur, baron
Henri de Rothschild.
Mich

Figure 5 Cartoon of Henri de Rothschild (1872–1947). Reproduced from a copy in the Rothschild Archive, London, with the permission of the owner, Frédéric Vincent. The Rothschild Archive, London.

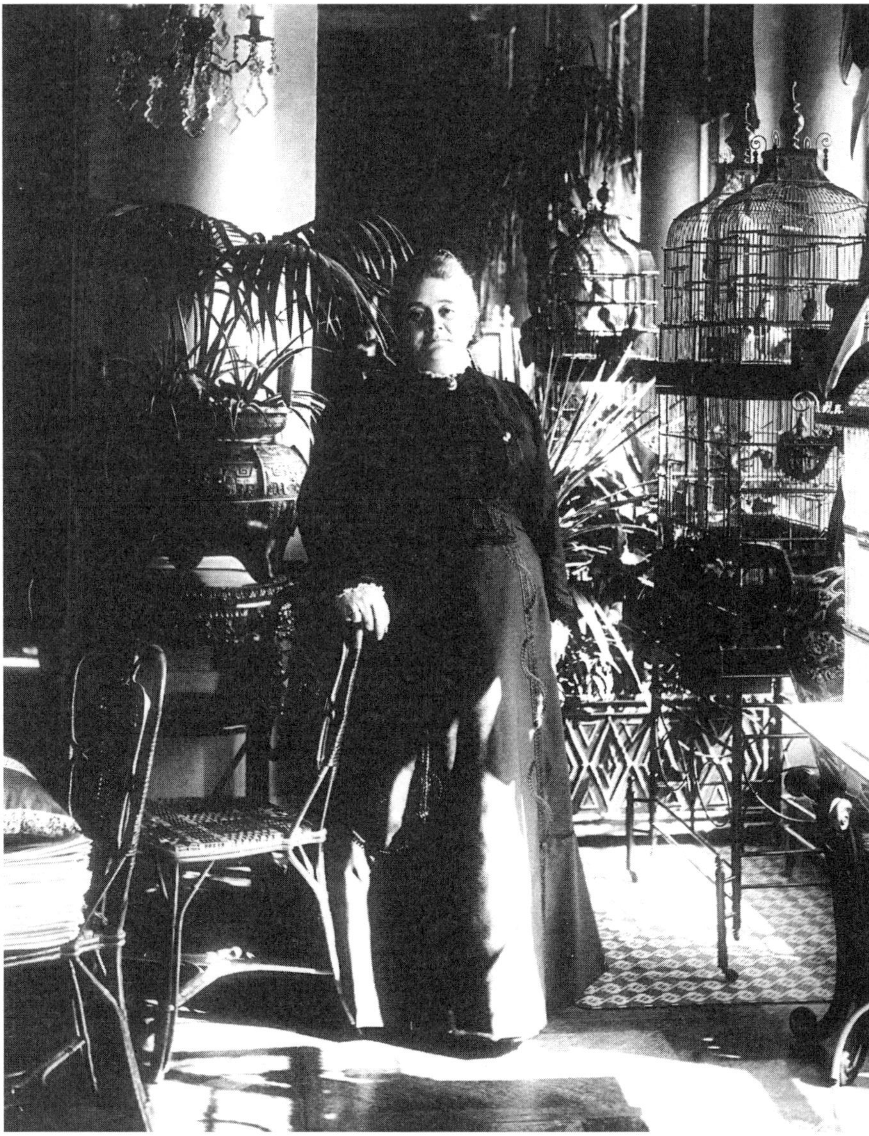

Figure 6 Photograph of Laura Thérèse de Rothschild (1847–1931, mother of Henri), photographed at Villa Madrid, Cannes, in 1922 by Charles Vincent and presented to The Rothschild Archive by his great-grandson, Frédéric Vincent. The Rothschild Archive, London.

Chapter 7
Rothschild Medical Service in World War I

Homo homini lupus[1]

> Like their neighboring enemies, "the Israelites … conceived of [their] God as a man of war," always on their side unless they were faithless, as they frequently managed to be.[2]

The ideology of "Gott mit Uns" is not a German invention. The Torah sets forth the laws of war, different categories of war, and reasons as necessary for justly killing the enemy. Perplexed Jews did not need to read Thomas Aquinas on the just war, for "the biblical and rabbinic laws of warfare are systemically presented in Maimonides' Hilkhot Melakhim."[3] The main theological problem (related to war) for Jews in modern history was finding a justification for serving in non-Jewish armies concerned with winning wars that had little to do with Jewish interests. Most scholars decided that having no choice in the matter, Jews had to serve in the armies of the countries in which they were citizens.[4] And enthusiastic citizens made courageous soldiers on opposing sides. Conditions of service varied according to the degree of enlightenment prevailing in various European belligerents, with discrimination increasing from west to east. During the Franco-Prussian war of 1870–71, there was no problem for qualified Jews like Jules Moch and Léopold Sée in becoming high-ranking officers in the French army, something not possible in the winning armies from across the Rhine. Of course German Jewish soldiers soon became as enthusiastic supporters of the army as were their gentile fellow citizens; to make sure that German Jewish soldiers had access to their God, the high command opened up the army to rabbis serving as chaplains. An illustration in the 5760 Jewish calendar of the B'nai B'rith Klutznick National Jewish Museum shows German Jewish soldiers praying during Yom Kippur. Jewish communities

---

[1] "Man is a wolf to man," cited by Freud, *Civilization and its Discontents* (New York, 1962), 58. Translation by James Strachey, who notes that the axiom is "derived from Plautus, *Asinaria*, II, iv, 88."

[2] R. J. Zwi Werblowsky and Geoffrey Wigoder (eds), *The Oxford Dictionary of the Jewish Religion* [ODJR] (New York, 1997), 718–19.

[3] Quotation is from ODJR, 718–19; and see Aviezer Ravitsky, "'Prohibited Wars' in Jewish Religious Law," at www.edah.org/backend/JournalArticle/Ravitsky-Final.pdf.

[4] ODJR, 718–19: "the principle of *dina' de-malkhuta' dina'* (the laws of the country are to be observed) implied the obligation to serve... ."

put up memorial plaques in synagogues to remind Jews of those who had died for the fatherland.[5] The constitution of the Bismarckian Reich had granted Jews full citizenship rights, which they had enjoyed in France since the Revolution accorded them this privilege along with other pariahs of the old regime.

One estimate puts the number of Jews in the world in 1914 at 16 million, most of whom lived in Czarist Russia, Austria-Hungary, and the United States. France with Algeria had only 180,000 Jews out of a population of 39 million; the U. K. had 270,000 Jews out of a population of 46 million; and the German Reich had 480,000 out of a population of 65 million. Jews went to war in 1914 as enthusiastically and mindlessly as Catholics and Protestants: the national imperative lured the citizen soldier into battle. *Der grosse Krieg* rightly enjoys an important niche in the mythology of Tsahal.[6] The number of men under arms on both sides was about 65 million, including 1.5 million Jews, or 2.3 percent of the total. Of the 42 million men of the allied forces, over 1 million (about 2.5 percent) were Jewish; of the 23 million in the forces of the central powers, 450,500 (about 2 percent) were Jewish. Out of about 13 million casualties, about 170,000 were Jewish, including perhaps 95,000 Russian, 40,000 Austrian–Hungarian, 12,000 German, 12,000 British, and 7500 French Jews. Forty thousand French Jews were mobilized.[7] It is often pointed out how keen German Jews were to defeat the enemy, though a high percentage of German Jewish soldiers were relegated to serving in the commissariat, the sanitary services, the medical and nursing corps, and as translators. "Of a population of 550,000 [sic] Jews in Germany, almost 100,000 served in the German army, 10,000 as volunteers."[8] Among other exploits, the winning of the Iron Cross, first class, a Prussian invention in 1813 and the highest German military decoration, may be cited as evidence of this group's derring-do. Ron Chernow says that 31,500 Jewish combatants won the Iron Cross, without giving a breakdown of first or second class.[9] Henri's mother, Laura-Thérèse de Rothschild, born in Frankfurt and married (1871) to the Parisian James-Edouard

5 In the Lois and Eli Schonberger gallery of The Jewish Museum in New York there is a memorial plaque from the Great Synagogue of Danzig: "1914–1918. Im Weltkrieg starben aus unserer Geminde für Vaterland. Deine Toten werden Leben (Jes. 26.19)." The plaque was among the contents of the synagogue shipped to the United States in 1939.

6 See Jacques Kupfer, *La Glaive de David. Aux sources de Tsahal dans la première guerre mondiale* (Paris, 1998).

7 See Philippe.-E. Landau, *Les Juifs de France et la Grande Guerre. Un patriotisme républicain 1914–1941* (Paris, 2008) and "Brève histoire des Juifs dans la Grande Guerre," in *Les Juifs dans la Grande Guerre* (Historial de la Grande Guerre, Péronne, Somme), catalog of an exposition in 2002.

8 Landau, *Les Juifs de France et la Grande Guerre*, 13.

9 Ron Chernow, *The Warburgs. The Twentieth-Century Odyssey of a Remarkable Jewish Family* (1993; New York, 1994), 171.

de Rothschild, experienced war on the German side in 1870–71 and then on the French side in 1914–18.

Thérèse de Rothschild in the Franco-Prussian War and World War I [10]

Thérèse spent a large part of her life devoted to medical philanthropy and charitable action. She won a gold medal at the *Exposition universelle internationale* of 1900 (Paris) for her charitable activities. During wartime she intensified her activity. Her first wartime experience was on the German side as a sort of medical aide in Frankfurt during the Franco-Prussian war. Her memories of that war included her experience in helping wounded soldiers in the hospital, where she became an active member of the bureau of correspondence, whose function was to write letters (in French or German) for wounded soldiers. The most abandoned prisoners attracted her attention. Thérèse believed that the wounded or sick captives in a country whose language they did not know had a basic right to special attention from hospital personnel. Not everyone agreed. Though she found it hard to believe, Thérèse reluctantly concluded that many people were narrow-minded and mean enough to criticize her kind gestures to these poor creatures. Having in no way neglected her fellow citizens, she was not intimidated and her conscience was untroubled by the harsh comments she heard.

For a while in Frankfurt both German and French wounded soldiers were kept in a large room on the premises of the society of agriculture; it was ideal in a way because of the space, ventilation, and light. Thérèse stayed there daily for hours with her mother, doing various tasks such as preparing compresses and dressings, repairing clothes, and cutting up food and generally looking after soldiers who were as helpless "as if they were children." It was difficult to exercise self-control when viewing the terrible wounds of some of the soldiers, but she succeeded, even to the point where she was able to stay by the beds when doctors or surgeons washed and dressed the wounds. Years later she still got a chill in remembering those wounds. Most wounds were probably multiple wounds from exploding artillery shells rather than from rifle shots or machine gun bursts.[11] She admired the heroic behavior of soldiers who were operated on without an anesthetic – not unusual in the case of surgery on the poor or military at this time. Thérèse admired the ability of men to exercise self-control in this situation. Some soldiers were so

---

[10] See Baronne James [Thérèse] de Rothschild, *Pages détachées du cahier d'une jeune fille* (Mâcon, 1925; first published in 1896), and Baronne James de Rothschild, *Souvenirs de la grande guerre 1914–1918* (Mâcon, 1927). This work is dedicated to Henri – praised for his war service – and his sister Jeanne – praised for her charitable work at the *Maternité* hospital after her post-war return to Paris.

[11] Albert Martin, *Souvenirs d'un chirurgien de la Grande Guerre* (Luneray, 1996), 207.

horribly mutilated that they just wanted to die holding the hands of Thérèse or her mother.

Thérèse was interested in a cultural comparison between the distinctive traits of character of German and French soldiers, which she extrapolated to their two nations. "In a small space, I was in the middle of two peoples."[12] Her biggest surprise may have been the discovery that many French soldiers were illiterate. She did not meet an illiterate German soldier. The Frenchman seemed much more excitable to her: the suffering German would not change expression and remain quiet while the Frenchman would curse his pain, complain or lose his temper, thus often making it difficult to dress his wounds. Why the difference? Thérèse thought it was the difference in physical nature between the two peoples, with the German race being calmer compared with the more nervous, refined French, who were consequently more sensitive to physical and moral afflictions. The French had an advantage in generally having an enviable good humor, a quality often lacking in Germans. Amiable and frank by nature, the suffering French displayed an insouciance and natural gaiety even in the German medical facility.

The citizens of Frankfurt who visited the prisoners were attracted to the French, a term including Algerians and other Arabs, whose brilliant sometimes strangely glittering eyes fascinated many visitors. These "wild children of the desert" were not an easy group to deal with. Suspicious that the medical personnel wanted to make them suffer – they were the enemy, after all – they sometimes exploded in shocking rudeness. The Muslim soldiers from Africa initially did not want wine but finally accepted it on being told that drinking the wine was medically prescribed as a remedy and was therefore not a sin. The prisoners provided a sort of innocent entertainment for locals (and perhaps vice versa), but those in charge also made minor attempts to introduce the captives to *Kultur*.

When the soldiers were moved from the center of Frankfurt to specially constructed barracks in the suburbs (a great green space in Pfingstwaide), the French and Germans were separated according to nationality into light wooden houses, each containing twenty beds. Thérèse and her mother did not like the new setup and left. Although it was not easy to get governmental permission to open up a kind of private military hospital, her mother succeeded in doing so with the help of their doctor. The mini-hospital took care of twenty-five German and French soldiers for the remaining six months of the war. It was another satisfying experience, enabling Thérèse to prattle on about the gratitude of the soldiers, attested by the letters she received. When the war was over, she returned to the family residence. These "tragic days were illuminated by a ray of happiness," for she had been "useful to ... fellow human beings during their cruel ordeals. And in the bottom of my soul there burned a lasting hatred of war, whose fatal and unjust hardships I had seen close-up."[13]

[12] Thérèse de Rothschild, *Pages détachées*, 308.

[13] Thérèse de Rothschild, *Souvenirs de la grande guerre 1914–1918*, 329.

Thérèse noted that the French and German soldiers got friendly enough with one another to play cards and checkers and to teach one another the rudiments of the other's language. This change from enemy to friend appeared strange to her, and it gave her an occasion to quote from the choir in *Die Braut von Messina* (1803) of her beloved Schiller. The common peoples might ooze pious sentiments to the effect that they did not hate one another and the other was not an enemy, but when the princes declared war, people had to massacre one another to establish order in the name of the law. Thérèse speculated on how peoples are not by nature enemies and, left alone, go about their peaceful activities. War is the fault of the "princes." For nearly half a century after the Prussian victory in 1871, she enjoyed peace in France, until the princes stumbled into the most murderous spectacle yet, thus giving her the opportunity to serve her fellow human beings once more.

Thérèse spent most of World War I at her summer residence, the château de Fontaines, in Gouvieux, near Chantilly, which was empty when the war came in 1914, except for four old English servants, who had worked in the stables for years. She managed to travel around a fair amount during the war, especially to see family members and to go to her hospital in Berck-sur-Mer. The war was a great time for charity-minded patriotic women. Much of Thérèse's wartime activity involved working in her small hospital in Gouvieux; named for James-Edouard, it had been founded as a dispensary–*Maison de secours* in 1888. In the same year she established a nursery in Gouvieux. *La Crèche Jeanne de Rothschild* cared daily for thirty working-class children, who had to be vaccinated. Medical and hospital care and welfare existed for the poor in French cities, though, as the Rothschilds showed, there was always need for more; in rural areas it was often up to private donors to provide services. (The *Assistance publique* had established some nurseries before 1900 for the children of married parents.)

In Gouvieux Thérèse saw the need for a dispensary offering free consultations and medications for the destitute as well as the need for a hospital to serve those requiring medical treatment and surgery but too poor to pay for such services. To run the hospital she called on the *Congrégation des Filles de la Sagesse*, an order of nuns whose different works included running the big hospitals of the French navy. Three sisters arrived on 22 October 1891, three days after Thérèse had hoped they would arrive, which would have been the feast day of Sainte-Thérèse. She was also kind to Protestants. From the time of the separation of church and state in 1905 until 1920, when the Hersent family picked up the tab, Thérèse paid the rent on the presbytery in town. Not that her good relations with Catholics and Protestants meant that she was any less Jewish. She did not permit mass to be celebrated in the hospital; nor did she allow crucifixes or other Christian signs in rooms. Some flexibility existed in extreme need, as, for example, in the case of a dying soldier allowed to clutch a crucifix. During 1891–95, there were 167 operations performed, including 162 patients cured, 4 improved, and only 1 death. The total statistics of Thérèse's establishments for the period included 2114 consultations, with 996 men, women, and children diagnosed as sick and 210 hospitalized. Thérèse died in 1931, and since the hospital provided important services to the community the municipal government bought it in 1932 for 150,000 francs.

A few months into the Great War, France found itself with only 235,000 military hospital beds for 275,000 wounded personnel; by the end of November there were 360,000 beds but 490,000 wounded soldiers needing hospitalization.[14] So every available hospital bed had to be pressed into service. With mobilization each hospital developed a military health department parallel to the existing civilian structure. Perhaps the temporary disorganization caused by this intrusion was compensated by the fact that the hospital system was put in touch with some important new methods. This is a familiar and probably good argument about the necessity and ability of military medicine to advance in both research and surgery.[15] Henri's friend the surgeon Pierre Delbet was a major figure in the debate over whether to amputate or conserve a limb and even invented an apparatus to help heal the limbs of wounded soldiers. Henri himself played a role in promoting a new treatment for burns. During the war about 3,000,000 French soldiers, according to one estimate, were wounded and hospitalized, half of them at least twice, many suffering from typhus, tuberculosis, or cholera.

Although France began training military nurses in 1909, the army had only a few mediocre male nurses available in 1914.[16] Georges Duhamel, an army volunteer surgeon, found nearly all the male nurses to be simple folk, driven by fear to laugh in the face of death.[17] Mobilization notices to 23,000 Red Cross nurses and volunteering eventually produced about 30,000 women who were qualified as military nurses.[18] The 1480 auxiliary hospitals were staffed by about 63,000 nurses, many of whom transferred to military hospitals, hospital ships, dressing stations, and surgical units. The availability of perhaps up to 10,000 nuns helped both the war effort and the post-war church, which had been crippled

[14] On French hospitals during World War I, see Nicole Rollin and others, *Les hôpitaux dans la guerre* (Paris, 2008).

[15] Nathalie Plazanet, *Inventaire des archives de la Guerre 1914–1918* (AP-HP, 603 Foss, Feb. 1989), 2. For the impact of the war on dealing with wounds, amputations, and therapy, see Sophie Delaporte, *Les médecins dans la Grande Guerre 1914–1918* (Paris, 2003).

[16] Katrin Schultheiss, *Bodies and Souls. Politics and the Professionalization of Nursing in France 1880–1922* (Cambridge, Mass., 2001), 158. Some sources just note that in 1914 there were ninety-six military nurses.

[17] Duhamel's literary success from the war was *Vie des martyrs 1914–1916* (Paris, 1917); in 1929 Hachette published an "édition définitive," with nineteen wood engravings by P. L. Guilbert.

[18] On the three French Red Cross societies, presided over by the marquis de Vogüé, see the Comtesse de Courson, *La Femme Française pendant la Guerre* (2d edn, Paris, 1916), 32–42. She claimed that by the end of 18 months, the three societies had supplied 180,000 "nurses." See also Françoise Thébaud, *La femme au temps de la guerre de 14* (Paris, 1986, 1994), 83–103, "Les anges blancs"; she points out that in 1914 the societies had a quarter million adherents with a capital of thirty million francs.

by anticlerical governments in a resolutely secular society. Conservatives fantasized that the asexual nun was the ideal nurse to avoid the probable romantic entanglements that would result from throwing secular nurses and men together, even in a medical environment.[19] The Rothschilds lost no time in making their hospital beds available. Thérèse paid for all hospital expenses without asking for reimbursement from the ministry of war. Five nursing sisters eventually worked at the hospital (twenty-one beds) in Gouvieux, pressed into military service as "auxiliary hospital no. 33," with Dr Ehrhart running the surgical department. The Alsatian Dr Vincent, the hospital doctor, was able to put his German to good use in convincing the invading Germans to refrain from violence in town. Thérèse happily reported that the "Senlis disaster," then exaggerated as "the French Louvain," was thus avoided, and so were "the atrocious crimes" that had been "committed by the enemy."[20] Chantilly, where the French army established its headquarters or Grand Quartier Général (GQG), in the *Hôtel du Grand Condé*, 3.5 kilometers from Gouvieux, also escaped the wrath of the invaders.

In August 1914 Thérèse and Jeanne (her mother refers to her as la baronne Léonino) returned to their residence at 42 avenue de Friedland in Paris before going on to spend six weeks at Dinard, near Saint Malo. Henri and family friends were already there. Finding seats on the train was not easy, but the family's railway connections enabled cooperative employees to liberate seats. The "elegant and worldly seaside resort" of Dinard had been transformed into a big wartime medical center. Thérèse and Jeanne volunteered to work for the *Service de santé militaire*, which gave them daily hospital duties. Though not in uniform, Thérèse assisted with the dressing of wounds and wrote letters for the soldiers. In the afternoon she went around to different towns in the area looking for provisions and useful items for the soldiers. Jeanne did much the same thing. As a doctor, Henri exercised a formal function in the hospitals. When her "eminent friend" Professor Letulle got a hundred children sent to Dinard, Thérèse helped with the expenses, for the municipal government could not pay for all that was needed. It was a busy six weeks.

After serving in Dinard, Thérèse stopped in Paris and then went on to London, where she happily met more family members, including her sister Emma and her grandchildren Nadine and Philippe. She returned to England at the end of 1914 and again in 1920. In March 1915 Thérèse went by train from Paris to Amiens, where she got special permission from the English authorities to continue by automobile to Berck. On the way she paid special attention to the organization of the British camps. It seems that there was often a medical lesson to be learned from the British – later she would scour the Scottish hospital at Royaumont. In

---

19 Margaret H. Darrow, *French Women and the First World War. War Stories of the Home Front* (Oxford, 2000), 146–51, and Thébaud, *La femme au temps de la guerre de 14*, 83–103.

20 Thérèse de Rothschild, *Souvenirs de la grande guerre 1914–1918*, 207.

June 1915 Thérèse set up at her residence in Gouvieux and, with a few absences, stayed there until the end of 1917.

The war was a constant worry, with the enemy nearby and her son, daughter-in-law (Mathilde), and grandson (James, "mon cher petit soldat") in the front lines. When the war broke out, James had been cruising for a month on Albert I of Monaco's yacht *Hirondelle*, then in the Azores. The prince was a good friend of Henri's. James enlisted before the age of eighteen, before completing the second part of his baccalauréat-ès-lettres, served first in the Balkans and then (1917–18) in France as a pilot with a combat squadron. He was lucky enough to return from the war, having earned the *croix de guerre* and the *croix de la Légion d'honneur*. He joined the family bank and lived (1896–1984) a modest Rothschild's life full of money, sport, hunting, and horses. Philippe and Nadine spent eighteen months of the war with relatives in England. Mathilde had little choice but to take them there after an official visit to 33 rue du Faubourg St-Honoré by Colonel Lucien Klotz of the military government of Paris. She returned to Paris to become a volunteer nurse at Henri's Paris hospital. After returning to victorious France in 1919 Nadine married Adrien Thierry and went on to enjoy the diplomatic life. It would be a totally different experience for the French Rothschilds during World War II, followed by their return to a country that had annulled their citizenship, seized their properties, and driven them into exile.

Running a Rothschild household during wartime was both exciting and difficult. French and foreign officers stayed at "Fontaines." So Thérèse met English generals, a Russian prince, and a Russian general, the latter of whom was questioned about his "quite original country."[21] Any hope for the return of peace and quiet was shattered by the German bombardments of 1918. And the family had to live without enjoying its great treasures. Family collections, including the library, were safely stored in Paris and at Mouton in the Médoc.[22] Thérèse's personal collection was considerable, though one rarely hears much about it. When her father (Mayer Carl) died in 1886, his collections of sixteenth-century German gold- and silversmith art, of enamels, wood and ivory sculptures, snuffboxes, French jewelry, and Italian art of the sixteenth to the eighteenth century occupied an entire townhouse in Frankfurt. Four daughters shared the inheritance; Mayer Carl disinherited his daughter Margaretha because she defected to the Christian camp on marrying the duc de Gramont in 1878. Thérèse's share of the collections enabled her to decorate three big salons of the residences in Gouvieux and Paris, as well as the library of the residence in the avenue de Friedland.[23]

---

21 Thérèse de Rothschild, *Souvenirs de la grande guerre 1914–1918*, 87.

22 Paris with its surrounding area was bombed on 31 January (63 dead and 207 wounded) and on 15 March 1918; 3 hospitals were damaged. Rollin, *Les hôpitaux dans la guerre*, 22.

23 "Les Rothschilds – Gouvieux-Chantilly 1880–1930," in *Bulletin de la Société historique de Gouvieux* (Oise), no. 4, 1992.

The Gouvieux estate escaped damage during the war, except for a big hole dug by a bomb that went off in the park and destroyed the chauffeur's house. And there was the nuisance of not having a telephone for medical purposes – she now found it a necessity rather than an infernal machine. (During the war the use of this piece of advanced technology was taken away from private residences.) Absurdly, the telephone was taken away from the hospital, but by appealing directly to Joffre, then commander-in-chief, Thérèse got service reestablished there after an investigation. There was a big advantage in being able to go straight to the top; she had also threatened to close the hospital if the telephone service were not restored.

For nearly two months in the summer of 1918 Thérèse and Jeanne went to the charming town of Fréteval (Loir-et-Cher), a few kilometers from Vendôme, where Henri had a small hunting property; he and his friends used to hunt there before the war. During her six-week stay, Thérèse soon began helping out in the local war effort. Soldiers, who received tobacco, drinks, and flowers, pleased her with their appreciation: "Merci, merci, grand'mère." Rejuvenated by her trip, she returned to Gouvieux on 24 July 1918. In October Nadine and Philippe showed up, only to be pressed into accompanying her on hospital rounds, much as Henri had done at Berck-sur-Mer. Thérèse forgot her old worries in the enjoyment of being back among her "good soldiers."

"The most perfect order" prevailed in the hospital in Gouvieux with the *Filles de la Sagesse* in command; by 1917 Sister Stylien had been in medical harness for 25 years. Thérèse was impressed by the fact that the soldiers obeyed the female nurses without any problems. Once installed back on her property, she relaxed by visiting nearby hospitals and ambulance units, including the auxiliary hospital (200 beds) at the abbey of Royaumont, in quest of ideas for the improvement of her own hospital.[24] The thirteenth-century royal abbey of Royaumont, founded in 1228 by Saint Louis, the best-preserved Cistercian abbey in France, was restored by the Gouin family, which had completed its purchase of the property by 1905, the year of separation of church and state. During the visit to Royaumont Thérèse's chauffeur got drunk; so she had to be driven home in the sole ambulance available at the hospital. It is curious that she does not identify this auxiliary hospital of the Scottish Women's Hospital Unit organized by Elsie Inglis (1864–1917; M.D.,

[24] *Ambulance*, a term that includes the personnel of the ambulance: nine officers, of whom six were doctors and one a pharmacist, three non-commissioned officers, and forty-eight nurses. Definition given by *Médecin Inspecteur général* Sieur, "Les organisations du Service de Santé aux Armées," in *Le Livre d'or des médecins morts pour la France 1914–1918* (Paris, n.d.), 28. See also Edmond Delorme (*Médecin Inspecteur général de l'Armée*), *Les enseignements chirurgicaux de la Grande Guerre. Front Occidental* (Paris, 1919). The formations increased in size as the war went on, and could be, as Antoine Prost says, "une vraie cité sanitaire." See Prost, "Le service de Santé militaire pendant la Première Guerre mondiale," in Annette Wieviorka (ed.), *Justin Godart. Un homme dans son siècle 1871–1956* (Paris, 2004, 2005), 150.

Edinburgh, 1892), founder of the famous "Scottish Women's Hospitals" and a pioneering figure in the early days of woman doctors. In the period 1915–19, the Royaumont hospital cared for 10,861 wounded soldiers in 600 beds. Inglis founded a second hospital in 1917 at Villers-Cotterêts (Aisne). Thérèse does not say if the Scots taught her anything.

Thérèse kept busy in Gouvieux. Keeping informed about military trains and medical convoys through a useful contact, she got to know the vicomte de Méré, the captain in charge of surveillance at the railway station, who facilitated her charitable acts, such as going to the station to pick up packages for the soldiers. She often paid for family members of the soldiers to visit and stay a day in the village. Wounded soldiers could read and smoke in a special room set up in the hospital. With a real professional interest acquired over a lifetime of experience with disease and suffering, Thérèse carefully followed some serious cases until recovery or, more likely, death. Her *Souvenirs* provided some quasi-clinical details. In her relations with the wounded, Thérèse had only one regret, namely that few of the departing soldiers accepted her invitation to come see her in the avenue de Friedland when they came to Paris. "Alas!" Perhaps the soldiers took class relations more seriously than Thérèse did. In June 1919 the ministry of war decided that it no longer needed the hospital in Gouvieux and, in spite of her efforts to keep it going, closed it down. She could console herself with figures, including the satisfying number of 492 wounded soldiers admitted and treated, most of them with her loving care.

The James-Edouard-de-Rothschild hospital in Berck-sur-Mer, militarily re-baptized as "Hôpital bénévole no. 22 bis," operating with 45 beds, received and treated 1076 wounded soldiers for a total of 14,705 days of hospitalization between 1914 and 1919. In the anti-German hysteria of the war, a German nurse (Lina), who had been employed for 30 years, was "taken away."[25] The director, Madame Bloch, impeccably French, was awarded the *Médaille de la reconnaissance nationale* at the end of the war. As far as Thérèse was concerned, the establishment in Berck was as successful as the hospital in Gouvieux because she made sure that they used the same methods. Of course medical techniques were pretty much the same, and no doubt she was thinking of general care of the patients, which is just as important as the surgery, indeed impossible to separate from it.

As a social eminence, Thérèse found herself playing an important role in the small communities in which she stayed. In Berck she participated in the establishment of a foundation for the Cazin hospital and was the leading founder of the *Asile maritime pour les marins et les pêcheuses âgées*. In 1915 she became president of the administrative council of the maritime asylum. This turned out to be fortunate for the area because during the war the inhabitants were deprived of their usual medical care. Thérèse managed to transform the asylum so that it could accept the sick inhabitants of Berck, who could no longer go to the militarized

[25] Thérèse de Rothschild, *Souvenirs de la grande guerre 1914–1918*, 153–4.

hospital in Montreuil-sur-Mer. Berck was a particularly busy place in 1914–16 because of convoys of sick people being sent there from areas invaded by the German armies.

Under the leadership of under-secretary of state Justin Godart the *Service de Santé militaire* was successful in supplying the army's medical needs but at a great cost to civilians.[26] In 1900 army horses had more doctors than the soldiers did: 1 veterinarian for 264 horses and 1 doctor for 421 men. By 1914 there were still only 1518 army doctors for an army of 600,000 (1/395), which meant that the army had to recruit another 700 doctors. Godart managed to swell the medical ranks to over 21,000 by the time of the armistice; and 19,474 of these doctors were reservists. In an army of 4.3 million there was a doctor for every 203 men; the British army got by with 1 doctor for every 376 men, which required mobilizing only 45 percent of civilian doctors. Eighty percent of France's 22,000 doctors were mobilized, leaving the civilian population with 1 doctor for every 14,000 people compared with 1 for 5777 in Germany and 1 for 2344 people in the U.K.[27] Thérèse was therefore making an important minor contribution to the solution of a serious civilian medical problem as well as doing her bit for the military medical effort. In one sense, Thérèse was continuing and extending her peacetime medical activities, which even extended to her playing a major role in the development of private nursing education.[28]

Armed with her long experience of working with nursing sisters, Thérèse continued her good relations with Catholics, even supporting the establishment of Catholic churches in Berck-Plage and Berck-Ville. Although she was not there to receive him, she purred with pleasure in praising a visit to the Berck hospital by the bishop of Arras, Msgr. Julien. Judging from her discourse, one supposes that Thérèse's relations with the social and political elites or men of power were on the friendly level of deferential equality, perhaps on both sides. Her relations with soldiers had to be different, no matter how friendly they might have been with her. In Berck and Gouvieux she met some black soldiers from the empire. These "simple souls," who were "like children" and called her *mémé* (*maman*), could conceal delicate feelings under their rough, gross exterior.[29] Her sympathetic remarks on French soldiers were not very different. Thérèse was pleased to have

26 Justin Godart (1871–1956), docteur en droit, sous-secrétaire d'Etat au Service de santé militaire, 1 July–29 Oct. 1915; 14 Dec. 1916–5 Feb. 1918, ministre du travail et de l'hygiène (Cartel des Gauches), ministre de la santé publique, 1932–33. The Ministère de l'hygiène, assistance et prévoyance, created in January 1920, became part of the ministry of work in 1924, with the Ministère de la Santé publique emerging only in 1930.

27 Lion Murard and Patrick Zylberman, *L'Hygiène dans la République. La santé publique en France ou l'utopie contrariée 1870–1918* (Paris, 1996), 563–5.

28 Thérèse supported and was the vice-president of the *Maison-école d'infirmières privées* founded in 1905; the founding committee met at her residence, 42 avenue de Friedland. Schultheiss, *Bodies and Souls*, 91.

29 Thérèse de Rothschild, *Souvenirs de la grande guerre 1914–1918*, 166–7.

discovered from personal experience that it was wrong to call the imperial soldiers "savages." One black soldier was allowed to ride around town with her; these joyful escapades astounded the native French, which also amused her.

In 1919 Thérèse was promoted to the rank of officer in the Legion of Honor for having devoted her medical establishments to the care of wounded soldiers. (The Legion of Honor was founded by Napoleon in 1802 for people who distinguish themselves from the rest of hoi polloi in civil or military service.[30]) She had been made a member of the Legion in 1913 for her works of charity, in particular her work at the James-Edouard-de-Rothschild hospital in Berck. On that occasion *L'Œuvre* treated "la dame James Amschel, so-called 'baroness' de Rothschild," to a nasty note from the acerbic pen of the well-known Parisian scribbler Urbain Gohier (pseudonym for Goulet, 1862–1951): each time the Rothschilds steal ten millions from the French people, they throw back a scrap of ten thousand, and the French weep in gratitude. Gohier did not approve of this trickle-down effect. Worse, her decoration came from the "Prussian" minister of education, the Protestant Jules Steeg. The anti-Semitic and anti-German feelings that reached a crescendo in the Dreyfus affair were still alive, virulently so in the case of the hatred directed against the Rothschilds. Gohier completed his political evolution in becoming a supporter of Vichy, when the pre-war anti-Semitism reignited, taking a murderous turn.

Henri in la Grande Guerre

Although the French Rothschilds were not so politically prominent as their English relatives, the family could boast of some modest political success. Maurice was elected deputy for the department of the Hautes-Pyrénées in 1919 and became senator in 1939; Edouard was also a senator. The political game was one of the few public activities in which Henri did not participate. Given his scale of activities, especially of a charitable nature, and his lavish style of entertaining, it is not surprising to find politicians and high-level bureaucrats frequently in his company. Nor were his friendships in high political circles of minor significance: Godart, a major figure in health politics and a supporter of feminism, was perhaps closest to Henri and his wife; Edouard Herriot (1872–1957), whose political views in the 1930s were anathema in the banking community, was a lycée classmate of Henri's, though one cannot make too much of that accident. Henri, a prominent figure in the Third Republic and an active medical supporter of the French imperialistic *mission civilisatrice*, had no difficulty in getting to see people at the top or in getting them to come to his social, medical, and cultural events.

Henri's medical philanthropy was heavily centered on Paris and, to a much lesser extent, Berck-sur-Mer. His interest extended to the empire in North Africa,

---

[30] For details on the awards, see http://www.ambafrance_gr.org/EVENEMENTS/legionhonneur.htm.

which had a substantial Jewish population, though their existence was not the main impetus for his action. It has been argued that there was a "symbiosis between French imperialism and the educational outreach of the Alliance Israélite Universelle," an organization supported by members of the Rothschild family. If Henri did not figure prominently in supporting French Jewish organizations taking up the burden of "the civilizing mission," he certainly had no hesitation in supporting the policy arising from "a French ideology of state secularism," whether or not he viewed it as "an alternative to Catholic foreign policy."[31] In the early twentieth century Henri established infirmaries or hospitals for local populations at Beni-Ounif, Colomb-Béchar, and Aïn-Sefra, in western Algeria – nearby Moroccans were optimistically considered in Paris as potentially Francophile. The Algerian medical adventure began in 1904, after his trip to the south of "our North African colony," which included a visit to the governor general (Charles Jonnart) to thank him for the facilities he had provided during the journey. Henri asked what he could do for Algeria. Jonnart suggested creating two medical facilities for "natives" near the Moroccan frontier, where Moroccans could be treated by French military doctors. Given the need for the French to cultivate good relations with the Moroccans, the medical venture would provide an excellent propaganda program to develop, in a peaceful way, French influence in a Morocco still teetering on the edge of the French imperial abyss. Henri paid for the hospitals after a study by civil and military authorities found the project a good idea. For over fifteen years he supplied the facilities with what the military doctors asked for. After 1920 instead of sending supplies every trimester, he gave the Algerian government a lump sum of money to buy them. On a visit to the south of Algeria in 1932, Henri was delighted to see his name on the pediment of a handsome Mooresque building in Colomb-Béchar.[32]

Henri's medical charity in Morocco was also part of the French imperial adventure in a more sinister context. In March 1907 Dr Emile Mauchamp was murdered in Marrakesh. Mauchamp had been sent by the ministry of foreign affairs to direct the town's dispensary, one of the French free dispensaries set up to give native care. Given that fact and his subsequent lionization in French political circles, it is highly probable that he was a government agent, certainly a government doctor. It may be that the crowd stoned him to death because of a rumor spread by the German consular agent that Mauchamp was a spy planning to set

---

31 Quotations are from Abigail Green, "The British Empire and the Jews: An Imperialism of Human Rights?," *Past and Present* 199 (May 2008): 178. Key works on these issues are Lisa Moses Leff, *Sacred Bonds of Solidarity. The Rise of Jewish Internationalism in Nineteenth-Century France* (Stanford, 2006); Michael M. Laskier, *The Alliance Israélite Universelle and the Jewish Communities of Morocco: 1862–1962* (Albany, 1983); and Aron Rodrigue, *French Jews, Turkish Jews. The Alliance Israélite Universelle and the Politics of Jewish Schooling in Turkey, 1860–1925* (Bloomington, IN, 1990).

32 Henri de Rothschild [HR], *La Lignée française de la famille Rothschild 1792–1942. Etude historique et biographique* (Oporto, 1942), 109.

up a radio post. His death furnished an excellent occasion for French meddling in Morocco with the aim of bringing it into the French imperial orbit, thus excluding other meddling European powers. Mauchamp was given a splendid funeral in his hometown of Chalon-sur-Saône; official France mourned and encouraged others to do so. He entered the Legion of Honor and got a statue. France, then enjoying a Clemenceau government, occupied Oujda, in northeast Morocco, near the Algerian border. In July 1907 eight European workers, of whom four were French, were killed in Casablanca. A French gunboat shelled the guilty city of about 20,000 people, killing hundreds. Moroccan sovereignty was about to come to an end, with the acquiescence of the other murderously inclined European powers.[33]

In early August Henri, amusing himself in Trouville, ran into the naval minister (Gaston Thomson, a deputy from Algeria), who seized the opportunity to ask him to go to Morocco immediately – it looks like the meeting might not have been accidental – to set up a hospital for an occupying French force. This secret mission meant that the Red Cross could not be asked to do the job. The governmental propaganda machine lulled the public into believing that France was undertaking a police operation, not a colonial war. Within 24 hours Henri had 280 packing cases of materiel ready to set up a hospital of 50 beds. Henri and two other doctors (Desjardin and De Sarl) from his polyclinic, two nurses and a cook set off by Sud-Express for Algeciras, the southern Spanish port, where they took a torpedo boat to Casablanca. Henri noted that the commandant was none other than the novelist Claude Farrère (Frédéric-Charles Bargone). Arriving on location, they set up the hospital (*Hôpital de Campagne pour le corps d'occupation de Casablanca*) and until the end of September lived in dreadful conditions. The Red Cross then took over. A cholera epidemic at the end of August hit officers and men badly. Henri boasted of having treated two generals for what he politely described as serious gastrointestinal problems. He paid for this entire imperial medical venture.[34]

In the evening of 15 June 1932 Henri de Rothschild entertained the audience at a medical and scientific meeting with an outline of his career. Godart, then minister of public health in Herriot's third ministry (3 June–18 December 1932), presided over the meeting.[35] Henri began with World War I, the greatest catastrophe in French history since the Revolution. Henri's first shock was mild; he found himself parked in a remote wooden hut on the grounds of the military hospital *Val-de-Grâce* with nothing to do. Henri made an appointment with Godart, who was

---

33 William A. Hosington, Jr., *Lyautey and the French Conquest of Morocco* (New York, 1995), 31. See also Thomas K. Park and Aomar Boum, *Historical Dictionary of Morocco* (1996; 2d edn, Lanham, 2006).

34 HR, *La Lignée*, 106–8. See Jonathan G. Katz, *Murder in Marrakesh: Emile Mauclair and the French Colonial Adventure* (Bloomington, IN, 2006).

35 See the introduction by Jean-Jacques Becker to 3d part ("La Santé"), in Wieviorka (ed.), *Justin Godart*. Godart was a eugenicist – who wasn't? – and a supporter of the development of sexology in France; see Alain Drouard, "Justin Godart et le développement de la sexologie en France," in Wieviorka (ed.), *Justin Godart*, 191–8.

then under-secretary of state for the military health service. The title of a low rank army doctor ("médecin aide major de 1e classe") did not disguise the baron Henri de Rothschild, M.D., and his friend Godart would ensure that his military potential would not remain unexploited.[36]

Like the prominent pillar of the Third Republic Edouard Herriot, Godart was from Lyon and a distinguished anticlerical of the Radical Socialist party.[37] This efficient and effective lawyer-politician was appointed to reform the disorganized *Service de santé militaire*, whose army doctors were notorious for their hostility to civilian medical men and women doctors.[38] Godart noted that commanding an "army" of 168,000 non-combatants was more a matter of organization than of medical science.[39] Georges Brouardel, nephew of Paul Brouardel, was among the advisers of the secretary on medical matters. Godart took over from *Médecin Inspecteur Général* Troussaint, under whose leadership low-level medical practice was aggravated by the army's imperviousness to civilian medical corps improvements in the treatment of wounds. Troussaint was determined to subject all non-military career doctors to army control at any cost. He had to resign.[40]

---

36 On 1 January 1918 part of the organization of army doctors was as follows:

288	médecins majors de 1re classe: A
91	médecins majors de 1re classe: C
475	médecins majors de 2e classe: A
891	médecins majors de 2e classe: C
29	médecins aides major: A
5,325	médecins aides major: C

The total number of army doctors on that date was 9208, dropping to 7589 by 1 September; there were also 1694 médecins auxiliaries. See Pierre Lefebvre (ed.), *Histoire de la Médecine aux armées* (Paris and Limoges, 1987), tome 3.

37 Godart later became known as a friend of Jewish causes: he was a supporter of the Zionist cause and a protector of Jews during Vichy; in 2004 his name was added to the "Righteous among the nations" (Yad Vashem, Jerusalem). See Wieviorka (ed.), *Justin Godart*, introduction.

38 Prost gives a superb introduction to "Le service de Santé militaire pendant la Première Guerre mondiale," in Wieviorka (ed.), *Justin Godart*, 145–56.

39 Under Godart's orders were 21,200 doctors, 3830 pharmacists, 5240 administrative officers, 127,400 male nurses, and 10,000 female nurses, making up the 168,000 personnel of the *Service militaire de Santé*. Usually ignored in accounts: about 113,000 titular stretcher carriers. See Léon Murard and Patrick Zylberman, "'Au dessus des individus et des groupements de politique pure' – Justin Godart et la Santé publique," in Wieviorka (ed.), *Justin Godart*, 169–70.

40 Godart's success in improving army surgery was recognized by at least one *Médecin Inspecteur Général*, Toubert. See Murard and Zylberman, in Wieviorka (ed.), *Justin Godart*, 169–90. Of course the system could be overwhelmed, as in April–May 1917 (Chemin des Dames, or the Nivelle offensive), when perhaps up to 100,000 soldiers were wounded in

Along with establishing civilian control of the military medical service, which involved cooperation with most of the medical inspectors (all generals), and making maximum use of civilian doctors, surgeons, and nurses, Godart introduced frontline evacuation hospitals (HOE or *Hôpital d'opération et d'évacuation*), mobile operating "rooms" (the famous "auto-chir"), and mobile x-ray units – the "petites Curies"; he was an early MASH man. In his appointments what counted was competence, not rank.[41] But real civilian control of the military medical decisions did not come until after the "désastre sanitaire" of Nivelle's offensive in April–May 1917, directly attributable to Nivelle's lack of medical preparation for large numbers of casualties along with his keeping top medical officers in ignorance of the planned offensive. Prost argues that the "emancipation" of the *Service de santé militaire* from the control of the general staff through integration was Godart's most important act as head of the service, something that could be done only by a skillful administrator who was also a working politician.[42]

Henri's official military record offers a skeletal account of his military career, but it is probably more accurate than some of the material in Henri's recollections years later.[43] His service during peacetime began in 1892, the year designating the contingent to which he belonged; he passed into the active army reserve in 1896, then into the "territorial army" in 1906, and ended up in its reserve in 1912. His *Conseil de révision* dumped him into the auxiliary service because he weighed over 100 kg, which made him unsuitable for active service. From 1898 Henri said he tried to get classified as a doctor in the active service but failed in spite

2 weeks; with 21 'auto-chir' and 427 surgical teams, the armies could not cope – e.g., on the 16, 17, and 18 April the HOE of Prouilly could operate on only 533 or the 1499 seriously wounded needing care. See Antoine Prost, "Le désastre sanitaire du Chemin des Dames," in Nicolas Offenstadt (ed.), *Le Chemin des Dames. De l'événement à la mémoire* (Paris, 2004), 137–51. There was rivalry between the traditional ambulance formations and the "auto-chir," with the advantages of the latter over the "hippomobile" usually being exaggerated. See Rollin, *Les hôpitaux dans la guerre*, 207. In Albert Martin's ambulance unit at Verdun for the period 28 February–8 April 1916 there were 4118 wounded, 1045 seriously – 245 of the 1045 died; by midnight on 28 February Martin had done 103 major operations. See "Rapport d'Albert Martin sur le fonctionnement intensif de l'ambulance 9/3 sous Verdun," in Martin, *Souvenirs d'un chirurgien de la Grande Guerre*, 205.

[41] André Pascal [HR], *Une dame d'autrefois. La Baronne Mathilde-Henri de Rothschild 1872–1926* (Lausanne, 1946), 287, note 1. Marie Curie, director of the army radiology services, trained radiologists, installed 200 permanent posts behind the lines, and introduced 20 of the "petites Curies." In the years 1917–18 over a million x-rays were taken. Thébaud, *La femme au temps de la guerre de 14*, 92. Murard and Zylberman, in Wieviorka (ed.), *Justin Godart*, 169–90, attribute to Godart the creation of "une chirurgie d'extrême urgence, – les fameuses 'auto-chir', ces ambulances motorisées qui transportaient rapidement le chirurgien vers l'avant."

[42] See Prost, "Le service de Santé militaire," in Wieviorka (ed.), *Justin Godart*, 155, on the decree of 11 May 1917.

[43] Ministère de la Guerre, archives administratives, 6Ye 12774.

of the intervention of several ministers. A large number of his colleagues were in the same situation; even hospital surgeons and professors (including *professeurs agrégés*) would have to be classified as nurses in wartime – something that no doubt pleased regular military doctors. Then a decree authorized a wartime change, allowing the doctors to come up before their *Conseil* again: Henri and others who appealed were then reclassified as *médecins auxilaires de deuxième classe* at the disposition of the ministry of war. So he began the war in October 1914 as "médecin lieutenant" and quickly entered what was his permanent rank, "médecin aide major de 1e classe." His physical condition and health were noted as good shortly before he became gravely ill. His sight was normal; he could ride a bicycle and a horse. He could go on campaign. The report noted his height of 1.71 m but not his weight, which was more than what it should have been: he had been assigned to a session on obesity back in 1893.

The laudatory reports on his service, after observing that this unusual soldier from a famous family was a well-known Paris doctor who spoke English and German, continued by noting his profound medical knowledge and his success in undertaking some delicate missions. One of these missions was to the newly Greek city of Salonica, important in the Allied Mediterranean strategy. In November 1915 the minister of foreign affairs (Briand) and the minister of war (Barthou) sent him to Salonica on a political mission. A military doctor (Kahn) and a military chaplain (Lévy) accompanied him. The mission, billed as military and sanitary in its aims, was minor in the grand scheme of things but not without local importance. The large Jewish community in Salonica (about 61,000 out of a population of 158,000 in 1913) "at this stage was largely for the Central Powers," though the politically connected and militarily mediocre General Maurice Sarrail and French troops soon became a powerful presence in the city. In addition to the importance of military and sanitary issues, there was then the matter of possibly having some impact on Jewish opinion. Perhaps not so far-fetched as it might seem at first glance, for down to the destruction of the Jewish community in World War II, "French remained the language of the cultural elite." Some thousands of Salonica's Jews who emigrated before World War II settled in Paris.[44]

When Henri began service he said he was in good health except for chronic albuminuria (proteinuria), which was a potentially big exception but seems to have been kept under control. Then he was stricken by a serious attack of uremia, which he attributed to an anti-typhoid shot given by André Chantemesse, who used his own famous method of vaccination.[45] In a letter to his commanding officer Henri got more specific in saying that he had a painful case of parenchymatous nephritis. Henri's letter of 7 September 1914 to General Marion stated that the cause might have been fatigue, a chill, or food poisoning – Dr Rothschild could not identify

44 Both quotations from Mark Mazower, *City of Ghosts: Christians, Muslims and Jews, 1430–1950* (London, 2004), 284, 290; see also 377 and 379.

45 "France Adopts Use of Typhoid Vaccine; In United States Army Fever Cases have been Greatly Cut Down by this Method," *The New York Times* (30 July 1911).

the etiology. The long-term consequence was that the future owner of Mouton Rothschild was restricted to Evian mineral water for the rest of his life. As he slowly improved, he got sent to convalesce at Dinard, where he was asked to set up a hospital of 600 beds but given few professional personnel to deal with the wounded arriving from the first battle of the Marne, a bloody clash producing thousands and thousands of casualties during 6–10 September 1914. Henri set up the hospital in the Casino Hotel and paid for the operation himself. In October he had to return to Paris because he was discharged as a result of an administrative error; he presumably should have been on sick leave. After the Salonica mission in 1915, Henri shows up on assignment at the military hospital Val-de-Grâce, where he was given a role in organizing the photographic museum of the *Service de Santé militaire*. He stayed there until May 1916, working in the archives and documents department as well as directing the photography department; he was under the orders of the *Médecin Inspecteur Général* Jacob, head surgeon and director of the hospital.[46] Henri, a keen photographer, was one of the doctors responsible for the publication in 1918 of the eight volumes of the splendid *Iconographie du Musée du Val-de-Grâce*.[47]

In 1916 Henri remained a busy doctor. After he completed an "ambrine mission" (investigating the efficacy of ambrine, a wax-based product, in treating burns), Godart sent him to the Italian front to study the evacuation of the wounded from high snow-covered areas. He met in Udine with the head doctor of the Italian armies and went on to Cortina del Ampezzo (1700 meters) to look at the operation of sled "ambulances" and medical personnel on skis. Back in France, Henri got sent to organize the health service of the civil population of areas of the Oise, the Somme, and the Aisne that the enemy had evacuated. During six months he headed the service from Noyon, which had been under German occupation for much of the war. The hospital in Noyon was run by the religious order of *Saint-Thomas de Villeneuve*. In a devastated zone Henri set up working places for poor unemployed women, clinics for infant feeding and medical care, and saw to the quick evacuation of urgent surgery cases. In 1917, after the French offensive at Malmaison, he became head doctor of the hospital in Soissons, specially organized for the treatment of burns and blister cases. On the day of the offensive, he had to be evacuated to the rear because the hospital was bombarded. At the beginning of 1918 Henri was named head doctor of the big hospital in Caen, which was designated to receive victims of gas attacks as well as burns and blister cases. In October 1918 the GQG sent him to organize a hospital in Laon, chief town in the Aisne, just evacuated by the Germans. Twenty-four hours after his arrival there, the armistice was signed on 11 November 1918. Demobilized in December

---

46 HR, *Une dame d'autrefois*, 276.

47 O. Jacob (ed.), *Iconographie du Muséee du Val-de-Grâce* (8 vols, Paris, 1918); "Archives et documents de guerre du Service de Santé militaire."

1918–January 1919, Henri entered into honorary army rank in 1925, though the formal date for the end of his service was 6 January 1930.[48]

By September 1914, about 400,000 wounded soldiers were already overwhelming the military medical service. The original plan for the *Assistance publique de Paris* to treat only military personnel having contagious diseases, including venereal ones, was abandoned, and by December 1916 there were 2234 wounded soldiers in Paris hospitals. Civilians, including children, were evacuated from hospitals and retirement institutions in order to manage a medical disaster.[49] Seventy surgical beds in Henri's Paris hospital were set up for the severely wounded, with Pierre Delbet as the head surgeon and Pierre Ehrhardt the head doctor. Between 1916 and 1918 Henri supplied to the appropriate organizations the materials necessary for treating burns and blister victims by the new ambrine method, which required gutta-percha and paraffin with the application apparatuses. Henri said he supplied half a million kilograms of ambrine between June 1916 and December 1918. For the last 200,000 kg the *Service de Santé militaire* supplied the paraffin, requisitioned by the ministry of national defense.

A New Method of Treatment for Burns

As a military doctor, Henri plunged again into pre-war work on the treatment of burns. The industrialization–mechanization of the war opened up opportunities for medical research and experimental treatment on a massive scale. Early in 1915 the method used to treat burns was already an advance on that introduced by Nageotte-Wilbouchevitch a few years earlier: the burn was first cleaned with a solution of hot water and peroxide (1/10 of the solution) and the surrounding integuments sterilized with alcohol or ether; then sterilized strips of taffeta were used to cover the wound; the dressing was changed daily. The advantage of the taffeta was that it came off the burnt area easily, thus providing a solution to the twin problem of pain and bleeding.

In May 1916 the dramatist Pierre Wolff (1865–1944) came to lunch chez Henri and Mathilde and told them an amazing story about a continuing medical miracle he had seen at the hospital in Issy-les-Moulineaux (suburb, southwest of Paris). Dr Jean-Marie Barthe de Sandfort, former navy doctor and an expert on mud baths and on thermal therapy at Dax in the Landes, claimed to have achieved a striking

48 *Who's Who in France. Dictionnaire biographique XX*e *siècle* (Paris, 2001) notes that Henri became sick from being vaccinated against typhoid fever, that he financed a military hospital in Dinard, and that in 1917 he was the head doctor of the hospital in Soissons. See HR, *La Lignée*, 127–30.

49 Rollin, "Les hôpitaux parisiens au coeur de la Grande Guerre," in *Les hôpitaux dans la guerre*, 20.

improvement in the treatment of burns.[50] Unlike an intrigued Mathilde, Henri, an expert on the treatment of burns, relegated the whole business to the category of charlatanism and refused to accompany them on a visit. A few days later other people brought up the subject again. So Henri asked Jacob for permission to check out the tale. Having already heard the tale, Jacob delegated Henri to investigate.

When Henri visited the military hospital of Issy-les-Moulineaux, he was surprised by the procedure and the therapeutic results obtained. Barthe de Sandfort was treating serious burns by applying a kind of translucent wax he called ambrine. The liquefied product was applied at seventy degrees centigrade over the burn by a brush or a pulverizing gadget. Then a thin piece of cotton wool saturated with ambrine was applied to the waxed burn. A layer of cotton covered the whole thing and was kept in place by strips of talatan. The dressing was flexible at body temperature. After twenty-four hours the dressing was replaced. The first striking result was that the procedure stopped pain. More important in the long run, the burn healed rapidly without leaving disfiguring scars of fibrous tissue and keloids.[51] Henri found it most astounding that the bandage could be easily removed. Presumably there was an antiseptic treatment of the wound, though Henri's general account does not mention a specific procedure or the new Carrel–Dakin treatment, a method of intermittent wound irrigation with Dakin's germicidal solution.[52] Carrel's method was soon replaced by that of Henri Gaudier, who introduced the technique of cutting out tissue, followed by closing and suturing the wound.[53] After reporting back to Jacob, Henri got permission to spend a month at Issy-les-Moulineaux studying the new burns treatment, in the hope of finding out how the wax worked and, a more delicate matter, exactly what the new substance was.

After three weeks Henri returned to *Val-de-Grâce*, where he was given a number of serious burns patients to treat with ambrine. A successful experiment led Jacob to send to Godart a report including a request for the use of ambrine on a vast scale. Meanwhile Barthe de Sandfort was not standing idly by: he invited Raymond Poincaré, the French president, to see the results of his treatment of burns victims at various stages of healing. Poincaré asked Godart to go see this remarkable mini-Lourdes in operation. After his visit to Issy-les-Moulineaux, Godart decided to use the ambrine method in all army medical units. But Barthe de

---

[50] See J.-M. Barthe de Sandfort, *Dax pittoresque et thermal; guide du médecin et du malade* (Paris, 1885) and *Guide du touriste et du malade* (Dax, 1886).

[51] Barthe de Sandfort, *Traitement des brûlures par la méthode du Dr Barthe de Sandfort; instructions pratiques pour l'application de l'ambrine* (Paris, 1916). He got coverage in *The New York Times* (19 April 1914) for his proposed cure of rheumatism, arthritis, and many other afflictions: immersion in a vat of wax at 120 degrees F; he demonstrated the near panacea himself.

[52] A. Carrel *et al*, "Traitement abortif de l'infection des plaies," *Bulletin de l'Académie de Médecine* 74 (3d series, 1915), 74: 361–8; H. D. Dakin also published the news in the *British Medical Journal* 2 (1915): 318–20.

[53] Guy Grenier, *100 ans de médecine francophone* (Québec, 2002), 158.

Sandfort insisted on keeping his formula and method of manufacture a secret. An indignant Godart asked Henri to deal with the refractory inventor, who was now suspected of degenerating into a potential war profiteer. Henri was just the person to handle this case, though at his own expense: he paid Barthe de Sandfort a lump sum and promised him ten percent on sales of ambrine after the war. Although "intractable and obstinate," Barthe de Sandfort had little choice because Henri had gotten all of the technical information about the product from Auguste Béhal, organic chemist, dean of the faculty of pharmacy in Paris, and director of the wartime department responsible for the organization of the production of chemical products. It turned out that the rare Far Eastern substances which supposedly entered into the manufacture of ambrine were limited to gutta-percha, which was dissolved in paraffin. Perhaps Barthe de Sandfort used latex from the Malaysian Palaquium Payena or some other Asian tree. The blending process had to be done at the temperature of dissolution of gutta-percha, 140 degrees centigrade. Paraffin melts at seventy degrees but burns in air at about 100 degrees; so the process had to be done in a closed autoclave. Producing large amounts would require a substantial investment.

Henri set up a factory, directed by Valensi, the pharmacist of his Marcadet polyclinic, to manufacture free ambrine for the army. He had earlier promised Godart that he would provide without cost to the state as much of the product as needed. Godart sent Henri to the GQG with the mission of teaching the new method of treating burns to doctors on the front; the *Médecin Inspecteur Général* Sieur expanded this task to ambulances, including evacuation hospitals. Henri began his routine of lecture and demonstration at Dunkerque and finished a year later in Elsaß, once again named Alsace. He published his lecture as an illustrated volume of 150 pages and then expanded the work to over 300 pages.[54] A leading expert on the treatment of burns, he brought out a major clinical and therapeutic work on the subject; Maurice Letulle, professor and pathologist, wrote an introduction.[55]

Those who survived the slaughter could look back later in appreciation of the work they did: Henri remembered working on the wounded under bombardment by German planes and in the tumult of gunfire and artillery barrages. He also marveled that his early experience in helping to treat patients at the Lariboisière hospital was a prelude to his war work, especially teaching fellow doctors the new way to treat burns. The medical story of the day about ambrine was that it worked

[54] HR, *Le Traitement des brûlures par la méthode cirique*. "Conférences faites à MM. Les médecins-majors des formations sanitaires des armies (mission du GQG)." See note 55 following.

[55] HR, *Traité des brûlures. Etude clinique et thérapeutique* (Paris, 1919). "Préface et étude histo-pathogénique, par le professeur Maurice Letulle." Letulle (1853–1929) was one of the big names in medicine in Paris: winner of the gold medal as intern, a member of the Academy of Medicine, Commander in the Legion of Honor, founder of the museum and library at the Boucicault hospital, he pioneered in the pathological anatomy of pulmonary sclerosis and played a leading role in the fight against TB and alcoholism.

miracles. I have seen no patient narrative casting doubt on the treatment; nor have I seen one confirming the medical miracle.

After the armistice (11 November 1918), Mathilde established a special department at Henri's polyclinic in Paris for the treatment of burns. There were few patients, though on several occasions the unit was useful. The wife of the French ambassador in "Russia," back in Paris in 1920, seriously burned her chest and arms by spilling a container of boiling water while she was in bed. The ambrine treatment gave her immediate relief and her burns healed without scars after about two weeks. Henri treated a more famous patient in 1923. Sarah Bernhardt was suffering from lumbar pruritus after an operation; her pain disappeared after the ambrine treatment. Like many medical treatments, the use of ambrine faded away, replaced by other substances and procedures. Ambrine still shows up on the Internet, though, as a wax made of resin mixed with paraffin.

The principle of ambrine treatment still underlay the procedure developed by Oliver Cope to treat victims of the Cocoanut Grove fire of 1942 in Boston: replacement of "the standard cleaning and débridement with ointment and protective dressing."[56] With that fire and World War II, medical discourse and practice changed as physicians faced "the imposing physiologic problems presented by the surgical care of burn patients" and "care during the shock phase." And "a burned patient's metabolic needs based on the amount of body surface burned" had to be estimated. Calculating accurately "the nature of the change in capillary lymphatic permeability produced by burn injury … became the basis for early supportive therapy with fluids and plasma for patients with severe burns."[57] More recently, a "revolution in burn wound care has been brought about by effective topical antimicrobial chemotherapy, early burn wound excision, and the development and use of effective skin substitutes."[58] These developments now make the ambrine treatment appear more miraculous than it did in 1916, but this is a type of common historical problem in trying to understand older therapies accepted by the medical profession but which we reject or at least regard as improbable.

---

[56] Review of John C. Esposito, *Fire in the Grove: The Cocoanut Grove Tragedy and its Aftermath* (Cambridge, Mass., 2005), by the editors in *Bulletin of the History of Medicine* 80 (2006): 610. A. S. Blumgarten, *Textbook of Materia Medica* (4th edn, completely revised, New York, 1927), 62–3, 139–40, gives much attention to Dakin's solution and the Dakin–Carrel method of the treatment of wounds, but he mentions only surgical or plastic paraffin as an excellent local application for burns because it excludes the air and coats the burn with a fine film that allows the growth of new tissue.

[57] "Memorial Minute: Oliver Cope 1902–1994," *The Harvard Gazette* (20 February 1997).

[58] Basil A. Pruitt, "Combat Casualty Care and Surgical Progress," *Annals of Surgery* (June 2006), 243: 715–29. For the career of a military surgeon (1872–1942), especially his experience in the Great War, see Prosper Viguier, *Un chirurgien de la grande guerre*, "présentation de Rémy Cazals" (Toulouse, 2007); see also Martin, *Souvenirs d'un chirurgien de la Grande Guerre*.

During the war basic foods and goods were in short supply and available only at high prices if at all. Henri proposed establishing a model dairy to furnish free milk to the military health personnel of Noyon and the sick they were caring for. There is no record of anything having come of it except a request from the medical inspector general to the general commandant of the third army. Henri's exalted title at this point was *Médecin Aide-Major, officier de liaison pour le Service Sanitaire civil des régions libérées*.[59] Noyon seems to have occupied a special place in Rothschild concerns during the war. Henri's papers contain dozens of documents on items sent in 1917 from the family enclave at 33 rue du Faubourg Saint-Honoré to Madame B. Aillon and others in Noyon. These items included clothing and household goods.[60] Corise, Henri's cousin, did her bit for military hospitals during the war. This included writing to tell him what things were needed to make hospitals function usefully. She emphasized the need for animal and agricultural products as well as medical supplies, including ambrine desperately needed by nurses for treating burns.[61]

After the war was over, helping wounded soldiers was to a great extent the responsibility of private organizations, though in France, unlike in Britain, there was "a robust veterans' movement" of "roughly 4 million men, or half of those who served."[62] Reminder of the score card for France: 1,400,000 dead, mostly young men, leaving about 680,000 widows (630,000, in some sources) and 760,000 "orphans" – children who lost their fathers – and more than 600,000 descendants with no support.[63] The number of French wounded has been conservatively estimated at about 1,100,000 with about 400,000 disabled. Sophie Delaporte's figures, published in 1996, indicated that out of some 8,000,000 men mobilized, there were 2,800,000 wounded, 300,000 mutilated, and 2,000,000 inflicted with at least 10 percent disability. But in her work published in 2003 she points out "a statistical problem," which can be summed up by admitting that we have to estimate the number of wounded at between 200,000 and 1,000,000 with the number of amputees being somewhere between 50,000 and the unbelievable figure of 800,000.[64] With the introduction of serotherapy to prevent gas gangrene, the need for amputations fell, with the incidence of this infection falling from

59 Q. G. A., le 18 août 1917, in RAL 000/930: 58-1, 172–82.

60 RAL 000/930: 58-1, 214.

61 RAL 000/930: 58-1, 186.

62 Jay Winter, "P vs C. The Still Burning Anger when the French Talk of the First World War, " *Times Literary Supplement* (16 June 2006): 3–4. Winter says that the "death toll in France was twice that of Britain's… One in six Frenchmen who served was killed; the figure is one in eight for the British army." Both countries lost a total of two million men (1914–18), four times the figure for World War II.

63 Pierre Guillaume, *Le rôle social du médecin depuis deux siècles 1800–1945* (Paris, 1996), 145.

64 Sophie Delaporte, *Gueules cassées de la Grande Guerre* (3d edn, Paris, 1996), 17; *Les médecins dans la Grande Guerre 1914–1918*.

16/100 to 4/100 among the "grands blessés des membres."[65] About 11 to 14 percent (10,000 to 15,000) soldiers were seriously wounded in the face – "les gueules cassées."[66] Some people who could afford to do so devoted the rest of their lives, or at least some years, to works of devotion and charity, whose ambitious aim was the "regeneration" of survivors of the trip back on the "ghost road."[67]

Marthe Brandès, who had played the first French Hedda Gabbler at the Vaudeville theater in December 1891 and was one of Henri's favorite actresses, left the stage for good in order to serve charitable organizations providing aid for wounded veterans. During a period of 8 years she headed an organization helping blind veterans (*L'Abri du Soldat Aveugle*) and then the soldiers who had been gassed and suffered from tuberculosis (*Les Amis des Blessés du Poumon*), of whom there were about 200,000.[68] Maurice Letulle was president of this organization, and Henri was its treasurer.[69] Nervous or mental effects of war on soldiers were certainly recognized though, as in the case of veterans of the last American war on Iraq, not at all adequately dealt with. Henri did his bit with the gift of his château and vegetable garden of four hectares in Arnouville (Seine) for these "blessés nerveux"; Justin Godart, omnipresent, became the honorary president of the group. Hundreds of veterans' associations targeting specific groups like railway workers or even political groups came into existence, totaling eventually over 3,000,000 members, with a *Confédération nationale* established in 1927.[70]

---

65 *Le Livre d'or des médecins morts pour la France*, 74. Jean-Jacques Schneider, *Le Service de Santé de l'armée française. Verdun 1916* (Metz, 2007), 16, says that 50 percent of the amputations and permanent handicaps could have been avoided. Schneider's work is a good source for figures (official statistics) on casualties, widows, orphans, and much more.

66 Delaporte, *Gueules cassées*, 33. The fine film *La chambre des officiers* (2001), directed by François Dupeyron, is about the experience of one of the "grands blessés de la face."

67 See the Great War trilogy by Pat Barker: *Regeneration* (1991), *The Eye in the Road* (1993), and *The Ghost Road* (1995), available in Plume (Penguin) editions.

68 In 1922 Godart judged France to be sick because of alcoholism and tuberculosis, the latter disease infecting 22.5/100,000 inhabitants, compared with 11/100,000 in England and Germany. Murard and Zylberman, in Wieviorka (ed.), *Justin Godart*, 170.

69 RAL 000/930: 58-1, 172–82. Letulle, an expert on tuberculosis, went along with Wallace C. Sabine on a mission for the Rockefeller Foundation to visit Parisian facilities for tuberculosis patients at the end of World War I. Maurice Lazard, secretary to Henri, also went along.

70 See the classic work by Antoine Prost, *Les anciens combatants et la société française 1914–1939* (3 vols, Paris, 1977). 1: Histoire; 2: Sociologie; 3: Mentalités et ideologies. Schneider, *Le Service de Santé*, 12–13, gives the official figures on the wounded. In 1918 the ministry of war gave invalid pensions to 2,000,000 wounded and 300,000 "grands invalides." The list of invalids included 56,000 amputees, 2585 blind, 4338 deaf, 14,502 mental cases, 15,000 *gueules cassées* ("*les baveux*"), and 65,000 *mutilés fonctionnels*, meaning having one or more dysfunctional organs.

Mathilde de Rothschild (la baronne Henri) in la Grande Guerre

Mathilde's war service interacted with Henri's in the development of the ambrine treatment of burns, but she also had a worthy individual medical service record. In her *Memories of the Great War* Thérèse devoted a short chapter to the hospital works of her daughter-in-law at the front.[71] Installed in Chantilly-Gouvieux, Thérèse could easily travel to her hospital in Gouvieux, which was about four km away from her residence. After early in 1918 she could also keep in touch with Mathilde, then in Aumont. Mathilde resembled many other society ladies who wanted to help care for the wounded but found themselves without formal medical qualifications. There were about 70,000 of these volunteers trained by the Red Cross societies. The *Société de secours aux blessés militaires*, according to Yvonne Knibiehler, also ran a diploma mill to deal with some of the estimated half a million women who joined the 6000 professional personnel in the war. Relations were not always smooth between the "femmes du peuple" and the *bourgeoises* and *aristocrates*.[72] Women like *les baronnes* James and Henri never mentioned this in their memoirs. Mathilde underwent some basic training for nurses and was soon armed with a *diplôme d'infirmière-major* in auxiliary hospital no. 21, Henri's polyclinic in Paris. There is no record that she made a nuisance of herself; quite to the contrary. Doctors complained when some of the women tried to exercise the same authority in their volunteer army medical work as they did in civilian society.[73] Mathilde's situation was unique: she had married into a family famous for its medical charity, and her husband was an army doctor. She soon became competent, useful, and, inevitably, well known in her new job.

Mathilde went with Pierre Wolff to see the results of Barthe de Sandfort's treatment of burns in May 1916. Her enthusiastic approval of what she saw led her to follow a course of instruction for a few weeks at the hospital in Issy-les-Moulineaux. A friend of Wolff's, Madame Van Cleef (the wife of the jeweler) also did the course. In June Mathilde went to see Godart with a tempting proposition. At her expense, she would organize, in cooperation with the *Service de Santé Militaire*, a hospital for the treatment of 250 burned and gassed soldiers, who would even be collected on the battlefield by her organization's ambulances. The great drawback

---

71 Thérèse de Rothschild, *Souvenirs de la Grande Guerre*, chapter 9.

72 Yvonne Knibiehler and others, *Cornettes et blouses blanches. Les Infirmières dans la société française 1880–1980* (Paris, 1984); between 1914 and 1920 the SSBM delivered 10,865 diplomas, taking either two or six months for two levels of training.

73 On nurses in the Great War see Darrow, *French Women and the First World War*, chapter 5, "White Angels of the Battlefield," and Margaret R. Higonnet (ed.), *Nurses at the Front. Writing the Wounds of the Great War* (Boston, 2001). In his play *Le plus grand amour* (Paris, 1920), 7, Henri (André Pascal) takes unfavorable note of women who did not do their bit in the war: Madame Morange says of Louise de Rouves "Elle s'est beaucoup dépensée pendant la guerre, mais ce n'était ni dans les hôpitaux ni dans les ambulances du front… "

in the treatment was organizational, not therapeutic. Wounded soldiers arrived too late at hospitals. It was probably Godart who had recommended the proven practice of the field hospital, adapted to special circumstances. If Godart gave his approval, personnel and some materiel would come from Henri's polyclinic. Henri would also supply the ambrine. Godart would have to supply beds, linen, furniture, household items, and drugs, as well as inform the GQG that Mathilde's group was an "official formation" with a specific mission. Godart was happy to give his consent for the establishment of the *Mission de l'Ambrine* at Compiègne.[74] Henri proudly noted that the woman who had been his companion for nearly 32 years sometimes went in an ambulance to the battlefield to treat wounded soldiers.

In May 1916 she was given formal rank as an army nurse (*Infirmière major*), attached to the French second army, which was under the command of Nivelle before his promotion to military commander in chief – his personal "Waterloo" would be the second battle of the Aisne in April 1917. With the approval of the GQG, she opened her Compiègne hospital in the convent of the *Assumption des Petites Soeurs des Pauvres*. Godart had agreed (or perhaps had even proposed) that she choose her own staff with herself as head, which she did. Madame Van Cleef became her indispensable collaborator as an army nurse in a hospital that soon expanded from 50 to 250 beds and moved to the *Orangerie de Compiègne*. Mathilde found Van Cleef to be a charming woman admired by everyone for her devotion to duty. To please the GQG, a young doctor (Ribaud) was assigned the agreeable task of being the head of the *Mission de l'Ambrine*. Godart visited the hospital several times and expressed his admiration for the work being done. The commander-in-chief of the French army also paid visits to award medals to soldiers, and he too could not help being amazed at the success of the treatment of burns with ambrine. Many French and foreign military and civilian doctors also came to become familiar with the new method.

While at Compiègne, Mathilde was fortunate in being able to get help from the American Elsie Anderson De Wolfe. In 1916 De Wolfe had spent four months at the St. Nicholas hospital in Issy-les-Moulineaux, where she saw the efficacy of Barthe de Sandfort's ambrine treatment. Returning to New York, she went on to raise money in large American and Canadian cities to establish dressing stations at the front and to buy vehicles to use as ambulances. In August 1914 there had been only eight ambulances for each army corps. Back in France, she spread the ambrine gospel in the hospitals of the American Red Cross. Accepting Mathilde's invitation to work at Compiègne, De Wolfe brought with her six Ford ambulances, which went right up to advance posts on the firing line to give first aid, select patients for treatment, and transport them to medical centers. (At Le Cercueil, in Meurthe et Moselle, 2000 patients were culled, cared for, and sent off to centers.) De Wolfe, following Mathilde's group when it evacuated to Aumont, ended up with the French tenth army, which in the summer of 1918 was placed under the command of the recalled Charles Mangin, flattered as "the butcher" and

[74] HR, *Une dame d'autrefois*, 286–8.

"le broyeur de noir" because of his eagerness to use Africans as cannon fodder in his notorious strategy of "guerre à outrance."

In July 1917, after the failure of the earlier Nivelle offensive, German bombardment forced a chaotic evacuation of Compiègne, with a scared population fleeing through its famous forest. A shell falling on the operating room of the *Mission de l'Ambrine* along with some further damage made it imperative to evacuate buildings. But the GQG had other things to think about. Fortunately on the second night of the attack an order was brought by General Clives, English liaison officer at the GQG, to evacuate the town with all the wounded. A train took the most serious of the 250 cases and others took ambulances and trucks in the direction of Villers-Cotterêts, towards the northeast of Paris. Mathilde had met Clives at Thérèse's summer place when the GQG was in Chantilly, and he had visited her ambrine operation several times. After 8 difficult days, when the family had no news of Mathilde and the group, the evacuees arrived at the bishop's palace in Meaux, 66 km from Compiègne and only 53 km from Paris. Much of Compiègne was destroyed, including the hospital where Alexis Carrel had done pioneer work on wound irrigation and had established a prototype of a frontline research facility.[75] "The krauts (*les boches*) are near Noyon,"[76] Mathilde lamented. It was a relief to get to Meaux, where the garden of the bishop's palace offered a bit of peace in the midst of disaster. She requested an audience with the bishop (Monseigneur Marbeau), who gave her a small cross he had blessed. She attended vespers, met a few friends, and relished a few hours of silent reflection before going on to Aumont. The banker Moïse de Camondo had turned the Château d'Aumont over to the army. Camondo's son Nissim died in aerial combat in 1917.[77]

Mathilde and her staff set up the new burns treatment facility at the Château d'Aumont, located between Senlis and Creil. They stayed there, not until the end of the great slaughter but until 1 December 1917, when the military ended Mathilde's "mission," two and a half years after she had left Paris to organize the unit. The wounded, far fewer in number, could easily be treated in the hospitals of Paris.

The state rewarded her leadership in the evacuation and reorganization of the burns treatment facility with the *croix de guerre* and the red ribbon of chevalier in the *Légion d'honneur*. Madame Van Cleef and Dr Ribaud also received these decorations. (Mathilde received two other decorations (*Médaille des Epidémies* and the *Brisques* or *Chevrons*) for her three years of medical work, nearly all in the war zone.) In going to rescue wounded soldiers on the battlefield, the trio came under fire but luckily escaped without physical damage. General Brissaud-Desmaillets, commander of the *Division bleue* or *L'Alsacienne* granted Mathilde's

[75] See Basil A. Pruitt, "Combat Casualty Care and Surgical Progress," *Annals of Surgery* 243/6 (June 2006): 715–29.

[76] HR, *Une dame d'autrefois*, 286.

[77] Camondo gave his furnished mansion and collection of eighteenth-century art to the *Union centrale des Arts Décoratifs* in Nissim's memory. The *Musée Nissim de Camondo* is in the Monceau quarter of Paris.

request to be designated as "godmother" of the division of the Blue Devils (*les diables bleus*). The general was proud to present decorations after the medical team faced heavy machine gun fire in driving twice onto the battlefield in their ambulances to rescue wounded *diables bleus*.[78] Mathilde gave herself a final reward. General Mangin, then head of the tenth army, permitted her to go along and relish the retreat of *les boches* as the French captured Laon, Nancy, Metz, and Straßburg. Her campaign ended in sad triumph, with any "hymn to the future" being a footnote to the "remembering of the dead."[79]

[78] HR, *Une dame d'autrefois*, 294–5.

[79] HR, *Une dame d'autrefois*, 294–5.

PART II
Rothschild's Hippocratic Theater

Chapter 8
The Doctor-Playwright

....For social history – for the history of culture, for the history of people's understanding of their own society – fiction occupies a privileged position.[1]

The *Journal 1887–1910* of Jules Renard (1864–1910), creator of the immortal Poil de Carotte, has long titillated the literary mind; it can also enlighten the historian of medicine, as Jacques Léonard showed in an essay analyzing what the journal tells us about French personal hygiene and even the beliefs and practices of doctors.[2] Some other perceptive historians like Roy Porter have enjoyed mining literary classics to illustrate the tributaries of medical history. Henri de Rothschild's literary output has not achieved the status of Jules Romains' *Knock ou le triomphe de la médecine* (1923) or even Shaw's *The Doctor's Dilemma* (1906), though some of his plays achieved a certain notoriety in their day and certainly an analysis of his "medical plays" is not without interest and significance in the historical development of twentieth-century medicine.

Although in recent years a few plays dealing with scientists, doctors, and even mathematicians have enjoyed success on the stage, it is difficult for us to grasp the popularity of plays about doctors in late nineteenth-century and early twentieth-century Paris.[3] François de Curel (1845–1929), a successful playwright, rich and secure on his estate in the Lorraine, remarked that because so many medical plays were on the Paris stage, a director friend of his was driven to refuse any play with a doctor in it. Diseases, remedies, and doctors (male and female) had been on the stage long enough, according to Curel's friend; it was time to move on to other subjects. Of course it would be difficult to get too serious about this, if it meant ignoring the plays of Aeschyles, Euripides, Sophocles, Shakespeare, Ibsen, Hauptmann, Gorki – just to name a few thespian monuments – all of whom found illness to be a vital dramatic subject. Often authors did not fully know what they were writing about until enlightened by medical experts. Curel registered

---

1 Keith Hopkins, cited in G. W. Bowersock, *Fiction as History. Nero to Julian* (Berkeley, 1994), ix.

2 Jacques Léonard, "Les soins corporals d'après le Journal de Jules Renard (1887–1910)," in *Médecins, maladies et société dans la France du XIXe siècle* (Paris, 1992), 261–73.

3 Paul Descoust, *La médecine au théâtre dans les temps modernes* (2d edn, Paris, 1906); see also François Helme, *Les Jardins de la médecine* (Paris, 1907), 181–94: "Le théâtre contemporain et la profession médicale – à propos de 'La nouvelle idole' de M. François de Curel." For literature in general rather than the theater, see Jean-Paul Thomas, *La plume et le scapel. La médecine au prisme de la littérature* (Paris, 2008).

surprise that Dr Paul Descoust recognized his play *La nouvelle idole* (1919) as a work in "medical jurisprudence"; Curel thought his play was only accidentally medical, the real subject being the capability of science, faith, and love to lead souls to the same high destination. This was a denial of the death of religion, killed by science, as well as of the thesis of the moral bankruptcy of science.[4] But to symbolize science Curel chose a doctor; though few doctors were really scientists, he argued that people believed in the miraculous powers of doctors as healers, much as primitive peoples accepted their sorcerer-healers. Another doctor pointed out that contemporary theater no longer considered the doctor as another piece of scenery but as a social power, the priest of the new religion, science, which was pretty much Curel's view. Doctors who commented on the play were grateful that Curel was not hostile to them; they found that most of the plays dealing with doctors were not favorably disposed to the medical profession. Since they also believed that the theater is a mirror of society, the image presented in the theater reflected the hostility to the profession of at least a substantial part of society; of course, this sociological fact gave hope, to Descoust at least, that the theater could also serve as a useful educational and even reforming instrument for the medical education of the masses.[5] Given the interest of people in popular science and medical issues, Curel noted that if his friend the director kept doctors off the stage, he risked having no more plays to put on.[6]

The New Idol may be Curel's masterpiece, as Lanson's classic history of French literature claims, but like many serious plays bristling with ideas, it has not enjoyed the stage life of some monuments of boulevard mediocrity.[7] The media attention given to recent unethical developments in medicine may change its representational history.[8] On a general level, according to Descoust, the play deals with two contemporary hot subjects in medical jurisprudence: the right of a doctor to experiment on a living subject and the right of a practitioner to have full liberty in hypnotizing a subject.[9] The drama is found in the experience of a young patient

---

4 See Jacqueline Lalouette, *La République anticléricale* (Paris, 2002).

5 Helme, *Les Jardins de la médecine*, 183, 181–94 (on Curel's play); see Descoust, *La médecine au théâtre*, 7–8, and part II on the plays of Zola, Brieux, and Louis Bruyerre tending to be educational and reform minded.

6 François de Curel, preface to Descoust, *La médecine au théâtre*, no pagination for preface.

7 G. Lanson, *Histoire de la Littérature française* (Paris, 1966), 1170–2. *La nouvelle idole* opened at the Antoine theater in March 1899 and had a run at the Comédie Française in June 1914.

8 See, e.g., Marcia Angell, "Drug Companies & Doctors: A Story of Corruption," *The New York Review of Books* LVI (15 Jan. 2009): 8–12. Criticism and Angell's effective reply are in the issue for 26 Feb. 2009: 45.

9 Descoust, *La médecine au théâtre*, 120–7. In Georges Duhamel, *Les Maîtres* (Paris, 1937), 178, professor Rohner refers to "the absurd laws" forbidding experiments on humans.

(Antoinette), who is supposed to die soon from tuberculosis – all the doctors who have seen her agree with this grim prognosis – and therefore appears to be a good subject in an experiment to produce a vaccine against cancer. Dr Albert Donnat, a brilliant Paris professor, injects cancer cells into the doomed orphan patient without anyone's consent. She is cured of the TB but the cancer soon takes over the role of killer. An added item of contemporary debate is introduced when it is revealed that she has been secretly drinking a little water from Lourdes every day. An excited press refers to fifteen to thirty patients who have been victims of Donnat's medical experiments; students get ready to kick up a fuss, and the dean asks Donnat to take a holiday. Of course there will also be legal consequences. His career is finished. Madame Donnat learns about Antoinette and arranges with the convent where she lives for the child to move into her household. She soon gets over her anger at her husband and also decides not to leave him for his friend the psychologist-hypnotist, who is in love with her. Antoinette figures out what Donnat did to her, forgives him, even boasting she is happy to sacrifice herself for the possible benefit of future victims of cancer – on a minor scale, she is imitating Jesus Christ. She also guesses that Donnat has injected himself as a guinea pig; both doctor and patient are sacrificed to the new idol. Commentators were grateful that the dangers of an occurrence of this sort of experimentation were less in France than in Germany and across the channel – a cultural prejudice not clearly explained by either Descoust or by François Helme, who also took a serious interest in Curel's play. Helme noted that much of the criticism of the medical profession came from doctors themselves. In his medical plays, Henri de Rothschild was sometimes accused of lese-majesty against his fellow doctors.

With thirty-eight plays to his credit, all of which, except one small item, hit the stage, André Pascal (the most common literary pseudonym of Henri de Rothschild) had a good claim to be a professional playwright. Henri described his productions as "works of psychology and observation." His first play was a one-act piece, *Le Secret professionnel*, put on for the *Congrès de la Tuberculose* in 1905 at the Châtelet by André Antoine, creator of the *Théâtre Libre* and advocate of a realist "slice of life" approach to the theater.[10] The play dealt with a topic much discussed in the medical world in the late nineteenth–early twentieth centuries: the professional (medical) secret. (I have not read a printed copy of this hard-to-find play but the undated typescript in The Rothschild Archive in London.) Karl des Fontaines is the quasi-Teutonic pseudonym Henri adopted for this effort.[11] *Le Secret professionnel* opens in the consulting room of Dr Paul Dupont, a famous specialist for nervous diseases. One thinks of Henri's friendship with Alfred Fournier, rival of Charcot: given the failure of the doctor in the play, it is tempting to suppose that the target was Charcot rather than Fournier. The professional secret is that the chauffeur of the woman the doctor's brother is about to marry has epilepsy. She

[10] René Peter, *Le Théâtre et la vie sous la Troisième République. Première Epoque* (Paris, 1945), 200.

[11] Karl des Fontaines, "Le secret professionnel," RAL 000/930: 58-1, 151.

dies in an accident right after the chauffeur gets the diagnosis from the doctor, who generously agrees to keep the secret while the chauffeur looks for another job. The suspicious fiancé-brother fails to get the doctor to reveal the diagnosis but he accuses him of killing Charlotte, his fiancée. It does not seem that this piece of corny melodrama enjoyed much success. It showed promise. Between 1906 and 1924 ten of Henri's plays went into production, nicely subsidized by the author. And he was the first author to make a major success out of putting the woman doctor on the Paris stage.[12]

Adrien Hébrard, the wealthy owner-editor of *Le Temps*, told Henri to stick to two subjects for his plays, both based in the real world he knew, namely the lives of doctors and rich people. The categories of physician and rich man, sometimes overlapping, are broad enough to allow the dramatist a pretty free rein. It is useful to keep in mind that in the evolution of the stage itself the director had "become one of the most powerful forces for renewal in the theater." Along with the emergence of this new force, one can detect a "shift away from theater conceived primarily as an aesthetic manifestation towards a more socially-motivated conception of the theater's role." [13] This is not to say that the so-called "boulevard theater" disappeared; far from it: the situation signaled by the immortal words "Ciel, mon mari" continued to keep people amused and filled the theaters, in spite of the intellectual and dramatic exhaustion of the genre.[14] Some writers see Henry Bernstein's plays as "the essence of the psychological, bourgeois, and boulevardier, rich, and necessarily popular theater in contrast to the art theater, necessarily poor and pure; for some people, it [Bernstein's theater] was [an example of] 'Jewified' (*enjuivé*) theater that had dominated the French scene since the dawn of the twentieth century."[15] The dueling Bernstein was a friend of Henri's and often encouraged his thespian efforts. The scientific and medical subject matter of some of Henri's plays, though hardly Shavian in emphasis or impact, can be seen as part of the move of the theater to assume a more socially responsible role. Of course the French theater produced *Knock* (1924; without a dissertation as preface), not *The Doctor's Dilemma* (1913). Still, we can say that two of the most famous plays

---

12 "André Pascal" for M. Pierre Plessis in the program for *La Vocation*, 1926–27 season. Staging by Jacques Baumer. Arsenal, Rf. 71.727.

13 David Whitton, *Stage Directors in Modern France* (Manchester, 1987), vii–viii.

14 See Olivier Barrot and Raymond Chirat, *"Ciel, mon mari!" Le Théâtre du Boulevard* (Paris, 1998). They note that Marcel Achard ground out a number every year, "light as a song," of course. Brigitte Brunet, *Le Théâtre du Boulevard* (Paris, 2004) lists among the "auteurs de boulevard" Marcel Achard (1899–1974), Jean Anouilh (1910–87), Marcel Aymé (1902–67), Henry Bernstein (1876–1953), Georges Courteline (1858–1929), Georges Feydeau (1862–1921), Robert de Fleurs (1872–1927), and Sacha Guitry (1885–1957).

15 See Georges Bernstein-Gruber and Gilbert Maurin, *Bernstein le magnifique* (Paris, 1988). For nearly eighteen years after 1917 Bernstein directed the Gymnase theater; in 1938 he took over the Ambassadeurs (now the Pierre Cardin theater).

of the first half of the twentieth century dealt with medicine; Henri's medical plays obviously do not fall into the same qualitative category but they were successful in their day and are not without considerable intellectual merit today.

In a preface to his last play, the four-act *Circé*, Henri coolly surveyed a lifetime's critical reception of his theatrical output.[16] Certainly, his thirty-eight plays had received their share of criticism, some of it spiteful and infected with an "irreductible bias": among the epithets thrown at him were "amateur," "mediocrity," and "plagiarist." He did not refer to the anti-Semitic complaint that the theater was being corrupted by Jews, who were as visible in Paris theater as they were in Hollywood filmmaking – and New York theater.[17] Like most successful writers, he shrugged off even the rudest criticism; nor did he allow critics to discourage him in his pursuit of theatrical success or destroy his love for the theater. But he had always been bothered by the suggestion from even friendly colleagues that his plays dealt too frequently with subjects taken from the medical world, even the more restricted area of pathology. He believed that this judgment was false. True, his play about medical ethics, *Le Caducée*, was often regarded as his best play because of its harshness and solid professional basis. And of course with his medical colleague Pierre Delbet he wrote *La Vocation*, another medical play that achieved a healthy notoriety in dealing with the woman doctor. But in between there was *Héritage*, which dealt with a major social problem, without proposing a solution and that may be why it was not so successful as some of his other plays. What the critics forgot in accusing him of being more doctor than playwright in writing plays was an entire repertory, based on the human condition, concerned with character and morals. In plays such as *La Rampe*, *Le Moulin de la Galette*, and *Pour être heureux* Henri claimed that medicine and the man of science had disappeared. In order to show his colleagues that he had made a clean break with medical subjects, he eventually looked for a subject in pure psychology, with a play based on "accurate, thoughtful observation."

This agonizing reappraisal must have gone on for some time as he considered different scenarios, carefully assigning them to different files. He finally chose file number three, the *Circé* dossier for which he confessed a strong predilection. Why it completely satisfied his personal tastes was more related to his knowledge of relatives or friends who had fallen into the Circean trap as well as to the construction of the play – how the material he had could be turned into a simple

16 André Pascal, *Circé* (Paris, 1929), I–XIV. The play is dedicated to André Antoine, "qui m'a fait la grande joie d'accepter la direction artistique du théâtre de la rue Pigalle et à mes fils James-Henri et Philippe de Rothschild." The second edition (1939) honored Marthe Régnier.

17 For a development of this idea, see Mary Louise Roberts, *Disruptive Acts. The New Woman in Fin-de-Siècle France* (Chicago, 2002), 10–17. Drumont added journalism to the professions corrupted by Jewish financing and management. Roberts notes that since women were prominent in both occupations, "Jew" and "new woman" were linked in nationalist anti-Semitic fantasies.

work based on life, without too much dependence on imagination or tricks of the thespian trade. In spite of his medical background, he was not tempted to deal in myths or their basis in reality. Circé was, after all, renowned for her knowledge of drugs and herbs, and the bad use she made of them was not unrelated to Henri's view of some unsavory aspects of contemporary medical practice. Anticholinergic intoxication counteracted by the flower snowdrop was not so interesting as the psychological dimension of the myth. So he decided to push the psychological study of his characters to the limit, showing them in action rather than indulging in monologues, which would have had the effect of masking the playwriting trick being used in the plot. He does not say that this approach was also more suitable to the entertainment business that most theater had become.

Bernstein's popular play *Le Voleur*, which opened at the Renaissance theater in December 1906 and had sold over 4000 copies by 1919, had a striking influence on Henri. The second act in particular convinced Henri that Bernstein's stature in the theater had allowed him to introduce a new conception of dramatic art. But this idea also paralyzed Henri because he thought that his play would be seen as an imitation of Bernstein's and therefore fail. So he shelved the manuscript. Henri does not say when he saw *Le Voleur*. Then in 1927 at the Gymnase theater he saw Bernstein's play *Le Vénin*, in which the playwright was even more artistically audacious than in *Le Voleur*.[18] This time Bernstein subjected the spectators to a second act of fifty-five minutes with only two actors. People loved it. Eager to enjoy some of the "Circean poison" himself, Henri returned to *Circé*. After eighteen months of work on the manuscript, he read it to friends, who told him that it was the best thing he had done.

Intent on anchoring his play in real life, Henri explained how the writing of *Circé* was inspired by what happened to a near relative of his on the Côte-d'Azur thirty years before. Believing he was hiring the services of a respectable whore, his relative was tricked into getting into bed with a minor in a classic hotel setup. This business required an expensive hotel, romantic dimness in the rooms, perjury-prone witnesses, and a naïve Rothschild. I suspect that the patsy was Arthur, whose relations with women were inclined to land him in a compromising situation with a Circean demimondaine of the Belle Epoque. A "friendly arrangement" in the presence of a notary got his relative out of danger of press coverage and, presumably, prosecution. The blackmailers earned three quarters of a million francs. Just to show that this example of female business was not an exception, Henri cited another case in which the son of friends of his got into legal hot water in a foreign country when the son's mistress took him to court over his supposed broken promise to marry her. In the legal battle, the family had to pay a bail of three million francs, which was returned when the son was acquitted. Legal expenses were considerable. Henri boasted that he could cite numerous similar examples. Mistresses and demimondaines were not rare in his circle, and some were daughters of Circe.

---

[18] Henry Bernstein, *Le Voleur* (Paris, 1907) and *Le Vénin* (Paris, 1928).

For the playwright hoping for originality there remained the matter of creating a new version of the duped male character. Henri wanted to avoid treating the victims of big-time blackmail as ninnies, as in Feydeau-type vaudeville; rather he thought that if blackmail were to be the pivot of a serious play, the victim had to be upgraded in character, intelligence, and social status, in effect a composite figure evoking three or four different types. So in *Circé* he created Pierre Bourdier, industrialist, financier, and owner-editor of a big newspaper (*L'Impartial*) to shoulder this heavy dramatic burden. Just to be sure that he was on solid psychological ground Henri got two professional opinions on the medical verisimilitude of his creation.

First, a psychiatrist friend, who often read drafts of his plays, assured Henri that his imagination had not led him too far from reality. Quite to the contrary. The friend had several patients resembling Pierre Bourdier. Their behavior was described in terms of frenzy or, more politely, excessive activity and amorous exaltation of a possibly violent and domineering nature, blossoming late in life in the case of males who for social or religious reasons had remained chaste up to their early forties. The psychosis unleashed (by a woman) in the patient could last for months, even years, though it usually disappeared as mysteriously as it had arrived. Another of Henri's medical colleagues who was in charge of a big private asylum in the Paris suburbs gave a similar description of the disease. This colleague noted that the malady usually struck highly intelligent men who were overworked – politicians, scientists, and artists were all vulnerable. The good news was that the affliction was not hereditary or contagious. So it was not farfetched to have Pierre Bourdier fall under the "fierce domination of Lydia Leroy," the Circe of the drama.

After working on *Circé* for two years, Henri had a nasty surprise. In spite of wanting to write a play about a non-medical subject, he found that it was impossible to ignore a lifetime of exposure to medical science and pathology. So once again the doctor became the collaborator of the playwright. Pierre Bourdier can be classified in psychiatric terms as an *obsédé*, suffering from an "erotic psychosis," a type precisely defined in psychiatric literature. B. J. Logre, yet another of Henri's highly placed medical friends, read the manuscript for a new version in 1939 and not only confirmed the fairly widespread nature of the disease but generously identified Henri II and Diane de Poitiers, along with Edward VIII and Wallis Simpson, as examples of the affliction in action. In the preface to the 1939 edition Henri identifies Bourdier as the alias of a high-ranking Parisian personality, a friend who told him his story in exciting detail – this was probably in late 1926 or early 1927.[19] Henri was so struck by the story that he used the material as the basis

---

19 André Pascal, *Circé* (Paris, 1939). Logre was identified by Henri as "an eminent psychiatrist, head doctor of the special infirmary of the *Préfecture de Police*." The preface to this edition was signed on his sixty-seventh birthday, 26 July 1939, at his estate in Lausanne. On obsession, see Jerome Burne, "The Time of the Single Mind," *Times Literary Supplement* (5 June 2009): 25, review of Lennard J. Davis, *Obsession. A History* (Chicago, 2009).

for the play, written in six months. But he was not satisfied with his psychological study, a "rigorous scientific 'dissection'" of Bourdier and Lydia Leroy, though his friends urged him to get it performed.

Looking back from 1939 over his most successful plays, including *La Rampe*, *Le Caducée*, *Le Moulin de la Galette*, and *Le Grand Patron*, Henri included *Circé* in the group of his best plays. He did not mention *La Vocation*, one of his most successful and controversial plays – perhaps the topic of woman doctors seemed unimportant in 1939, though Nazi policy had begun thinning their ranks in the Reich. The other plays were set in milieus of characters whose moral and mental states were unfamiliar to the general public. Though obviously different groups of people would prefer certain plays to others, it would be difficult to find a majority of people voting in favor of one play in particular as the author's best. Henri was convinced that *Circé*, a play that carried the psychological dissection of character to an extreme, could be placed among a handful of his best plays because the psychological study was developed in and by the dramatic action rather than, as in the other plays, by dialogue. Following the advice of "one of the great masters of contemporary theater" (probably Bernstein), Henri did not give the play a happy ending, which would have meant trying to please the public with an "illogical and artificial ending with the characters restored to virtue and happiness." The hero sacrifices wife, children, home, and social position – everything – for Lydia. Nor was Bourdier allowed the luxury of killing himself in order to give the author an easy exit. Instead Henri introduced what he said is a theatrical novelty, "moral suicide … and oblivion." In both versions (1929 and 1939) of the play Bourdier just leaves home, though he has a revolver in his pocket – perhaps just in case the author is wrong.

After rewriting the text twice in three years, he had a new version in 1928, and the play, starring Constant Rémy and Vera Korène, opened for a successful run on 9 March 1929. Critical reception was generally very favorable. Henri, half-satisfied with the play, thought he could improve it. But the 1930s was a difficult decade for him, especially 1936–39, when illness prevented him from working at all. Only in April 1939 could he start writing again, beginning with some small items or booklets and revising *Circé* while waiting for his old energy to return so he could begin a new work. At the same time Vera Korène, then a member of the *Comédie Française*, asked permission to perform the play while on tour. Henri says that she got the third edition, an entirely new work in dialogue and construction, with the old second act and nine characters eliminated. Bourdier was given the age of fifty instead of forty-six and Leroy made thirty years old instead of twenty-six. The principle may have been "the older, the sillier" or, in the case of Bourdier, the sicker if in love. He had no worries about the revised play, for with the looming threat from the Third Reich, a new drama was about to begin for the Rothschilds, with years of exile in Portugal for Henri.

Chapter 9
Doctor-Charlatans in Contemporary Society (Circa 1900)

To fall ill: an old notion that doesn't stand up before the facts of current science.[1]

The term charlatan has fallen from its old pedestal of quasi-respectability into the gutter of pure quackery. The word charlatan entered into French and English from Italian, but charlatans in early modern Italian states practiced the licensed occupation of peddling medicines as well as delivering healthcare ("simple forms of medicine") to a "wide sector of the population." Medical tribunals licensed charlatans in the Kingdom of Naples and the Papal States. Of course they were not doctors, and in 1632 one physician defined them as "people who appear in the square and sell a few things with entertainments and buffoonery." So even if the term is "a constructed category" popular with historians, the degradation of name is not a recent development.[2] Even in the eighteenth century it carried a pejorative patina, though "it was used interchangeably with 'empirique' [empiric] ... for a self-styled physician." Not quite all charlatans "in early modern France were primarily glorified dung peddlers."[3] In 1833 the *Gazette médicale de Paris* published a long and apparently waggish, anonymous defense of general as well as medical charlatanism.[4] Nowadays we may be tempted to think of charlatanism as "the creation of professionalism," excluded from medicine because charlatans are not subjected to medical authority and operate outside the professional rules based on exclusive claims of expertise and objectivity.[5] In 1833 the *Gazette*'s author was not interested in the assessment of medical therapies but in defining charlatanism in a new way as the application of industry to medicine and in praising the great

---

[1] Jules Romains, *Knock* (Paris, 1924), 80.

[2] Quotations and information from David Gentilcore, *Medical Charlatanism in Early Modern Italy* (Oxford and New York, 2006), 1–3.

[3] Matthew Ramsey, *Professional and Popular Medicine in France 1770–1830. The Social World of Medical Practice* (Cambridge, 1988), 133. On *Dreckapotheke* see Harry W. Paul, *Bacchic Medicine. Wine and Alcohol Therapies from Napoleon to the French Paradox* (Amsterdam, 2001), 1–24.

[4] "Du charlatanisme en général et du charlatanisme médical en particulier," *Gazette médicale de Paris* 1 (1833): 713–15.

[5] See Evelleen Richards, "The Politics of Therapeutic Evaluation: The Vitamin C and Cancer Controversy," *Social Studies of Science* 18 (1988): 653–701, and *Vitamin C and Cancer. Medicine or Politics?* (London, 1991).

advantage of "medical industrialism."[6] Making millions from selling a drug is a good thing, for, after all, what medical practitioner could buy a château after only a few years' work? Science is an excellent thing, but without industry it is impotent. Since industry in medicine is what one condemns as charlatanism, the general introduction of the industrial spirit into medicine would cause the prejudice against charlatanism to disappear. Looked at through this linguistic lens, charlatanism becomes a quality worthy of widespread emulation.

In the beginning years of the Bourgeois Monarchy (1830–48), our anonymous commentator saw industry flooding medicine, with the spirit of competition multiplying marvels. Three cheap medical newspapers had appeared, "marking a new era in medical journalism." Without industrialism (charlatanism), science would never have been capable of such an achievement. Not that this medical industrialism was an easy business. Establishing a reputation, creating customers, and opening commercial outlets were all risky, difficult tasks. Here was a spectacle of modernity one had to admire, the charlatan at the top of the wheel of fortune taking pity on the scientist left at the bottom and becoming his protector. Not that the author hoped that everyone would agree with this seemingly perverse argument. The "honest industrials," then numerous in the medical business, would perhaps appreciate this recognition of their "independent genius," which had shown them "the shortest route to fortune." Charlatans were no longer quacks, false pretenders to knowledge, though they were still vendors of medicine. Nor were they itinerants or mountebanks. Pliny the Elder's sally "medicine is an art of the charlatan" had been given an entirely new meaning, announcing the coming triumphs of pharmaceutical products and patent medicines.[7]

Jacques Léonard pointed out that charlatanism was a useful and sometimes amusing treatment adopted by some Belle Epoque doctors in their treatment of difficult hypochondriacs, re-baptized as neurasthenics. In *Knock* (1923) Jules Romains gave a brilliant satirical theatrical treatment of the subject: the hero, Knock, was able to build a flourishing medical empire by convincing an entire rural community that it was sick. "Every well person is a sick person who doesn't know it."[8] In 1911, when there were 25,000 physicians practicing in France, Henri de Rothschild gave a rather long talk on the doctor in contemporary society, a topic that had become of general interest as the public and political roles of the doctor impinged on the daily lives of more and more people.[9] An important part of his

[6] On the evolution of the pharmaceutical industry, see W. F. Bynum, *Science and the Practice of Medicine in the Nineteenth Century* (Cambridge, 1994), 164–8.

[7] "Du charlatanisme en général et du charlatanisme médical en particulier," *Gazette médicale de Paris* 1 (1833): 713–15.

[8] Jacques Léonard, "Le Malade imaginaire de Molière à Jules Romains," in *Médecins, maladies et société dans la France du XIXe siècle* (Paris, 1992), 275–83.

[9] Henri de Rothschild [HR], *Le médecin dans la société contemporaine. Conférence à la salle des agricultureurs le 2 mars 1911* (Paris, 1911). Pamphlet of forty-seven pages.

talk was about what we call "problem doctors." In the year 2000 about 3300 of the 676,000 doctors practicing in the United States had their licenses revoked or restricted by medical boards in the different states and territories. The difficulties of the defrocked doctors ran the gamut of human problems: mental disease, criminal behavior, unethical sex (with patients), stupidity, ignorance, sloppiness, laziness, disorganization, drug abuse, and senility. The position of problem doctors is not desperate: according to the rehabilitation industry, only about 15 percent of them cannot be educationally saved by organizations such as Colorado's Institute for Physician Evaluation.[10] A century ago few people even recognized the existence of such problems in the medical profession, and the subject was hardly treated at all in the Paris Faculty of Medicine, except under the rubric of legal medicine. As dean, Paul Brouardel opened up the faculty to the subject so that students could get a systematic treatment of the principal ethical rules a physician must follow.[11] According to Henri, the subject was more important than ever in the early twentieth century: the new charlatans (real doctors) had arrived.

Chance plays a large role in medicine, as it does in science, and nowhere was this more evident to Henri than in the recruitment of the new model medical army. Entry into a career is often determined by chance: the paternal example – "the country doctor who follows in his father's footsteps" – or family influence in childhood – such as that experienced by Henri himself. Not only personal taste enters into career choice. Why do young people take up medicine? What is the motivation for accepting the burden of this difficult career? Many young people feel an irresistible urge to answer the call to a life of curing the sick. Can one say that most practitioners were born to be doctors? Henri, slightly infected with optimism, said so, though this does not preclude a certain number of persons from becoming doctors just for the money. No reason to hide this bad news. It was a sign of the profession's confidence in itself and also of the public's trust in doctors that Henri could deal with ethical problems outside the Hippocratic confessional. So these greedy doctors turned one of the liberal professions, undoubtedly the noblest of them all, into a real industry. The term medical industry was then shocking to the ideal medical conscience. Sometimes Henri reassured listeners or readers on this potentially alarming issue by declaring that there were only a few black sheep in the medical flock; on other occasions he would change emphasis and even his opinion by asserting that the bad eggs made up too numerous a group to ignore, painful though it was to recognize such people as doctors. This was recognition of the danger of being caught in an illogical position. Why spend so much time on a

[10] Abigail Zuger, "A Program's Goal: Evaluate and Rehabilitate Problem Doctors," *The New York Times* (3 July 2001), D5. The bad doctor pays for his own rehabilitation. Sidney Wolfe, director of the Public Citizen Health Research Group, thinks the program is a good idea but points out that few states have programs for rehabilitation.

[11] See Paul Le Gendre and G. Lepage, *Le Médecin dans la société contemporaine – conférences de déontologie* (Paris, 1902), and P. Le Gendre and H. Ribadeau-Dumas, *La Vie du médecin. Déontologie et jurisprudence médicale* (Paris, 1920).

subject if it was not important? And once he had conceived of malpractice as the subject of a play, it was not easy to deny its importance. The theater is the forum of truth as play.

Henri believed that to take on the subject of the doctor in contemporary society was a vast but doable program. In half a century therapeutic medicine had extended its empire to horizons undreamed of in the mid-nineteenth century. Everyone knew about the revolution in surgery brought about by the application of Pasteurian methods: the patient's probability of dying from infected surgical wounds, puerperal fever, or septicemia had been largely banished by the institutionalization of antisepsis and asepsis. Endoscopy had opened up the body for a non-surgical diagnosis of disease in organs such as the larynx, stomach, and bladder, while radiology had "made surgical diagnosis more rapid and more exact by allowing the surgeon to recognize with absolute certainty the site and nature of the most diverse lesions."[12] No patient was now likely to escape the doctor without being told of his wretched condition. Henri rounded up the usual sciences to explain why medical care had improved, though he does not provide any statistical evidence; the generation that saw the fall in mortality from transmissible diseases and concomitant introduction of vaccines and serums assumed an obvious connection. We can afford to see that the fall in mortality is not so simply explained and allow ourselves a certain luxury of doubt. For the doctor living in the new medical dawn of the twentieth century it was all too simple: bacteriology and biochemistry made it possible to establish the cause and nature of diseases and to prepare the weapons to conquer them. Better still, these sciences furnished the means for public health to take effective preventive measures against the spread of contagious diseases. Similar praise could be lavished on such "accessory sciences" as electrotherapy, radiotherapy, radium therapy, and warm-air medication. Though of recent vintage, these medical sciences had tremendously expanded the art of curing.

So far, so good. The trouble was that this vast encyclopedic body of knowledge had to be incorporated into the already overloaded educational program for training doctors. The "inevitable consequence" was to accelerate medical specialization. By the early twentieth century, the epidemic of specialization had clearly infected the medical profession. Henri did not seem too happy about someone devoting himself exclusively to one branch of medicine, because most physicians need a wide knowledge of all the medical sciences. It takes a lifetime to master one of them. But to become "the perfect practitioner" was no longer scientifically possible, if it ever had been. So ignorance made new bedfellows, with doctors and surgeons collaborating in the hope of offering the best possible care for the patient. Henri still wondered how medical students could possibly run through their program in the short time available – five years for courses, practical training, hospital training in internal medicine, surgery, and obstetrics. Though possibly a smaller proportion of prodigies among students mastered the modern medical corpus than had mastered the *Corpus Hippocratum*, there did exist an elite medical

12 Léonard, "Le Malade imaginaire de Molière à Jules Romains."

corps, classified according to their scientific qualifications and their success in competitive examinations for positions. Indulging in the medical metaphor, Henri saw the medical corps as an army whose mission is to protect society against disease. And this army has its clearly defined hierarchy: leaders, officers, and soldiers.

Henri concocted his own quasi-literary typology of practitioners: the Balzacian category of country doctor;[13] the garden variety of family doctor; the head of a school (an intellectual rather than institutional accolade); and the Moliéresque trade of charlatan. Fortunately, the selection process that produces doctors gives the patient serious guarantees. Selection involves rejection. Out of 2000 students enrolled each year in the Paris Faculty of Medicine, among those submitting to the *concours des hôpitaux* only 600 made it to the *externat des hôpitaux*, 60 to the *internat*, 7 to the position of physician or surgeon in the hospitals, and every 3 years 8 doctors ascended to the *agrégation*. Henri noted that the physician's professional duty includes moral obligations, chief among which are devotion and abnegation. No profession demands more abnegation than that of the doctor, accurately described as a secular confessor. Classification had not completely replaced consolation.[14] Unfortunately, this rigorous training combined with competitive examinations did not prevent some doctors from becoming charlatans. Quite to the contrary, the superbly trained doctor became a great charlatan if his moral fiber did not prevent him from falling into temptation.

Who was this new charlatan? Henri's original view was that, contrary to common belief, the doctor can and does become a charlatan when, lured by filthy lucre, he is cynical and clever enough to convince the public that he is the only competent person in a matter and that his colleagues are incapable of providing services comparable to his. He added, unconvincingly, that in most cases charlatans are simply ignorant incompetents using illegal and immoral means to attract a credulous clientele or one that is badly informed on scientific issues. He did not note that this judgment might include a large part of the public, and probably explains the charlatan's success. But it is difficult to escape the argument, implicit in Henri's talk, that modern medicine creates the real charlatan, with considerable help from the patient. The worst of the charlatans were the doctors whose intelligence and know-how (*savoir-faire*, which possibly has a slightly pejorative taint) are not guided by high moral principles. As physicians, they gave their patients too many appointments, prescribed useless remedies, recommended hydrotherapy, massage, and electrical treatment in order to jack up their incomes. As surgeons, they did unnecessary surgery, including serious surgery with frequent fatal consequences, all rewarded with high fees, even small fortunes sometimes. Henri did not wish to

---

13 See the 4th edn of Honoré de Balzac, *Le Médecin de campagne* (1833; Paris, 1974) with a preface by Emmanuel Le Roy Ladurie. "Etablisssement du texte et notes de Patrick Berthier."

14 See Jan Goldstein, *Console and Classify. The French Psychiatric Profession in the Nineteenth Century* (Cambridge, 1987; Chicago, 2001).

dwell on these freaks of science – happily rare exceptions, he insisted – while at the same time giving them considerable exposure. He would be equally unconvincing on this defense in discussing his play *Le Caducée* (1921).

The patient makes the doctor. A doctor cannot become a great charlatan by treating the ignorant and unfortunate, more likely, we assume, to be found among the poor, who are unable to get good medical information or to find absolutely reliable doctors with good scientific credentials. No, that's not at all the pool of patients exploited by our doctor-charlatan. Henri was often astounded to find that rich people of high social standing became the easy victims of charlatans, even fake doctors. One of his stories featured a dentist who, calling himself a medical doctor, practiced medicine, including surgery – with unfortunate results. Even when the patient dies, the family ends up paying fees that "would probably not have been given to a prince of science."[15] The basic problem, as Henri saw it, was the social evolution of the medical profession into a trade, nearly into an industry, with the emphasis on profits, not on the care of the sick, who were put in constant danger by either too little or, worse, too much treatment. All this becomes more astounding when we remind ourselves that it is one of the best-known figures on the Parisian medical scene making this indictment, someone with a profound knowledge of that scene as well, not excluding some of the kind of knowledge possessed by the more proletarian Dr Destouches (Céline) in Montmartre.

Charlatanism was not an exclusively French speciality, though it seemed that it had made striking progress in France as well as abroad. Henri was particularly intrigued by Samuel Pozzi's report on charlatanism in the United States, where medical rackets seemed remarkably well developed. American newspapers advertised the latest medical marvels, including non-surgical removal of the appendix and even resurrection of dead patients. Seeing is believing: artistically manipulated photographs helped seduce the epistemologically naive. Pozzi claimed that in the United States the profession was infested by two species of pseudo-medical sects: the osteopaths and the Christian Scientists, the latter of which had developed to the point of becoming a threat to public health.[16] Although the French charlatans were not so advanced as their American colleagues, firmly established on the medical fringe, French newspapers advertised medical services claiming to cure incurable diseases. Henri thought that fraudulent claims to cure baldness or remove corns is one thing, not terribly serious or expensive, but to traffic in the treatment of serious and contagious diseases is another matter, deeply immoral and a danger to society as well as the patient. Both the cynical industrialist who makes the "medicines" and the doctor who "prostitutes his degree" in pushing them are criminals, partners in crime.

Henri's indictment of charlatans covered three main points, apart from his reminder of the income lost to legitimate practitioners as a result of the activity of

---

15 Léonard, "Le Malade imaginaire de Molière à Jules Romains."

16 S. Pozzi, "Hôpitaux et chirurgiens aux Etats-unis," in *Actualités médico-chirurgicales – Polyclinique Henri de Rothschild* (Paris, 1911), 131–64.

the charlatans. Diseases that can be treated easily when detected early become more difficult to cure by the time the patient gets to see a serious doctor; some diseases kill the sufferer, quicker with the charlatan's nostrums than with the orthodox doctor's treatments, sometimes because the latter is called in too late; and in the case of transmissible diseases, the sick person keeps on needlessly spreading the infection to others. An anecdote illustrated the danger of charlatanism to the sick person and to society. What better disease to cite in this case than syphilis? Since Henri's medical interest in treating syphilis was well known and also because he was a well-advertised philanthropist, people wrote to him asking for help. A young man in the early stages of this disease asked Henri for a hundred francs to pay a doctor who guaranteed a cure in fifteen days. The miracle medicament was not "606" but "monkey serum," whose preparation and efficacy were set forth in impressive detail by the doctor offering the cure. Henri convinced the syphilitic to go to one of his medical friends, who applied the "rational and classical treatment" without cost to the patient. As Fournier told Henri, there was no legal remedy allowing a third party to intervene in such cases, and in a way the doctor was legally helpless when faced with such medical frauds.

Every profession confronted by a crisis, real or imagined, which is usually produced by its own success, imagines a golden age in the long ago when its members lived in harmony and prosperity. Henri looked back fifty years to when there was a relatively small number of doctors and surgeons who distributed their patients equitably among themselves. Growth spoiled everything. The profession, apparently so financially rewarding, attracted so many students that even with a high failure rate in the faculty, the profession became overcrowded. The historian, addicted to comparative observations, may remark that it's 1848 all over again with its surplus of educated men. Economists may preach the advantages of competition, but this Rothschild thought that it had gotten completely out of hand in early twentieth-century Parisian medicine. Doctors were more common than wine merchants and tobacco shops, with a doctor for every two buildings in some quarters. Difficult for new doctors to make a living in such a jungle. The result was a continual struggle to entice patients from colleagues, which led to the commercialization of medicine by doctors unencumbered by moral scruples. Methods used to sell industrial services and products were used to attract clients: flashy publicity and regular, systematic advertising in brochures and newspapers. The press could also be useful in publishing friendly or at least non-critical articles. And profitable alliances with other professions such as pharmacy worked well. Even hotel managers could be valuable agents.

Another of Henri's anecdotes illustrated his argument. A rich American – a valuable analytical category in French social theory – wanted to consult a leading light of the medical faculty in Paris. The professor agreed to see the prospective patient at the *grand hôtel parisien* where he was staying. After two unsuccessful attempts to get past the hotel personnel, who lied that the American was out, the wily professor used the card of a well-known businessman to get through to the sick client's room. This comedy took place because the hotel administration had a contract with another doctor who monopolized the medical services needed by the hotel's guests to the profit of both doctor and hotel. We assume that the professor did not have a contract with another hotel.

And here Henri comes to the heart of the matter: the financial arrangements of the medical profession, its fees. Fees in the end are a matter of ethics or deontology, an impressive Greek-derived word that dates in French and English from the early nineteenth century. The word was born in the period when the professions themselves started flowering. The need for professional rules to govern professional behavior was clear in the Hippocratic oath, but that venerable doctrine certainly required a great deal of interpretive commentary and extension in a modern medical education with its standardized production of faculty- and clinically-trained professional doctors. Specialization was in part a way of taking care of a surplus of doctors as well as a surplus of knowledge, but this professional development also necessarily introduced ethical questions concerning referral of patients and fee splitting, an illicit practice given a patina of respectability in French as *dichotomie*, whose usage dates from 1907. Noting that the practice was of fairly recent origin, Henri declared that it should be forbidden or at least declared to be an immoral medical practice. With the growth of the number of specialists and more specialization being encouraged by the breakdown of general disease categories like hysteria into several specific diseases, the practice of splitting fees was threatening to become a normal practice.

The simple mechanism of the practice encouraged the spread of an attractive income-generating device. The family doctor and the doctor in the provinces sent patients to specialists in Paris; of course it was also possible to see specialists of renown in faculty cities like Lyon and Bordeaux, though those in Paris thought themselves, rightly in many cases, to be the leaders in their fields. Once paid, the specialist sent between one quarter and one half of his fee to the referring doctor. What were the consequences of this practice? First, the patient paid more than he should. Henri did not think that this was the most serious consequence. Damage to the patient's pocketbook could be minor compared to damage to his (or, more likely, her) body. Doctors nearly always referred their patients to the specialists giving the biggest kickbacks. These generous fellows were not necessarily the best surgeons. So according to Henri's grim observation, a patient could end up as a cripple or even die as a result of an inopportune or badly done operation.

The worst consequence of the system was that it encouraged surgeons to do unnecessary operations and doctors to undertake unneeded or useless procedures. Knock's principle prevailed in some doctor–patient relationships. The referring doctor is not innocent in this business. Having an interest in recommending a procedure, he declares it indispensable. So, many patients who could be cured by a minor medical treatment end up in a hospital for the profit of the collaborating doctors. In other cases, inaction could have unfortunate consequences for the patient. A greedy doctor might prolong an inefficacious treatment for profit instead of sending the patient to a surgeon for an urgently needed operation. In cases like appendicitis it might be too late when the patient finally gets competent attention.

One is tempted to wonder how all these medical crimes and mistakes Henri waxed eloquent about could ever be separated from normal medical practice. Or how many honest mistakes and normal human errors got attributed to the medical immoral practice of *la dichotomie*. Not easy questions to answer, as we know all too well a century later, when we are plagued by similar problems. It is testimony to Henri's intelligence and sense of medical ethics that he was a pioneer in dealing with the issue publicly.

Henri easily understood that when material interests are at stake, the human conscience becomes flexible, and it was improbable that all 25,000 French doctors were paragons of Hippocratic virtue, indifferent to the lure of comfort and luxury. Practitioners of fee splitting argued that the referring doctor must be reimbursed for the monetary loss he suffers as a result of the patient's cure by surgery, which obviates the visits to the doctor that would have taken place without the surgical cure. "Strange reasoning!" exclaimed Henri. The patient is not a form of capital for the doctor, who has a moral duty to cure his patient as quickly and cheaply as possible rather than use the patient as a cash cow for as long as possible. Curing the patient is the only justification for a doctor to recommend an operation, whose sole responsibility is that of the surgeon, who alone should be remunerated. Henri claimed that in many cases doctors hesitated to send their patients to a surgeon as soon as they should, so that they could keep collecting fees for as long as possible. The consequences were often devastating for the patient, who could even die in some cases. Such crimes could only be prevented by the doctor's conscience, which could be helped by an exclusion of the practice from medically ethical behavior.

Charlatanism, variously defined, was a commonly discussed subject in medical circles in the early twentieth century, with the publication of the journal *Revue de déontologie* beginning in 1903.[17] Interest in the subject did not abate after the Great War. The excessively prolific medical scribbler of Romanian origin, Petre Trisca, scoured the literature in order to publish in 1922 a work regurgitating or recasting, sometimes with sweeping panache, the arguments already made by doctors Brouardel, Michaut, Lévy, Le Gendre, and Rothschild.[18] It was pretty well accepted that some charlatans were practicing medicine legally. How many was a subject of debate, especially given the impossibility of coming up with figures on this nebulous issue. Drawing on Michaut's work, Trisca pointed out

[17] *Revue de déontologie et d'intérêts professionnels médicaux* ("organe mensuel de l'Association corporative des étudiants en médecine de Paris"). See, e.g., Michaut, "Les illégaux de la médecine," *Revue de déontologie* (août 1905), and Alexandre Leroy, *De la répression du charlatanisme médical* (thesis, Paris Faculty of Law, 1907).

[18] Petre Trisca, *Prolégomènes à une déontologie medico-sociale* (Paris, 1922), "Charlatanisme," 333–9; preface and introduction by P. Cibrié and Victor Balthazard. See Paul Le Gendre, "La vie du médecin, déontologie et jurisprudence médicales," in Emile Sergent and others (eds), *Traité de pathologie médicale et de jurisprudence appliquée* (Paris, 1920).

that charlatanism often resulted from relations between doctors and pharmacists as well as other businesses, notoriously the mineral water business – he might have mentioned the wine industry too. Michaut had drawn attention to the notorious examples of two Parisian medical societies receiving revenues from mineral water companies and manufacturers of some ostensibly medical products. Trisca agreed with the harsh judgment of Michaut that too many scoundrels and too many bourgeois idiots were invading the medical profession, all too easy to enter. Paul Cibrié, president of the union of doctors of the department of the Seine, protested, in a friendly preface, that Trisca was inclined to overemphasize faults committed by a few doctors. Trisca admitted that doctors were not always responsible for the commercial use of their names. Using two examples, Brouardel had warned against "involuntary charlatanism." In one case a grateful journalist told the news of his cure by a certain doctor, and in another case a pharmacist advertised the fact that a doctor recommended a specific medicament, which was legal according to a decision handed down by the Tribunal of the Seine. In his commentary, Victor Balthazard seemed more eager to advertise the fact that all French doctors were opposed to the bureaucratization of medicine, that is, becoming employees of the state, though he admitted that Trisca was right in saying that in an agricultural country like Romania the patient-starved doctor has to be a civil servant with a salary.[19]

Charlatanism on the stage: Dr Canulard

A century after its proclamation in the *Gazette*, we see the medical charlatanism of the 1830s being practiced as normal medicine by the famous doctor Canulard (Plague), hero of a satirical play by Julien Teppe.[20] The play opens with the doctor calculating the profits of his medical activity for the week: injections, infrared and ultraviolet radiation treatments, and, above all, writing prescriptions. Medicine as a money machine. He is cynically deciding to increase the number of prescriptions for Tulard's inferior pharmaceutical products, in order to forestall the druggist's predicable complaints, when his companion Norma enters crying in pain. But the "great doctor" has no idea of what medication to give her, though he refuses to poison her with some therapeutic novelties that came in yesterday: they are nothing but expensive rubbish. No new Golot sinapisms (mustard plasters) or other useless products for Norma. Fortunately for Norma, the doctor remembers that the concierge cured her own similar pains with a cataplasm of flax flour and potato starch. When a suffering male patient calls to inquire about trying a traditional cataplasm, the doctor goes into a medical froth, denouncing this old

---

19 An important figure in the history of forensic medicine, Victor Balthazard (1872–1950) was the author of the classic *Précis de médecine légale* (Paris, 1906; 6th edn, 1943).

20 Julien Teppe, *Les Histrions au miroir ou les morticioles tels qu'ils sont* (Paris, 1931). "One act satirical play."

fashioned, laughable, empirical nostrum, an old woman's or, worse, a concierge's remedy. Instead, Canulard prescribes the new expensive Golot sinapism, the latest achievement in modern therapy, producing a quick and powerful effect. Meanwhile Norma's crisis has passed. A farce of mistakes follows, all based on mistakes in a prescription for a detested patient. Norma gets her lover to write a prescription to ruin the skin of a society beauty she hates and goes off to see the concierge. As she is leaving, Canulard invites her and some of her friends to a clinic the next day to see operations done by his colleague: five fibrous tumors, two cataracts, and three cancers. A good time is promised.

Life is beautiful, scene three promises, but for the doctor only it turns out. An exasperated patient, discovering too late that in his search for a doctor he had found a third rate actor, receives a lesson on the modern doctor, who patronizes the latest pharmaceutical creation and launches it with high praise as if it were a perfume or a dress. Deciding what remedy will be in vogue for the season, the doctors give it an appealing symbolic name – an enema might be called "Rêve de vase." The astounded patient cannot believe that doctors are vulgar shopkeepers or "amateurs ironiques": a doctor is not a banker or a grocer; medicine is a true calling, a priestly function. An incredulous Canulard explains to this simple young man how he became a doctor. Not being bright enough to get into the *grandes écoles*, bored by law and the arts, he could only become a lawyer or a politician (a deputy), both professions open to the first idiot to come along. In the medical competitive examinations a professor swaps support of a colleague's student for the support of his student by the colleague. Not having your patron on the jury could be fatal to success, as Henri de Rothschild observed about his own failure to pass the *internat* examination. Canulard likes a profession that allows him to indulge his penchant for sadism and bad acting.

Canulard declares it an illusion to believe that the modern doctor will try to cure you. Doctors are born scribblers, always busy writing memoirs and that sort of thing, while leaving aside the prosaic questions of health. "Yes, we doctors need more and more science." So they devote themselves to the fabrication of statistics, hold congresses, and make prophecies. Their careers are helped by the fact that people have short memories or are very credulous. No problem then in enjoying public praise and honors, while non-licensed practitioners are punished by the law. Doctors pass for the martyrs of science. "Look at the faculties: if medicine enjoyed a surplus of virtues and special talents … would the number of doctors in France have increased from 15,000 in 1900 to 30,000 in 1930?" Soon there would be more doctors than patients.

The patient's discourse on vocation is extremely unpleasant for the modern doctor, generally a fatuous or greedy person. Bluff has replaced everything. Canulard's portrait is beginning to resemble that of the wine expert. An unbeatable "puffisme" drives the new sawbones to declare himself tops as he goes from success to success with science inscribed on the end of his banner. The fact that a patient may have been ruined personally and financially by a doctor is of no interest to Canulard, for after all that is how a doctor becomes rich and famous.

Mention of the word human by the patient causes our quack to laugh. “A human doctor! That’s the limit!” How could anyone possibly believe that a doctor is a man? “Ambitiosa est medicina,” observed Pliny the Elder. The heavy satire of the theater had its basis in the more moderate discourse of the profession itself.

Charlatanism on the stage: *Le Grand Patron*

At the same time that Teppe’s play was being generally ignored, another play about the medical profession created a big splash in the world of Parisian theater. *Le Grand Patron* by André Pascal (Henri) opened to a large number of favorable reviews in February 1931 at the Comédie des Champs-Elysées.[21] If the doctor had become a figure in the news, it was partly due to the popularity of the famous play *Knock* by Jules Romains, with Louis Jouvet in the role of Knock. The charlatanism praised in the *Gazette* in 1833 as a fruitful interaction of medicine and commercialism culminated in the brilliant medical empire built by Knock, who, as we have seen, added a new element, the apparently well person eager to be diagnosed as a sick patient ready to be cured by the latest medical magic. In 1931 Jouvet left Paris on a long trip, and though the play continued, some space was opened up on the Paris scene for a new play about the medical profession. Critics still remembered Henri’s play *Le Caducée*, which the author now looked back on as a portrait-satire of contemporary medical morality. The dramatic action of *Le Grand Patron* takes place in the family of a well-known surgeon, and most of the characters are physicians. On one level the play deals with the financial difficulties of doctors constrained by laws and rules written for another age; worse, the doctors’ taxes had substantially increased without their fees having changed much since 1914. Yet many doctors were flourishing, even though they might have been charlatans who were crippling patients and ripping them off in unnecessary treatments. Charlatanism allied with a venal or mercenary outlook had become prominent in medicine – a development strongly deplored by the protagonist, “le grand patron” himself, a great surgeon-professor. The dramatic irony of the play stems from the professor’s unwitting involvement in a colossal medical racket. One reviewer misleadingly referred to “le grand patron” as professor Knock. And the play was staged not in Henri’s own new Pigalle theater but in the Comédie des Champs-Elysées, where Louis Jouvet had played Knock.[22]

Although this approach again violates Eagleton’s canon forbidding the analysis of plots, here is the story. The well-known surgeon and researcher

---

[21] HR, *Le Grand Patron*. “Pièce en 3 actes et 4 tableaux. Représentée pour la première fois sur la scène de la Comédie des Champs-Elysées, le 5 février 1931.” See André Pascal [HR], *Théâtre* (7 vols, Paris, 1931, VII). The plays in these seven volumes were staged in the period 1921–31.

[22] Jacques Baumer staged the play. The sets, designed by Paul Colin, were built in the ateliers of Henri’s Théâtre Pigalle. See André Pascal, *Moi, je...* (Paris, 1931).

professor Raymond Volnys, member of the Academy of Medicine, sixty years old, is happily married to Thérèse, aged thirty-six, loyal wife and spendthrift social butterfly. He is about to give a paper at the Academy on his successful experiments on the regeneration of monkey bones; of course the implication of the paper is that another great medical advance for humanity is in the works. Doctor Berthaud, the surgeon's "chef de clinique" and popularizer of the professor's work, wants to marry Gisèle, Volnys's daughter, who is kept busy doing work for her father and does not have a dowry. She intends to continue her sacrifices for papa, a great man. Volnys is nearly universally detested by colleagues and by fellow members of the academies of medicine and of surgery for his brilliance, arrogance, and intolerance of money grubbing and fee splitting by physicians. Just the sort of fellow that hubris loves to visit. Volnys attributes the death of a patient he operated on to a late referral by his colleague Le Roy, recognized by everyone else as a good physician. Le Roy points out that people are not too eager to be sent to surgeons for operations, especially since certain doctors are notorious for recommending unnecessary surgery, with the patients ending up crippled and massacred by charlatans. Not of course by Volnys, who never sees these unfortunates except to repair the damage done by other doctors.

When it comes to doctor–patient relations, Volnys believes that many doctors lack the authority and energy to impose their will on the patient – essential for the successful functioning of medicine. He is obviously thinking of the patient who needs a surgeon but is reluctant to go to one; the difficulty with his view is that the medical charlatans succeed only too well in imposing their view. Le Roy quickly points out that it is professors like Volnys who, by always crying charlatanism and venality, have given the public the idea that doctors cannot be trusted. Implacable, Volnys replies that his action is justified because charlatanism and venality are the scourges of the time. Le Roy then tells Volnys he should not blame practicing doctors if their patients sometimes believe that they are being trapped by someone more interested in milking them than curing them. This *dialogue de sourds* continues until Le Roy has to go fight the daily battle with his patients; Volnys remains intransigent, oozing virtue, remote from the daily struggles of practitioners like Le Roy. A defense of Le Roy by Dr Alix, Volnys's sixty-year-old friend, does not change the professor's beliefs.

Next Alix tells Thérèse why Le Roy looked shattered in leaving. Surprised, she points out that her husband sends patients to Le Roy. Volnys says he is wrong to do so, for Le Roy is a weak person led by his patients. Alix quickly replies that this is not a correct analysis: Le Roy knows his patients whereas Volnys just examines and operates on them. Alix emphasizes the difficulty of getting a patient to accept a necessary operation. Nine times out of ten they would rather accept the advice of a hairdresser than consult a capable and honest doctor. Next, in a general discussion at dinner, one guest defends non-medical cures, but her example of the prowess of a Hungarian medium is topped by Volnys's example of one of his patients who went to the United States to get a sprain cured by an osteopath. The professor does not distinguish between the two charlatans.

Volnys is also blind to the slavish situation in which he keeps his daughter Gisèle. When Alix suggests that Volnys sell his collections of medals and coins to furnish a dowry for her, we discover that they have already been sold to pay for the dinners, receptions, and gifts that are part of the package coming with a young bride. The wife got an emerald for her birthday. Then there are the professor's research expenses, not all of which are covered by the annual 1500 francs provided by the faculty of medicine for laboratory expenses. A monkey costs more than 1000 francs. He is lucky that he can exploit Gisèle, who does leatherwork, including bookbinding (held in high regard by Henri), at night to earn her own spending money.

Mlle Le Prince (the villain), a guest who won at the poker game, plays up to Volnys by declaring people to be dumb because they refuse to consult specialists on health and on money. She had no hesitation in letting Volnys operate on her to save her life. Now she would like to help him. Her keen business eye has diagnosed his problem of negative cash flow. Posing as one of Thérese's friends, she wants to offer him a way out of his money troubles. When Volnys serves up the quaint view that scientists – and he counts himself in their ranks, thus distinguishing himself from ordinary practicing physicians – cannot worry about business and money, she replies that worry now seems unavoidable as a result of all the expenses the medical researcher incurs as physician and laboratory man. She easily turns the "oldie" Volnys, in spite of some protests on his part, into the very model of a modern medical man. His salary is about 200,000 francs, only one tenth of what it would be if he did not refuse to enter into "illicit schemes." Scandalized at this pitiful amount, she offers the money he needs to meet his budget, including money for research and happiness for his wife. After some hesitation and worry about not consulting a lawyer before signing an agreement, he suddenly accepts when she says that if he doesn't sign up within 48 hours, she will get professor Barbier. Volnys declares that his colleague already makes too much money from his excessive operations. Le Prince has hooked a front man for her organization.

What is this setup in which "le grand patron" unwittingly becomes the chief charlatan, enjoying a sinecure as president of the board of directors of a banking and insurance cooperative intended to serve the medical profession? The *Crédit médical*, as it is called, will make loans to young doctors setting up practices, supply information to doctors on the wealth of their patients, and take care of money matters for them, including the collection of debts. There are plans to build a 10 million franc sanatorium for the numerous doctors who are victims of tuberculosis. The less rich are not forgotten: low-income people will get a 20 million franc surgical clinic where payment of 40 francs a day will cover everything. Volnys is unhappy with the chief source of the company's profits: the pharmaceutical industry. That industry is worth hundreds of millions but needs reorganization, perhaps by channeling their products to patients through the medical network – one of Le Prince's areas of expertise. This is not a simple matter of petty dealings between doctors and "distributors of rubbish" (Volnys's phrase), for the pharmacists make 300 percent profit on their products. But

Volnys seems uninterested in the whole business until Barbier's name comes up. Accepting the deal gets him 75,000 company shares with a return of 20 percent and 200,000 francs annually in director's fees. Research and household bliss would be generously funded.

This manna has fallen not a moment too soon. Thérèse reveals to her husband that she thought that he was as rich as his colleagues, who have their estates, several automobiles, and hunting domains. Perhaps here, as in many of his plays, the author was parodying the popular image of himself. A discussion over spending has come about because she discovered that Volnys has sold his beloved Utrillo and Renoir to buy her birthday emerald. The shocked Thérèse is afraid that people's talk about this new poverty would have a negative influence on patients. But he replies that things will be fine if spending is not increased. And modern painting hardly interests him now. Thérèse also tells him that people say his lack of patients can be blamed on his rigid character. But the problem with money is not over because she has already blown the 40,000 francs he gave her for household expenses. Worse, her dressmaker's bill of 60,000 francs, a year overdue, must be paid now. Perhaps Thérèse should be his office manager, for she told Le Prince that the cost of her operation was 15,000 francs, three times Volnys's low fee. He is shocked, but Thérèse points out that Le Prince expected a higher bill. When Volnys rushes off to operate on a patient in pain, Thérèse hopes for another 15,000 francs. A hopeless case, for the surgeon has promised to operate without charging a fee.

At the beginning of the second act, Volnys is a happy man because he has just spent two hours in his laboratory with his monkeys. The experiments on reconstituting their tibias were a total success, with the happy creatures now capering about. The author held a rosy view of animal experimentation, a view typical in France but not in England. Volnys is now ready to communicate his results to the *Société de Chirurgie* the following month. With the arrival of Alix and Barbier his world begins to crumble. *Crédit médical* is in financial difficulty, with Le Prince suspected of malfeasance. His colleagues fear that the reputation of the faculty and the Academy of Medicine will be sullied if it is true that Volnys is the head of the company. When Volnys is summoned to appear before an examining magistrate (*juge d'instruction*), Gisèle and Berthaud call in a lawyer, another character successfully treated by Volnys ten years before, who manages to keep the professor's name out of the press for a few days and gets the dossier from the magistrate, a friend of his. Henri did not paint an edifying picture of either press or justice.

The only way out, it seems, is for Volnys to pay for the shares he was given and then have his case dismissed for lack of evidence. This is of course legal nonsense necessary for dramatic movement; in law Volnys would still be responsible as a sort of CEO. Sending the professor to jail would ruin the theme of the play. To round up 750,000 francs and save the honor and reputation of faculty and academy, all of Volnys's few friends and some of his many enemies are asked to contribute to this worthy cause. Volnys is humiliated enough to plan suicide. Thérèse reveals that she cannot sell her jewels because they are fake; she sold the real ones to pay gambling debts. She may have rejuvenated an aging professor but she looks like a bad matrimonial investment at this point, and wife and stepdaughter quarrel. Thérèse's real vice turns out to be her inability to see her husband's overweening pride, which is aggravated by her cavorting in high society. But soon she sees the light and promises to reform. Reconciled, the two women rush off to save the great man from killing himself.

Act III takes place in the professor's country house (near Pontoise), one thing he has not had to sell yet. By this time the press smells blood, and is eager to get the dirt on the people behind Le Prince, whose exposure is not enough to keep readers interested for long. Volnys is convinced that he is ruined, though the campaign to raise his ransom is well underway. A piece of irony unfolds when salvation comes to depend on several hundred thousand francs from Barbier, whom Volnys believes is a swine, jealous of always having had to play second fiddle to "le grand Patron." Barbier also married into money. But Barbier can only contribute 50,000 francs because his daughter requires an immediate large dowry. A squabble follows between the two doctors; Volnys begins to look more like the wretch people think he is. When the property is besieged by a flock of journalists and others, everyone assumes that they want to hear about the scandal at *Crédit médical*. Instead, the invasion resulted from the news that Volnys has won the Nobel Prize in physiology or medicine – curiously given for surgery in the play. This is a deus ex machina worthy of *Tartuffe*, as one critic noted. Volnys is saved by a million with a few hundred thousand left over to pamper a sobered Thérèse and to buy a few more monkeys. Barbier gets back his measly check, and after a typical pre-crisis exchange he says that he won't be speaking to Volnys again. He is wrong. Suddenly humanized by universal recognition and the Nobel bonanza, Volnys tells his colleague that in his next communication to the Academy he will talk about Barbier's work, not his own. Volnys quickly regains his old ego for the interview and photo session with the press. *L'Intransigeant* is appropriately prominent in the latter part of the play. And a *reporteresse* is a sign of the greater opening of the professions to women. The play ends with the great man boasting of having been first in the *externat des hôpitaux*, the *internat*, the *concours des hôpitaux*, and the *agrégation*. The reporters provide a counterpoint chorus of "Ahs!"

In the play's preface, which is non-Shavian in length and spirit, Henri pointed out that the ethical rules governing the medical profession prohibited doctors from profiting in a material way from their personal contribution to a commercial enterprise. But given the cost of living and the heavy taxes on professions, it was not surprising to find the rule being ignored. And since salaries had not changed much in the previous quarter century, the activity seemed justified even if unethical and illegal. Aggravating the doctor's situation was the existence of certain charlatans whose success in attracting clients could be blamed on naive and ignorant patients, who provided a convenient target towards which Henri could direct blame for this medical mess. Patients tended to see wealth as a sign of professional worth, thus increasing the importance of appearances or the mise en scène. Their guilt was soon reduced by his condemnation of the secret actions of certain surgeons, often of debatable professional worth, in securing profitable patients. So the situation of a career surgeon, not entirely unlike that of Volnys, was not difficult to imagine. For dramatic purposes, Volnys's situation required the existence of additional problems. It seems that many factors contributed to the perceived declining economic status of doctors not willing to play the new game. (It was not so new as Henri believed.) The play does not try to solve the problem of what an older doctor should do in the face of a changing medical economy; rather it exposes the problem through the character of professor Volnys, whose third of a century of work and sacrifice seemed about to end in disaster.

On the basis of personal observation over thirty years or so, Henri had concluded that many scientists and artists were just "big children" knowing little outside their profession. Hence in money matters they often got exploited by convincing swindlers. As a rich man, Henri had a lot of experience with them. In the portrait of Volnys, Henri wanted to give a general psychological portrait of the scientific man. "The character of a scientist is always somewhat complex. Scientific specialization nearly always implies naïveté and credulity, immoderate pride or excessive modesty."[23] Henri's sweeping judgment seems to cover most of the medico-scientific community. He thought the true scientist to be, at least in France, a modest fellow.[24] But it being more interesting for the dramatist to deal with the exception, he made Volnys a proud fellow. Hubris then took its course, with sundry events turning the hero's life topsy-turvy just at the peak of his glory. Drama required the tragic events to happen to the surgeon believing himself infallible. By definition, great tragedies on the stage can happen only to great people. Henri did not believe himself to be an infallible playwright. He was aware that his psychological profile of Volnys was open to criticism. Was Volnys an egoist? Only if pride implies egoism, or the notorious *culte de soi-même* – presumably a reference to the Barrèsian *culte du moi* rather than to dandyism à la Baudelaire. Henri was convinced that it is psychologically impossible to suffer from pride without being an egoist. Dramatically the scheme worked.

Henri believed that plays could be an effective way of discussing social dangers, that is, threats to the bourgeois society that he and some lucky French citizens enjoyed, perhaps less in 1930 than in 1914. In this play he decided not to deal with one danger – minor though it may now seem – that of doctors splitting fees. Henri saw it as a burning problem, but said that he was not qualified to deal with it; he boasted of always refusing to treat the subject, being willing to accept

---

[23] Léonard, "Le Malade imaginaire de Molière à Jules Romains." Sartre, *Situations*, II, 230, made a similar observation about great men: cited in *Le Grand Robert de la langue française* (2d edn, Paris, 2001), 5: 3–4.

[24] La Fontaine would probably have disagreed: "Se croire un personnage est fort commun en France / C'est proprement le mal français." *Fables*, VIII, 15, cited in *Le Grand Robert*, 5: 3–4.

the fact that his refusal was "to the profit of those ... little qualified to appreciate its dangers."[25] Besides, this issue was being kicked around years before World War I. In *Le Caducée* (1921) he denounced the common "courtage médico-chirurgical," – the system of kickback from surgeons to doctors who sent them patients. Henri still believed in the right of the incompetent public to ignorance on the subject, as perhaps on all medical subjects. A man of his time, he held that these purely professional controversies would not benefit from being made public. The public merely supplied the paying patient. Not entirely consistent on the issue, Henri praised a recent public airing of the matter by his "cher maître et grand ami" in *L'Echo de Paris*. He also seems to have forgotten his treatment of the subject in a speech, expanded in a pamphlet back in 1911. No matter what position he took on fee splitting, he was bound to irritate some group of doctors, and at this point Henri wanted to have as many friends as possible, especially in the Academy of Medicine.

Another social danger, ripe for treatment, could be dealt with by the author without fear of irritating colleagues: speculation in financial or industrial operations by ignorant and credulous people looking to double (at least) their investment capital. The number of people infected with speculative fever was so striking that Henri dubbed it a passion or, worse, a fashion, like cocktail parties, the tango, negro music (jazz), and nudism – all fads from the USA and South America. Henri regretted that he had seen friends lose two thirds of their assets as a result of following the advice of unscrupulous advisers or well-informed friends or inventors of genius or even brazen speculators. No one wanted to follow the advice of well informed and honest professionals. He believed it was possible to distinguish one group from the other. After a long career of austerity and honesty, Professor Volnys turned, at the age of sixty, to speculation, though the author let him escape from danger with more of his fortune than a more didactic emplotment would have required.

Critical reaction to *Le Grand Patron* was overwhelmingly favorable, with some critics gushing that it was the best play Henri had written in a quarter century of playwriting, even better than *Le Caducée*. In fact *Le Grand Patron* was so good that Henri was accused of plagiarism. In 1930 he finished a play called *Moi*; unfortunately that was also the title of a play by Labiche being revived at the Comédie Française. Friends told him to avoid the silly title of *Moi ... je*; so he chose the title of *Le Grand Patron*, a cliché full of the right messages, including irony. Albert Wuarin and Roger Ducos claimed that Henri's play resembled in subject, scenario, and characters a play called *Les Conquérants*, written in 1913 and swallowed up by the Great War and not revived after. Convinced that the accusation was nonsense, Henri refused to reply to their letter to him and rejected their idea of an arbitration of claims to be done by the president of the *Société des*

[25] Léonard, "Le Malade imaginaire de Molière à Jules Romains."

auteurs et compositeurs dramatiques. The archival trail ends there.[26] Few good writers escape the flattering accusation of plagiarism, and he provided a more tempting target than many other scribblers.[27]

As was often the case, some critics could not resist the banal temptation of playing with Henri's writing plays as André Pascal, "a transparent mask." And too many critics played with the equally stale issue of his being an amateur playwright, though nearly everyone admitted that after a quarter century of writing plays, including a number of striking successes, he was as professional a playwright as a writer who wrote for a living. Of course it was always possible to give more credit to the actors than to the author, and Henri coyly pretended to go along with that when called on stage at the end of *Le Grand Patron*, though the enthusiastic audience gave him as much credit as the actors. Robert de Thiac observed that most of Henri's plays had been criticized excessively because of his *personalité* – we might use the word persona, that is, Henri's being a notorious Parisian personality.[28]

Criticism concentrated on two points. Some critics saw the denouement, Volnys's winning the Nobel Prize, as an easy deus ex machina, a gimmick. But the public loved it, recognizing the brilliance of a "coup de théâtre." The denouement can be seen as an essential part of the success of the play, a bourgeois drama written according to the old canon: good solid literary workmanship, that is, composition and balanced construction, all based on a serious study of the subject. Emile Mas found the play to be based on a late nineteenth-century dramatic model.[29] It had a plan, expounded a subject, and developed a plot to arrive at a more or less plausible denouement. Henri seems to have appreciated though not have imitated the work of Pirandello, who had no interest in Henri's plays. According to the critics, the public wanted clear, logical, living drama uncomplicated by advocacy of ideas or theses, by fake lyricism, or by complex psychology. In a certain sense, critics damned Henri with faint praise for not being modern; the public loved him for not advancing dramatic practice, let alone theory.

The second major criticism made by critics centered on the psychological profile of Volnys. James de Coquet, writing in *Le Figaro*, found Henri guilty of taking liberties with the laws of psychology because the character of Volnys contained contradictory traits. Human, one is tempted to say, but the critic found

---

26 "Un cas de propriété littéraire," *Volonté* (4 juin 1931), in Arsenal, Rf. 71.742. But see *Moi, je...* . "Représentée pour la première fois sur la scène de la Comédie des Champs-Elysées, le 4 février 1931." The play is dedicated to his friend Léopold Marchand, who wrote some plays with Colette. Like Colette, he went on a cruise to Norway with Henri on the *Eros*.

27 In RAL 000/930: 58-1, 172–82, there is evidence of Henri's sensitivity to the possibility of plagiarism concerning his play *Le Moulin de la Galette* as he carefully establishes the chronology of composition of the works involved.

28 Arsenal, Rf. 71.742

29 Arsenal, Rf. 71.742.

it implausible that a great, proud, intolerant, intransigent, highly moral surgeon would at the same time behave with such incredible thoughtlessness. Was this "a diagnostic mistake" on the part of the physician playwright? With our view of the contradictory elements of many personalities and special tensions of the medical personality, we might not think so. As for Volnys's acceptance of Le Prince's business deal, he had a choice of accepting what seemed like a good honest deal or of continuing his economic decline. Whatever one may think of these factors, the author had a psychological escape route; he explained in his preface how he viewed great men: part genius, part child, not likely to behave according to a normal model of rationality. Scientists and artists are generally "big children" who know little of real life and will not behave according to some model of rational behavior derived from an artificial bourgeois psychology. This is a pathological case. Madame Gérard d'Houville, also writing in *Le Figaro*, found the character of Volnys completely plausible in what Jean Bastia called a "Fantaisie clinico-théâtrale." And Edmond Sée found the play to be "a perfect study of character."[30]

In a condescending, bizarre commentary in *Le Temps*, Pierre Brisson declared that Henri's play would have been even more successful in a neighborhood theater before a simple, non-demanding audience rather than in the "petite salle" of the Comédie des Champs-Elysées. Brisson was convinced that André Pascal was a popular author but didn't know it. Brisson was trying to be funny, but he was less amusing than Pierre Veber, who liked *Le Grand Patron* and thought that the author was finally going to make some money.

[30] Arsenal, Rf. 71.742.

Chapter 10
Medical Ethics: *Le Caducée*

> In all circumstances the doctor must respect the principles of morality, honesty, and devotion that are indispensable to the exercise of medicine.[1]

In 1922 a realistic interpretation of Henri de Rothschild's play *The Risk* (*Le Caducée*) at the Strand theater in London received eleven curtain calls at the end of the third and final act. True, the actors were remarkable – Arthur Bouchier and his wife, Kyre Bellew, and the bilingual Carmen Nesville, but so was the subject: medical malpractice. In London, as in Paris, the play stirred up a fuss that must have been welcome to the theater. Though the play's medical villain was French and his victim was a frivolous American bourgeoise, Londoners were inspired to write letters to the press about the play's dreadful subject, which was obviously not entirely irrelevant to London medicine. Henri had written the play in 1910 for the Odéon national theater, where André Antoine was then director, and published it in 1912. A much revised version was staged in Paris at the Renaissance theater on 5 February 1921 and then revived in June at the Gymnase for a successful run. A final much revised version of the play was published in 1928. Between 1910 and the 1920s the situations of physicians and women (including women doctors) had changed so much that a play written before World War I would have seemed hopelessly "old hat" on the post-war Paris stage. Henri noted that certain personalities had a different mentality: some of the *femmes du monde*, for example, had been nurses in the war, which had produced new behavior and language in the medical milieu; the women's experience would have given them a perspective on life that they could not conceivably have had before. Yet the subject of the play was even more relevant than before the war, and medical ethics was certainly generally thought to have acquired a new importance.[2]

Le Caducée had been slated to open at the Odéon during the season of 1911–12. But when Henri decided to delay a production of his play *Crésus* at the Vaudeville,

---

1 *Le code de déontologie médicale*, Titre I, article 3; the code (1995) is cited in Martin Winckler, *C'est grave, docteur? Ce que disent les patients, ce qu'entendent les médecins* (Paris, 2002), 195–222.

2 André Pascal [HR], *Le Caducée* supplement to *La Petite Illustration* no. 51,11 juin 1921 (revised and corrected text, Paris, 1928). *L'Illustration*, which published a supplement for the theater after 1899, gave coverage of the theater and criticism; it was aimed at a well-to-do public, more family oriented than the *Revue des Deux Mondes*, which every two weeks offered its rich, cultivated public a critique of a selection of plays in Paris. See Hélène Lebel, *Le Théâtre à Paris (1880–1914): reflet d'une société?* (Villeneuve d'Ascq, 1996).

the director of that theater agreed to put on *Le Caducée* instead. Antoine, the director of the Odéon, did not object because Henri offered him another play. As it turned out, the Vaudeville never put on *Le Caducée* because the director Paul Porel got cold feet when the cast became alarmed at its "violent and combative character." Porel succeeded in getting Henri to withdraw the play, though not until the author had discussed the matter with friends, including Gaston Calmette, editor of *Le Figaro*, and Henry Bernstein.[3] When *Le Figaro* published Henri's account of his adventure, Porel replied that the problem was that Henri's candor and ardor in treating purely professional issues made the script a *pamphlet* rather than a play. (The word *pamphlet* in French refers to "a short satirical, vehement work; the word is often used pejoratively."[4]) The astonished Henri thought that nothing was better suited to the stage than a treatment of these exciting and serious moral questions concerning the doctor's morality and conscience. The author turned out to be right.

Henri was resigned to seeing his play only in the pages of *la Petite Illustration* when Antoine told him that it had been a mistake to withdraw the play from the boulevard and that he would put it on at the Odéon. (Boulevard refers to the kind of plays usually put on in the theaters of the Grands Boulevards – light, traditional, and popular comedy; vaudeville, but subversive of bourgeois morality.) But directors changed at the Odéon while the play was in rehearsal, and though the new director, Gavault, ratified his predecessor's agreement with Henri, the outbreak of war in 1914 put an end to plans for an opening. So it was not until 1921, due in no small part to the pressure of Henri's friends, that the revised version was staged, at the Renaissance theater, and then was given three performances at the Gymnase.[5] The money taken in at a public performance was given to the *Fondation Curie* for the benefit of the *Œuvre de la protection des enfants libérés* (Alsace-Lorraine) and the *Œuvre du Radium* (*Institut du Radium*). For the performance labeled "couturières" there were numerous invited doctors in the audience, including many of the big medical names in Paris: Roux, Letulle, Tuffier, Grumberg, Hartmann, Emery, Cunéo, Bastard, Picot, and, of course, Delbet.[6] Many of the big guns in theater and criticism attended, among them Sarah Bernhardt, Marthe Brandès, Cora and Marie Laparcerie, Robert de Fleurs, and Henry Bernstein. Another performance was given for the press. The president of the republic attended a performance given for 400 members of the *Congrès de l'histoire de la médecine*. General critical

---

3 Paul Parfournu (dit Porel) wrote *L'Odéon, histoire administrative, anecdotique et littéraire du second Théâtre français* (2 vols; I: 1782–1818; II: 1818–53; Paris, 1876–1905).

4 *Trésor de la langue française* (Paris, 1986), 12:842.

5 See Joan Littlewood, *Baron Philippe. The Very Candid Autobiography of Baron Philippe de Rothschild* (1984; New York, 1986), 23–9, for an amusing account of the rehearsing for the play and Philippe's help in modifying scenery and costumes.

6 "Couturières" is the rehearsal before the dress rehearsal ("la générale") and named for the "dressmakers" or "seamstresses" who make the last adjustments to costumes.

approval and considerable public interest in the play led to a successful run at the Gymnase.

What was *Le Caducée* all about?

The play opens in the richly appointed surgery of Dr Armand Revard. His Renoir is worth eighty million francs. A few rich doctors had become part of the bourgeois landscape by the 1920s. French doctors could, for example, read with envy that William J. Mayo owned a 75 ton boat, which had cost $100,000, with 11 cabins, several salons, a library, and an operating room.[7] Revard's old friend from medical school days, Charles Durieux, then buried at Loudéac, deep in Brittany, comes to see him.[8] Durieux has taken a rich châtelaine to see the great professor Godfroy, who confirms Durieux's opinion that there is no point in subjecting her to an operation to try to solve her health problem. Revard scorns this consultation of the 65-year-old Godfroy, who abstains on principle from doing questionable surgery. Although Godfroy is a professor of clinical medicine and a member of the Academy of Medicine, Revard classifies him as a fossil and jocularly adds that Durieux should have brought his châtelaine to him. Durieux is surprised that Revard has become so famous since they last met six years ago, when Revard was preparing for the *internat* and the *agrégation* examinations in order to get an official teaching position. But ten years of penury was enough for Revard, and after his two *patrons* were inconsiderate enough to die, he decided, at the age of thirty-five, to move into private practice, for without *patrons* to help him there was little hope of obtaining an official position. (This may be another reference to Henri's *patrons* having also died before he could succeed in the *internat* examinations.) Durieux, surprised that things have not changed since he was a student, cites two cases to show that Revard too would have succeeded had he persevered. But Revard sees the cases as minor exceptions to the general system of favoritism permitted by the official medical elite to cover up the functioning of the system of clientelism that prevails.

How did Revard get to be a great Parisian surgeon, which seems prima facie a more difficult task? Quite a bit of good luck was involved, though his mind was obviously prepared to seize opportunity when it presented itself. Given the sad fate that the author reserved for Revard, it is important to keep in mind that Revard was a skillful surgeon. "A surgeon who knows his trade can still make a place in the sun for himself." Especially in Paris, where sick people, better informed than in the past, are no longer impressed with fancy academic diplomas and high sounding titles. A man who is going to have his belly opened now asks not for diplomas or decorations as proof of a surgeon's skill but for solid statistics on the success of

---

7 *La Chronique médicale* 28 (1923): 377.

8 The Vilage Loudéac is next to Querrien, where the Virgin appeared for the first time on 15 August 1652 and is now a sort of mini-Lourdes receiving 80,000 to 100,000 pilgrims each year to celebrate the Assumption.

the doctor's operations. Durieux comments that in the doctor's trade, it's luck that counts, but Revard emphasizes the Pasteurian wisdom of knowing how to profit from chance and how to play your cards after luck visits you. "Succeed in a few delicate and bold operations, save a half dozen important people in finance, politics, and the arts. That's how in our time a surgeon can assure his future." In his own case Revard was lucky enough about eighteen months earlier to be present when a young girl was hit by an automobile and to be able to save her life by intervening quickly. During visits to his patient, Revard met her uncle, Constantin Leroux, a well-known businessman and financier, who liked the doctor well enough to spread lavish praise of him everywhere he went, that is, in the social circles in which a doctor wants to be praised. Chic patients and people who count – politicians and the nouveaux riches – were soon coming from all over Paris to see Revard. His office on the avenue des Gobelins (13th arrondissement) was not a smart enough address for a doctor hoping to treat the upper classes; so in order to keep contact with his new clientele he had to move to a more ritzy quarter.

One might wonder if Henri was using an incident in the life of the anatomist Vicq d'Azyr (1748–94) as the model for this transformation of Revard's life. After having being denied the use of the faculty amphitheater in which to teach his course in comparative anatomy and losing out to Portal (supported by Buffon) in an attempt to get the chair in anatomy at the *Jardin du Roi*, Vicq d'Azyr's fortune was changed by a happy accident. One day he was able to take care of a woman who had fainted while passing his house; she turned out to be the niece of the famous naturalist Daubenton. Doctor and patient married, and from then on Daubenton used his influence to see that the talents of Vicq d'Azyr were allowed to flower brilliantly in research, publication, and employment. He even succeeded Buffon in the French Academy.[9] In spite of attacks from faculty doctors, Vicq d'Azyr, a successful establishment man, can hardly be compared with Revard, except for the career-transforming accident.

Revard gets another lucky break when the countess d'Orsant, on the recommendation of the uncle (eventually revealed as "wicked") comes to see him because she is wasting away in "the hands of abominable charlatans." After carefully examining the patient, Revard recommends an operation, which the "exquisite and delicious creature" lets Revard do. After a few weeks the countess is rehabilitated, and Revard, now widely known as a doctor who worked a miracle, rises to the dangerous status of medical savior. Like surgeons, patients believe in the effective power of surgery over any other medical treatment. Revard begins to meet the elegant *tout Paris* in the countess's salons. Even more dangerous for Revard is the fact that he now earns three times more than the best known old fogies of the faculty of medicine. But the cost of his medical theater is high. The luxury required by his up-market trade costs him 40,000 francs a year in addition to the license fee and taxes. Revard's explanation of how he manages to pay for

9 Story in J. E. Dezeimeris, *Dictionnaire historique de la médecine ancienne et moderne* (4 vols, Paris, 1828–39), volume 4.

all this plunges us into the seamy side of medical practice. The theatrical device by which the playwright reveals this to us is a secretary's entering with a letter from Dr Lambert about the Rumanian female patient he sent to Revard last week. Revard tells the secretary to telephone Lambert to tell him that the operation costs 6000 francs, a sum that perks up Durieux's ears. Since this is the first case that the doctor has referred to Revard, Lambert will get a generous commission of 50 percent of the surgeon's fee. Subsequent referrals will earn Lambert 30 percent of the fee.

Durieux is shocked to find his friend practicing fee splitting, of which patients are ignorant. Revard's spin on the practice is that he just helps doctors starting out, who need the money; encouraging them is different from the fee splitting condemned by the professional medical code, which does, however, permit the surgeon to charge for aides and the attending physician or family doctor. Revard notes that this virtuous theory succumbs to a corrupt practice because patients rarely discuss the surgeon's fee but refuse eight out of ten times to pay the others involved in the operation, though the consulting doctor has at least as much responsibility as the specialist because he recommends the operation and picks the operator. But to Revard's reasonable explanation of fee splitting in Paris, where the struggle is hard, Durieux answers with a total rejection of the practice in any form.[10] A bouquet-bearing servant, followed by Revard's longtime "petite camarade," the actress Fernande de Ligny, interrupts them.

During their conversation it emerges that Durieux met Fernande chez Revard in the bad old days in the avenue des Gobelins. The "king of surgery" – Fernande's accolade – gives a silver fox fur to his woman. This stunning item cost two appendix operations. Durieux wonders if he will ever be able to give his wife such a gift. Perhaps, if he makes enough money from an anti-infection serum that he is working on. Revard's interest perks up and, on discovering that the serum is to be tested in the laboratory of one of the medical professors, he denounces the poverty of the faculty and hospital laboratories. He offers to let Durieux test the serum in a model asylum having all the latest equipment. Is this a sly reference to Henri's establishment? Revard adds that if the serum works, he will spread the good word. Eager to profit from six years of research, Durieux agrees to the scheme. In the interests of good drama and medical ethics, the gravy train is soon derailed.

Revard owes 623,000 francs to Leroux, the "wicked uncle" who started him on the road to fortune. (Leroux paid the contractors 315,000 for Revard's asylum, 110,000 for the apartment, and the rest for cash loans.) A first note for 100,000 francs (15 percent interest) will be due in 4 months. Leroux needs his money to launch a *couturière*. Leroux consoles the shocked Revard by telling him that it was a true tour de force to have spent hardly 600,000 francs in order to install a surgeon in a setting worthy of his talent and in less than two years create a pool of rich patients. As a reward for his services, Leroux used Revard's name in advertising.

---

10 Revard cynically notes that it is easy to fool a suffering patient with useless promises, and so on. *Le Caducée*, 33.

Consequently, *Le Cri d'alarme* attacked the doctor as a vile commercial operator, a shameful fee splitter, and a charlatan. Fortunately for Revard, salvation is at hand with the entry into his pool of patients of Jessie Watson, a rich American hypochondriac, daughter of the marquis d'Avranches. She is married to the "lift king" of New York.

Jessie was recruited by the comtesse d'Orsant, née Duran and so only an aristocrat by marriage. The countess tells Revard that if he knows how to handle the American, his fortune is assured. Although she is full of energy and is the picture of good health, Jessie is exhausted by the duties and pleasures imposed on her by New York obligations and Paris social rounds. In our day she might have been diagnosed as suffering from chronic fatigue syndrome or even fibromyalgia (said to afflict some six million American women). And, as in the case of the modern diseases, there was medical disagreement over Jessie's case, and though one of the opinions is suspect, we have to recognize that the patient thought she was sick. She recites an impressive list of symptoms: inability to sleep, frequent stomach pains, which travel upward to her chest and threaten to suffocate her, and have been torturing her for two months; her nerves seem concentrated in a suffocating ball; everything seems in a knot. Revard is not old fashioned enough to diagnose madame's disease as hysteria. His examination is rather painless: eyes, reflexes, tests with mallet and pin; some vague conclusions expressed in quasi-medical jargon ("légère inégalité papillaire, exagération des réflexes, diminution de la sensibilité ... zone d'anesthésie"). The anxious patient asks "do I need an operation?" The doctor, though a "virtuoso of the scalpel," merely keeps his options open with the reply, "not at this time." Nowadays we would want to know if the patient was disappointed in not needing an operation. As curious as it may seem to the healthy patient, the sick patient often prefers surgery to other treatments. The definitive diagnosis is a mild "asthénie centrifuge." The patient wonders what it is, but the doctor wisely prescribes treatment instead of explaining the inexplicable. To improve her general condition, Revard prescribes "névrosthéniques" injections and a systematic cure by colored rays of electric light. Thus her "nervous centers" will be acted on efficaciously. The treatment by colored rays emanating from a screen is regulated for the intensity of the electric current, specified by the doctor.[11] The colors used for the particular "névrosthénisante" action in this case have a strong aesthetic lure for the patient: among the different colors, she loves the blue. After a week's exposure to colored rays, she will be ready to take a dose of ultra-violet rays. The ray-man is a student of Revard's; so the business is kept in the closely associated professional family. Normal practice.

Revard is a successful doctor who knows how to keep his patients happy. Jessie exclaims "What a beautiful way to treat illnesses!" Revard replies that the

---

[11] Georges Duhamel, *Les Maîtres* (Paris, 1937), 189, describes a patient being treated in the hospital to "des essais de bains lumineux." The patient, a good-looking, chubby young woman, inspires Professor Rohner to punctuate his observations with some risqué remarks.

"modern practitioner must treat his patients with the latest and most efficacious therapeutic methods." By this time Jessie is falling in love with the doctor, as becomes painfully evident later when she nearly faints on hearing d'Orsant's expression of love for Revard. In order to keep her abreast of new systems of treatment – she "adores medicine" – he signs her up for a journal he edits, *le Chirurgien Mondain*, which popularizes his ideas. The next day the doctor sees her at the *Institut photo-thérapeutique*, where he is present for her first ray bath before giving her an injection.

Le Caducée presents another type of doctor, one who gives a different kind of physical examination – thorough. Jessie tells Revard that professor Godfroy, the doctor of the marquise d'Avranches, palpated her with his enormous hands and during the auscultation he was breathing like a seal. All this torture after the indignity of having to wait in his proletarian office and then to get only a prescription to take baths! Revard notes with ironic amusement that Godfroy is faithful to traditions of the old medicine. We learn later from Godfroy's conversation with the marquise that the old doctor wants her to go back to her husband in New York as soon as possible. This was probably more a moral judgment on the presence of a young married woman alone in Paris and a wife's marital obligations than a subtle way of stating the Viennese prescription of "penis normalis dosim repetatur," though one cannot completely exclude the latter possibility. On hearing that her regular American doctor recommended an operation, Godfroy threw his hands in the air and exclaimed that the fellow must be crazy. Great doctors had no need to cultivate a winning bedside manner.

When Revard later meets Fernande, he ecstatically tells her that this amazing neurasthenic American woman came to tell him a lot of laughable nonsense and that he fobbed off one of his treatments upon her. This makes it easier for us to accept the panegyric of "le père Godfroy" a while later: "an ace … an old-fashioned honest surgeon! Nothing in common with this Revard."[12] Maybe not, but Jessie says that she feels great since Dr Revard has been taking care of her. Her mother remarks on Jessie's clear eyes and the healthy glow to her cheeks, though she hardly finds the time to eat and sleep. The marquis is amused by his daughter's worship of medical prowess.

In Godfroy, Henri gives us a caricature of the ancient medical patriarch, a type still flourishing in the twentieth century. He boasts that the practices of his professional conscience mesh poorly with contemporary practices. The respect of traditions, a virtue for Godfroy, is becoming rare in the medical profession though, martyr to the cause, he still tries to inculcate this notion in his apparently refractory students. During the course of a reception, the painter Vernet asks the professor if it is possible to visit his medical establishment for documentation on a painting of a surgeon operating in a clinic. Godfroy replies that he never lets outsiders into his domain; he would never pose professionally for a painter or photographer. This view would certainly have surprised the giants of the French

[12] *Le Caducée*, 104–5.

scientific and medical world, but it is consistent with Godfroy's *Weltanschauung*. He has a passionate conversation with a layman about hunting woodcock rather than surgery because he "avoids talking about professional questions with people who are incapable of understanding them." As in the play *La Vocation*, Henri gives vent here to his irritation with the continual medical chitchat in Parisian social circles. The marquise agrees with Godfroy. He is a rare bird in a period when "so many doctors chose exactly those who understand nothing of medicine to speak to them about an interesting case or a miraculous operation."[13] This praise gives Godfroy the opportunity to launch into a discourse providing a capsule history of the social development of the medical profession during his lifetime.

Godfroy's basic belief concerning the practice of surgery is that the sole medical concern must be the cure and relief of the patient along with the teaching of students. In his mind there was no possibility of a conflict here. The grave nature of a major operation, involving considerable bleeding, excludes any presence other than medical in the operating room. And though nearly everyone else is behaving with no conscience and even less virtue and has made cowardly concessions to modern "unhealthy curiosity," this 65-year-old professor intends to defend the ancient Hippocratic fort. Jessie is also taken aback by this outburst. The marquis approves. Revard appears on the periphery of the group while Godfroy is in full flow.

The professor ingeniously argues that the public's interest in seeing what goes on in surgery is a logical development of a pre-1914 passion on the part of a perverted public for violent sports. The Great War gave people more than they asked for. One of the results of the conflict, as Henri observed on several occasions, was the greatly increased presence of women in medicine. Godfroy praises their devotion and sacrifices, but now that peace has returned, women should return to *Küche, Kinder und Kirche*. Women are no longer needed to take care of the sick; they have a more important role in maintaining the married household while the breadwinner is restoring the prosperity of the ruined country. His young medical colleagues could do their part by following the advice he gives at the beginning of his course each year: indulge in no flashy publicity but work in splendid silence, for that is how great character and strong minds are formed. It is with relief that we hear Revard's ironic "bravo!" as he penetrates the group to declare that medicine is an apostolate.

Revard represents the new generation of doctors that Godfroy has imagined in order to hate. And no doubt there were some Revard-like types wielding the scalpel in Paris. The important social point about the Revard type is the new ascendancy of the doctor. Vernet growls about their irritating over-presence everywhere in society. Another character sees the doctor as occupying a new social role. The new doctor is old abbé writ large. Doctors "have taken in the boudoirs of pretty women the role that the abbés of the eighteenth century had with our grandmothers."

[13] *Le Caducée*, 107–8.

Vernet regrets even more that they have often become "the secular confessors of our wives and daughters."[14]

Revard deals with the split in the medical profession in a more interesting way than Godfroy, or at least he clearly identifies an old problem that had become more serious ethically in modern times. In his entrance speech to the group he regrets that "certain colleagues are ignorant of the true significance of our glorious caduceus." There is a discussion of the two different emblems called by the same name, one associated with Asclepius having one snake and the other associated with Hermes (Mercury) having two intertwined snakes and sometimes wings at the top. (Hermes began with two white ribbons on a stick but deceived eyes found snakes.) Revard deals with the one-snake wand and Godfroy, picking up on the remark that Mercury is the god of commerce, slips in an observation on doctors who have a flexible conscience. But it is Revard who lectures the group on the two emblems, emphasizing that the medical emblem has the mirror of truth at its top and gives its followers the satisfaction of having served humanity while avoiding the worship of Mercury. "The true scientist, truly worthy of the name of doctor, will never hesitate between the two emblems." Revard's gush of fine-sounding hypocritical talk enchants his listeners. Godfroy leaves, muttering "Quel cabot!" He sees Revard as a phony actor.

Revard continues his act by agreeing to let Vernet come to his establishment to do his painting for the salon show coming up. The women ask to come too, and Revard agrees. The word amphitheater now seems all too appropriate. Dr Javelin, Revard's associate, is disgusted with the circus-like atmosphere of the clinic, in particular with the invasion by the "femmes du monde." The circus expands when reporters show up to see an actress recovering from a bullet wound. Fernande handles the reporters before rushing off to a rehearsal. But the irreverent reporters from *Le Cri d'Alarme* and *L'Eveil* give a devastating view of what the medical community thinks of Revard. "The genius surgeon," the "great magician" is laughed at. The brother of one of the reporters is a hospital intern, whose colleagues split their sides laughing at the bluffer Revard. Damage control to save the skills if not the character of the protagonist seems in order, and Henri soon provides it.

After Revard presents Vernet and a gaggle of his visitors to the reporters, d'Orsant praises the doctor's dexterity and sang-froid. Vernet praises his rapidity, measured with a chronometer. A hilarious account of a pyloromyotomy, for someone presumably diagnosed with pyloric stenosis, is centered on the procedure's being timed down to the fifth of a second. The trick wins over even the most skeptical reporters. D'Orsant has only to give the final accolade as the "modern magician" prepares to leave, though not without another brief speech. (A minor mystery intrudes when Revard ignores the information that the patient in room 23 is in critical condition.) Revard declares that "in our time of scientific popularization, it is good, even necessary, to initiate the public into the mysteries of modern surgery." Madame de Clessy gives a typical patient's viewpoint in noting that she

14 *Le Caducée*, 105.

finds Revard charming, which means that she rejects all of the bad things that her doctor said about Revard. A gay ending to this gathering presages tragedy. In an establishment with photographic and film studios, it is easy to please people with a group photograph. The spectacle of the "femmes du monde" in nurse's uniforms provokes general gaiety, which is counterbalanced by the disgruntled Javelin. He does not want to get blamed for what happened in room 23; though he gave the patient an injection of camphorated oil, it is Revard's case – a dirty business Javelin calls it. He is on the point of quitting.

So in spite of the medical establishment's low opinion of him, Revard is riding high. When a cabinet minister is introduced to Revard, he addresses the doctor with a title of distinction. But "monsieur le professeur" is not a professor. Revard explains to the astonished politician that he is not part of the "official school" but is an independent. The quick-thinking minister declares that Revard's place should be in the faculty of medicine; he also approves of Revard's independence. This approval signals the probability of Revard's being elevated into the Legion of Honor, thus rewarding his independence with official recognition.

At the root of Revard's problems is his debt to Leroux; his fix is aggravated by the failure of the clinic to generate enough income to cover expenses. The secretary tells Dr Javelin that expenses are more than twice the clinic's income. Perhaps this disastrous financial situation explains Revard's base act of refusing to operate on a child for the 2000 francs the mother had scraped together towards the 8000 francs stipulated earlier as the price of the operation. He had done an appendix operation for 600 francs a week before. Revard boasts that six times out of ten he operates free for the advertising value of the charitable act. As he and d'Orsant discuss his financial quandary, it comes out that he is collecting 10,000 francs a month from Jessie (as a patient); d'Orsant observes that if the doctor had listened to the patient, he would have admitted her to the clinic long ago. Revard regrets that she is in good health while noting that an attack of acute appendicitis could occur at any time. This attack is highly probable because any profits from the serum developed by Durieux are at least six months away. And the straight-dealing Durieux has to be handled carefully.

The result of a bad medical decision slowly unfolds, bringing with it the destruction of Revard's career and his suicide. He operates on Jessie, who, we have guessed, turns out to be the patient in room 23; the patient's critical and deteriorating post-operative state can be made known to Revard by room number only, not name, according to house rules. It seems contrived but the theatrical effect is good. Jessie's operation comes about as the end of developments precipitated by a telegram from her husband telling her to come home immediately. Worried about interrupting her treatment and agitated over leaving Paris (and Revard), she gets a little pain like the one she had six weeks ago. She sees Revard and the countess d'Orsant, who help her evade the marital command by arranging a trip with d'Orsant to the villa of the countess in Saint-Cloud, from where she can easily go to Revard's nearby clinic to receive electrical stimulation. A judicious combination of the mundane and the medical: careful watching of her symptoms and rest rather than a potentially dangerous ocean crossing is the doctor's prescription. All this is done through d'Orsant because Revard cannot give advice going against the husband's wishes. D'Orsant points out that Revard took responsibility for Jessie's health, but the subterfuge has no medical justification because Revard believes that Jessie is as fit as a fiddle.

The operation on the healthy patient turns out to be medically disastrous and financially unnecessary. Leroux manages to sell the serum formula to a Swiss company for 50 percent of profits and 500,000 francs cash, a sum that takes care of all problems, with the lion's share of the money going to Leroux. Durieux agrees to the plan for 10,000 francs in cash and 10 percent of the profits. He also agrees to negotiate with Revard on future discoveries. The ghastliness of all this wheeling and dealing is illustrated when personnel of the clinic remind Revard that the patient in room 23 is getting worse while the doctor is fending off Leroux and convincing Durieux to sign away most of the fruits of his labors. When the patient is reported as pale, agitated, and having a low temperature and rapid pulse, Revard orders the operating room made ready: artificial serum, adrenaline, camphorated oil, and containers of hot water have to be available. He finally rushes off to room 23 when the patient hemorrhages. "Fichtre! C'est grave!"[15] The plot thickens when Jessie's parents show up demanding to see their daughter; after learning of the operation, the marquis threatens to go to the police. Revard justifies his actions by stating that he was called to see madame Watson because she was very sick, nervous, agitated, and suffering from internal pains. Revard admits that so far he has given no justification for the operation, a possibility mentioned incidentally to Jessie, but he goes on to claim that there were undeniable symptoms of peritonitis, whose source he was unable to detect at first – "appendix, gall bladder ... well, in many cases, a precise diagnosis is hardly possible."[16] Surgery seemed in order. The marquis wants Godfroy to come in on the case. Revard refuses; he himself is handling the post-operative complications.

While the patient is dying, the doctors squabble over responsibility and ethics. Javelin is quitting because he is fed up with being an accomplice in needless operations, done three times out of five for money rather than medical necessity. Javelin predicts Jessie's death, which will make Revard a killer because she had nothing wrong with her except "imaginary pains," which were exploited by Revard in order to seduce her into concluding (or agree with her) that her serious state required the operation.[17] Revard does make a good point in asking Javelin if he imagines that doctors can always make an accurate diagnosis and operate with the certainty of succeeding, though this question does not change Javelin's mind concerning Revard's crime. And Javelin refuses to leave before assisting in a vain effort to save Jessie's life. Revard recognizes that the death of a rich patient in

[15] *Le Caducée*, 213.

[16] *Le Caducée*, 224.

[17] *Le Caducée*, 236.

suspicious circumstances means that the jig is up.[18] Jessie's death was a successful piece of theater, no doubt because of the skill of the actress in dying and perhaps also the audience's perception that they are all potential patients who might die in a similar situation.

Revard decides to disappear for a few days after d'Orsant tries to convince him to weather it out. "After all, it's one of those unfortunate cases that can happen to any surgeon."[19] She offers to defend him, even in the press. But before Revard can leave, professor Godfroy appears to hand down judgment. Revard is demoted from the status of colleague: "our profession does not recognize your 'trade'." Accused of murder, Revard repeats the question he asked Javelin: has the professor always operated with certainty of success?[20] It's a good question even if asked in bad faith. The crushing professorial non-reply is that in his department he has always practiced with absolute honesty and never permitted this most repugnant of masquerades. After a scathing review of Revard's actions, Godfroy says that there is proof of Jessie's having written a check for 60,000 francs payable to Revard, then endorsed by d'Orsant (Revard's "beater"), and cashed by Leroux. This is an affair for the state prosecutor, with Godfroy as eager witness – scandal or not. Jessie was not Revard's first victim but she will be his last.

Godfroy dangles an out for Revard. He can disappear, leave France. Revard replies that this is crazy, but Godfroy reveals the existence of a letter Jessie wrote to Revard saying that she loves him, though he made her suffer, and that she knows that if he gets to read this letter she will be dead. At the end of his tether, Revard tells Godfroy that he understands. The professor leaves. This revelation explains why the marquis would be willing to remain silent if Revard disappears. For professional reasons, Godfroy is willing to accept Revard's escape from justice. Revard is still a doctor: "there is no higher title than doctor of medicine."[21] Its prestige must be safeguarded. No cases of corruption can be tolerated in the ranks because of the great danger of young doctors becoming infected. So when a black sheep shows up, it must be slaughtered, or sent out to the hills far away. This hardly solves the ethical problem, but at least the victims would not be French or, at least, they would remain unknown to the profession. So out of deference to the members of the profession and out of respect for Revard's title of doctor, Godfroy reluctantly lets Revard disappear.

Revard accepts the offer he can't refuse but he has other plans, involving the ultimate sacrifice for the profession. In the interest of science he chooses to exit in an expiatory act of self-experimentation. Before the death drama began, Durieux had delivered to Revard two flasks of different sizes, one containing the famous serum and the other containing the extremely poisonous toxin from which it was prepared. Durieux is not sure how the toxin works. A rabbit sacrificed for the

---

18 "Je suis foutu!" *Le Caducée*, 239.

19 *Le Caducée*, 244.

20 *Le Caducée*, 251.

21 *Le Caducée*, 239.

progress of science died fifteen minutes after receiving a dose of one drop per kilo. Five cc of the serum totally neutralizes the poison. After Godfroy leaves, Revard tears up the contract selling Durieux's serum, burns Jessie's letter, and pours the serum down the sink. He then injects five cc of toxin into his left arm, looks at his watch, and starts taking notes. On coming back for the signed contract, Leroux is told that a conclusive and necessary experiment is underway and will take only a short time. When Revard tells Leroux about the source of the 100,000 francs used to pay off the note, the death of the exploited patient, and the lawsuit in the works, Leroux replies that a good lawyer always successfully defends even the most unskilled of doctors. Revard then denounces Leroux, who goes off to deal directly with Durieux. That attempt fails. Durieux comes in as Revard is showing signs of poisoning but is alert enough to confess his last crime, the unnecessary and fatal operation on "la petite Watson." A martyr to the end, Revard writes down his symptoms. In repentant mood, he gives Durieux a letter for Javelin, who had just left, eyes full of scorn and hatred. Then a note for Fernande. A professional to the end, Revard's last words are for Godfroy. "I understood … I understood everything!" Salvation achieved, he dies with an enlightened if not clear conscience.

What was the reaction of the Parisian medical community to *Le Caducée*? There are two answers to this question: one is fictive and one is true. Paul Veyne argued that "Men do not find the truth; they create it, as they create their history."[22] We might say something similar about fiction, which has been consecrated as a valuable source of historical knowledge. The withdrawal of the play after the author frightened a rather timid group of actors with his reading in December 1911 led to speculation in the press about pressure from the medical community. Certain medical bigwigs, supposedly upset by the subject, got Henri to withdraw the play from production. One story related that some famous doctors, on learning of Henri's "bellicose intentions," went to ask him to withdraw or modify the play.[23] Henri's ironic question concerning this misinformation was not without its danger for the medical profession, though neither reporter nor doctor took up the subtext: do the "great doctors" recognize "themselves in the charlatans." A variant of this story identifies the protesting actors as members of the faculty of medicine. When Charles de Lagrille asked about this scoop by a fellow reporter, Henri denied that the reported event had occurred. Quite to the contrary: a group of doctors from inside and outside the faculty completely approved of the play. In 1910, when it appeared that the Vaudeville theater would stage the play, Henri was easily able to invite a group of "maîtres de la science médicale," including Pozzi, Segond, Dieulafoy, and Delbet – his former teachers and friends – to give their approval after a reading of the play. The doctors easily followed Henri's interpretation

[22] Paul Veyne, *Did the Greeks Believe their Myths?*, quoted in G. W. Bowerstock, *Fiction as History. Nero to Julian* (Berkeley, 1994), 11, note 9.

[23] Article by R. T. in "Les Théâtres," Arsenal Rf. 71.727. Newspaper clipping, with no source or date given.

that he was just attacking bad doctors, rare creatures in the profession he insisted optimistically. And of course the play had its medical heroes, who brought honor to science and honesty to their noble profession.[24]

And the play did not give rise to any problems at the *Salle des agriculteurs* in March when Henri spoke to his colleagues on the weighty topic of "Le médecin dans la société contemporaine." It could be argued that the author was following the earlier advice of Farabeuf on ethical behavior. When Pierre Delbet was given a gold medal commemorating his nomination to the surgical chair in the faculty, Farabeuf declared in an accompanying speech that it is a "useful and even necessary work to stigmatize certain condemnable practices engaged in by certain doctors hungry for money, luxury, fame, and honors."[25]

Critics and spectators did not necessarily come to the same conclusion as the doctors. Henri hoped that the play would create a stir in the medical world and stimulate excitement among critics and theatergoers. He was not disappointed, though he did not escape being surprised by unintended consequences and by how quickly rumors started flying. Henri denied that the play dealt with the illegal practice of fee splitting, as some people said.[26] They might be forgiven for this mistake, for the play does present an egregious example of the practice. Henri explained away the potential paradox by noting that Revard was a charlatan and therefore unrepresentative of the medical profession. A reasonable claim, though a rather facile dismissal of a thorny ethical issue in the practice of medicine – an issue handled skillfully in the play.

A way out of the quandary was to shrink the pool of criminal doctors to "a few." This was the not uncommon strategy employed by Robert de Beauplan, who brandished the rhetoric of good and evil in *La Liberté*.[27] Fortunately, no one seems to have thought of the metaphor of the bad apple that spoils the barrel. De Beauplan made a more interesting point about the play by comparing it with the neo-classical treatment of doctors by Molière and company: they turned the charlatan into a buffoon. Comedy, not tragedy. Robert de Fleurs asserted that playwrights used doctors chiefly in comedy but kept surgeons in reserve especially for drama. De Fleurs found in *Le Caducée* the striking autopsy of "a sinister category of arriviste sawbones."[28] There is an important difference between Léon Daudet's treatment of doctors and Henri's. Maurice de Waleffe noted the colorful extravagance of

[24] The play was dedicated to the memory of Farabeuf, faculty professor of anatomy, "who taught 30 generations of physicians, whose work and science had taken French surgical art so far," and to G. Dieulafoy, professor of clinical medicine.

[25] Farabeuf, "Discours ... 6 juillet 1910 à l'hôpital Necker ... remise d'une médaille d'or au professeur Pierre Delbet, en souvenir de sa nomination à la chaire chirurgicale de la faculté de médecine de Paris," quoted at the beginning of *Le Caducée* (1912).

[26] "... Une pièce ... qui est, en quelque sorte, un réquisitoire dialogué contre la 'dichotomie'. See pp. 237–8 above.

[27] Quoted in *La petite Illustration* 51 (11 juin 1921).

[28] Robert de Fleurs, in *Le Gaulois* (7 février 1921), Arsenal, Rf. 71.727.

Daudet's portrait, which lacked, however, the nuances of *Le Caducée*.[29] And, as some great novelists discovered to their sorrow, the ability to write a successful novel does not translate easily into the ability to write a good play. In *Le Caducée* the charlatan, who was a real scientific physician, became a criminal. Nothing could be more serious. "Irony … gave way to anguish," as de Beauplan so nicely put it. Science (misused), greed (the doctor's), and hope (the patient's) corrupted medicine (a noble profession). Of course a play could always end on an optimistic note. At the end of *Le Caducée* Dr Revard's conscience is awakened as he dies in Faustian innocence with the meaning of the Hippocratic Logos fully revealed. De Fleurs thought that the last act was weakened by Revard's killing himself in order to avoid legal battle; if Revard had died for professional honor, he would have appeared as "an expiatory martyr of science," and so the last act would be more satisfying intellectually and, in this view, better drama.[30] But since Revard used a medical experiment as a means of suicide, he was a martyr. There are easier ways for a doctor to die. And death seems a sensible solution to his legal problems. It is not easy to change one part of the play without messing up another. The author knows best. G. de Pawlowski exaggerated a point in saying that the play was "an interesting work of propaganda, written by a person of good faith"– and of independent means.[31] There is little evidence to back up Louis Schneider's opinion that the play would have the same polemical impact in surgical circles that Eugène Brieux's *La robe rouge* had on the magistracy. It may be, as de Fleurs said, that the surgeon transformed his profession into a trade whereas it must be exercised as a sacerdotal function. Of course modern surgeons, who successfully marry the two activities, are likely to be puzzled by the argument that one excludes the other, a proposition that is itself an interpretation of creative theatrical ambiguity.

People addicted to non-theatrical reality could always see in Dr Revard the name of the famous surgeon (not named in the texts I have seen) who had been the protagonist in a drama not totally different from that in *Le Caducée*, but we should remember that the original unrevised play preceded the historical event. It was easier to conflate play and reality than Henri had originally thought, though the pre-war draft of the play had been stimulated by what he called "one of those mysterious and terrible dramas" little talked about except vaguely in the press and more often than not hidden from the public. The play was then in a sense a quick rough sketch of an event the author himself had witnessed. A medical tragedy had led Henri to do what he always thought should be done: write a play set in the medical world. No doubt he recognized that he had dredged up a scabrous subject; the important thing was that he would enlighten the public through the theater. If the public did not know already, it would learn that most surgeons, personifying the professional conscience, respected their art and felt their responsibilities. The problem was the others, the scoundrels of the scalpel ("les apaches du bistouri"),

[29] Maurice de Waleffe, in *Comœdia illustré* (20 février 1921), Arsenal, Rf. 71.727.

[30] Robert de Fleurs, in *Le Gaulois* (7 février 1921), Arsenal, Rf. 71.727.

[31] G. de Pawlowski, in Arsenal Rf. 71.727; no source given; dated 21 mars 1921.

ambitious, greedy, bold, careless, and cynical doctors. To denounce them and their practices was a service to humanity, especially to that part of humanity Henri diagnosed as neurotic women. These impressionable creatures were the easy prey of the medical "apache" because they were easily disarmed by the doctor's eloquence, dumbfounded by his knowledge, and conquered by his reputation.[32] These then were the ideas propelling Henri into finishing the play that one of his admirers called "an exciting incursion into an environment whose 'underside' is unknown to us."[33] And it was an excellent example of what Fernand Gregh called "le pathétique moderne."[34]

Le Caducée gave a pathetic form to that elusive abstraction, the doctor's conscience. De Waleffe believed this to be a serious enough issue to declare that the sick people of Paris – *le grand public* – should all see the play. Doctors were the only people having the power of life and death over their fellow human beings without the need to account to anyone. The power to pronounce death sentences had been taken away from magistrates of the assize courts and given to a jury in order not to deaden the professional judge's sensibility. But "the privilege that justice gives to the accused, modern medicine refuses to the innocent [the patient]." De Waleffe did not think that Henri had found a solution to the problem; so he gave it to him. Completely turn around professional practices by having surgery put under the control of several experts for pre-operative advice. This would be comparable to the procedure for committing a person to a mental asylum. Surgeons, well known for belief in their own infallibility, might be offended, but in a system where the judge had an interest in the verdict, he could not be allowed to pick the jury. The problem, as de Waleffe saw it, was not so much in dealing with doctors as with surgeons. One could always consult a second doctor without the first doctor knowing about it. But once a patient was admitted to a clinic for surgery, only one weak human being made the decision to cut or not to cut. De Waleffe managed to extract himself from this frightful situation only by insisting, like Henri, that most Parisian surgeons "remained perfectly incapable of succumbing to this criminal temptation."[35] It did not sound any more convincing in the critic's analysis than in the play. Both playwright and critic might have benefited from a light dose of anxiety-creating ambiguity on the issue of unnecessary surgery. Cosmetic or aesthetic surgery did not yet seem ripe for the playwright's pen. And certainly the idea of women as a group being victims of the surgeon's scalpel was even more remote, though *Le Caducée* raised the idea incidentally.

---

32 Larito, "L'histoire du '*Caducée*'," in *Le Gaulois* (2 février 1921), Arsenal, Rf. 71.727.

33 Larito, "L'histoire du '*Caducée*'," in *Le Gaulois* (2 février 1921), Arsenal, Rf. 71.727.

34 Fernand Gregh, clipping dated 6 février 1921; no source given; Arsenal, Rf. 71.727.

35 Maurice de Waleffe, in *Comœdia illustré* (20 février 1921), 13, in Arsenal, Rf. 71.727.

In an introduction to *Le Caducée* in 1912 Henri stated that he believed the play to be about morals and character, only incidentally about doctors.[36] Still, he could not get away from the fact that he had paraded a number of medical types on the stage to give their opinions on professional ethics and practices. These were related to serious contemporary social problems while also being controversial scientific issues. Henri's reason for choosing to give an accurate portrait of the medical world was simply that the doctor had come to occupy a leading role in French society. And it was the duty of an "independent dramatic author" who had "the advantage of belonging to the medical corps" to expose any abuses of medical power or lapses in professional ethics of which he was aware. Otherwise he would be hurting all the innocent and competent "true doctors" loyally and conscientiously exercising their profession.

So *Le Caducée* was not an attack on "true doctors." The hero (Miltonic style) of the play, Dr Revard, though a real doctor, had to be seen as an exception in the profession, a professional man of the scalpel who had transformed his profession into a trade.[37] Worse, he was a charlatan who seriously competed with "true doctors," who were represented by Godfroy, the austere and moral surgeon, and two other types, Durieux, the scrupulous country doctor, and, after he saw the light, Javelin, the honest assistant. The great doctors of the day agreed with Henri. Dieulafoy declared the play "not only useful but necessary."[38] Delbet had no problem in promising his friend that he would write a preface to the play. Assaulted by all this medical approval of the play, one might be tempted to think that it was too friendly to doctors. But as we have seen, *le petit public* had another interpretation of the play.

Gossip about the play was inseparable from gossip about Henri, "une personnalité des plus Parisiens." Antoine declared that the brilliant success of *Le Caducée* permanently buried the Parisian legend of the frivolity of the author, the rich dabbler in the theater. It was now impossible to contest the fact that Henri was a serious author. The public's skepticism about his talent was no longer justified, if it ever had been. Robert de Fleurs, a voice of cultural authority, praised the play's "powerful dramatic interest" and the author's "remarkable scenic gift." The critical babel predicted that *Le Caducée* would be "one of the sensational events of the theatrical season." Baron de Rothschild could be described as "one of the most active and happiest" of authors, though one who was appropriately shy enough to try (unsuccessfully) to avoid a special ovation for the author at the performance *couturières*.[39]

---

36 *Le Caducée* (1912), "Avant-propos" and "Introduction," i–xiii.

37 "Il représente sans exagération, le type de ces professionnels du bistouri, heureusement rares, qui ont transformé leur profession en un véritable métier ... " *Le Caducée* (1912)., "Introduction," xi.

38 *Le Caducée* (1912), "Avant-propos" and "Introduction," i–xiii.

39 *Le Gaulois* (6 février 1921) and *Annales* (20 février 1921), Arsenal, Rf. 71.727.

Chapter 11
The Female Doctor's Dilemma: *La Vocation*

Doctors don't change diapers. [1]

In a pioneering study of "Seven who made a revolution," Thomas Bonner made the reasonable claim that the seven women who began studies in the 1860s for a medical degree at the University of Zurich "made possible the greatest victory won by medical women in the nineteenth century." In spite of many problems, the pedagogical experiment succeeded so well that other Swiss universities (Bern, Geneva, and Lausanne) also accepted female medical students; by 1907 about a thousand women were studying medicine in Swiss universities, "a number greater than the rest of Europe combined."[2] The presence of women in European universities, mainly in Switzerland and France, and to a lesser degree in Belgium and Germany, was one half of a new educational phenomenon, what Natalia Tikhonov described as the "appearance [1870–1910] of two new categories of students ... foreigners and women."[3] Tikhonov put forward the idea of a "Zurich model," an "open" university popular with foreigners, one that favored feminization. Most of the foreigners were from Eastern Europe, with Jewish students from the Russian Empire the dominant category. Of course, as Tikhonov points out, in Western Europe as a whole, foreigners and particularly foreign women remained marginal compared to the student mass.[4]

Most discussion of medicine in France is centered on Paris with its prestigious faculty of medicine. An enormous amount of historical work has been done on French student populations, but it is just as well to face up to the sober fact that when it comes to women as students in medicine and as graduating doctors we are dealing with small numbers. In the period 1870–1900 for Paris, out of a total of 14,529 doctors who graduated, only 1538 were foreigners, including 172 women;

---

1 Perri Klass, *A Not Entirely Benign Procedure. Four Years as a Medical Student* (New York, 1994), 179.

2 Thomas Neville Bonner, "Rendezvous in Zurich. Seven who Made a Revolution in Women's Medical Education, 1864–1874," *Journal of the History of Medicine and Allied Sciences* 44 (Jan. 1989): 7–27.

3 Natalia Tikhonov, "Migrations des étudiants et féminisation de quelques universités européennes à la recherche d'une convergence," in Harmut Rüdiger and Peter and Natalia Tikhonov (eds), *Universitäten als Brücken in Europa* (Frankfurt am Main, 1993), 43–53.

4 See Tikhonov, "Migrations des étudiants et féminisation de quelques universitiés européennes à la recherche d'une convergence," in Rüdiger and Peter and Natalia Tikonov (eds), *Universitäten als Brücken in Europa*, 43–9.

28 of a total of 200 women were French.[5] After 1905 the Paris faculty turned out more French than foreign women medical doctors. Out of the total for the entire period, over 16 percent of the graduates were foreign and less than 4 percent were female. Henri de Rothschild noted nostalgically that in the Paris faculty back in 1890 there were only 3500 students, among whom were a few women – he was guessing: one official total student count was 4319. World War I caused a steep drop in the number of women in medical schools, but in the 1920s the number rose to new heights. In 1921 *La chronique médicale* proclaimed the "feminine invasion of the University of Paris".[6] By 1927 in Paris the number of female medical students was up to 832. And in 1927–28, 47 French and 9 foreign women received the degree of doctor of medicine from French faculties. In 1900 there had been 87 women doctors practicing in France, mostly in Paris; by 1928 the *Annuaire médical* identified 556 women practicing medicine in France, of whom 314 were in the department of the Seine.[7] When he was nearing the end of his medical career in the late 1930s Henri thought regretfully that 35 percent of the medical students were female, which seemed to interest him more than the fact that 20 percent of the students were foreigners.[8] For the Paris faculty in 1935 George Weisz gives a total figure of 4067 students, of whom 22 percent were women.[9] By the 1930s the male doctors were more alarmed about competition from foreigners than from women.

In the Théâtre de la Michodière, on 10 May 1927, Henri, behind his thespian mask of André Pascal, spoke to a joint meeting of two large groups, the Paris Lyceum Club and the *Automobile Club féminin*, both of which were presided over by the duchess d'Uzès, née Mortemart. Enthusiasm for the automobile was one of the common bonds between the duchess and Henri and Mathilde. Henri spoke about his play *La Vocation*. Translated as *The Dilemma*, the working title of the play had been "La doctoresse." The play, which he wrote in collaboration with the surgeon Pierre Delbet, was the talk of the town because of its treatment of the role of the woman physician in modern society. To introduce Henri's talk, the critic Edmond Sée spoke informally about André Pascal's plays, and after both discourses, four

---

5 Pierre Moulinier gives a figure of 201 women graduating as doctors, including 41 externs and 3 interns, during the same period. See www.barthes.ens.fr/clio/dos/genre/com/moulinierprem.pdf.

6 *La chronique médicale*, 28 (1921): 214.

7 Melina Lipinska, *Les femmes et le progrès des sciences médicales* (Paris, 1930), 174–5.

8 Henri de Rothschild [HR], *Croisière autour de mes souvenirs*. II: *Mes maîtres et mes amis à la faculté et dans les hôpitaux* (Paris, 1936), 9–10.

9 George Weisz, *The Emergence of Modern Universities in France, 1863–1914* (Princeton, 1983), 246; see chapter 7 for discussion of numbers of students. On medical education, see Weisz, "Reform and Conflict in French Medical Education," in Robert Fox and George Weisz (eds), *The Organization of Science and Technology in France 1800–1914* (Cambridge, 1980), 61–94.

well-known actors and actresses interpreted a few scenes from some of Henri's major plays. A gala event.[10] Though Henri spread large on the Paris medical scene and was known as a playwright, this particular talk stemmed from a mini-scandal in the Parisian theater. The trouble resulted mostly from the interpretation given by a number of male and female medical students to some provocative dialogue on women doctors in *La Vocation*, which began a successful run at the Théâtre de la Renaissance in November 1926. A lively success gave rise to nasty polemics. Showing considerable skill in planning, medical students staged incidents during the performance to protest against the anti-feminist opinions developed, with some virulence, by Dr Gerbier, an incidental character whose importance was enhanced by his status of professor in the faculty of medicine. Reports on the protests differed in their estimation of seriousness. "Incidents au Théâtre de la Renaissance" was a title promising readers of *Comœdia illustré* (4 Dec. 1926) more than it delivered, except some overheated prose about the "noisy events": loud whistling, shouting, exclamations, interpellations accompanying Gerbier's dialogue, all culminating in a few blows with some students' dresses torn during a scuffle in the staircase. The police, called in to help theater personnel, took the protestors away to the police station, thus permitting the spectators to enjoy the play in peace. A large part of the audience enjoyed participating in the melee to show their support for play and authors. The protests probably contributed to the play's success when the press brought it to the attention of many people who might not otherwise have been interested.

La Vocation dealt with a great issue of the day. *Excelsior* (17 Nov. 1926) noted that professional women were in fashion as the subject of plays during the season of 1926–27. Doctors and lawyers were the two groups attracting attention at the Athénée and the Renaissance theaters. G. de Pawlowski thought that there had not been so many doctors on the stage since Molière (*Le Journal*, 20 Nov. 1926). An analytical summing up of the play's action and ideas is a useful way to begin a discussion.[11] A playwright named François Mareuil is married to Irene Farrel, a physician who had promised before marriage not to practice medicine. But not being able to break her previous oath to Asclepius she now has a large practice taking up most of her time, which means she pays little attention to her seven-year-old daughter, Germaine. And when love has fled, separate bedrooms are the rule, and even separate entertaining of guests. Robert Kemp thought that the diverse matters

[10] André Pascal [HR], *La femme médecin dans la société moderne.* "Conférence faite au Lyceum club le 10 mai 1927." The scene played from *La Vocation* came from the third act, a husband–wife conflict, rather than a scene dealing with a social issue; then the witty consultation scene in *Le Caducée*, which appears to have been most popular; the new version of the third act of *La Rampe*; and finally a snippet from *L'Affaire Juliette*. The audience was full of aristocrats, intellectuals, doctors, and medical faculty professors with their wives. *Le Gaulois* (5 Nov. 1927), in Arsenal, Rf 71.747.

[11] Also neatly and critically done by Robert Kemp in *L'Intransigeant* (14 Nov. 1926), Arsenal, Rf. 71.727.

treated here came under the rubric of feminism, a word with nasty implications in the play. And Professor Gerbier, Irene's old faculty teacher, is the vehicle of a vigorous and titillating anti-feminist discourse, though of striking unoriginality he boasts. Irene gets called to treat an emergency case, which turns out to be the sick mistress of her husband, who is with her when Irene arrives. Though the shocked doctor is tempted to let her competitor die, she does her duty and saves the patient, who is also acting in Mareuil's current play. Irene has no interest in the real theater; she spends her days and nights in the theater of life and death. She and the mistress eventually have an interesting chat. Irene decides on a divorce. No Corneille-like monologue or internal debate or Molière-type farce here. The discussion between Irene and François stalls over the custody of Germaine. The husband perversely thinks that Irene wants custody just to spite him, which is not completely false. And to wound François in the heart of his paternal ego, she leads him to think that he might not be Germaine's father. This is a lie, but it eventually drives the neurasthenic François crazy and leads to his suicide, in spite of Irene's attempts to kiss and make up.

Irene's medical office is on the first floor of a small Parisian town house. At the beginning of the play a potential conflict between her professional and married lives is signaled in the catty remark by her mother-in-law that the house lacks the true feminine touch and in a lament by her husband that he alone has to raise their daughter because Irene does not have any time to be a mother. Her husband is a sick patient Irene can safely ignore. François had hoped that she would be more than a wife, specifically that she would help him as a writer: being more subtle than men, women can be useful in finding the *mot juste*, in finding the perfect expression, of even men's thoughts.

Though the practical consequences of a married woman being a doctor are played out from beginning to end in the duel between Irene and François, the high-level theoretical debate over women in medicine is an affair between Professor Gerbier and his "dear student," Irene. Gerbier is among the small elite at the peak of medical science, including membership in the Academy of Medicine, and he exudes the authority of his "high scientific position." Candole, dramatic collaborator of François, appreciates at least one of Gerbier's virtues: he doesn't overwhelm people by publicizing his discoveries or miraculous cures. Gerbier is the opposite of "the hammy doctor" who, in Henri's play *Le Caducée*, is incarnated in the surgeon Revard. Gerbier only talks about medicine with those who can understand it; in *Le Caducée* Godfroy has a similar horror of medical shoptalk with non-professionals, in this case the Parisian upper crust who treat medicine as a hot topic of social gossip. Henri's exasperation with the social elite's fascination with the medical world and their eternal social chitchat about doctors is given free rein in the creation of these two great doctors. The creation of these characters also turns out to be a good way to attack the different medical cults, often cultivated by the *médecins-cabotins* (doctors as ham actors), which Henri found to be the subject of conversation among *le tout Paris*. Gerbier will have none of it. The downside of his attitude is not discussed in the play, though Candole denounces doctors who prefer patients to remain in ignorance of the treatment they receive: such doctors prefer "the ideal case, the miraculous operation, the self-advertising lecture – what pretentious bores!"

Gerbier's remark that a few years earlier he would not have accepted Irene as a student opens up the discussion of women in medicine. A stupefied Irene replies that she has never heard him say anything against female medical students. Gerbier adopts a safe bureaucratic defense in noting that his role is simply to teach the students assigned to him by the faculty or the *Assistance publique*, not to lecture on this issue. But Candole and Irene insist that the reluctant Gerbier state his opinion of the woman doctor. He begins with the confession that he is not a feminist but tarts up this remark by adding that he admires women too much to masculinize them. The subtext is that the process of becoming a doctor defeminizes women. Gerbier is aware of a generational change. The polite rituals of the older generation seem ridiculous when performed for a woman who has the nape of her neck shaved and shows her knees. His anthropology being even weaker than his sociology, Gerbier does not see these changes as new mating rituals.

The core of his concern is the preservation of the family – the thing that "fucks you up" according to a *Granta* classic cover some time ago. Gerbier's cruel syllogism begins with the family as the basis of society, next asserts that women are the soul of the family, and, as conclusion, ineluctably imprisons women in it as its savior. When women exercise a profession, the social armature weakens. Biology determines all. Anatomy is social destiny for Gerbier: the human species enjoys a physiological inequality of the sexes. The professor thinks of the response of "savages" to claims of female equality – a couple of punches. This academic fantasy leads Irene to remark that men have been odious in their abuse of power. Which leads to Gerbier's good theatrical reply that women have abused their weakness. The female is after all a creature of sensibility and intuition, not logic; her intelligence leads to "les femmes savantes." Molière had settled the issue. A paradox, Irene exclaims.

Not for Gerbier, however. Seventeenth-century learned women were dilettantes; modern women use learning to grow rich. Irene corrects her *maître*: women want to gain a living and above all to be independent. Deaf to the female voice, Gerbier continues to pontificate, blaming women's blindness and pride for the end of the historical intimate male–female communion defining western civilization. Women scorned their admirable social role, which earned them the homage of men. Gerbier is an all too successful portrait of a phallic colossus who sees women as wanting to have the advantages of both sexes. He perhaps descends to absurdity in declaring that a man cannot be expected to kiss a hand that has just probed a wound. But his basic claim is clear: the profession of medicine is the last that a woman should consider.

Irene believes that medicine is the first occupation that women should think of since it demands the most sensibility and compassion. Gerbier sees these qualities as more those of the nurse than the doctor, who must show compassion but remain master of his sensibility. The implication is that men are better than women at this. There are some things that were not meant for women to do. So the prudish Gerbier feels embarrassed when he has to explain certain physiological or pathological mechanisms to young women, who are less embarrassed – if at all – than he is. And he has never forgotten the pretty woman he saw opening a cadaver's skull to expose the brain. Not a woman's work, and though she married one of Gerbier's colleagues, he insisted that the woman lived in an association with a fellow physician rather than in a marital union and though she became a mother, she was never maternal. A fine distinction between the biological and the social by Gerbier, the self-designated "retardaire en sociologie." He admits that he doesn't understand contemporary social evolution, though it makes him uneasy. Still, the changes cannot be stopped. Gerbier even admits a possible justification for feminism. Better for a woman to ignore the social duties of her sex by exercising a profession than to ignore them while spending a life in frivolous pursuits such as riding, bridge, and dancing. Irene is somewhat mollified by this churlish concession to the "esprit nouveau." Gerbier is consoled by the example of Irene's noble ideal as well as the fact that her marriage, to a man happily ignorant of medical practice, is one that permits a married woman to combine profession and family life. The professor is in for a shock.

A fair amount of *La Vocation* might be classified as comic relief, or it certainly seems funny to our hardened hearts. But the comic also carries its didactic burden. One critic found it incongruous that the play begins as vaudeville and ends as drama. Theatrical genres should not be mixed. This is hesitation, always a danger on stage. Art should not imitate life. At the end of the first act, La Rivière, the treasurer of the dispensary headed by Irene, tells the *doctoresse* that she is charming and, in her white coat, even seductive. But the sweet and most desirable of women tests her suitor's declaration of love with an offer to get divorced and marry him. His ardor cools rapidly. Irene uses this occasion to praise her marriage with François because it gives her total independence to practice her profession. Her husband enjoys the same privilege. Neither is jealous because they both have confidence in each other's loyalty. Irene had earlier declared that a *doctoresse* is a secular nun. Her virtues will soon be sorely tested and found wanting, at least long enough to incubate disaster.

At the beginning of the second act we enter the bedroom of the actress Madeleine Colombier, François' mistress, whose illness offers the occasion for the authors to inflict some medical knowledge on us as the actress sweats, coughs, and gasps for breath during an acute crisis. Madeleine's mother is not happy that a woman doctor responded to the emergency. She doesn't trust them because they don't know as much as real doctors, who must be male. Worse, seeing Mareuil's distress on Irene's arrival, the mother concludes that the *doctoresse* is the mistress he dropped for Madeleine and will kill her daughter. "A jealous woman is capable of anything." When she tries to stop Irene from treating Madeleine, Irene states that as a doctor she has only one aim, to save her patient. Since Madeleine accepts treatment, Irene saves her patient by bleeding her. After the brutal drama is over, a professionally exhausted and emotionally drained Irene tells the mother that

Madeleine's regular doctor will follow the patient's convalescence. A serious doubter of medical competence, the mother exclaims that Dr La Porte could not even cure her sciatica. Irene is firm, for she cannot follow this case without committing a "serious impropriety," moral and professional.

In a later discussion with François, Irene confesses to having wanted to kill Madeleine but boasts that, like a soldier under fire, she did her duty. Gerbier later commends Irene on her magnificent medical and moral behavior. Doctors frequently agree on such matters. It turns out that Irene really acted without thinking much about the horrible situation and only considered later that she might have let Madeleine die. To François it all seems like another piece of boasting by Irene, whose most powerful feeling is pride, or rather vanity. Everything in her life has been based on this ancient vice. Irene begins to look human after all, but that is the problem for François, who wants an ideal wife, like you find in the theater. We find out that Irene concluded that the promise she had made not to practice medicine after marriage came to seem a monstrous demand in light of all the work she had done to become a physician. She does not refuse new patients because a doctor's duty is to the sick and, by implication, takes priority over marital responsibilities. François is not impressed by this moral blather, for after all, "in Paris there are more doctors than patients." Nor can he reach his wife, who is serene in the ecstasy of her calling – *la Vocation*.

In the opening of the third act François' collaborator and mother, Candole and Madame Mareuil, are nattering away about love, marriage, and Irene's suitability as a wife for François. Madame Mareuil puzzles over how a man can fall in love with a woman who has such a profession! And for her son, "so refined, so sensitive," to fall for a woman who spends her life handling cadavers passes her understanding. Candole is able to view the matter with the detachment of a bachelor who knows life through the theater. Marriage is like politics: "liberté, égalité, hostilité." But Madame Mareuil remembers the great girls of yesterday, the graceful, subtle, polite women whose faces were bare of makeup and whose legs were covered. Irene cannot find time to look after her daughter; in fact, since Germaine has no mother and François has no wife, the couple should get divorced.

The recriminations between husband and wife eventually touch on sexual relations. François has never forgotten the first time a telephone call pulled Irene from his arms. She boasts that in spite of a full schedule she has never turned him down. The disgruntled François rejects the compromise of quarreling during the day and screwing at night. Too much like animals. Not that the couple has much time together to quarrel, but absence is worse. François is also jealous of his wife's being in her office with male patients. He also complains about her lack of carc when he was sick. This may be more a case of mental distress than a physical problem, but Irene says that it's all theater. Nor does Irene accept the idea that Madeleine restored François' self-confidence by showing genuine interest in him and his work; the actress just wanted a good role. And this is knowledge gleaned from the patient's bedside. It may be that Irene shuts herself up in her feminist vanity, immune to François' blandishments, but she leaves him seriously wounded. Finding herself betrayed, with the loyalty she depended on destroyed, Irene strikes back with a devastating lie: the hint that she too enjoyed extramarital comfort, perhaps even conceiving Germaine as a result. At thirty-five, she realizes that she still wants love, unshared by a mistress, and that she can still attract men.

The critic Robert Kemp thought that if Irene had forgiven François she would have shown the moral victory of feminism as well as avoided a lot of tedious rehashing of their dull life together, or rather not together.[12] But the play is an attempt to lay out in detail the effect of the wife's medical practice on family life. Not to mention the fact that playwrights had no stomach for the moral triumph of feminism. Kemp could not understand why Irene would tell such a devastating lie, which is totally out of character and even in contradiction with the cool, intelligent Irene of the earlier part of the play. Perhaps only critics would not be shattered in meeting their spouses with lovers. Nor does the irrational course of life follow the logician's handbook.

Irene explains the unfolding tragedy in professional terms, an act that seems somewhat out of character, but she might have changed her mind on having an intimation of the abyss just ahead. Unable to get any response from her husband on a generous offer not to divorce him, Irene sadly concludes that a woman who enters a male profession is perhaps led to display the bad characteristics of the two sexes. This perverse idea, though understandable in the case of the trapped Irene, conforms to Henri's view of the professional woman. Irene also insists that Germaine is really François' daughter and converts to a *bonne maman* type, and they agree to live happily ever after in the old style of their early-wedded bliss. The unreality of this situation is shown by Irene's promise to give up her practice. François says it's too late. He is between two abysses. Either Irene told a terrible lie – now a double lie – or she didn't lie, in which case he sees himself without wife and child, his genetic patrimony gone up in smoke. "The only parent one can be sure of is the mother," François tells Irene. François is ready for the last act of the play, "life with my wife the doctor."

In the final action of *La Vocation* Professor Gerbier is brought in to try to save the situation, chiefly by diagnosing the trouble with François. He does not know of the lie, which Irene hides from him as long as possible. Earlier the non-sociologist analyzed modern society; now the non-psychiatrist analyzes the development of François' mental aberration. In making a diagnosis, Gerbier declares, the doctor often proceeds like a *juge d'instruction*, the investigating magistrate in France's *étatiste* judicial system. The neurasthenic François was a bit depressed and a bit of a hypochondriac but still worked successfully as a dramatist. Now he is obsessed with heredity. He quizzes Gerbier on parental instincts, which doctors know through animal psychology – useful, the professor explains, for its maximum of simplicity. François wants to know if a child separated from its parents for some years would still recognize them. Gerbier replies with Oedipus. Not encouraging news for François. Nor does Gerbier believe that one can love any child as much

12 Arsenal, Rf. 71.747.

as one's own. All of Gerbier's discourse is based on the assumption that the father is sure of his paternity. All that remains is for François to express his opinion that certainty is an act of faith he cannot be sure of. Now he has two obsessions: the paternity of Germaine and the certainty of human knowledge. This is Pyrrhonism, observes Gerbier, who bases his certainty on observation and verification of facts by the senses without worrying about metaphysical absurdities. François leaves in a fog of doubt about the paternity of Germaine. The only reality left is the self, now a suffering machine. Recognizing a probable suicide, Gerbier warns Candole not to leave François alone.

The play has to end. Closure occurs with François' contrived suicide. He tricks Candole into carrying a message and shoots himself. But the end does not come before a final reckoning in medical and personal ethics for Irene, with the master's condemnation when his astute questioning of an evasive Irene uncovers the lie. At last Gerbier understands why François became ill. So much for the educational or civilizing value of the cult of science, Gerbier laments on finding one of his favorite students wallowing in turpitude. Her only possible defense is temporary insanity: "J'étais folle." Gerbier exposes Irene's character, rather unfairly it might be argued, as basically flawed, for one only acts according to one's nature even in anger or moments of madness.

Gerbier piles it on, seeming to enjoy giving a lesson to a fallen pupil. Even worse than a doctor's injection of a fatal substance into a body was Irene's injection of an idea into her husband's mind, thus destroying his creative faculties. "You are the doctor who kills, and your victim is your husband." Irene is wrong in thinking that the crisis will pass, Gerbier insists. The only possible treatment is putting him in a place where he will be isolated in total quiet, which would perhaps reestablish his mental equilibrium. The cure is unnecessary. On learning that her husband is dead, the guilty *doctoresse* shrieks and collapses into a chair. Curtain.

This convenient ending, a bullet as deus ex machina, displeased some critics, none more than Robert Kemp. Finding the first two acts successful, he was completely puzzled by the last two acts. It seemed to Kemp that the authors did not have enough time (or expertise, he might have added) to end with a psychiatric session, which the critic would have found interesting.[13] He did not add that it would have been a play too much, a play within a play. Still, the authors did open themselves up to this criticism: Irene experiences her moment of *folie*, François is neurasthenic and eventually a *demi-fou*, while Gerbier notes his own incompetence in psychiatry. One choleric commentator exclaimed that Irene is a monster and her husband an imbecile.[14] And so, if one follows the Kempian critique, the authors would not have had to try to do two things at once. The Kempian problem of how to connect the subject of feminism to the second subject of Irene's "poisonous lie" is not so easily solved, though perhaps a psychiatric session would have usefully obscured if it had not solved the problem.

[13] Arsenal, Rf. 71.747.

[14] Arsenal, Rf. 71.747.

After the play opened, the critics, who flattered themselves as guides of the public, rushed into print with their praise and criticism. Both authors and directors received advice on what was wrong with the play and how it could be improved. In The Rothschild Archive (London) there is an anonymous document of several pages (in several versions) analyzing the play's problems and giving suggestions for improvement.[15] This document states that the chief problem was the view of the critics, though it was hardly expressed by the public, that *La Vocation* was an anti-feminist play, indeed an all out general attack on feminism itself. The vehicle of this assault was the theories of Gerbier, furnishing the basic principle on which the social structure rests, all of which he expounded provocatively in the first act: an ardently and cogently argued paternalism, typical of the French medical community. Although medical students might shout in protest, the public, probably including a large number of women, expected Gerbier's thesis to be proven in the manner of a syllogism. The play led the public down the wrong road because a misleading signpost had promised a demonstration of feminism as a social law, that is, a refutation of the outmoded views of Gerbier. The anonymous commentator diagnosed a misunderstanding between authors and the public. (One has to wonder how rare this is and what it has to do with the success of a play.)

But how does the public form a critical opinion? Mr Anonymous argued that in this case the public was guided by journalists and critics who refused to see the exact significance of the drama and often made an effort to lead the "sheep" astray. Instead, the commentators generalized as much as possible concerning feminism and ended up by emphasizing an imaginary dualistic structure of the play, summed up in the classic judgment "There are two plays in one." The public was wrong to accept this judgment, well, partially wrong at least. Though this "error," originating with lazy critics, was merely a venal sin, the authors were guilty of a double and more damnable mistake. First, they had not made clear what their real subject was, the key idea of the suitability of a woman being a practicing doctor. Second, their protagonist or leading character was too superficial to provide the center of gravity around which the other characters developed in order to illustrate the character of the *doctoresse* through reflection and contrast. In the first act, generalizations and secondary ideas obscured the thesis; the act should instead have been only a framework, avoiding any hint of an archaic and reactionary crusade against feminism. The disastrous consequences of Irene's pursuit of a medical career were explained only in a dialogue by the trivia of material existence, whereas for the main character the consequences needed to be explained by a "psychic and sensorial analysis of the deformation of her character and her state of mind." Mr Anonymous further insisted that Irene's psychological disequilibrium should have given unity to the play. It was supposedly not clear that the play did *not* deal with feminism in general – an ambiguous concept in itself – but with women doctors. This criticism seems a bit ingenuous, for the entry of women into the practice of medicine was one of the most striking and important developments of feminism.

15 RAL 000/930: 58-1, 40.

Rewriting *La Vocation* could involve an interlocutor's giving crushing replies to Gerbier's patriarchal opinions. The real thesis of the play had to dominate the action, with the clear conclusion being that if feminism is supportable in certain cases, medical hyper-feminism must be subordinated to the subject – the woman doctor. The anonymous commentator, obviously a professional in the world of the theater, showed the technical method of achieving these results, namely replacing feminist ideas with those of the woman doctor. Gerbier needed to be shown as an old backward idiot on feminism but right about women doctors. (Given the mentality of the period, this seemed like good advice but now appears to us as an absurd contradiction.) Gerbier's interlocutor could be Candole, whose bohemian socialist and democratic mind could easily accommodate the extra baggage of feminism. These modifications would ensure that the public would *not* expect a demonstration of anti-feminism in the play.

The modifications of Irene's character needed to show that her problem did not arise from medical studies – *pace* Gerbier – but from the *practice* of medicine. Practicing medicine is harmful to the female organism because it suppresses woman's sensibility, sweetness, and intuition. The female physiological state, in its normal condition, conserves all the little female defects, namely all the mean feelings of pitiless hate and jealousy, which are always ready to explode into action on any shock to the nervous system. The commentator recommended showing Irene's lack of pity and compassion in a refusal, for example, to give a proper dose of morphine to a patient. Henri took this idea into account later. The continuous spectacle of human misery and suffering leads to the destruction of the essential female character. One version of the commentator's notes ends on a universal solution to all these problems: "women must vote." They would have to wait a long time in France for the political patriarch de Gaulle to solve this problem.

In criticism, as in all human activities, there is a fair amount of bad faith. Some critics complained of *naïvetés*, a somewhat infantile construction, and salon-like speeches too long for the stage. One critic who shot these arrows still found the play to be good theater, especially the second act. We all enjoy an amorous disaster in someone else's family. Nozière (pseudonym) denounced "the dangerous mania of critics who rewrite a play."[16] Critics seemed to think that they had a professional duty to judge Henri's plays severely. Nozière regretted that people were suspicious of his looking at Henri's world in a friendly light. But some careful critics like Paul Sabatier had a high opinion of the play as a sound, logical, beautiful work, as one would expect in a play written according to the traditional rules.[17] Insofar as the public thought about these high matters, it agreed with Sabatier. In the end what counted for the theater and actors, though not necessarily for these two authors, was the reception of the play by the public. Paul Reboux did not hesitate to describe

[16] Nozière was the pseudonym of Fernand Weyl (1874–1931), drama critic of *Gil Blas*, playwright and prolific writer.

[17] Arsenal, Rf. 71.747.

the public as amused, interested, and moved by the play.[18] Nor did the public have any hang-ups about dealing with the work of André Pascal; unlike some critics, the public spoke of him with a "cavalier indifference." They did not seem to mind that so-called social plays always dealt with rich people. Quite to the contrary, they were fascinated by a different world inhabited by another social species. The critic sometimes had an interest in establishing their expertise by inventing faults in the work of the upper classes or of a non-professional writer (more applicable to Delbet than to Henri, though Delbet scribbled much in his technical field). Experts should stay on their own turf. This law was amusingly illustrated by an account in *Le Cri d'alarme* (28 Nov. 1926) describing the playwrights Henry Bernstein and Pierre Wolff going to a hospital to amputate a leg.

Delbet, a big name in surgery, was a favorite target of critics attempting to be witty about his debut as a dramatic author. (Delbet also made a name for himself in ceramics, where it was more difficult for critics to be witty.) Clément Vautel hoped that after putting so many patients to sleep, Delbet would not also cause theater audiences to nod off.[19] His collaboration with the author of *Le Caducée* gave *La Vocation* more than dramatic interest. Georges Drouilly thought that the play had a deep social significance, enhanced by the exposé of truths from the experimental domain.[20] Henri too described *La Vocation* in terms of social observation and evolution rather than, as was erroneously said, a "laboratory play." Delbet was attacked more than Henri, probably because he taught so many students, who were surprised to find him as co-author of a play in which a professor subscribed to the social ideas of an anti-feminist fogy.

One critic joked that students came to rag their professor's evening courses, something that would have been difficult to do in the instructional setup of hospitals and clinics.[21] His students enjoyed shouting out during the play: "hang Delbet" and, even worse, "Au Sénat, le retardaire!" This was perhaps a reference to the Senate's opposition to giving women the right to vote. Delbet's post-mortem comments did not improve matters. It may be doubted that the authors took pains, as Delbet claimed, not to upset anyone. Basically, it seems that Delbet agreed with Gerbier that young women should do something other than medicine. Of course he had excellent female students, "but women, you know..."[22] Fortunately he did not finish the sentence. In an age of linguistic *pudeur* in newspapers, some student comments on Delbet's putative views could not be printed. *L'Ere nouvelle* (5 Dec. 1926) played a sour note in arguing that judging the incident by the value of the work, it was all a lot of noise for nothing. The authors themselves were the issue:

---

18 Arsenal, Rf. 71.747.

19 Arsenal, Rf. 71.747. Clément Vautel (pseudonym of Clément-Henri Vaulet (1875–1954), novelist and playwright, author of the popular *L'amour à la parisienne* (Paris, 1927).

20 Arsenal, Rf. 71.747.

21 Arsenal, Rf. 71.747.

22 Arsenal, Rf. 71.747.

one a famous surgeon and the other a famous doctor of great influence, which is an interesting if incomplete explanation of the social froth that the performance produced. Nor can it be assumed that the opinions of the two "old-fashioned" authors were unique. Georges Drouilly noted that the origin of the play was in long conversations between Henri and medical professors, whose ideas stimulated Henri to prepare a draft of *La Vocation*.[23]

An article in *Paris Midi* (4 Dec. 1926) on the disturbance during the performance of *La Vocation* began with a novel point, namely that medical students, male and female, came to the theater to defend (noisily) the play's heroine, Dr Farrel, against the attacks of the anti-feminist professor, Dr Gerbier. This simplification makes a good point about the positive side of the students' protest. Drouilly noted with approval that the play was not a special trial of women doctors but something better, the trial of excessive feminism, which was doing so many bad things, creating havoc everywhere. Henri put the matter more politely: "feminism is on trial. We [the authors] ask the question 'should a woman doctor marry or not?' And if she gets married, should she continue to practice?"[24] In an interview in *Le Figaro* (4 Nov. 1926), Henri was unambiguous in his opinion on feminism. "The modern woman is really evading, more and more, her natural role as mother and wife in order to practice male professions, without perceiving that she loses daily her natural grace along with our idealist respect and even our consideration." The writer for the newspaper, R. Cardinne-Petit, liked this male lament so much that he underlined "the tragic consequences for the emancipation of women": households destroyed and children behaving according to their instincts, along with other contemporary horrors, all imagined by this unhistorical writer as novelties of the modern age.

Taking up this popular issue, Pierre Sabatier, writing in *Le Monde illustré* (27 Nov. 1926) grew solemn about "the most sensitive problem of modern social life": can a woman, without compromising her role of wife and mother, take up "a masculine career that assumes her independence and makes her the working equal of her husband?" Sabatier recognized that the question had already been answered affirmatively by the existence of an increasing number of female lawyers and doctors, in addition to other women in less brilliant but equally demanding and worthy professions. These workingwomen were perfect associates and devoted mothers. So Sabatier concluded that it would be risky to draw from the play any clear conclusions on the feminist issue. Sabatier might have pointed out that in France women were doing much better in the medical profession than in the legal profession, which was the reverse of the situation in the USA. In 1935 women made up over fifteen percent of the law-student population and nearly twenty-two percent of the medical-student population in France. One has to take into account the influx of foreign women students in French medical faculties, of course, but

23 *Le Gaulois* (15 November 1926), in Arsenal, Rf. 71.727.

24 *Le Figaro* (4 Nov. 1926) in Arsenal, Rf. 71.747.

that makes the French medical faculties even more remarkable, at least from this limited point of view.[25]

Some commentators, such as André Antoine, found it surprising that the uproar created by *La Vocation* had not occurred over the entry of women into the legal profession, subject of the popular play *Maître Bolbec et son mari* (1926).[26] Why did not law students kick up a fuss at the Athénée theater? Even after one takes into account the volatility of the student population in the crowded Paris Faculty of Medicine, it is a bit of a puzzle. Was the medical faculty more sensitive than the law faculty? Or was it the nature of the play, a *comédie dramatique* like *La Vocation* being a more serious vehicle of opinion than a light comedy? Nor did the army protest its representation in *La Carcasse*; nor did the *amazones* get excited over *Mademoiselle Jockey*. Making the matter more puzzling for some critics was the fact that Irene was irreproachable – meaning she was a monster for others – while the flirtatious heroine Maître Bolbec inspired much less confidence. Perhaps Henri and Delbet had managed to insult both women and science, in a play that was more serious than amusing. It took a female expert on the subject to work out an interesting explanation within the general context of feminism.

Few women had the opportunity to pontificate like men in the national press. Colette Yver, a prolific writer and translator whose subjects ranged from saints and warriors to the beatitudes, was a striking exception. This "Catholic feminist" produced many bestsellers during fifty years of scribbling.[27] Her opening salvo in the affair of *La Vocation* established the general context of the squabble and put the literary gang in their reactionary place. Yver elevated the woman doctor to the saintly status of "prow-figure on the bow of the feminist warship." In the battle of ideas being fought it was not odd therefore that this figure should receive the first blows. And of course the literary friends of social theses often attacked *la doctoresse*. Yver's article in *Le Gaulois* (17 Dec. 1926) was entitled "Are women doctors necessary?" She took note that the question was already answered in practice. More than 700 French women were enrolled in the Paris Faculty of

---

[25] Regina Markell Morantz-Sanchez, *Sympathy and Science. Women Physicians in American Medicine* (1985; Chapel Hill, 2000), 314; and Weisz, *The Emergence of Modern Universities in France, 1863–1914*, 246.

[26] Arsenal, Rf. 71.747.

[27] Yver wrote on Saint Bernadette and Joan of Arc; *Le mystère des béatitudes* was in its 35th edition by 1947 and *Le vote des femmes* in its 12th edition by 1932. Her *Princesses de science* (Paris, 1907), translated as *The Doctor's Wife*, deals with professional–maternal conflicts in the medical profession, allowing the triumph of the maternal when the woman gives up her career to look after hubby. In *Les Cervelines* (Paris, 1908), the brainy woman is Jeanne Boerk, a pathology student who rejects love and peace to seek bitter fame (Anna Akhmatova's notorious dilemma) in Paris. *Les Dames du Palais* (Paris, 1920) submits the woman lawyer to the same maternal laws; then as a sort of summing up, *Femmes d'aujourd'hui; enquête sur les nouvelles carrières féminines* (Paris, 1929) does much the same for all the professions open for women, particularly after the Great War.

Medicine. There was no area in Paris where a few women doctors did not practice. And even in the provinces the woman doctor was slowly appearing on the medical scene. Yver predicted that there would be more; she might have been pleasantly shocked to find out how many there would be three quarters of a century later. And there was, she argued, nothing to the illogical argument that female modesty was an obstacle to a medical career: in addition to the existence of midwives and nurses, including nursing sisters, the historical role of the woman healer made this position untenable. So the idea of the woman doctor had been integrated into the customs of the times; she was, grosso modo, accepted by the people.

Yet from the viewpoint of social utility, Yver did not believe that female doctors were needed. What then explained this new vocation? What was attracting women to medicine, "la plus intelligente des sciences"? It was less the idea of social good than women's ardent desire for personal development, for an important role in society. Males had no need to fear *la doctoresse* as a social danger. Though she did not have figures to prove her case, Yver argued that looking at the practical side of things, woman doctors did not survive as independent women but married and often gave up practicing medicine. This is vintage Yver. In her novel *Princesses de science*, the brilliant *interne* Thérèse Herlinge gives up her profession after the death of her baby shows that career and motherhood are incompatible.[28] Even Irene Farrel tried to save her marriage by offering to give up her career. Yver explained this development by a variety of factors ranging from husbands' demands to women's "natural wisdom" in seeking happiness and love. No doubt renouncing a career based on an ardent scientific passion was a difficult decision, often heart-rending even if kept secret. "Could the most generous of husbands be asked to do such a thing?" Yver ended her article by admitting that feminists would devour her because what she said essentially reduced women to a small role in the modern world. She need not have worried about the appetite of the feminists. "Une petite bourgeoise," writing in *Le Temps* (16 Dec. 1926), remarked that French feminism was a moderate enterprise and the problems raised by the play came from the fact that Irene was a wicked woman. Of course it seems a trifle simplistic to reduce the play to a husband's misfortunes produced by a modern Jezebel. But the "petite bourgeoise" made one good point, namely that women doctors should be no more offended by *La Vocation* than the army had been by its representation in *La Carcasse*. Being misrepresented on the stage is one of the privileges of an elite profession.

If women were becoming doctors and lawyers to further their personal development, this activity certainly included one of the most elusive and most pursued of human aims, the achievement of happiness. And that aim would include work, an essential ingredient of the Rothschild ideology. Interviewing Henri on

---

28 Françoise Mayeur, *L'Education des filles en France au XIXᵉ siècle* (Paris, 1979), 147, gives a brief analysis of *Princesses de science*, ending on the grim note that for Yver "a woman can rise to the intellectual level of a man but at the price of sacrifices that mutilate and destroy her."

"the social question," Jules Huret asked him if he thought that riches produce happiness.[29] After all, people believed that with his billions Henri must be the happiest of men. Henri replied that if a fortune did not have some advantages it would not be so eagerly pursued but that basically the only true happiness is in work. He gave a good Rothschild answer, which applied with equal insight to Irene. Perhaps the idea would have seemed far-fetched to Henri, though many of his friends were also hard workers – actresses, for example. Rothschild women were not idle and were often happy, but they did not work in the same sense that Henri's granddaughter does as the head of one of the world's great wine companies.[30]

It may seem strange to us that the claim could be made back in 1927 that women were getting a monopoly on the medical profession. An enrolment of more than 800 young women – the figure was also expressed as nearly a thousand – in the medical faculty provided the statistical basis for male anxiety. Of the dozen or so women in medical studies back in 1890, when Henri began his medical studies, only two succeeded in the difficult examinations permitting them to become hospital interns. Nearly forty years later a certain number of women candidates succeeded in winning places in every competition for the hospital *externat* and *internat*. Only the highest prize remained unattainable, holding an official teaching position in the Paris Faculty of Medicine. Henri morosely conceded that the day was not far off when this last bastion of male medical privilege (the *agrégation*) would fall to madame la professeur.[31]

In speaking to the noble and bourgeois clubwomen, Henri insisted that Delbet and he had not raised the serious and disturbing problem arising from the existence of the female physician in order to express their personal opinions. The plot did it. The playwrights, disclaiming any intention of attacking feminism in general – though the temptation to do so was not easy to resist – emphasized the play's attack on an attempt by women to monopolize the medical profession. And even this attack could be defended as text-driven, the result of the demands of the script, rather than stemming from any personal opinions of the authors. The development of the play dictated to the authors not only their character's denunciation of Irene's practice of medicine but the nature of the personality of the female physician as well as the role that she played in the home as wife and mother. This ingenious explanation made sense, especially as complex emotions and actions of the characters were explained in Henri's jargon-free language. If Irene had not created a professional life outside her home in order to care for a large clientele, if the life of her husband François had not thus been made intolerable, and if she had not turned over the raising and education of their daughter to François, then "the violent drama that had so tragically upset her household would never have been

[29] Arsenal, Rf. 71.747.

[30] The daughter of Philippe de Rothschild (thespian mask: Philippine Pascale) during part of her fruitful acting career was also a member of *La Société*, *La Comédie Française*.

[31] Pascal, *La femme médecin*, 30–1. He did not use the linguistic innovation of 'madame la professeur.'

launched."[32] Events were the result of the necessarily realistic emplotment of the play.

Henri boasted that André Pascal found it easy to develop Irene Farrel's character. After all, he had been concerned for years with the role of the female physician in modern society. He had been a physician for more than twenty-five years when *La Vocation* opened. Many times he had exchanged ideas on "this serious question" with colleagues who were among the biggest names in French medicine. He had also studied his female colleagues at close range, probing their character, their professional mentality, and their sensibility. Perhaps the females showed an equal curiosity in the medical personality of Henri de Rothschild. And he had met on more than one occasion some "éminentes doctoresses" at the bedside of sick patients. Discussion with most of his colleagues corroborated the social and moral observations gathered by André Pascal in this impressive "dossier." Male doctors completely agreed in "unreservedly admiring the devotion, sacrifice, and even the real professional competence of their female colleagues," but they all also agreed that the practice of medicine was not generally a profession for women and especially not for a married woman. This condescending admiration and turf-inspired jealousy had to be reconciled with the reality of the practice of medicine. Henri admitted that in light of the constantly growing number of female medical students and the substantial lists of clients of a good number of *doctoresses*, this discordant opinion of the male doctors might surprise many people.[33]

In considering the theme of the play, a believer in the sanctity of medicine might argue that one of the most important and shocking things about this play was that it was by two of the best known names on the Parisian medical scene. In July 1925 Henri read the chief scenes of the play to his friend Delbet when they were on a cruise in the Baltic. (He did not mention that it was on his yacht *Eros*. Everyone knew.) The year before, Henri had spoken at length to Delbet about the subject of *La Vocation*, and "the eminent surgeon had adopted without reserve the thesis of his colleague." Delbet was also fully satisfied with the opinions expressed, in the first act, by Dr Gerbier concerning woman doctors. Moreover, on more than one occasion Delbet himself had publicly defended the same theories. Delbet's commentary on Gerbier's ideas was so interesting and he showed such mastery in the statement of his arguments that Henri asked that they go over the text together so that it could be improved by the addition to the dialogue of Delbet's terse and biting repartee, improvised "with so much finesse and wit." So "one of the happiest medico-literary collaborations was born," and over a period of a few weeks the two doctors revised the play. The play quickly attracted hordes of curious people and hostile students after it opened in the fall of 1926.[34]

In the first act of *La Vocation* the contentious social and sentimental issues were the subject of moderate and courteous debate between Professor Gerbier,

---

32 Pascal, *La femme médecin*, 29–32.

33 Pascal, *La femme médecin*, 29.

34 Pascal, *La femme médecin*, 42–4.

Dr Farrel, and a male friend of her husband's. Henri emphasized that in writing the scene the authors expressed themselves with absolute sincerity and good faith. He thought that it was of considerable importance that the authors treated only the social and sentimental side of the problem, deliberately leaving aside the professional or technical issues traditionally associated with the admission of women to medical practice. The important point for Henri and Delbet seemed to be the argument that even the most extreme feminist would find it difficult to argue that a busy female physician could be a good wife and mother. Like most doctors, the authors believed that a single woman had no problem in practicing medicine. But they attempted to show that once the *doctoresse* married, which implied that she would want to keep the home happy and peaceful, she had no choice but to give up her clientele and at most limit her medical work to scientific research and laboratory work. Henri noted that in the post-war period that sort of activity could be as profitable as taking care of patients – the income of doctors was not high.[35]

This theatrically proposed restriction on the professional liberty of the married woman doctor was put forward with a great deal of caution. Not only did the idea clash with an effervescent feminism in general but with a growing interest of women in the medical profession. Then there was a general social issue, frankly recognized by Henri in his speech to the women's clubs. Society needed "intelligent and well-trained female doctors" among its medical personnel. All doctors were aware of the fact that a number of women refuse to be examined and cared for by male doctors. These same women never hesitate to consult a woman doctor. For Henri there was a great importance in having a sufficient number of female doctors available to detect and treat disease early enough in women patients to prevent them from dying unnecessarily. The woman doctor, aware of her professional duties, could also be an ideal counselor for families, whether rich or poor. No matter what the social status of a family, the mother and children were infinitely more likely to confide in a woman doctor than in a male doctor. "Only a fool would want to preach a crusade against the female physician."[36] It should not be forgotten that this eulogy of the role of the female doctor applied only to the single woman.

Much to the surprise of its authors, *La Vocation* appeared to critics to be two plays in one. It seemed at first that the play was going to develop the thesis that feminism could be demonstrated as the unfolding of a social law, but in reality the plot revealed itself as only a sentimental adventure. So there was a structural division in the play between the anti-feminist first act and the family drama of the following three acts. The authors had missed an opportunity to link all four acts through an analysis of Irene Farrel's "psychological disequilibrium," which "could have been illustrated by the very inhuman attitude she adopted, as a result of her

35 Pascal, *La femme médecin*, 32–3.

36 Pascal, *La femme médecin*, 34.

profession, in everyday situations."[37] Henri readily admitted that the criticism was fair. In the first act some of Gerbier's dialogue dealing directly with "feminism in general" should have been restricted to women doctors. Gerbier should have delivered fewer lines against feminism and more against them. Gerbier's model sallies included lines like "Of all the professions, medicine is the last one a woman should dream about," and "Isn't it taking unfair advantage to want me to kiss the hand that just probed a wound?" In these two cases, Gerbier was grappling directly with the subject of the play: "medical hyper-feminism," which Henri viewed as unpleasant and redoubtable.[38]

Henri regretted that he and Delbet had not done more to draw attention to Irene's mental instability, which was shown in the play by the fact that she was consumed by anger, vanity, and pride. But they did show the dire consequences of this mental unbalance for the family. For her patients Irene might have been self-sacrificing, but to her husband she was cruel enough to hint that another man had sired their daughter. The character of an unbalanced woman (in plays) was not new to Henri. His play *Le Talion* featured an actress who lied naturally when she went into paroxysms of rage, and *La Vocation* was developed from *Le Talion*, which played over 100 times at the Théâtre Marigny in the spring of 1914. *La Vocation* did not follow the "method" of making concessions to the public, a gimmick so "dear to the English and the Americans," especially the latter group, who "want the darkest tragedy always to end in reconciliation, with a return to happiness. The cinema has adopted in a systematic way this type of denouement. If it [theater] can accommodate itself to such an artistic conception, the theater, and especially my plays, can be damaged by it."[39] Recently film seems to be coming round to Henri's way of thinking.[40] The history of Irene's mental evolution was of some importance in understanding the tragedy. This young woman of a good family who became a medical doctor was of excellent temperament, refined and sensitive; she was transformed and, indeed, her mind was warped by the exercise of her profession. So her vengeful acts and her husband's madness only served to show how her profession had deformed "the heart and mind of this woman, who had been transplanted to an ultra materialistic environment as a result of her studies and then her job." Irene's "psychological deformity" was "the consequence of her medical studies." The dreaded scenario could be avoided only if the married *doctoresse* abandoned her patients for home and family.[41]

---

[37] Pascal, *La femme médecin*, quoting, without identifying, one of the three critics (Antoine, André Rivoire, and Edmond Sée).

[38] Pascal, *La femme médecin*, 36.

[39] Pascal, *La femme médecin*, 17.

[40] Even "the king of the happy ending," Steven Spielberg, fell into a sad ending in *A.I.* It may be *The Sweet Hereafter* from now on. Kristin Hohenadel, "'Happily Ever After' Fading Fast from Film," *The New York Times* (Sunday, 13 Jan. 2002), RA 13–18.

[41] Pascal, *La femme médecin*, 36–7 and 38.

Still, Henri was not condemning the study of medicine for women, since it had a certain educational value, though it was severely limited in the end. What he insisted on was the "important transforming role of medical practice on the female organism." This terminology seemed to legitimate a debatable diagnosis. How exactly did the practice of medicine act on the female psychic and sensory state? Henri used strong language in answering this question, much as Gerbier had. Medical practice works in the most detestable way: it suppresses the essential quality of woman, her femininity, namely her sensibility, her gentleness, and her intuition. The loss of these fine feminine qualities is not compensated for by an increase of intelligence, or reasoning power, or common sense. Indeed, woman's physiological condition is an obstacle to such growth because it ceaselessly counterbalances and destroys the development of intellectual qualities. The female doctor's sensibility is dulled by the endless spectacle of human poverty and suffering. Pride and a desire not to show moral inferiority lead her to neglect to take account of the role of pain in sickness, merely discussing it as if it were "a problem in analytical geometry, to be solved by establishing an equation between clinical observation and a cure." In the action of *La Vocation* Irene's character showed itself in her indifference to the madness of François and her taking care of her ill husband as if he were any other patient, at least until Gerbier showed the chronic nature of the illness. "The female doctor retains intact" feminine defects such as vengeance, "which are always ready to erupt in a woman subject to the influence of the least nervous shock." In the third act Irene, confronted with "a brutal event of normal life, acts like any ordinary woman rather than like a superior person, an intellectual. Her senses immediately dominate her brain; moreover, her harshness and toughness reinforce her vanity, evident in her already formed opinion that she is the equal of the male." So she ended by carrying out a "diabolical vengeance, more vile and more cruel than could have been imagined by a normal woman, one used to a healthy and regular life."[42]

"Cruelty is in fact one of the characteristics of the female doctor." The basis Henri offered for this astonishing statement was the observations he and his colleagues made "demonstrating irrefutably that the practice of medicine not only dulls the sensibility of women but develops in most of them, in a quasi-pathological way, this inhuman feeling, this particular form of voluptuousness called cruelty." (All that is missing here is a reference to the Nietzschean conceit of "the voluptuousness of the martyr.") The male doctors saw or imagined the professional behavior of their female colleagues so different from their own that it became the subject of specific discussion. Henri delivered a few examples with commentary to add empirical substance to the shocking psychological profile he had developed, though not before he had established a clear professional difference between doctors and nurses. The woman whose action requires use of the verb *traiter* (giving treatment) is a doctor; the one whose action is encoded by *soigner* (taking care of) is a nurse. Nurses, both the hospital and home varieties, display,

42 Pascal, *La femme médecin*, 38–40.

nearly without exception, kindness, compassion, and pity. But Henri warned his audience not to forget that nurses obey the orders of the doctor in charge of the case and that their responsibilities are limited to working hours, which end when they return to private life, resuming their roles of "affectionate and tender wives and mothers."[43] The *doctoresse* is a different creature.

At this point Henri returned to his obsession with the idea of a loss of emotion and sensibility by the woman who, "scalpel in hand," lived for years in contact with so much of the ugliness of life. So most female doctors, showing a lot less pity than men – a certain amount of wiggle room was allowed by admitting to numerous exceptions to the judgment – treated their patients with "a certain brutality, a certain contempt for physical pain." In this the women doctors resembled midwives, which provided a curious comparison with a group socially inferior to the medical profession. And then, finally, a long promised if general example. At the hospital, a female medical student would stitch up a wound and lance an abscess or a whitlow without using an anesthetic, whereas no matter what the status of the male physician, he would always spare his patient any unnecessary suffering. It seems that Henri had been thinking for some time about cruelty as a distinguishing characteristic of the woman doctor. On more than one occasion, in the course of discussions with his female colleagues, he asked them what they would do if "a poor devil addicted to morphine," used to taking 40 to 50 cc daily and therefore a human wreck, came to them for a prescription to get the drug he had been weaned from for some hours. They all replied that they would refuse to write a prescription. Neither Henri nor any of his male colleagues would have refused to give a prescription to the poor devil, in order to assuage his suffering and perhaps to prevent a suicide.[44] One may speculate that the female doctors were giving the answer they thought "correct," the one that any male doctor would give, and that if they had known the "correct" reply, they would have given it. Or they may have had some therapeutic gambit in mind.

"Irene's terrible vengeance is the logical corollary of her profession," meaning the exercise of medical practice by a married woman.[45] Fortified by this male logic, Henri and Delbet concluded that it was useful to show in *La Vocation* the moral danger to which contemporary girls and young women would be exposed if, driven by a strong inclination for medicine, they nourished the otherwise noble ambition of entering medical practice, in spite of having or planning to have a husband and children, which she would be obliged to leave alone at home. So the stage and the professional world of the woman doctor were curiously conflated, to the disadvantage of the *doctoresse*.

Henri finished by insisting in his talk to the clubwomen that *La Vocation* was not an anti-feminist play. The aristocratic and bourgeois women of the two famous clubs of Paris listening to him seem to have seen his point, or at least were polite

43 Pascal, *La femme médecin* 40–1.

44 Pascal, *La femme médecin*, 41–2.

45 Pascal, *La femme médecin*, 42–3.

enough to listen to him without protest. But that was part of the female code of behavior too. Henri accepted the working woman as "one of the exigencies of our time," which required of nearly all women some daily work when they wanted to improve the wellbeing of loved ones. Feminists could rest assured that André Pascal supported the effort of any working woman who wanted to rise above the typical mediocrity of daily life.[46]

[46] Pascal, *La femme médecin*, 42–3.

Conclusion
The 1930s: Medical Götterdämmerung

> The faithful question for the human species seems to me to be whether and to what extent their cultural development will succeed in mastering the disturbance of their communal life by the human instinct of aggression and self-destruction.[1]

If in 1900 one had asked Parisians who was the most prominent Jew in Paris, some of them would have replied Henri de Rothschild. The virulent anti-Semitic journalist Raphaël Viau, who was for a time one of the literary henchmen of Edouard Drumont, the king of French anti-Semites, explained why.[2] Henri de Rothschild was not only eminently representative "of a race we take for granted as atavistically harmful to ours, he was also young, a good shot, and rich." So Henri was the best possible target in the war against the Rothschilds, who themselves were the leading representatives of the Jews. Viau failed to note that Henri was the best Jewish target for anti-Semitic journalists because he was often referred to as the "quintessential Parisian." This could have been for Viau a good illustration of the potentially corrupting influence of Jews in French society, particularly in the Third Republic, though use of this idea might have indicated that it was too late to do anything about the decadence of "the French race." The concept of Jewish racial identity, one of the favorite propaganda weapons of anti-Semites, was a by-product of the adoption of racial language by Jews that enabled them to take part in an intellectual discourse about race. As the concept of race developed in the European mind after the 1820s, Jewish intellectuals defined and defended themselves by using a common idiom.[3] The gestation of this climate of opinion is not easy to grasp, but a brief consideration of the salient features of the French scene throws some light on the evolution of the situation of the Rothschilds, Henri in particular, as well as the position of French Jewish doctors in France by the 1930s.

---

[1] Sigmund Freud, *Civilization and its Discontents* (New York, 1962), 92. A translation of *Das Unbehagen in der Kultur* (1930) by James Strachey.

[2] Raphaël Viau, *Vingt ans d'antisémitisme 1889–1909* (Paris, 1910), chapters 6 and 10; Bertrand Joly, *Dictionnaire biographique et géographique du nationalisme français 1800–1900* (Paris, 1998), 401–2.

[3] Lisa Moses Leff, "Self-definition and Self-defense: Jewish Racial Identity in Nineteenth-Century France," *Jewish History* 19 (2005): 7–28. This issue of the journal is devoted to "Racial self-fashioning in comparative perspective." See also Jay R. Berkovitz, *The Shaping of Jewish Identity in Nineteenth-Century France* (Detroit, 1989).

Jews – all 40,000 of them – had become full French citizens in 1791–92 as a result of the democratic *Gleichschaltung* of the French Revolution. Christianity having become a political triviality, there was also no reason to exclude Protestants (0.16 percent of the population) from the new democratic dispensation. France became a model of emancipation for other countries, often after being encouraged by imperial bayonets. Ralph Schor enthusiastically sees French Jews casting themselves "in the national cultural mold" and becoming "one of the most assimilated European communities."[4] It has been calculated that 171 Jewish deputies, senators, ministers, army generals (25), prefects, and magistrates served the Third Republic (1870s–1940). The assimilation of these "state Jews" did not involve their abandoning the "religious-ethnic community," that is, they "maintained strong ties of Jewish identity and association." This view rejects "the stereotype of assimilated Jews as necessarily distanced from their origins and religious-ethnic community."[5] Of course one has to take into account that the "heavy price" of citizenship was the surrender of Jewish "communal autonomy and rabbinic jurisdiction in civil affairs."[6] Not many Jews regretted the bargain. In a desperate attempt to deal with "the Jewish problem" in establishing "the identity of France," Braudel took refuge in the tattered concept of civilization, giving Jews a possible dual identity as the possessors of two civilizations, the one to which they become perfectly assimilated and the "inner civilization" they leave, though not completely.[7]

After emancipation Jews could be defined as a people rather than a religion, and this is a subject best left to the practitioners of the *Wissenschaft des Judentums*.[8] In France Jews were tempted to follow the national foible of defining themselves

---

4 Ralph Schor, *L'Antisémitisme en France pendant les années trente. Prélude à Vichy* (Bruxelles, 1992), 11–12. Unlike fellow Moslems, Algerian Jews became French citizens in 1870, thanks to the Crémieux decree of 24 October. Adolphe Crémieux was minister of justice in the government of national defense, 1870–71.

5 Pierre Birnbaum, *The Jews of the Republic. A Political History of State Jews in France from Gambetta to Vichy* (Stanford, 1996). Translated by Jane Marie Todd. See the review by Paula E. Hyman in the *Journal of Modern History* 70 (1998): 198–9. A stronger case for the assimilationist view is presented by Schor, *L'Antisémitisme en France pendant les années trente*.

6 Jay R. Berkovitz, *Rites and Passages. The Beginnings of Modern Jewish Culture in France, 1650–1860* (Philadelphia, 2004), 89. See the review (online) by Ronald Schechter in *H-France Review*, 5/57 (May 2005). See also Michael Graetz, *Les Juifs en France au XIXe siècle. De la Révolution Française à l'Alliance Israélite universelle* (Paris, 1989). Tranlated from Hebrew (1982) by Salomon Malka.

7 Fernand Braudel, *L'identité de la France. Les hommes et les choses* (Paris, 1986), 193.

8 See the articles on "Jew, Who is A? Controversy" and "Jewish Identity" in R. J. Zwi Werblowsky and Geoffrey Wigoder (eds), *The Oxford Dictionary of the Jewish Religion* (Oxford, 1997). Modern reproductive technologies have made Jewish identity a more complex matter: see Judith Berck, "When Science Aids Reproduction, Some Parents

intellectually, but during the Belle Epoque they added a republican patina to their identity, which fueled the myth of the Judaized Republic. The Dreyfus affair left Jews with a curious conflation of state and Republic, symbolizing a delicate balance between *raison d'Etat* and the rights of man. The Jewish tragedy in Vichy was therefore a double betrayal by the Republic and the state.[9]

When anti-Semites wished to find evidence of the malign influence of Jews in the Third Republic, it was easy enough to pick a target. By the 1890s the Jewish population, still one of the smallest groups of Jews in Europe, had grown to about 75,000, partly due to emigration from Alsace after the German annexation in 1871.[10] In addition to the contingent of Jews serving the state, prominent Jewish names could be found in most areas of French life, whether the big industries such as Citroën, department stores such as Galeries Lafayette, and the banks. Yves Lequin has emphasized that in the 1890s the visibility of the Jewish community was not so much a matter of the vast number of poor, working-class Jews but of the big banking and finance families such as Herz, Reinach, Bischoffheim, Pereire, Finalys, Lazard, and Rothschild – all heavily influential in the community; in Paris these names stood for the control of about a third of the world of finance.[11] A master myth was born. With annual family profits supposedly equal to the income of 450,000 bureaucrats, the Rothschilds provided a handy symbol of Jewish power: "the kings of the republic," according to a prolific right-wing author, Henri Coston.[12] In a certain sector of smart society it was chic to be anti-Semitic, though few bigots would be bold (and nonsensical) enough to proclaim, as Gyp did in court in 1899, that their profession was anti-Semitism.[13] Across the channel, anti-Semitism "was an unthinking feature of the English middle class milieu," or so it

Wonder What It Takes To Be Jewish," *The New York Times* (1 July 2006), online at www.nytimes.com/2006/07/01/us/01religion.html.

9 Perrine Simon-Nahum, "La République des Juifs," in Vincent Duclert and Christophe Prochasson (eds), *Dictionnaire critique de la République* (Paris, 2002), 371–7.

10 Graetz, *Les Juifs en France au XIXe siècle*, 12, notes that about the year 1800, French Jews numbered 45,000 and by 1900, about 100,000, whereas the number of Jews in Germany was 600,000 and 250,000 in England.

11 Yves Lequin, "Dreyfus à l'usine? Le silence d'une mémoire," in Pierre Birnbaum (ed.), *La France de l'Affaire Dreyfus* (Paris, 1994), 390. Though there are now several independent Rothschild banks, the old family name still provides valuable publicity. An advertisement in *Le Monde* (2/3 août 2005) for the finance company Edmond de Rothschild makes the point: "private banker ... independent family group ... banker over generations ... stability of its teams and permanence of its name."

12 See Simon-Nahum, "La République des Juifs," in Duclert and Prochasson (eds), *Dictionnaire critique de la République*, 371–7.

13 Gyp (nom de plume of Sibille-Gabrielle de Riquetti de Mirabeau, 1849–1932) was a rabid rightist writer and sometimes an amusing caricaturist. Willa Z. Silverman, *The Notorious Life of Gyp: Right-Wing Anarchist in fin-de-siècle France* (New York, 1995).

is often argued.[14] And there is little argument about anti-Jewish feeling across the Rhine.

Drumont first made Henri the target of an anti-Semitic campaign in 1896, as a result of the notorious "affair of the Forêt du Lys," a hunting ground (near Chantilly), owned by Henri. In May 1896 four poachers hunting pheasants at night were caught by Henri's gamekeepers. Shots were exchanged: one poacher (Mazille Cahon) was killed, one was wounded but hid and managed to escape, as did the two others. Drumont, sniffing out a big story here, assigned Viau to cover the affair by visiting the neighboring villages of Coye-la-Forêt and Lamorlaye as well as surrounding areas. The aim of this inquiry was to produce a series of sensational articles against the Rothschilds, dealing in particular with Henri, "not the least" of the tribe. Drumont was able to write up a sob story in the *Petit Pontoisien* about Cahon, the poor woodcutter killed while hunting rabbits to feed his old mother. This journalistic sleuthing turned up some interesting socio-economic information, namely, the claim of the villagers that Henri was a usurper in their midst, a rich intruder who prevented them from using the land for farming; and why should he have all the game for himself? The *Petit Pontoisien*, notoriously hostile to Henri, carried on its campaign along these lines until about 1900.

At the end of three days Viau's journalistic probe ended in a nasty surprise for him: he discovered that Cahon had been a "sinister, violent drunkard, feared by everyone in the area, living for many years off poaching and robbery."[15] A widower at the time of his death, he had been a notorious wife-beater. He lived with his mother, his daughter, and two granddaughters, whom he whipped when necessary. In spite of having this information and knowing that all the poachers had had guns and fired on the gamekeepers, Viau kept fiscal faith in Drumont and wrote a series of articles sympathetic to the poachers. Given the mores of the period on dueling, Viau expected Henri to challenge him to a duel; he was annoyed that Dr Rothschild did not. Unlike duel-loving Dr Clemenceau, who had an inconclusive exchange of shots with Drumont, Henri did not fight duels; nor did he emulate Dr Virchow, who joked he would duel Bismarck with scalpels as weapons. Viau later confessed that Henri was right to ignore him. Edouard de Rothschild (1868–1949) did fight a duel and lived to tell the tale. Protocol required duelists to aim to miss if using pistols and to stop if the opponent was wounded in a sword duel. In the Third Republic dueling supposedly had a specific function in the social game, namely to give the dueler some notoriety that would help him rise in society, or at least this may have been what journalists hoped for in their frequent duels. Nor can we ignore the role of the amorphous concept of honor.[16]

---

14 Nicholas Murray, *Aldous Huxley – An English Intellectual* (London, 2003), 168.

15 Viau, *Vingt ans d'antisémitisme 1889–1909*, 121–2.

16 See Jean-Noël Jeanneney, *Le duel. Une passion française 1789–1914* (Paris, 2004), and François Guillet, "La tyrannie de l'honneur. Les usages du duel dans la France du premier XIXe siècle," *Revue historique* CCCVIII/4 (Oct. 2006): 879–99.

In 1900 Drumont asked Viau to start a new campaign against Henri. Anti-Semitism was also a standard topic for increasing circulation of tabloid newspapers and perhaps increasing the income of journalists. One of Henri's cars ran into a coach. Henri was not in the car but that did not stop Viau from following Drumont's bad advice to write an aggressive article against the car's owner. Drumont hoped to boost his paper's sagging circulation with tales of a duel against the Rothschilds. Viau was again disappointed because Henri did not rise to the bait. No offer of a duel except in court. A fortnight after the article appeared, Drumont and Viau were prosecuted for libel in the ninth *Chambre correctionnelle* in Paris; plaintiff Henri de Rothschild asked for damages to the tune of 30,000 francs. Drumont and Viau were each fined 10,000 francs and *La Libre Parole* had to pay for the insertion of the guilty verdict in 20 newspapers costing 100 francs for each insertion. This ill-conceived venture cost Drumont, Viau, and the paper a total of 22,778 francs plus legal fees. Viau needed a different kind of job. Even after going over to Jules Guérin's corrupt anti-Semitic enterprise, he ended up as a near pauper for a while.

Later in the year 1900 Viau saw Henri with his medical colleagues come to the "black village" of an ethnographical exhibition on the Champ de Mars. Viau had taken the job of secretary-general of the affair. Henri was there with fellow doctors to examine Sudanese and Senegalese people and take samples of their fluids in order to test the theory that these Africans urinated blood as a result of some exotic disease. The subjects were paid for their fluids and troubles. Not being able to meet Henri, Viau contented himself with a number of amiable bromides on his former enemy: he was friendly, seemed tired or sad, he did not say much, he gazed at the subjects for a long time, and he was polite; above all, he was happy with the samples. Viau never had occasion to see Henri again.[17]

In the 1930s the old quarrel about France being swamped by immigrants reemerged with increased and heavily anti-Semitic virulence. Braudel pointed out that large-scale immigration to France is fairly recent. In 1851 foreigners made up only 1 percent of the population, rising by 1914 to less than 3 percent (1,100,000). By 1931 the percentage had risen to 6.6, about 2,700,000; by 1976 anti-immigrant voices were able to complain of the historically high number of 3,700,000 immigrants, about 7 percent of the population. The French Jewish population grew from about 75,000 at the time of the Dreyfus Affair to about 260,000 by the mid-1930s. Between the two world wars about 150,000 Jews entered France from Central and Eastern Europe, the old Ottoman Empire, the Balkans, and North Africa. The Jewish population in England grew from 60,000 in 1880 to 300,000 in 1914. Poor Russian and Polish Jews "saturated a predominantly middle class and anglicized Jewish population." In 1905 the Jewish population of London was about

[17] Viau, *Vingt ans d'antisémitisme 1889–1909*, 121–2. See also Viau, *Ces bons Juifs!* (Paris, 1898), for a reprint of the articles from *La Libre Parole*.

144,000, of whom about 120,000 lived in Stepney.[18] The cultural identity of the new French immigrants, based on geographical origin, religious practice, and Yiddish, made them appear as conspicuous clusters in the 3rd and 4th arrondissements of Paris. They were also strikingly poorer than the older Jewish community. By 1936 the new Jews had the misfortune to be labeled culturally pro-German and dubbed ex-enemies who spoke French badly. Robert de Rothschild initially thought that the new Jews should lie low – love France or leave it – and not endanger the comfortable situation of the old integrated Jewish community. This emphasis on patriotism led him and rabbi Jacob Kaplan to support the right wing *Croix de Feu*. By 1938 Robert realized he had deluded himself and that all Jews would be "put in the same sack" by the anti-Semites.[19] It seemed like a replay of the 1890s with a more vulnerable cast of victims and a more reality-based xenophobia. Drumont had babbled ad nauseam about the German origin of French Jews.

The New Jewish Doctor

French physicians were conspicuous in denouncing the foreign invasion, in particular the arrival of medical students from Eastern Europe, which began with general Jewish immigration in the 1880s. It has been argued that in both France and Germany a new outlook on wellbeing developed during World War I, with a need for medicine to move from an emphasis on individual health to concern for the health of the nation, the race. This was the general context of the history of medicine in the 1920s and especially the 1930s, though it was not exactly new.[20] After 1898 more and more foreigners took the degree of *doctorat de l'Université*, which required jumping fewer bureaucratic educational barriers, but was of course useless for a career in France, where the *doctorat d'Etat* was required. Dentistry proved mildly attractive to Frenchwomen, or it may be it looks that way because the medical profession was not welcoming. "The most virulent of all professional campaigns waged against foreign Jews was, however, that led by the *Confédération des Syndicats Médicaux* (CSM), the association of French doctors, together with its student affiliates."[21] Back in 1914 Léon Daudet had denounced the presence of too many Jews in the Paris Faculty of Medicine – "les Hébreux de la Faculté."[22] From

[18] Braudel, *L'identité de la France. Les hommes et les choses*, 186–7. On England, see David Feldman, *Englishmen and Jews. Social Relations and \Political Culture 1840–1914* (New Haven, 1994).

[19] Schor, *L'Antisémitisme en France pendant les années trente*, 12, 210, 256.

[20] See the superb comparative analysis by Susanne Michl, *Im Dienste des "Volkskörpers". Deutsche und französische Ärzte im Ersten Weltkrieg* (Göttingen, 2007).

[21] Vicki Caron, *Uneasy Asylum. France and the Jewish Refugee Crisis, 1933–1942* (Stanford, 1999), 29.

[22] Léon Daudet, *Devant la douleur* (1914), second volume of his *Souvenirs et polémiques*, "édition établie par Bernard Oudin" in the collection "Bouquins" (Paris, 1992),

the 1920s on the CSM became obsessed with the "medical plethora," an excess of foreign medical students, ranging from over twenty percent (Paris) to over one third (Strasbourg), totaling about twenty-one percent of medical students in 1934. Most of these students were Jewish, and a large number of them were from Romania, a hotbed of anti-Semitism and a country where there were Jewish student quotas in universities.[23] The foreigners threatened French jobs and would likely lower the moral standards of the profession, at least according to the judgment (1930) of Victor Balthazard, expert in legal medicine, professor and dean of the Paris medical faculty, and Dr Paul Cibrié.[24] The shady morals of these Jewish doctors supposedly led them to engage in illegal practices, such as performing abortions and abusing drug prescriptions for patients. Many also stooped to quackery. In 1930 three percent of the doctors practicing in France and eleven percent of those in Paris were foreigners.[25] (In pre-Nazi Germany about thirteen percent of the medical profession was classified as Jewish, though in large cities the percentage could be as high as fifty.[26]) After 1933 a series of laws increasingly restricted the practice of medicine in France to French citizens and subjects and residents of the empire and protectorates. Student strikes in 1935 encouraged politicians to pass laws making it extremely difficult for foreigners to practice medicine.[27] The logical, perverse culmination came in 1940–41 with laws requiring French paternity for practicing doctors and even an act denaturalizing anyone who had been naturalized since 1927. In 1941 a limitation, with some exceptions, of two percent of the number of practicing doctors in defined medical areas was established for those doctors classified as Jewish. Finally, all French nationals who had left France without official approval had their property confiscated and their citizenship cancelled.[28]

164; Toby Gelfand, "25,000 Medical Students: The Medical Thesis in the Nineteenth Century," unpublished paper, 2–3.

[23] Donna Evleth, "The 'Romanian Privilege' in French Medicine and Anti-Semitism," *Social History of Medicine* 11 (1998): 213–32.

[24] Caron, *Uneasy Asylum*, 29.

[25] Caron, *Uneasy Asylum*, 29–30. According to Pierre Guillaume, *Le rôle social du médecin depuis deux siècles 1800–1945* (Paris, 1996), 280, out of the 27,000 practitioners in France and the empire in 1941, about 6000 were of foreign origin, including 900 in Paris. Xavier Vallat (Commissioner-General for Jewish Affairs in Vichy (1941–42), estimated that 12.5 percent of doctors and 9.3 percent of dentists in France were Jewish.

[26] Robert Jay Lifton, *The Nazi Doctors. Medical Killing and the Psychology of Genocide* (New York, 1986), 36.

[27] For the connection of medical students with Action Française, see Françine Muel-Dreyfus, *Vichy et l'éternel féminin. Contribution à une sociologie politique de l'ordre des corps* (Paris, 1996), 305.

[28] Caron, *Uneasy Asylum,* 29–32, 323–4, 326; Guillaume, *Le rôle social du médecin*, 279.

Jews were the principal victims, and prominent among them one finds Henri de Rothschild, who lost property, citizenship, and his medical licence.[29]

Rejection by the Academy of Medicine

One of Henri's last plays, *Le Grand Patron* (1931), was not about the medical profession (France's 20,000 or so physicians), according to James de Coquet, but about something quite different, the Academy of Medicine.[30] It is not easy to separate the academy from the profession, and certainly Henri hoped that his medical career would be crowned by his election to that prestigious body. Scene xii of act I of the play is a dialogue between the medical hero and academy member, Professor Volnys, and his good friend Dr Tavernier, a candidate for election to the Academy of Medicine. Tavernier is surprised to learn that Volnys has already promised Dr Rivière to vote for Marnier, Rivière's brother-in-law. Rivière, the doctor looking after the academician who died, was able to take action before anyone else. The seat had been vacant for only 48 hours. Tavernier's virtuous prudence appears to have doomed his candidacy. Volnys tells Tavernier that campaigns start when a sick member's temperature reaches 40 degrees. A speedy Rivière telephoned Volnys an hour after Dutilier's death. Tavernier says that next time he will be just as ruthless as his opponents. Volnys then holds out hope for his friend. It is not the promise of a member to vote for someone that counts but the way the promise is given. Volnys quotes a famous wit of the illustrious company: "Members of the academy take engagements for politeness, and the candidates take politeness for engagements." Volnys promises to vote for Marnier only in the first round of voting; so he can vote for Tavernier in the second round and even the third. Tavernier, surprised but grateful, leaves as Volnys tells him to keep absolutely quiet about their conversation. If a third candidate emerges Volnys could easily change his mind. His friend replies that with Volnys at least one knows where one stands. Volnys himself could be dead before the election, he tells his friend. So who knows what will happen. The professor lights up his second cigarette during the scene and returns to his office as Tavernier leaves with some hope and little assurance.

Henri must have been thinking of his own stinging defeat a year before in a campaign for election to the Academy when he wrote this scene about Tavernier's run for the Institute. Having run a typical, shameless campaign himself, he knew what he was writing about. The scene in the play is a sanitized version of his own failure to get elected. Going up against Jean Charcot (1867–1936), Henri took three rounds of voting to lose. In the first round he had the most votes (47), in the second he had the same score as Charcot (48), and in the third he lost by four votes

[29] On Vichy anti-Semitism in the professions, see Donna Elveth, "The Ordre des Médecins and the Jews in Vichy France," *French History* 20 (2006): 204–24.

[30] *Le Figaro* (8 février 1931), in Arsenal, Rf. 71.742.

(46 to 50). There were two minor candidates who were knocked out in the second round. Volnys knew what he was talking about when he explained how a member could change his vote between rounds. In going up against Charcot, Henri had the bad luck to have, on the surface at least, a strong opponent, though if one looks at their respective careers in medicine, Charcot was a far weaker candidate than Henri. As a popular candidate, Charcot was hard to beat. Henri's maneuvers nearly carried the day. Perhaps he tried too hard. Jean, the son of the great neurologist, carried heavy patriarchal baggage. Sovereign of Salpêtriére, Charcot *père* had been a member of the academies of sciences and of medicine. Jean followed in his footsteps: a degree in medicine in 1895, intern in the hospitals of Paris, head of the clinic of nervous diseases of the Paris Faculty of Medicine, connection with the Pasteur Institute, and, inevitably, the winner of gold medals. (Henri also had won a couple of gold medals, including one from the Academy of Medicine in 1898 for his work *L'allaitement mixte et l'allaitement artificiel*.) Charcot was president of the Yacht club de France from 1913 to 1936, the year in which he went down with his ship in a hurricane twenty miles north of Reykjavik. Retired after a long period as captain of the *Pourquoi Pas*, he had the bad luck to be on ship as the head of a special mission. Henri lived on, sick and in exile during World War II, for another decade after Jean Charcot died.[31]

The campaign of Charcot versus Rothschild got known as the battle of "name against money." An amusing, sometimes ironic account – more at Henri's expense than Charcot's – of the triple-voting waltz with all the gory details appeared in *Candide*, which lived up to its name and reputation. The following remarks follow that account unscrupulously. The vacant seat was in the *Section des membres libres* of the Academy, the section Clemenceau called the "Section des malades." Dr Clemenceau was a member of this less prestigious section of the Academy. So Henri, now nearly sixty years old, modestly knocked at the smaller door to the Academy: not the tradesmen's entrance but certainly not the grand portal reserved for the great men of medicine elected as regular members. The "purs" or uncommitted in the Academy encouraged other candidates untainted by fame and money to apply for the spot Henri wanted: Trillat received thirteen votes in the first round. Charcot was already a member (*membre libre*) of the Academy of Sciences; perhaps he wanted to follow his father in becoming a member of both academies. Having earlier declared he was not a candidate, Charcot was open to some criticism after changing his mind, and he got it from Dr Bouquet right in the corridors of the Academy of Medicine. Several months of political activity preceded the election. Such agitation had not been seen in the ossified world of the academies since the physicist Edouard Branly beat Marie Curie in an election to the Academy of Sciences in 1909.

[31] *Index biographique des membres, des associés et des correspondants de l'Académie de médecine 1820–1990* and *A la mémoire de Jean-Baptiste Charcot 1867–1936* (Paris, 1936), Eloge by Dr Henri Meige.

It became clear to the members that no one had the votes to be elected in the first round. This provided a temptation to the forces of the *Assistance publique* to meddle by asking Mourier to become an outside candidate. Not that anyone expected him to win. He could at most get a few votes in the first round and then give his support to Henri. This was one scenario imagined by the pro-Rothschild contingent. "L'assistance privé," according to *Candide.* Mourier's reward for participating in this maneuver would be Clemenceau's chair in the next election. (Clemenceau had died in November 1929.) The trouble with this scheme was that if Henri were elected, the chair of "the tiger" would nearly certainly be reserved for Charcot. Mourier would fall between two stools, according to *Candide*. Interest in the election attracted ninety-six voters, a rare turnout in the rue Bonaparte.

Charcot's support was organized by Dr Souques, a power in the office of the Academy and its longtime secretary. This inside support was probably decisive in favor of Charcot. Henri's most powerful supporter was Emile Roux, the director of the Pasteur Institute (IP). Rumor had it that Henri promised to give three million francs to the IP if he were elected. This seems a little crude. Not that *Candide* thought that Roux could be bribed; he had, after all, given the 100,000 francs of his Osiris prize to the IP. Perhaps discussions had been broached over a gift for laboratories. Both candidates had connections with the IP, Charcot as an attaché and Henri as a one time lecturer. It is hard to know if this business made much difference in the outcome. One thing that might be noted is the mutual medical interest of Henri and Roux. Much of Henri's work had centered on the prevention of infant diseases through ensuring safe and nutritious infant feeding. Roux and he were united in a germ warfare alliance.

Henri's personal campaign was embarrassingly intense. Every Tuesday he came to the gallery, which exhibited the busts of dead great doctors, and stood near the table where members signed in. He shook hands, gave out some tickets for his theater in Pigalle, invited some people to hunt at Vaulx de Cernay, or nonchalantly took down an address to which a golden pheasant would be delivered the next day. (Charcot hated hunting as a cowardly pursuit.) Henri's daughter, Nadine, classified as charming by *Candide*, sometimes helped out in this delicate business of soliciting votes without appearing to. In addition to putting in an appearance on the rue Bonaparte, she presided over dinners given in honor of big shots in the Parisian medical tribe. She probably won over a few votes but not enough.

Another action Henri took attracted attention and perhaps jealousy and scorn. Candidates presented their qualifications in a pamphlet of sorts, whose bad quality was exaggerated by *Candide* as four or five sheets of ordinary school paper with the information only typed up. This model contrasted with Henri's fifty-eight-page "magnificent pamphlet handsomely printed on Japan paper and presented in an impressive gray cover."[32] Perhaps Henri ought to have presented a typical CV

[32] *Exposé des titres et travaux scientifiques du Docteur Henri de Rothschild* (Saint-Ouen, 1929).

to impress the members; given his interest in printing, binding, and fine editions, such a shabby strategy would have been painful for him.

The contents of the pamphlet provided more amusement for *Candide*. Anyone who has read a few curricula vitae or concocted a CV will be inclined to cast an indulgent eye on Henri's production. It must be said that his achievements were considerable, even in the area of scientific publication. With "charming modesty" he noted his passion for biological sciences, particularly those rendering immediate service to humanity – a nice Pasteurian note here to describe his early years in medicine, when he did so much work on infant feeding. *Candide* recognized that he analyzed his medical and veterinary experience with an admirable candor. How to describe his funding of medical research? The prose was a bit stilted but not overly egoistic. In fact the account looks too modest and somewhat distorted. Being able to support research, he did medicine in order to be better able to discern the most interesting topics and the people most capable of studying them. This may be the way he viewed things in 1930, but back in 1900 it looked like he was doing medicine because he was interested in becoming a physician. He confesses that his medical role was always more of a supporting than an intellectual nature. This again goes too far and shows us how disappointed he was in at least not having got more recognition in the medical field. Most doctors would have been happy to be so disappointed. But Rothschild goals were high. "It is in the choice of scientists [to support] that I have been able to render some services" was a sad epitaph to a life as a physician. *Candide* may have been right in saying that this apparent charming modesty was what was required of candidates, the homage that pride paid to power.

In listing his charitable medical works, Henri found it more difficult to feign modesty. The list included the excellent *gouttes de lait*, the Picpus polyclinic, the hospital in the rue Marcadet, and even the popular restaurant. And as a railway "administrator" he had been able to hand out free travel passes to deserving scientists. He also mentioned other charitable activities but without much emphasis, as if he knew that they should not be mentioned at all. So much work in vain to get into the "Section des malades" of the Academy! The man whose family name was on three hospitals in Paris never even made it into the category of *membres libres* of the Academy of Medicine. This all seems rather minor now: in the 1930s and early 1940s much medical behavior would be far worse than voting against a Rothschild.

"The Gathering Storm"

The 1930s appear to have been a difficult or at least radically changing period for some traditional Rothschild interests. A change in the statute of the *Banque de France* in 1936 deprived Edouard of his post of regent, which he had inherited from his father Edmond; the post had been a family fixture since the heady days of Alphonse. Nationalization became a popular political fix for the economy with the advent of the Popular Front: in 1937 the "family railroad" (*Société des chemins de fer du Nord*) folded into the new S.N.C.F., but the pain of loss was assuaged with 270,000 shares of the new company, and the old Rothschild firm took flight as an instrument for managing real estate investments. In 1940 the Belgian government bought the Belgian branch of the railroad.[33] Not that any of this affected Henri directly, and it is difficult to speculate on any mental stress that these events caused, especially because he had serious physical problems, which always manage to monopolize one's mind.

In the mid-1930s Henri took up residence in Switzerland, near Lausanne; some have speculated that his inspiration was fiscal, others that his purpose was to find a healthier environment than Paris for his aging, suffering body. He was still afflicted with uremia, a nasty condition in which inefficiently operating kidneys produce excess urea and other nitrogenous compounds in the blood. He was also rumored to have fallen ill as a result of a visit to China during a cruise in 1935 and advised by his doctors to live in Switzerland, and this is the account he gives in one of his final works. In March 1935, on arriving in China, he experienced severe earaches and disorders of the sympathetic nervous system. He deteriorated in China. After treatment by specialists back in France, he got worse and vegetated three and a half months in his bedroom. Doctors told him that in order to recover he would have to spend two to four years in Switzerland. So on 2 August 1936 he established himself on a small estate near Lausanne. He improved slightly. In 1940 he followed medical advice to change climate and altitude. Doctors advised him to benefit from a temperate and even climate in Portugal. Two months would speed up his recovery.[34] With the Nazis in full control of an anti-Semitic Germany, perhaps Henri feared that Switzerland would also become a dangerous place for Jews, especially for Rothschilds. So he went off to Salazar's Portugal, which had an obvious political and geographical advantage over Switzerland when one was escaping from the Nazis. His longtime friend Marthe Régnier was also there. At first at least, he stayed in a small villa near the sea and not far from Lisbon. In getting set up in Portugal, Henri was able to call on help from the *Banco Espírito Santo*: his friend Ricardo Espírito Santo offered to do what was necessary to get him established, including the difficult task of finding a suitable residence. Ricardo was also able to facilitate the process of getting governmental permission to equip Henri's small automobile with a charcoal-burning gazogene.[35] Before the war Henri had added to his French properties by buying an estate near Hyères (Var), next to the vast Domaine de Mauvannes of the actress Simone Berriau;

---

33 Dreyfus, *Pillages sur ordonnances*, 215–17.

34 Henri de Rothschild, *La Lignée française de la famille Rothschild 1792–1942. Etude historique et biographique* (Oporto, 1942), 131.

35 Letter to Ricardo from Henri in Carlos Alberto Damas and Augusto de Ataíde, *O Banco Espírito santo; una dinastia financeira portuguesa* (Lisbon, 2004), I (*1869–1973*), 183. The letter is headed Villa Sagres, Elvassida m. de Albuquerque, Estoril, le 14 sep. 1942.

Admiral Darlan took over Henri's house during the war. After the allies liberated France, Henri was able to visit Paris, the old "paradise of his dreams"; he used to stay at the hotel Raphaël, whose classic style with a terrace overlooking the city he no doubt appreciated. On 10 October 1947 Henri died at Castel Beau Cidri (Jouxtens), his estate near Lausanne, where he had resettled after his return from Portugal in April 1946.[36] A lifetime smoker, he had been living with a damaged heart for years.

The words on the Berck hospital plaque for Nathaniel also seem appropriate for Henri. "Les justes, même morts, sont toujours vivants, leurs œuvres perpétuent leur souvenir."[37]

---

36 The name Castel Beau Cidri is also written Castel Beau Cèdre. See "Les Rothschilds – Gouvieux-Chantilly 1880–1930," in *Bulletin de la Société historique de Gouvieux* (Oise) 4 (1992): 164. The phrase "paradise of his dreams" is a modification of the last line, "Vers le paradis de mes rêves," in Baudelaire's poem "Le vin des amants."

37 "The righteous, even after death, are still living in their works perpetuating their memory."

Bibliography

Archival Sources

Archives de l'Assistance publique-Hôpitaux de Paris. Includes the "Fonds Iconographique" *Les établissements hospitaliers Rothschild* and the "Fonds Iconographique" *Berck*. Both inventories done by Stéphanie Le Toux.

Archives et documents de guerre du Service de Santé militaire. *Iconographie du Muséee du Val-de-Grâce*, edited by O. Jacob (8 vols, Paris: Editions scientifiques. Aristide Quillet, 1918).

Archives Nationales: Centre des archives du monde (CAMT), Roubaix. 132 AQ 7, 301, 324, 5914.

Archives de Paris. Perotin/8/Roth/77/1 1-100.

Bibliothèque de l'Arsenal (at the end of 2004 the département des Arts du spectacle was transferred to the Bibliothèque nationale de France, site Richelieu).

Plazanet, Nathalie, *Inventaire des archives de la Guerre 1914–1918* (AP-HP, 603 Foss, Feb. 1989).

Service historique de la Défense, armée de terre ("Ministère de la Guerre, Archives administratives," 6Ye 12774).

The Rothschild Archive. London, 000/930: 58-1; 221 files.

The Rothschild Family Tree (London: The Rothschild Archive, 2000).

Printed Sources

Barthe de Sandfort, J.-M., *Dax pittoresque et thermal; guide du médecin et du malade* (Paris: Dentu, 1885).

------*Traitement des brûlures par la méthode du Dr Barthe de Sandfort; instructions pratiques pour l'application de l'ambrine* (Paris: Laboratoire de l'ambrine, 1916).

Bergeron, Jules, and Marjolin, René, *Rapport sur les résultats obtenus dans le traitement des enfants scrofuleux à l'hôpital de Berck-sur-Mer* (Paris: Grandremy et Henon, 1866).

Bourneville, D.-M., "Visite aux œuvres du Dr H. de Rothschild," *La revue philanthropique* 20 (1906–07): 485–7.

Brouardel, Paul, *La profession médicale au commencement du XXe siècle* (Paris: Baillière, 1903).

Budin, Pierre, *Femmes en couches et nouveaux-nés – Recherches cliniques et expérimentales* (Paris: Doin, 1897).

-----,"Ligue contre la mortalité infantile," *La revue philanthropique* 15 (1904): 231–6.

-----, "La ville de Paris et la mortalité infantile" (lecture given on 4 December 1903 in the *mairie* of the 4th arrondissement...), *La revue philanthropique* 14 (1903–04): 381–416.

Calot, François-Jean, *Berck. Ses méthodes de traitement et son climat idéal pour les malades* (1914; 4th edn, Maloine, 1929; 5th edn, Maloine 1933).

-----, *L'hôpital de Henri de Rothschild à Berck-sur-Mer* (Paris: Masson, 1900).

Caron, A. *La puériculture ou la science d'élever hygiéniquement et physiologiquement les enfants* (2d edn, Rouen: Baillière, 1866).

Carrel, Alex, *et al*, "Traitement abortif de l'infection des plaies," *Bulletin de l'Académie de Médecine* 74, 3rd series (1915): 361–8.

Cazin, Henri, *Les établissements hôspitaliers à Berck-sur-Mer* (Paris: Asselin et Houzeau, 1885).

-----, *De l'influence des bains de mer sur la scrofula des enfants* (Paris: Asselin et Houzeau, 1885).

Daudet, Léon, *Devant la douleur* (1914), second volume of his *Souvenirs et polémiques*, "édition établie par Bernard Oudin" in the collection "Bouquins" (Paris: Laffont, 1992).

Delbet, Pierre, *Fondation Henri de Rothschild. Rapport de M. le professeur Pierre Delbet* (Paris: n. p., 1919).

Delorme, Edmond (*Médecin Inspecteur général de l'Armée*), *Les enseignements chirurgicaux de la Grande Guerre. Front Occidental* (Paris: Maloine, 1919). Imprimerie et librairie centrales des chemins de fer, 1919).

Desprès, Armand, *La chirurgie journalière* (1877; 3rd edn, Paris: Baillière, 1888; 4th edn, 1894).

Devraigne, Louis, *Vingt-cinq ans de puériculture et d'hygiène sociale* (Paris: Doin, 1928).

Dezeimeris, J.-E., *Dictionnaire historique de la médecine ancienne et moderne* (4 vols, Paris: Béchet Jeune, 1828–39).

Dieulafoy, Georges, *Clinique médicale de l'Hôtel-Dieu de Paris 1896–1897* (Paris: Masson, 1898).

Dluski, Bronislas, *Contribution à l'étude de l'allaitement maternel* (thesis, Paris Faculty of Medicine, 1894).

Duclaux, Emile, *Le lait, études chimiques et microbiologiques* (Paris: Baillière, 1887; 1894).

Emery, E., "La méthode d'Ehrlich," *Actualités Médico-chirurgicales* 2nd series (1912): 20–52.

Fosseyeux, Marcel, *Les grands travaux hospitaliers,1903–1911. Hôpital maritime de Berck-sur-Mer, 1861–1911* (Paris: Berger-Levrault, 1911).

La Fondation de Rothschild, 1852–1952 (Paris: Astra, 1952).

Hooper-Blackler-Kalopothakès, Marie, *Troubles et lésions gastriques dans la dyspepsie gastro-intestinale chronique des nourrissions* (thesis, Paris Faculty of Medicine, 1894).

Icard, Séverin, *L'alimentation des nouveaux-nés. Hygiène de l'allaitement artificiel* (Paris: Alcan, 1894).

Index biographique des membres, des associés et des correspondants de l'Académie de médecine 1820–1939 (Paris: Masson, 1939)..

Labarthe, Paul, and others, *Dictionnaire populaire de médecine. Usuelle d'hygiène publique et privée* (2 vols, Paris: Marpon et Flammarion, n.d.; 3d edn, 1890).

Le Gendre, Paul, and Lepage, G., *Le Médecin dans la société contemporaine – conférences de déontologie* (Paris: Masson, 1902).

-----, "La vie du médecin, déontologie et jurisprudence médicales," in Emile Sergent and others (eds), *Traité de pathologie médicale et de jurisprudence appliquée* (Paris: Maloine, 1920).

Leguay, Emile, "Inauguration de l'hôpital Israélite à Paris," *Annales de la charité*, 8 (1852): 375–81.

Lemaire, A., "Les régimes de nourrissons," *Le Progrès médical* 27 (5 juillet 1930): 1190–6.

Lesage, Adolphe, *Le Traitement des gastro-entérites des nourrissons et du choléra infantile* (Paris: Masson, 1906).

Lévy-Solal, Edmond, *La Puériculture* (Paris: Editions Leroux, 1919).

Lorreyte, Gaston, *Contribution à l'étude du traitement de l'hérédo-syphilis par l'injection d'arséno-benzol au cours de la grossesse* (thesis, Paris Faculty of Medicine, 1911).

Loze, Henry, *L'Hôpital Nathaniel de Rothschild à Berck-sur-Mer* (Paris: Masson, 1908).

Lucas-Championnière, Just, *Chirurgie antiseptique. Principes, modes d'application et résultats du pansement de Lister* (2nd edn, Paris: Ballière, 1880).

-----, *Statistique des opérations faites ... mai 1887 à mai 1889* (Paris: Coccoz, 1889).

-----, *Le passé et le présent de la méthode antiseptique* (Paris: no imprint, 1899).

Marfan, A.-B., "Nécrologie – Variot (1855–1930)," *Le Nourrisson* 18 (1930): 206–08.

-----, *Traité de l'allaitement et de l'alimentation des enfants du premier âge* (1899; 1903; 1906; 4th edn, revised and expanded, Paris: Masson, 1930).

Martin, Albert, *Souvenirs d'un chirurgien de la Grande Guerre* (Luneray: Bertout, 1996).

Maygrier, Charles, *Les Consultations de nourrissons* (Paris: Masson, 1903).

-----, *La Consultation des nourrissons à la Charité de 1898 à 1901* (Paris, n. p., 1901). "Extrait de *L'Obstétrique* (15 mai 1901)."

Métayer, Léopold, *Les injections intra-musculaires de sublime à doses rares et élevées dans la syphilis; comparison avec le calomel et l'huile grise* (thesis, Paris Faculty of Medicine, 1899).

Metchnikoff, Elie, *Quelques remarques sur le lait aigri* (1904), from the *Essais optimistes* (Paris: Maloine, 1907).

Mignon, A., *L'évolution du Service de Santé pendant la guerre 1914–1918*, I, 625–7. *Le Service de Santé pendant la guerre …* (4 vols, Paris: Masson, 1926).

Nageotte-Wilbouchevitch, Marie, *Traitement antiseptique des brûlures* (thesis, Paris Faculty of Medicine, 1893).

-----, *Atlas manuel de gymnastique orthopédique, Traitement des déviations de la taille* (Paris: Masson, 1903).

-----, *Traitement des déviations de la colonne vertébrale et de l'insuffisance respiratoire* (2nd edn, Paris: Baillière, 1937).

Nicaise, Edouard, *L'antisepsie dans la pratique de la chirurgie journalière* (Paris: Baillière, 1896).

Nobécourt, Pierre, "Leçon d'ouverture – chaire de clinique médicale des enfants" (6 Jan. 1921), in *La Presse médicale* (19 février 1921).

Le Nourrisson. Revue d'hygiène et de pathologie de la première enfance, 1913–1960.

Péan, Jules-Emile, *Ovariotomie; l'ovariotomie, peut-elle être faite à Paris avec des chances favorables de succès?* (2nd edn, Paris: Germer-Baillière, 1869).

Pegoud, Albert, *De la valeur des courants continus dans le traitement des tumeurs fibreuses de l'utérus* (thesis, Paris Faculty of Medicine, 1881).

Pinard, Adolphe, *Du fonctionnement de la maternité de Lariboisière et des résultats obtenus depuis 1882 jusqu'en 1889* (Paris: Steinheil, 1889).

-----, *La puériculture du premier âge* (Paris: Colin, 1904).

-----, *Stéphane Tarnier, 1828–1897* (Paris: Maretheux, 1898).

-----, and Wallich, V., *Traitement de l'infection puerpérale* (Paris: Steinheil, 1896).

Pozzi, Samuel, "Hôpitaux et chirurgiens aux Etats-unis," in *Actualités médico-chirurgicales – Polyclinique Henri de Rothschild* (Paris: Doin, 1911), 131–64.

-----, *Quelques observations à propos du pansement de Lister appliqué aux plaies d'amputation et d'ablation de tumeurs* (Paris: Delahaye, 1876).

Py, Louis, *La puériculture en France à l'heure actuelle* (thesis, Faculty of Medicine, Toulouse, 1913).

Regaud, Claudius-François, 'Radiumtherapy', *Encyclopaedia Britannica* (1943), 18: 908.

Revue de déontologie et d'intérêts professionnels médicaux ('organe mensuel de l'Association corporative des étudiants en médecine de Paris'), 1903–05.

Revue d'hygiène et de médecine infantiles et Annales de la polyclinique H. de Rothschild, 1902–11.

Ribadeau-Dumas, H., *Déontologie et jurisprudence médicale. Déontologie* by P. Le Gendre, and *Jurisprudence médicale* by H. Ribadeau-Dumas (Paris: Maloine, 1920).

Rilliet, Frédéric, and Barthez, Ernest, *Traité clinique et pratique des maladies des enfants* (3 vols, Paris: Baillière, 1843); 2nd revised and expanded edition, 1861; 3rd edn, expanded by Barthez and A. Sanné, published by Alcan in 1891.

Roger, Henri, *Seméiotique des maladies de l'enfance ... leçons* (Paris: Asselin, 1864).

-----, *Recherches cliniques sur les maladies de l'enfance* (Paris: Asselin, 1872–83).

Rosier, L., "Hospice israélite de Paris," *L'Illustration, Journal Universel* (29 mai 1852): 363–4.

"Les prix Henri de Rothschild," *La revue philanthropique* 19 (1906–07): 648.

"Les Rothschilds – Gouvieux-Chantilly 1880–1930," *Bulletin de la Société historique de Gouvieux* (Oise) 4 (1992).

Rothschild, Henri de (including pseudonym André Pascal). A superb illustrated bibliography is easily available online:

The Rothschild Archive online site: http://www.rothschildarchive.org/ta/.

Research Forum: The Rothschild bibliography: Henri de Rothschild (1872–1947): http://www.rothschildarchive.org/research/?doc=/research/articles/bib_514.

Rothschild, Henri de. The online general catalog of the Bibliothèque nationale de France lists 163 items: http://www.bnf.fr/.

Rothschild, Thérèse de (*la baronne* James), *Pages détachées du cahier d'une jeune fille* (Mâcon: Protat frères, imprimeurs, 1896; 1925).

Rothschild, Thérèse de, *Souvenirs de la grande guerre 1914–1918* (Mâcon: Protat frères, imprimeurs, 1927).

Sieur, Marcel, "Les organisations du Service de Santé aux Armées," in *Le Livre d'or des médecins morts pour la France 1914–1918* (Paris: Baillière, n.d.).

Soranus' Gynecology, translated by Owsei Temkin (Baltimore: The Johns Hopkins University Press, 1956).

Tarnier, Stéphane, *De l'asepsie et de l'antisepsie en obstétrique .. leçons professées à la clinique d'accouchements* (Paris: Steinheil, 1894), collected and edited by Dr J. Potocki.

-----, *Recherches sur l'état puerpérale et sur les maladies des femmes en couches* (thesis, Paris Faculty of Medicine, 1857).

-----, *De la fièvre puerpérale observée à l'hospice de la Maternité* (Paris: Baillière, 1858).

-----, *Mémoire sur l'hygiène des hôpitaux de femmes en couches* (Paris: Parent, 1864).

Terrier, Félix, *Statistique des opérations pratiquées à l'Hôpital Bichat (service des consultations et service hospitalier) pendant l'année 1892 [–93, 1898–99](Paris: Bataille* and then *Alcan*, 1893–1900).

Trisca, Petre, *Prolégomènes à une déontologie medico-sociale* (Paris: Alcan, 1922).

-----, *La protection du nourrisson et de la maternité en Allemagne* (Paris: Baillière, 1926).

Trousseau, A., *La Fondation ophtalmologique Adolphe de Rothschild* (Paris: Fondation Rothschild, 1905).

Variot, G., *La mortalité infantile et l'ignorance des mères* ("Conférence … réouverture des cours de l'Institut de Puériculture, le 16 novembre 1916").

-----, *Traité d'hygiène infantile* (Paris: Doin, 1910).

Victor, Henri-A., *La maternité de l'hôpital de Rothschild. Son fonctionnement jusqu'en 1930* (thesis, Paris Faculty of Medicine, 1931).
Viguier, Prosper, *Un chirurgien de la grande guerre*, "présentation de Rémy Cazals" (Toulouse: Privat, 2007).

Secondary Sources

Aisenberg, Andrew, *Contagion, Disease, Government, and the "Social Question" in Nineteenth-Century France* (Stanford: Stanford University Press, 1999).
Barrot, Olivier, and Chirat, Raymond, *"Ciel, mon mari!". Le Théâtre du Boulevard* (Paris: Gallimard, 1998).
Beauvalet-Boutouyrie, Scarlett, *Naître à l'hôpital au XIXe siècle* (Paris: Belin, 1999).
Berkovitz, Jay R., *Rites and Passages. The Beginnings of Modern Jewish Culture in France, 1650–1860* (Philadelphia: University of Pennsylvania Press, 2004).
-----, *The Shaping of Jewish Identity in Nineteenth-Century France* (Detroit: Wayne State University Press, 1989).
Bernstein-Gruber, Georges, and Maurin, Gilbert, *Bernstein le magnifique* (Paris: J. C. Lattes, 1988).
Birnbaum, Pierre, *The Jews of the Republic. A Political History of State Jews in France from Gambetta to Vichy* (Stanford: Stanford University Press, 1996). Translated by Jane Marie Todd.
Bonner, Thomas Neville, *Becoming a Physician. Medical Education in Britain, France, Germany, and the United States, 1750–1945* (New York: Oxford University Press, 1955).
-----, "Rendezvous in Zurich. Seven who Made a Revolution in Women's Medical Education, 1864–1874," *Journal of the History of Medicine and Allied Sciences* 44/1 (Jan. 1989): 7–27.
-----, *To the Ends of the Earth. Women's Search for Education in Medicine* (Cambridge, Mass.: Harvard University Press, 1992).
Brieux, Eugène, *Les Avariés* (Paris: P.-V. Stock, 1909).
-----, *Les Remplaçantes* (8th edn, Paris: Calmann-Lévy, 1907).
Brunet, Brigitte, *Le Théâtre du Boulevard* (Paris: Nathan, 2004).
Bynum, W. F., *Science and the Practice of Medicine in the Nineteenth Century* (Cambridge: Cambridge University Press, 1994).
Caron, Vicki, *Uneasy Asylum. France and the Jewish Refugee Crisis, 1933–1942* (Stanford: Stanford University Press, 1999).
"Du charlatanisme en général et du charlatanisme médical en particulier," *Gazette médicale de Paris* 1 (1833): 713–15.
Contrepois, Alain, "The Clinician, Germs and Infectious Diseases: The Example of Charles Bouchard [1837–1915] in Paris," *Medical History* 46 (April 2002): 197–220.
Cordier, G., *Paris et les anatomistes au cours de l'histoire* (Paris: I. A. C., 1955).

Courson, Comtesse de, *La Femme Française pendant la Guerre* (2nd edn, Paris: Thielleux, 1916).

Crépin, Michèle and Guy, *Un hôpital crée une ville. L'hôpital maritime de Berck-sur-Mer, Assistance publique – Hôpitaux de Paris de sa création jusqu'en 1920* (Berck: Cahiers du Musée de Berck, série histoire No. 1, 1999).

Damas, Carlos Alberto, and de Ataíde, Augusto, *O Banco Espírito santo; una dinastia financeira portuguesa* (Lisbon: Centro de Estudos da Historia do BES, 2004), I (1869–1973).

Daremberg, Georges, *Les grands médecins du XIXe siècle* (Paris: Masson, 1907).

Darrow, Margaret H., *French Women and the First World War. War Stories of the Home Front* (Oxford: Berg, 2000).

Debré, Robert, *L'honneur de vivre. Témoignage* (Paris: Hermann et Stock, 1974).

Defrance, Henri, *Nouveaux hôpitaux, maisons de santé, maternités, etc.* (Paris: Massin, 1930).

Delahaye, Marie-Claude, *Tétons et tétines – histoire de l'allaitement* (Paris: Trame Way, 1990).

-----, *Bébés au biberon – petite histoire de l'allaitement* (Paris: Hoëbeke, 2003).

-----, and Lett, Didier, *Une histoire de l'allaitement* (Paris: Editions de la Martinière, 2006).

Delalande, Nicolas, *La genèse d'un parcours philanthropique: les Rothschild et le cas de l'hôpital israélite (1852–1914),* "Mémoire de maîtrise, histoire contemporaine," (Paris, I Panthéon-Sorbonne, 2003).

Delaporte, Sophie, *Les Gueules Cassées: les blessés de la face de la Grande Guerre* (Paris: Noêsis, 1996).

-----, *Les médecins dans la Grande Guerre 1914–1918* (Paris: Bayard, 2003).

Delavault, Robert, *L'Asepsie un demi-siècle avant Pasteur: Ignace Semmelweis 1818–1865* (Paris: L'Harmattan, 2007), in the collection *Médecine à travers les siècles*.

Deroin, Emmeline, *La Maternité de Paris de 1850 à 1900,* "Université de Paris V. Ecole de sages-femmes Baudelocque. Mémoire de fin d'études de sage-femme" (Paris, 2005).

Descoust, Paul, *La médecine au théâtre dans les temps modernes* (2nd edn, Paris: Boulanger, 1906).

Duhamel, Georges, *Les Maîtres* (Paris: Mercure de France, 1937).

-----, *Vie des martyrs 1914–1916* (Paris: Mercure de France, 1917, 1929).

Duker, Abraham G., *Jews in World War I,* reprinted from *Contemporary Jewish Record* (New York: American Jewish Committee, c. 1939).

Dupont, Michel, *Dictionnaire historique des Médecins dans et hors de la Médecine* (Paris: Larousse-Bordas/HER, 1999).

Ellis, Jack D., *The Physician-Legislators of France. Medicine and Politics in the Early Third Republic, 1870–1914* (Cambridge: Cambridge University Press, 1990).

Evleth, Donna, 'The Ordre des Médecins and the Jews in Vichy France', *French History* 20 (2006): 204–24.

-----, "The 'Romanian Privilege' in French Medicine and Anti-Semitism," *Social History of Medicine* 11 (1998): 213–32.

Faux, Sabrina, *Aspects médicaux et sociaux du traitement de la tuberculose à Berck-sur-Mer, 1880–1940* (Paris, University of Paris VII, "Mémoire maîtrise Histoire," 1992).

Fäy-Sallois, Fanny, *Les nourrices à Paris au XIXe siècle* (Paris: Payot, 1980).

Ferguson, Niall, *The House of Rothschild. The World's Banker 1449–1999* (2 vols, New York: Viking, 1999).

Fette, Julie, "Pride and Prejudice in the Professions. Women Doctors and Lawyers in Third Republic France," *Journal of Women's History* 19/3 (2007): 60–86.

Fèvre, Marcel, "Etienne Sorrel (1882–1965)," *Bulletin de l'Académie de Médecine* 151 (1967): 38–46.

Fontanel, Béatrice, and d'Harcourt, Claire, *L'épopée des bébés, une histoire des petits d'hommes* (Paris: Editions de la Martinière, 1996).

Fouchou-Lapeyrade, Joseph, *Contribution à l'étude de la coxalgie par la radiographie* (thesis, Paris Faculty of Medicine, 1906).

Fuchs, Rachel G., *Abandoned Children. Foundlings and Child Welfare in Nineteenth-Century France* (Albany, N.Y.: SUNY Press, 1984).

-----, *Poor and Pregnant in Paris: Strategies for Survival in the Nineteenth Century* (New Brunswick, N.J.: Rutgers University Press, 1992).

Galzy, Jeanne, *Les Allongés* (Paris: Gallimard, 1975).

Gelfand, Toby, "Medical Nemesis, Paris 1894: Léon Daudet's *Les Morticoles*," *Bulletin of the History of Medicine*, 60 (1986): 155–76.

-----, "25,000 Medical Students: The Medical Thesis in the Nineteenth Century," unpublished paper.

-----, "The Rothschild Hospital of Paris: Between Autonomy and Assimilation", unpublished paper.

Gentilcore, David, *Medical Charlatanism in Early Modern Italy* (Oxford and New York: Oxford University Press, 2006).

Genty, Maurice, *Les Biographies médicales*, 2nd series, "Les Maîtres d'aujourd'hui" (Paris: Baillière, 1930–36).

Gilman, Sander L., *Jewish Frontiers. Essays on Bodies, Histories, and Identities* (New York: Palgrave Macmillan, 2003; paperback, 2004).

Goetz, Christopher G., Bonduelle, Michel, and Gelfand, Toby, *Charcot. Constructing Neurology* (New York: Oxford University Press, 1995).

Goldstein, Jan E., *Console and Classify. The French Psychiatric Profession in the Nineteenth Century* (Cambridge: Cambridge University Press, 1987).

Gourevitch, Danielle, *Le mal d'être femme: La femme et la médecine dans la Rome antique* (Paris: "Les Belles Lettres," 1984).

Graetz, Michael, *Les Juifs en France au XIXe siècle. De la Révolution française à l'Alliance Israélite Universelle* (Paris: Seuil, 1989). Translated from the Hebrew by Salomon Malka.

Grancher, Joseph, Comby, J., and Marfan, A.-B., (eds), *Traité des maladies de l'enfance* (5 vols, Paris: Masson, 1897; 2nd edn 1904–05).

Green, Abigail, "The British Empire and the Jews: An Imperialism of Human Rights?," *Past and Present* 199 (May 2008): 175–205.

Green, Nancy L., *The Pletzl of Paris. Jewish Immigrant Workers in the Belle Epoque* (New York: Holmes & Meier, 1986).

Guillaume, Pierre, *Le rôle social du médecin depuis deux siècles 1800–1945* (Paris: association pour l'Etude de l'histoire de la Sécurité Sociale, 1996).

Helme, F., *Les Jardins de la médecine* (Paris: Vigot, 1907).

Higonnet, Margaret R. (ed.), *Nurses at the Front. Writing the Wounds of the Great War* (Boston: Northeastern University Press, 2001).

Huguet, François, *Les professeurs de la faculté de médecine. Dictionnaire biographique* (Paris: CNRS Editions, 1991).

Hyman, Paula E., "Acculturation of the Jews in Nineteenth-Century France," in *The Emergence of Jewish Artists in Nineteenth-Century Europe* (New York: Merrell Publishers and The Jewish Museum, 2001), 31–9.

Katz, Jonathan G., *Murder in Marrakesh: Emile Mauclair and the French Colonial Adventure* (Bloomington, IN: Indiana University Press, 2006).

Kernahan, Peter J., "Causation and Cleanliness: George Callender, Wounds, and the Debates over Listerism," *Journal of the History of Medicine and Allied Sciences* 64 (Jan. 2009): 1–37.

Kevles, Bettyann Holtzmann, *Naked to the Bone. Medical Imaging in the Twentieth Century* (New Brunswick, N.J.: Rutgers University Press, 1997).

Knibiehler, Yvonne, "Allaitement," in *Dictionnaire de la pensée médicale*; ed., Dominique Lecourt (Paris: Presses Universitaires de France, 2004).

-----, and others, *Cornettes et blouses blanches. Les Infirmières dans la société française 1880–1980* (Paris: Hachette, 1984).

Kupfer, Jacques, *La Glaive de David. Aux sources de Tsahal dans la première guerre mondiale* (Paris: Laurans, 1998).

Landau, Philippe-E., *Les Juifs de France et la Grande Guerre. Un patriotisme républicain 1914–1941* (Paris: CNRS Editions, 1999, 2008) and "Brève histoire des Juifs dans la Grande Guerre," in *Les Juifs dans la Grande Guerre* (Historial de la Grande Guerre, Péronne, Somme), catalog of an exposition, 24 Sept. to 15 Dec. 2002.

Larcan, Alain, and Ferrandis, Jean Jacques, *Le Service de Santé aux Armées pendant la première guerre mondiale* (Paris: Editions LBM, 2008).

Laskier, Michael M., *The Alliance Israélite Universelle and the Jewish Communities of Morocco: 1862–1962* (Albany: SUNY, 1983).

Latour, Bruno, *The Pasteurization of France* (Cambridge, Mass.: Harvard University Press, 1988), 29–30. Translation by Alan Sheridan and John Law.

Lawrence, Christopher, "'A Time to Heal': The Diffusion of Listerism in Victorian Britain," *Bulletin of the History of Medicine* 74 (2000): 618–19.

-----, *Medical Theory, Surgical Practice: Studies in the History of Surgery* (Wellcome Institute Series in the History of Medicine; London and New York: Routledge, 1992).

Lebel, Hélène, *Le Théâtre à Paris (1880–1914): reflet d'une société?* (Villeneuve d'Ascq: Presses Universitaires du Septentrion, 1996).

Lefebvre, Pierre (ed.), *Histoire de la Médecine aux armées* (Paris and Limoges: Lavauzelle, 1987), tome 3.

Lefèvre, Marine, *Rothschild. Chronique d'un hôpital pas comme les autres, 1743–1999* (Paris: Collection Assistance publique-Hôpitaux de Paris, 1999).

Leff, Lisa Moses, *Sacred Bonds of Solidarity. The Rise of Jewish Internationalism in Nineteenth-Century France* (Stanford: Stanford University Press, 2006).

-----, "Self-definition and Self-defense: Jewish Racial Identity in Nineteenth-Century France," *Jewish History* (2005), 19: 7–28.

Léonard, Jacques, "Le Malade imaginaire de Molière à Jules Romains," and "les soins corporals d'après le *Journal* de Jules Renard (1887–1910)," in *Médecins, maladies et société dans la France du XIXe siècle* (Paris: Sciences en Situation, 1992), 261–73, 275–83.

Lequin, Yves, "Dreyfus à l'usine? Le silence d'une mémoire," in Pierre Birnbaum (ed.), *La France de l'Affaire Dreyfus* (Paris: Gallimard, 1994).

Lipinska, Melina, *Les femmes et le progrès des sciences médicales* (Paris: Masson, 1930).

Lise, Caron, *L'hôpital maritime de Berck-sur-Mer: des origines à 1914* ("Mémoire de maîtrise," institution not listed, 2000/01).

Littlewood, Joan, *Baron Philippe. The Very Candid Autobiography of Baron Philippe de Rothschild* (New York: Ballantine Books, 1986).

Lucien, Guy-Marie, *Cent cinquantenaire de l'internat des hôpitaux de Paris* (thesis, Paris Faculty of Medicine, 1952).

Mahnke, C. Becket, "The Growth and Development of a Specialty: The History of Pediatrics," *Clinical Pediatrics* 39 (2000): 705–14.

Margadant, Jo Burr (ed.), *The New Biography. Performing Femininity in Nineteenth-Century France* (Berkeley: University of California Press, 2000).

Markell Morantz-Sanchez, Regina, *Sympathy and Science. Women Physicians in American Medicine* (1985; Chapel Hill: University of North Carolina Press, 2000).

Mayeur, Françoise, *L'Education des filles en France au XIXe siècle* (Paris: Hachette, 1979).

Meige, Henri, *A la mémoire de Jean-Baptiste Charcot 1867–1936* (Paris: Yacht club de France, 1936).

Mialaret, Jacques, *Paul Poirier, 1853–1907* (Paris: Masson, 1965).

Michl, Susanne, *Im Dienste des "Volkskörpers". Deutsche und französische Ärzte im Ersten Weltkrieg* (Göttingen: Vandenhoeck & Rupecht, 2007).

Moulin, Anne Marie, *Le dernier language de la médecine. Histoire de l'immunologie de Pasteur au Sida* (Paris: Presses Universitaires de France, 1991).

Moulinier, Pierre, www.barthes.ens.fr/clio/dos/genre/com/moulinierprem.pdf.

Muel-Dreyfus, Françine, *Vichy et l'éternel féminin. Contribution à une sociologie politique de l'ordre des corps* (Paris: Seuil, 1996).

Murard, Lion, and Zylberman, Patrick, *L'Hygiène dans la République. La santé publique en France ou l'utopie contrariée 1870–1918* (Paris: Fayard, 1996).

Nagai, Nobuhito, *Les conseillers municipaux de Paris sous la Troisième République 1871–1914* (Paris: Publications de la Sorbonne [Université Paris I – Panthéon – Sorbonne], 2002).

Paul, Harry W., "Collecting Chardins: Charlotte and Henri de Rothschild," *The Rothschild Archive* ("Review of the year April 2004 to March 2005"), 21–6.

Pennington, T. H., "Listerism, its Decline and its Persistence: The Introduction of Aseptic Surgical Techniques in Three British Teaching Hospitals, 1890–99," *Medical History* 39 (1995): 35–60.

Picard, Jean-François, "American Patronage and French Medicine", http://picardp1. ivry.cnrs.fr/.

Pinell, Patrice, *The Fight Against Cancer: France 1890–1940* (London and New York: Routledge, 2002). Translated by David Madell.

-----, "La Ligue contre le cancer," in Annette Wieviorka (ed.), *Justin Godart. Un homme dans son siècle 1871–1956* (Paris: CNRS, 2004, 2005), 163–8.

-----, "Pédiatrie," in *Dictionnaire de la pensée médicale* (ed.), Dominique Lecourt (Paris: Presses Universitaires de France, 2004), 853–7.

Porter, Roy, *The Greatest Benefit to Mankind. A Medical History of Humanity* (New York: Norton, 1998).

Prost, Antoine, *Les anciens combatants et la société française 1914–1939* (3 vols, Paris: Presses de la Fondation nationale des sciences politiques, 1977).

-----, "Le désastre sanitaire du Chemin des Dames," in Nicolas Offenstadt (ed.), *Le Chemin des Dames. De l'événement à la mémoire* (Paris: Stock, 2004).

-----, "Le service de Santé militaire pendant la Première Guerre mondiale," in Annette Wieviorka (ed.), *Justin Godart. Un homme dans son siècle 1871–1956* (Paris: CNRS, 2004, 2005).

Quétel, Claude, *History of Syphilis* (Baltimore: Johns Hopkins University Press, 1992), 137. Translated by Judith Braddock and Brian Pike.

Ramsey, Matthew, *Professional and Popular Medicine in France 1770–1830. The Social World of Medical Practice* (Cambridge: Cambridge University Press, 1988).

Regaud, Jean, *Claudius Regaud (1870–1940). Pionnier de la cancérologie, Créateur de la Fondation Curie. Chronique de sa vie et son oeuvre* (Paris: Maloine, 1982).

Remy, Jean-Robert and Gabriel, *A Corps prisonniers, âmes libres. Berck.* (Lille: Mercure de Flandre, 1928; 2nd edn, Bresle, 1928).

Risse, Guenter B., *Mending Bodies, Saving Souls. A History of Hospitals* (New York and Oxford: Oxford University Press, 1999).

Roberts, Mary Louise, *Disruptive Acts. The New Woman in Fin-de-Siècle France* (Chicago: University of Chicago Press, 2002).

Rodrigue, Aron, *French Jews, Turkish Jews. The Alliance Israélite Universelle and the Politics of Jewish Schooling in Turkey, 1860–1925* (Bloomington, IN: Indiana University Press, 1990).

Rollet, Catherine, *Les enfants au XIXe siècle* (Paris: Hachette, 2001).

-----, and Morel, Marie-France, *Des bébés et des hommes. Tradition et modernité des soins aux tout-petits* (Paris: Albin Michel, 2000).

Rollin, Nicole, and others, *Les hôpitaux dans la guerre* (Paris: Le Cherche Midi, 2008).

Romains, Jules, *Knock* (Paris: Gallimard, 1924).

Schneider, Jean-Jacques, *Le Service de Santé de l'armée française. Verdun 1916* (Metz: Editions Serpenoise, 2007).

Schor, Ralph, *L'Antisémitisme en France pendant les années trente. Prélude à Vichy* (Bruxelles: Editions Complexe, 1992).

Schultheiss, Katrin, *Bodies and Souls. Politics and the Professionalization of Nursing in France 1880–1922* (Cambridge, Mass.: Harvard University Press, 2001).

Simon-Nahum, Perrine, "La République des Juifs," in Vincent Duclert and Christophe Prochasson (eds), *Dictionnaire critique de la République* (Paris: Flammarion, 2002), 371–7.

Sussman, George D., *Selling Mother's Milk – The Wet-Nursing Business in France, 1715–1914* (Urbana, IL: University of Illinois Press, 1982).

Bertrand Taithe, *Defeated Flesh. Welfare, Warfare and the Making of Modern France* (Manchester: Manchester University Press, 1999).

Teppe, Julien, *Les Histrions au miroir ou les morticioles tels qu'ils sont* (Paris: Editions de la Caravelle, 1931).

Thébaud, Françoise, *La femme au temps de la guerre de 14* (Paris: Stock, 1986, 1994).

Thomas, Jean-Paul, *La plume et le scapel. La médecine au prisme de la littérature* (Paris: Presses Universitaires de France, 2008).

Tikhonov, Natalia, "Migrations des étudiants et féminisation de quelques universités européennes à la recherche d'une convergence," in Harmut Rüdiger and Peter and Natalia Tikhonov (eds), *Universitäten als Brücken in Europa* (Frankfurt am Main: Peter Lang, 1993), 43–53.

Vergez-Chaignon, Bénédicte, "Le Médecin," in Jean-Pierrre Roux and Jean-François Sirinelli (eds), *La France d'un siècle à l'autre. Dictionnaire critique* (Paris: Hachette, 2000).

-----, *Le Monde des médecins au XXe siècle* (Bruxelles: Editions Complexe, 1996).

Walton, John, and others (eds), *The Oxford Medical Companion* (Oxford: Oxford University Press, 1994).

Weindling, Paul, "From Isolation to Therapy: Children's Hospitals and Diphtheria in Fin de Siècle Paris, London and Berlin," in Roger Cooter (ed.), *In the Name of the Child. Health and Welfare, 1880–1940*, (London and New York: Routledge, 1992).

Weisz, George, *Divide and Conquer. A Comparative History of Medical Specialization* (New York: Oxford University Press, 2006).

-----, *The Emergence of Modern Universities in France, 1863–1914* (Princeton: Princeton University Press, 1983).

-----, "Reform and Conflict in French Medical Education," in Robert Fox and George Weisz (eds), *The Organization of Science and Technology in France 1800–1914* (Cambridge: Cambridge University Press, 1980), 61–94.

Werblowsky, R. J., and Wigoder, Geoffrey (eds in chief), *The Oxford Dictionary of the Jewish Religion* (New York: Oxford University Press, 1997).

Whitton, David, *Stage Directors in Modern France* (Manchester: Manchester University Press, 1987).

Wieviorka, Annette (ed.), *Justin Godart. Un homme dans son siècle 1871–1956* (Paris: CNRS, 2004, 2005).

Winckler, Martin, *C'est grave, docteur? Ce que disent les patients, ce qu'entendent les médecins* (Paris: Editions de la Martinière, 2002).

Winter, Jay, "P vs C. The Still Burning Anger when the French Talk of the First World War," *Times Literary Supplement* (16 June 2006), 3–4.

Yver, Colette, *Princesses de science* (Paris: Calmann-Lévy, 1907).

-----, *Les Cervelines* (Paris: F. Juven, 1908).

-----, *Les Dames du Palais* (Paris: Calmann Lévy, 1920).

-----, *Femmes d'aujourd'hui; enqûete sur les nouvelles carrières féminines* (Paris: Calmann Lévy, 1929).

Index

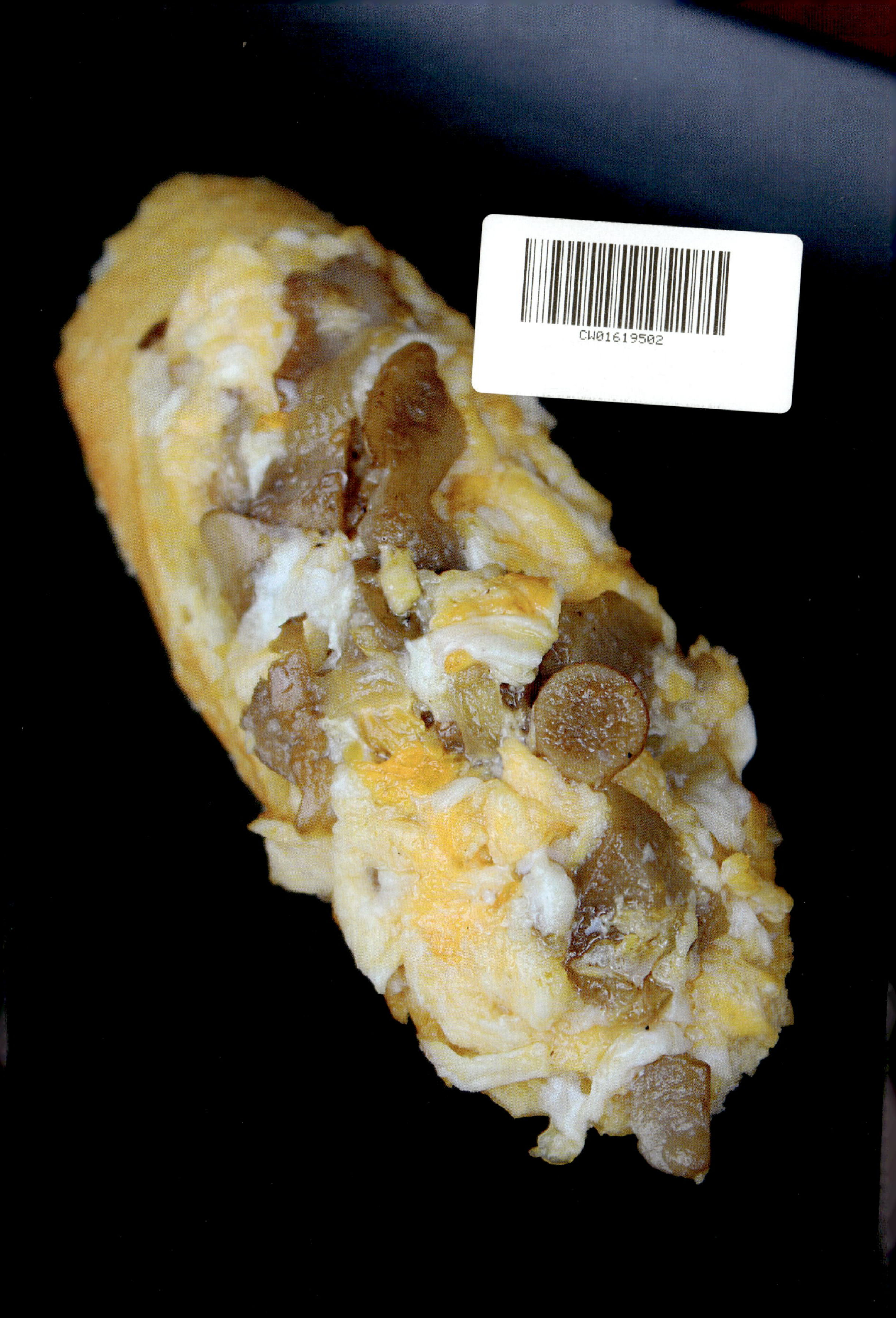

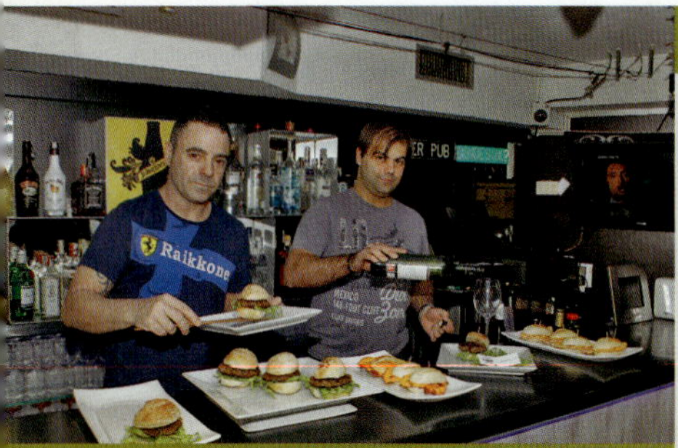

Maria Lezo, 1
ERRENTERIA
943 51 61 04
facebook.com/aker.errenteria

AKER

Los errenteriarras **Mendeku y Jesús** llevan desde 1992 al cargo de este local que, a pesar de ofrecer pintxos de día y retransmisiones de partidos por las tardes, sigue siendo una cita ineludible las noches de los fines de semana por su buen ambiente, su música actual y variada, y su **atractiva carta de Gin-tonics** con más de 15 ginebras premium.
Ahora, y **tras su remodelación total, el Aker se reinventa** y amplía su oferta hostelera abriendo todos los días desde las 8:00 de la mañana, y ofreciendo un sinfín de tostas, hojaldres, encurtidos e ibéricos, regados por excelentes caldos y aperitivos.
Es de destacar su **trío de pintxo-potes**, pues en este bar se ofrecen **los jueves, los viernes y los sábados, de 7 de la tarde hasta fin de existencias**. Estos tres días, mientras dura el pintxo-pote, podremos elegir entre 3 ó 4 pintxos de esta atractiva barra.

Otros pintxos:

- *Crêpe de chipirón en su tinta*
- *Croquetas de foie*
- *Pulguitas variadas (tortillas, etc...)*
- *Mini fajita mexicana*
- *Falso paté de manzana y nuez*
- *Ensaladilla de primavera*
- *Crêpe de puerros y gambas*
- *Taco de vaca con cebolla caramelizada y foie*

Raciones:

- *Patatas bravas y Patatas ali-oli*

Milhojas de ventresca sobre cama de verduritas y antxoas del Cantábrico

Ingredientes:

Masa quebrada de hojaldre
3 láminas de ventresca
2 antxoas del Cantábrico
1 boquerón
Mayonesa
Perejil

· Para el pisto:
Calabacín
Cebolla
Pimiento verde
Pimiento rojo
Tomate natural
Aceite de oliva

Elaboración:

Para el pisto: Picamos finamente el calabacín con su piel, la cebolla, el pimiento verde, y el pimiento rojo y los ponemos a pochar en una sartén con aceite de oliva a fuego muy suave. Mientras se va haciendo, pelamos el tomate y lo picamos en daditos. Cuando el resto de las verduras están medio pochadas, añadimos los daditos de tomate y seguimos rehogando hasta que el conjunto esté bien blandito. Salpimentamos y reservamos.

Final y presentación: Abrimos por la mitad la pasta quebrada, como si de un bocata se tratara, y la rellenamos, primeramente con una cucharada generosa de pisto. Sobre el pisto colocamos 3 láminas de ventresca. Sobre ellas, las dos antxoas del Cantábrico y el boquerón. Cerramos el milhojas y lo coronamos con un puntito de mayonesa antes de espolvorearlo con perejil fresco recién picado.

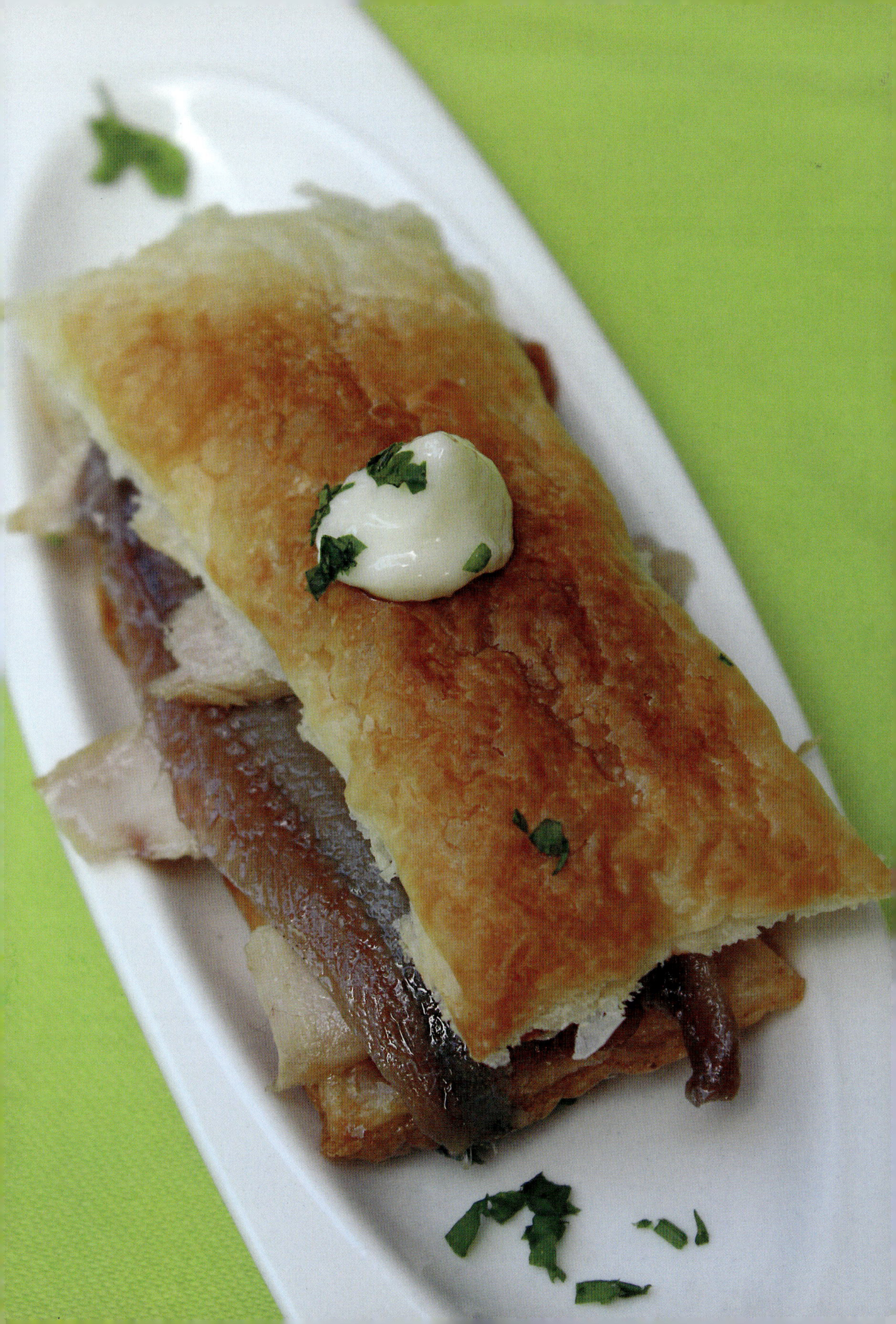

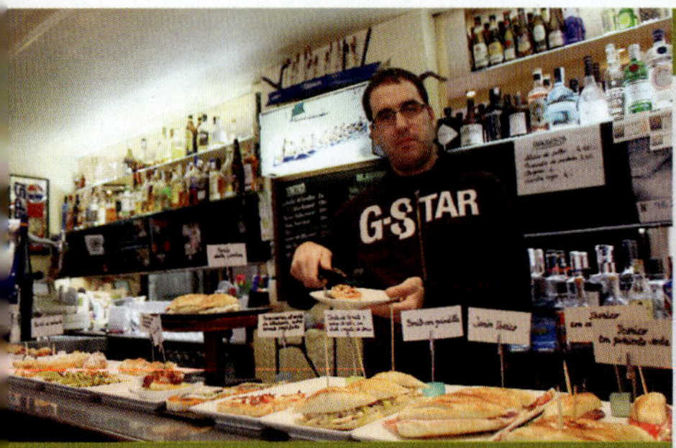

ALAI

Ipar kalea, 8
ZARAUTZ
943 01 05 46

Tras pasar una temporada al frente del bar Zazpi, de Kale Nagusia, **Helena Pedros e Iñigo Intxauspe** se hicieron con este bar, que llevaba abierto 20 años y en el que han cumplido ellos otras dos décadas en enero de 2014. Alai es un bar de toda la vida con terraza en Musika Plaza que abre todos los días a las 9 de la mañana para ofrecer **Desayunos, Pintxos, Platos combinados, Sandwiches, Hamburguesas de ternera y de pollo, Raciones y Cazuelitas** como Morros en salsa de txakoli, Pimientos rellenos de kabratxo, Alcachofas con jamón, Champiñones en salsa, Callos... Alai cuenta también con una amplia selección de vinos, aunque **en lo que más destaca es en su variedad de Gin-Tonics**, con más de 50 ginebras premium y alrededor de una docena de tónicas diferentes. También cuenta con una carta de **Vermouths premium** así como una **carta de cafés especiales.**

Otros pintxos:

- *Champiñones en salsa*
- *Pimiento relleno*
- *Morro*
- *Revuelto de champiñones*
- *Croquetas*
- *Revuelto de setas*

Raciones:

- *Pulpo a feira*
- *Pimientos del Padrón*
- *Embutidos ibéricos*

Miniatura de codorniz al whisky con patatas

Ingredientes:

Pechuga de codorniz
Huevo de codorniz
Patata
Sal
Aceite de oliva

• Para la salsa de whisky:
Aceite de oliva
Ajo
Whisky
Maizena
Caldo de carne

Elaboración:

Para la salsa de whisky: Partimos un diente de ajo en tres trocitos y lo ponemos a dorar. Cuando coja color lo retiramos y añadimos un chorro generoso de whisky. Lo dejamos reducir. Mientras, en una taza, diluimos una cucharada de maizena en caldo de carne, lo mezclamos bien y lo añadimos al whisky. Dejamos que hierva todo junto durante unos 5 minutos y lo retiramos del fuego, sin triturarlo.

Hacemos la pechuga y el huevo de codorniz a la plancha y elaboramos unas patatas fritas caseras delgaditas.

Final y presentación: Disponemos en un plato la pechuga y el huevo de codorniz junto a las patatas fritas y regamos el conjunto con la salsa de whisky.

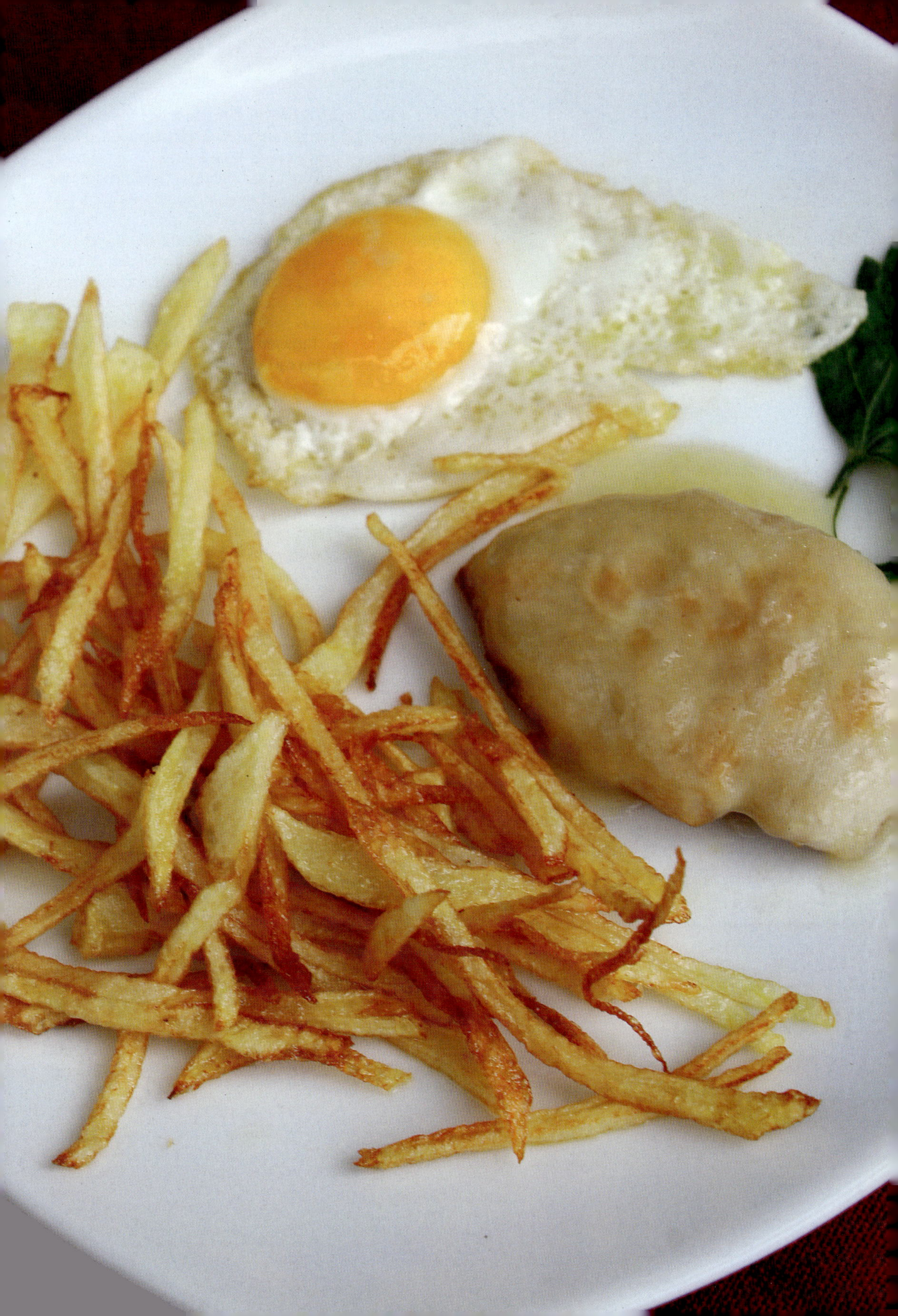

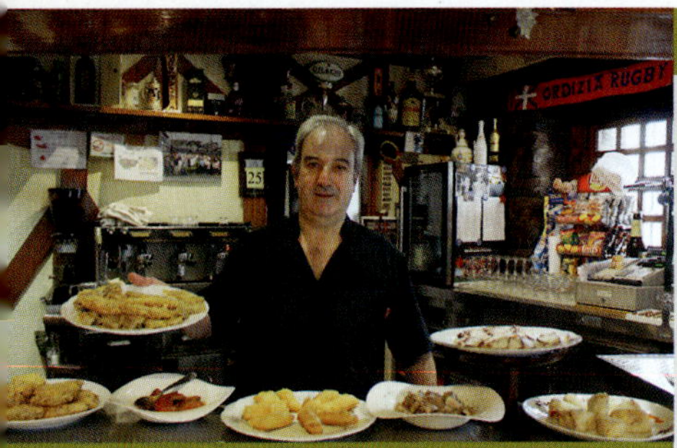

Urdaneta, 27
ORDIZIA
943 88 00 23
www.aldasorotaberna.com

ALDASORO

Cuesta creer que **Juan José Martínez de Rituerto Arregi** no sea un cocinero experimentado, pero así son las cosas. Juanjo se había dedicado toda la vida al mundo de la empresa hasta que hacia 2010 cambió de registro y se hizo con este veterano local que supera ampliamente los 70 años de antigüedad. Una vez hecho a su nuevo hábitat, apañándose en su pequeña cocina y con la inestimable ayuda y la simpatía en sala de **Mª Jose**, su mujer, este lazkaotarra ha convertido este bar de barrio en una de las referencias culinarias de la capital gastronómica del Goierri. **Juan José ofrece una cocina casera que juega con el mercado y el producto, y ha recuperado los platos de casquería casera que se habían perdido con el tiempo**, tanto los más tradicionales como las versiones más actuales de los mismos. Recientemente ha sido renovado el comedor, convirtiéndose en una sala mucho más acogedora.

Otros pintxos:

- *Manitas rebozadas*
- *Morros rebozados o en salsa*
- *Oreja salteada con jamón y pimiento rojo*
- *Bacalao a la plancha, rebozado o con tomate*
- *Morcilla de Ordizia o Mondeju*
- *Pimientos rellenos de bacalao*
- *Tortilla de patata*
- *Boquerones caseros*
- *Carrilleras de rape*
- *Vertical (brocheta de champiñón y gamba)*

Milhoja de patata confitada, mermelada de piquillo y mollejas de cordero

Ingredientes:

Mollejas de cordero
Agua
Vinagre
Patata
Cebolla
Aceite de oliva

- **Para la mermelada de piquillo:**

1 lata de pimientos del piquillo
Azúcar moreno

- **Para decorar:**

Crema de piquillos
Aceite de perejil

Elaboración:

Para las mollejas: Limpiamos de telilla y grasa las mollejas y las dejamos 24 horas en la nevera con agua y un poquito de vinagre. Al día siguiente, quitamos el agua y las ponemos en una cazuela con agua fría hasta que ésta empiece a hervir. Quitamos la espuma y las pasamos por el grifo. (A este proceso se le llama *blanquear*). Antes de preparar el pintxo, las salteamos ligeramente.

Para la patata y la cebolla confitada: Cortamos la cebolla en Juliana y la patata en rodajas y las confitamos en aceite de oliva a 50-60° por espacio de una hora aproximadamente.

Para la mermelada de piquillo: Quitamos las pepitas a los piquillos y los ponemos a pochar con el propio jugo de su lata. Cuando llevan media hora, añadimos una cucharada de azúcar moreno y dejamos que reduzca un poco. Seguidamente, los aplastamos con un tenedor.

Final y presentación: Hacemos el milhojas empezando con una capa de patata, una de cebolla, otra de patata, otra de mermelada, y coronamos con las mollejas salteadas. Decoramos con un poco de crema de piquillos y aceite de perejil.

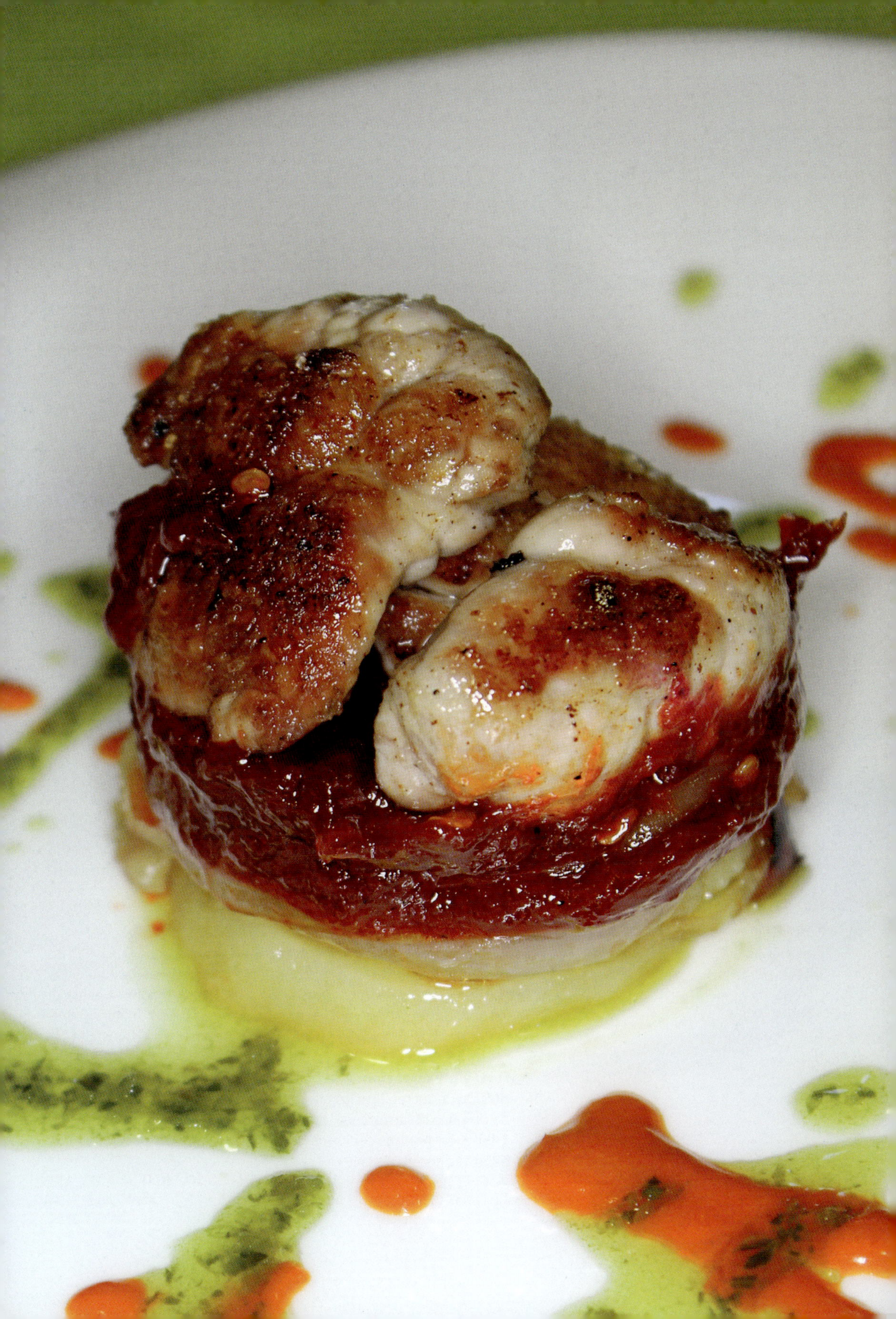

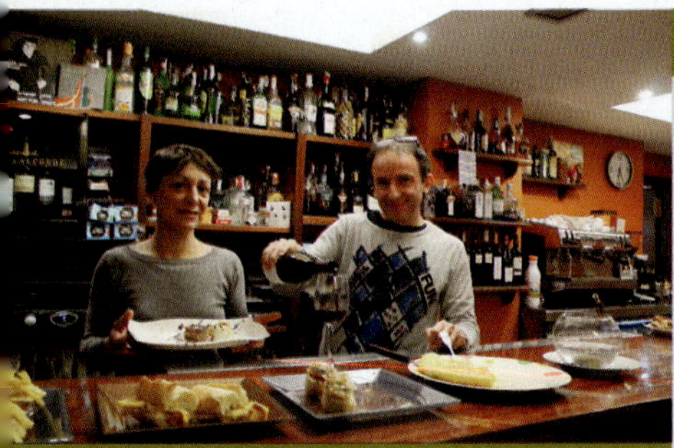

ALKORTA

El Alkorta es un bar de sabor dulce. Por una parte, antes de ser bar, hace ya muchos años, este local dirigido por **Ana Etxabe y Rikardo Zengotita** albergó a la pastelería Alkorta. Por otra parte, los dulces se cuidan especialmente en este bar que ya desde las 8 de la mañana ofrece repostería casera y dónde entre sus postres destacan las **tartas caseras** (de manzana, de frambuesa, de pera...), así como la exquisita Pantxineta elaborada por Ana, siguiendo la receta de su padre, Antxon, quien llevó en su tiempo la Pastelería Nikolenea en Zumaia. Eso sí, los amantes del salado disfrutarán igualmente con la cocina casera del Alkorta, su **menú diario**, sus especialidades como Ensalada de frutos de mar, Bacalao frito, Secreto ibérico, Chuletillas de cordero... así como sus pintxos, sus **platos combinados**, sus ricas **hamburguesas caseras servidas con pan de verdad** (de buey, de pollo, vegetal...) y sus originales **pizzas artesanas.**

Erdi Kale 7
ZESTOA
943 14 86 06

Otros pintxos:

- *Tortilla de patata*
- *Lengua rebozada*
- *Bacalao con cebolla*
- *Pimiento verde con antxoa*
- *Sardinas del Cantábrico sobre tostada*
- *"Inconprendido"*
- *Pulpo a la gallega*

Raciones:

- *Calamares caseros*
- *Tempura de langostino con crujiente de amapola*

Cochinillo deshuesado con arroz cuatro delicias

Ingredientes:

Cochinillo
Cuerno de croissant
Escamas de sal
Reducción de Módena

- **Para el arroz:**

Arroz
Guisantes
Zanahoria
Tortilla
Gamba

Elaboración:

Asamos el cochinillo a la manera tradicional, aplicando el tiempo adecuado a la potencia del horno.

Dejamos enfriar el cochinillo y lo deshuesamos. Vamos encajando los trozos deshuesados en una fuente de horno y finalmente cubrimos la carne con la piel del cochinillo. Reservamos en la nevera para que quede una masa compacta.

Para el arroz: Elaboramos una tortilla francesa. La troceamos en pedacitos pequeños y la reservamos. Picamos la zanahoria, y las gambas y las salteamos junto a los guisantes. Añadimos el arroz, lo rehogamos un rato y adjuntamos el agua. Dejamos hervir alrededor de 16 minutos y lo retiramos del fuego.

Final y presentación: A la hora de servir el pintxo, cortamos una porción de cochinillo y lo calentamos en el horno. Lo acompañamos de un poco de arroz y varias rodajas de cuerno de croissant. Finalmente, decoramos con unos hilos de reducción de Módena y unas escamas de sal.

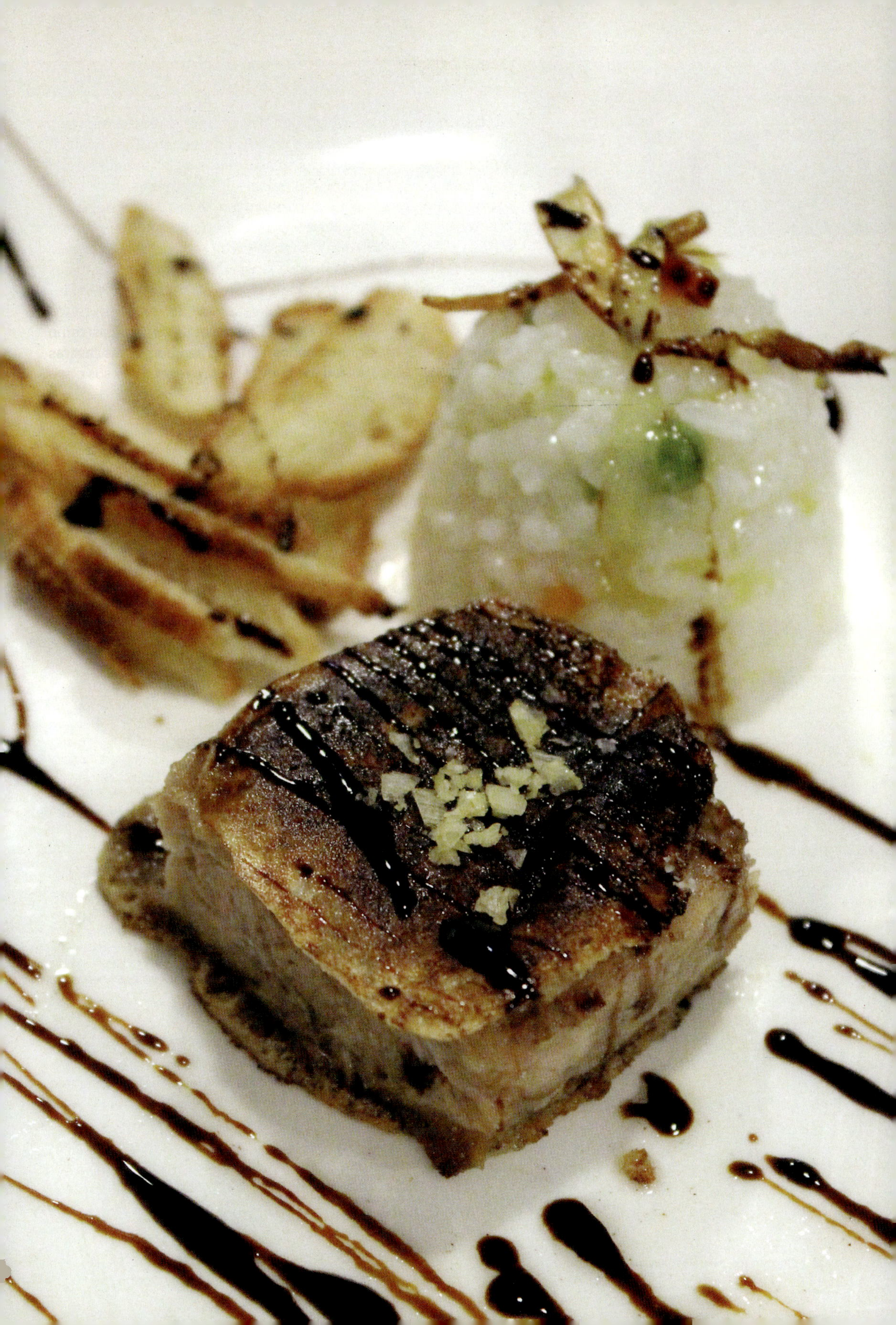

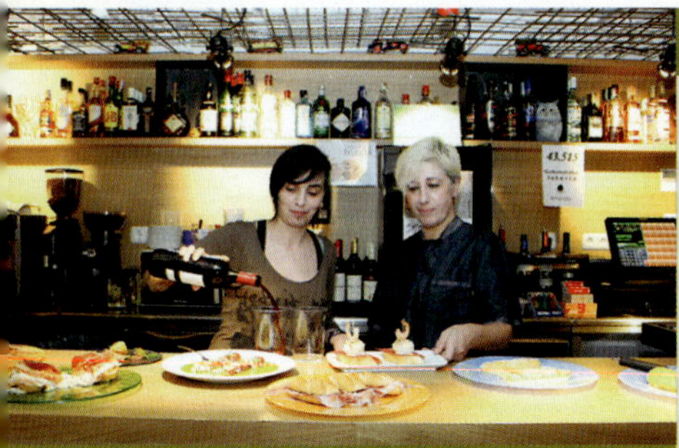

AMAIUR

Beotibar, 5
TOLOSA
659 24 54 69

El local que durante décadas albergó al mítico Zarauztarra se ha dotado de nueva y dinámica vida desde que el 15 de julio de 2014 fuera reinaugurado por **Maite Campos y su hija Erika Morales** que además de reformarlo de arriba a abajo y dotarlo de una apariencia actual y elegante, **han renovado por completo su oferta gastronómica**. Como buena gallega, Maite domina a la perfección el pulpo, que se sirve a la gallega o a la vinagreta, así como cualquier producto del mar, principalmente **los txipirones, que se sirven de diferentes maneras, todas ellas con gran éxito**. Han cobrado gran fama las hermosas **Hamburguesas, de 180 gramos**, elaboradas con carne adquirida a Patxi Otxua y servidas con pan hecho al momento. Asimismo, las **ensaladas** gozan de una gran aceptación, principalmente la de foie. **Los sandwiches, los bokatas, las pastas y los arroces** completan la oferta de este local que abre todos los días a partir de las 10 de la mañana, salvo martes.

Otros pintxos:

- *Espárrago con jamón y queso y crema de puerro*
- *Berenjena con bacon, queso y crema de jamón y hongo*
- *Tomate relleno de ensaladilla*
- *Pintxo moruno*
- *Tortillas variadas*
- *Pulpo a la vinagreta*
- *Pulpo a la gallega*

Raciones:

- *Patatas con tres salsas (brava, rosa, ali-oli)*
- *Txipirones a la plancha*

Txipirón relleno

Ingredientes:

1 txipirón limpio ó 2 (según tamaño)
Cebolla
Puerro
Pimiento rojo
Pimiento verde
Jamón ibérico
Harina
Huevo
sal
Pimienta
Aceite de oliva
Aceite de girasol
Tomate natural
Perlas de Caviaroli

Elaboración:

Picamos muy finamente la cebolla, el puerro, el pimiento rojo y el pimiento verde, y los pochamos en una sartén hasta que queden muy blanditos. Añadimos sal y un poco de pimienta.

Cuando las verduras están en su punto, añadimos el jamón ibérico muy picado y las patitas del txipirón. Dejamos hacerse todo unos dos minutos más, para que los dos últimos ingredientes incorporados suelten su jugo.

Ponemos todo en una manga pastelera, y rellenamos el txipirón en frío.

Rebozamos el txipirón relleno en harina y huevo y lo freímos en aceite de girasol muy caliente. Lo freímos muy poco tiempo, sin llegar a minuto y medio, ya que de freírlo demasiado, hay riesgo de que se seque o se endurezca en exceso.

Final y presentación: Servimos el txipirón en un platillo, acompañado de unas cucharadas de tomate natural, unas perlas de Caviaroli y un chorrito de aceite de oliva.

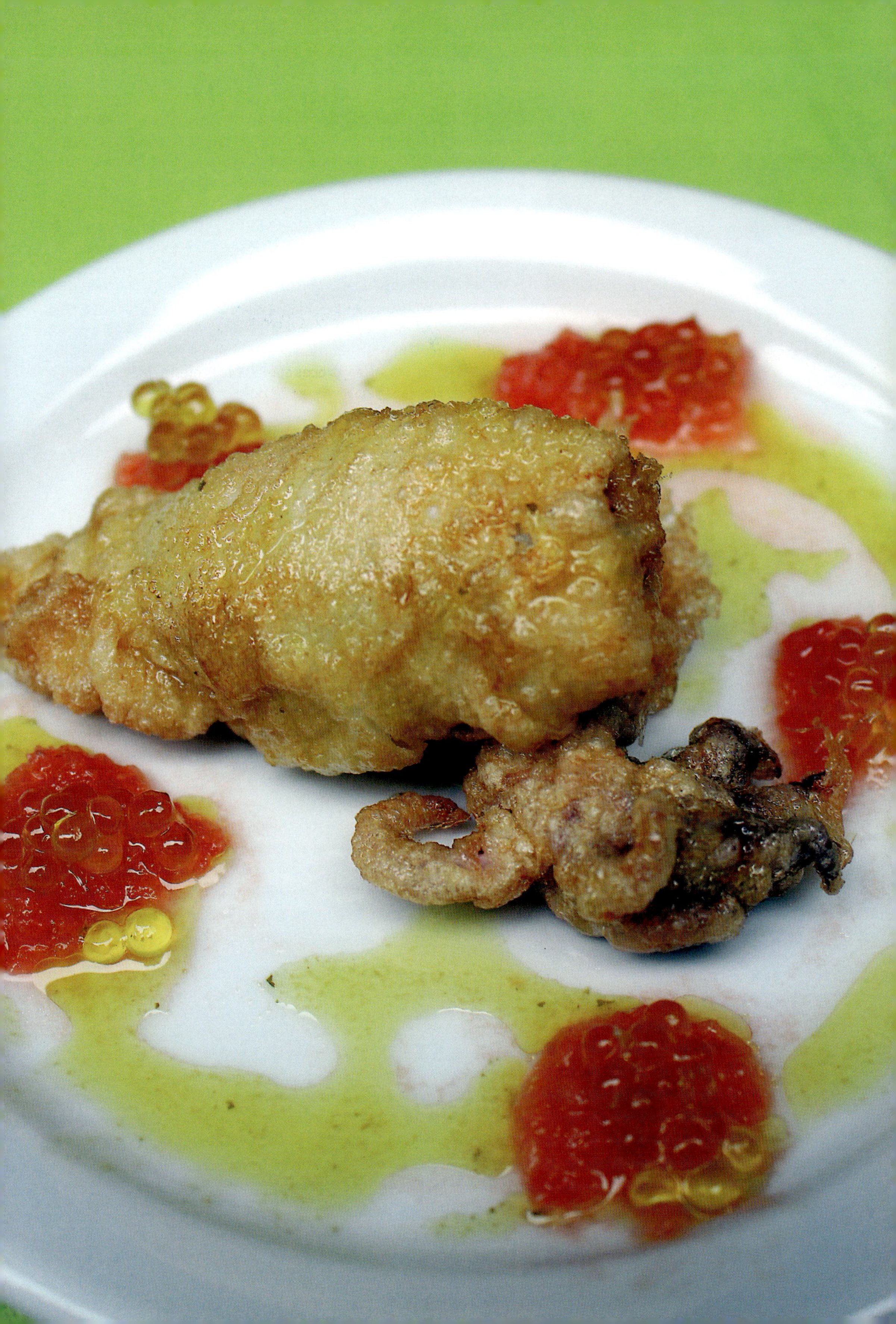

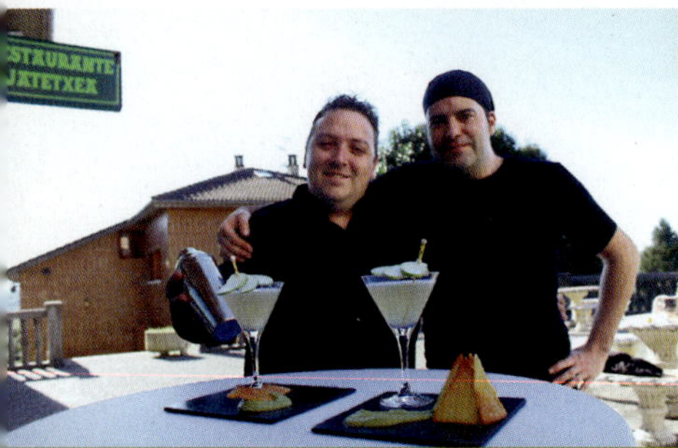

AMETZAGAÑA

Situado en un entorno natural, con entrada directa al Parque Ametzagaina, y a tan sólo 5 minutos del centro de Donostia, el Complejo Ametzagaña ofrece **dos espacios muy diferenciados**: Por una parte, el restaurante, con un gran **salón de banquetes**, ideal para la celebración de eventos, con una capacidad hasta 330 personas, en el que se ofrece un **Menú de fin de semana**. Por otra parte, el **Coffee & Lounge Bar**, al que puede acudirse todo el día para tomar un café, una infusión o un buen gin tonic, y donde pueden saborearse **todo tipo de raciones, bocadillos o hamburguesas a partir de las 7 de la tarde**. Los viernes, además, puede disfrutarse de una cena ligera acompañada de monólogos. El Complejo Ametzagaña es el lugar ideal para acudir en familia pues, además de estar rodeado de zonas verdes, cuenta con parque de juegos y un amplio aparcamiento. Este complejo cuenta además con una **coqueta Pensión de 40 habitaciones** con precios que oscilan entre los 40 y los 60 euros por habitación doble.

C° de Uba, 61 (Intxaurrondo)
DONOSTIA
943 45 63 99
www.ametzagana.com

Otros pintxos:

- *Variedad de tortillas rellenas*
- *Minis de ibéricos*
- *Crujiente de langostino*
- *Txapela de champiñón con hongos*
- *Minicroquetas variadas*
- *Tosta con crema de patata y triguero con pulpo y aceite de pimentón dulce*

Raciones:
- *Alitas de pollo a la barbacoa*
- *Buñuelos de bacalao*

Nachos de Idiazábal, guacamole de guindillas de Ibarra y Margarita de manzana

Ingredientes:

• Para los nachos:
300 g de queso Idiazabal

• Para el guacamole:
3 aguacates maduros
200 g de guindilla fresca de Ibarra
3 txalotas
3 limones verdes o Limas
Aceite
Sal

• Para el margarita de manzana:
3 Cl tequila Reposado
3 Cl licor de manzana Blanca de Navarra
6 Cl mosto de manzana
1 manzana verde
Coctelera
Cubitos de hielo
Pizarra para emplatar
Palillos
Copa de cóctel

Elaboración:

Para los nachos: Cortamos el queso Idiazabal en lonchas de 4 mm de grosor y a su vez los cortamos con forma triangular. En una sartén antiadherente a fuego muy fuerte colocamos los triángulos de queso y los dejamos que se doren durante minuto y medio. Acto seguido llevamos la sartén a una fuente con agua y hielo para poderlo separar con facilidad. Reservamos.

Para el guacamole: Lavamos las guindillas y las secamos bien. Las ponemos en un sauté a fuego suave con abundante aceite. Cuando vemos que están tiernas las despepitamos, hacemos con ellas un puré, y reservamos. Pelamos las txalotas y las picamos en brounoise. Pelamos los aguacates y hacemos un puré al cual añadiremos la brounoise de txalotas, el puré de guindillas, el zumo de limón y una pizca de sal.

Para el margarita de manzana: En la coctelera introduciremos el tequila, el licor de manzana Blanca de Navarra y el mosto, y exprimiremos un limón verde o lima. Completamos con hielo, cerramos la coctelera y agitamos bien, hasta notar la coctelera bien fría. Abrimos la coctelera y vertemos nuestro cóctel en la copa. Para decorar, cortaremos finamente 3 rodajas de manzana verde, las uniremos con un palillo largo y las pondremos sobre la copa.

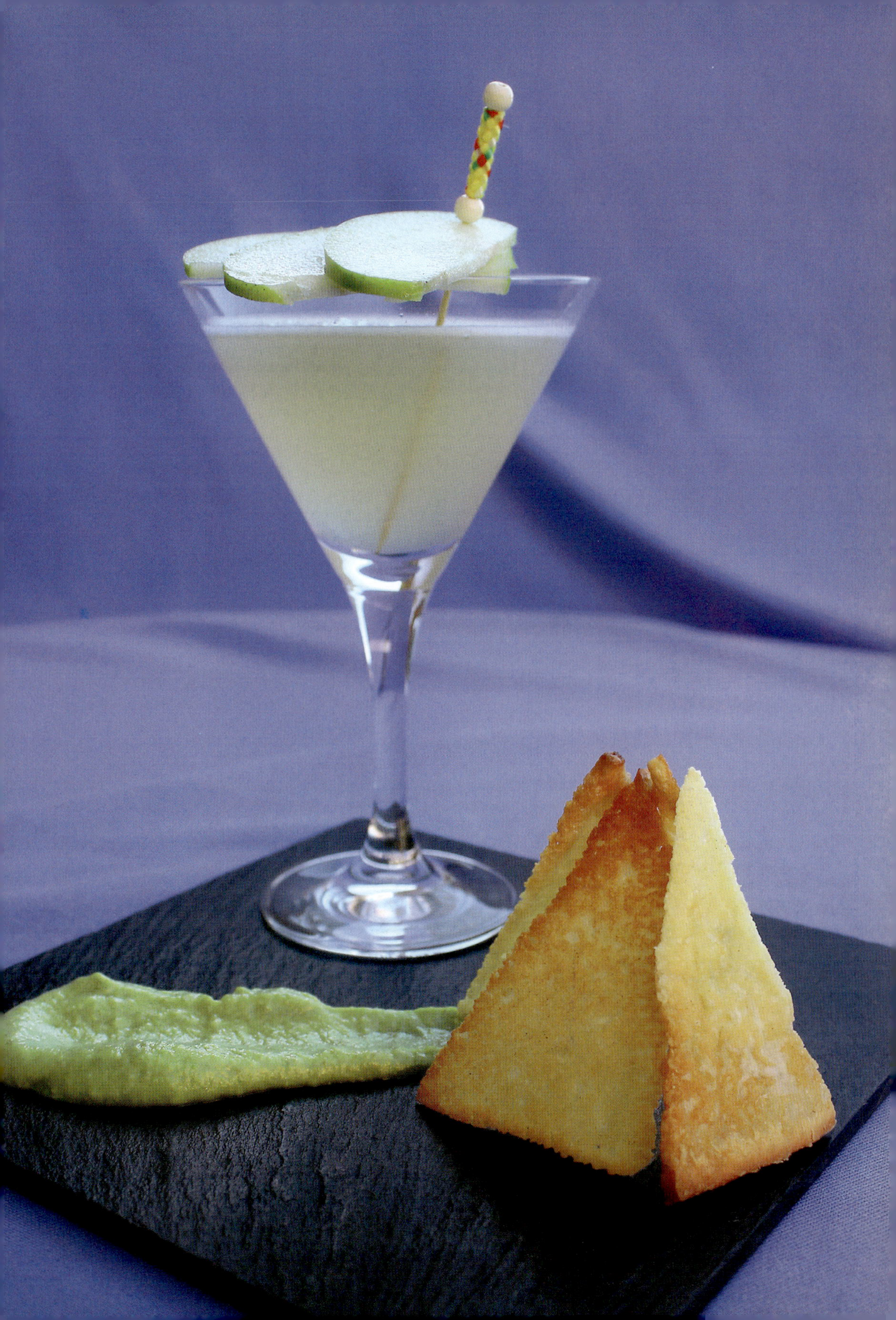

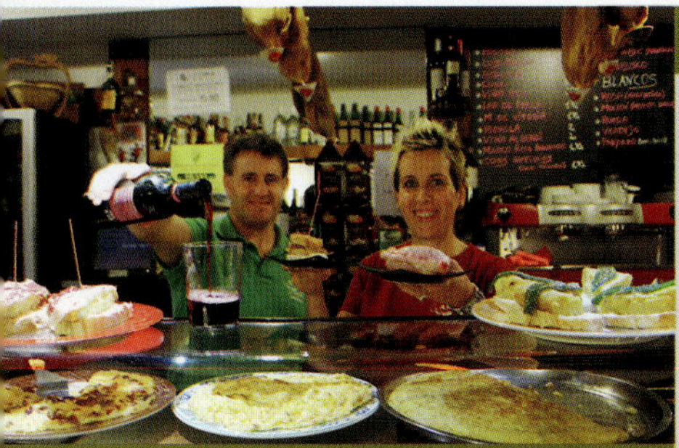

Ipeñarrieta, 18
URRETXU
943 72 58 87

APAIN

Si algo no se le puede negar a **Margari Arruti,** es su capacidad para ofrecer continuamente nuevas opciones a la clientela en este local que ha mejorado de manera espectacular desde que se hizo con él allá por 2006 y en el que cuenta a día de hoy con la impagable ayuda de **Axier Zubillaga**. Por una parte, la oferta de barra cuenta con una **gran oferta de pintxos y cazuelitas** como las solicitadas Manitas de cerdo albardadas o los exquisitos Caracoles en salsa de tomate y piquillos. Otra original propuesta es su **gran variedad de ensaladas** (cerca de diez diferentes) con un precio realmente ajustado y un tamaño espectacular, por lo que se convierte en una opción ideal para compartir. Por otra parte, Apain destaca por su excelente **menú del día, con más de 30 platos a elegir**, su menú fin de semana y el **Menú especial Apain para dos personas**, un auténtico festín. Apain ofrece, además, **dos pintxo-potes**, los viernes por la tarde y los domingos por la mañana.

Otros pintxos:

- *Tortilla de patata XXL (32 huevos)*
- *Oreja de cerdo rebozada*
- *Manitas de cerdo rebozadas*
- *Callos*
- *Lengua rebozada*
- *Foie a la plancha con cebolla o jamón*
- *Caracoles (en temporada)*
- *Albóndigas caseras*
- *Bacalao en salsa verde*
- *Alitas de pollo adobadas*

Criadillas rebozadas

Ingredientes:

Criadillas
Cebolla
Harina
Huevo
Pan rallado
Sal
Pan
Aceite de oliva

Elaboración:

Con la ayuda de un cuchillo afilado y de nuestras manos, quitaremos la película exterior de la criadilla.

Cortamos la criadilla en lonchas delgaditas, de 5 ó 6 milímetros de grosor aproximadamente.

Pasamos las rodajas de criadilla por harina, huevo y pan rallado y las freímos en aceite de oliva hasta que adquieran un agradable color dorado.

Cortamos la cebolla en Juliana y la freímos en aceite de oliva a fuego bajo hasta que se caramelice

Final y presentación: Sobre una rodaja de pan casero colocamos una rodaja de criadilla rebozada, una capa de cebolla caramelizada y una segunda rodaja de criadilla, ensartando todo el conjunto con un palillo de brocheta.

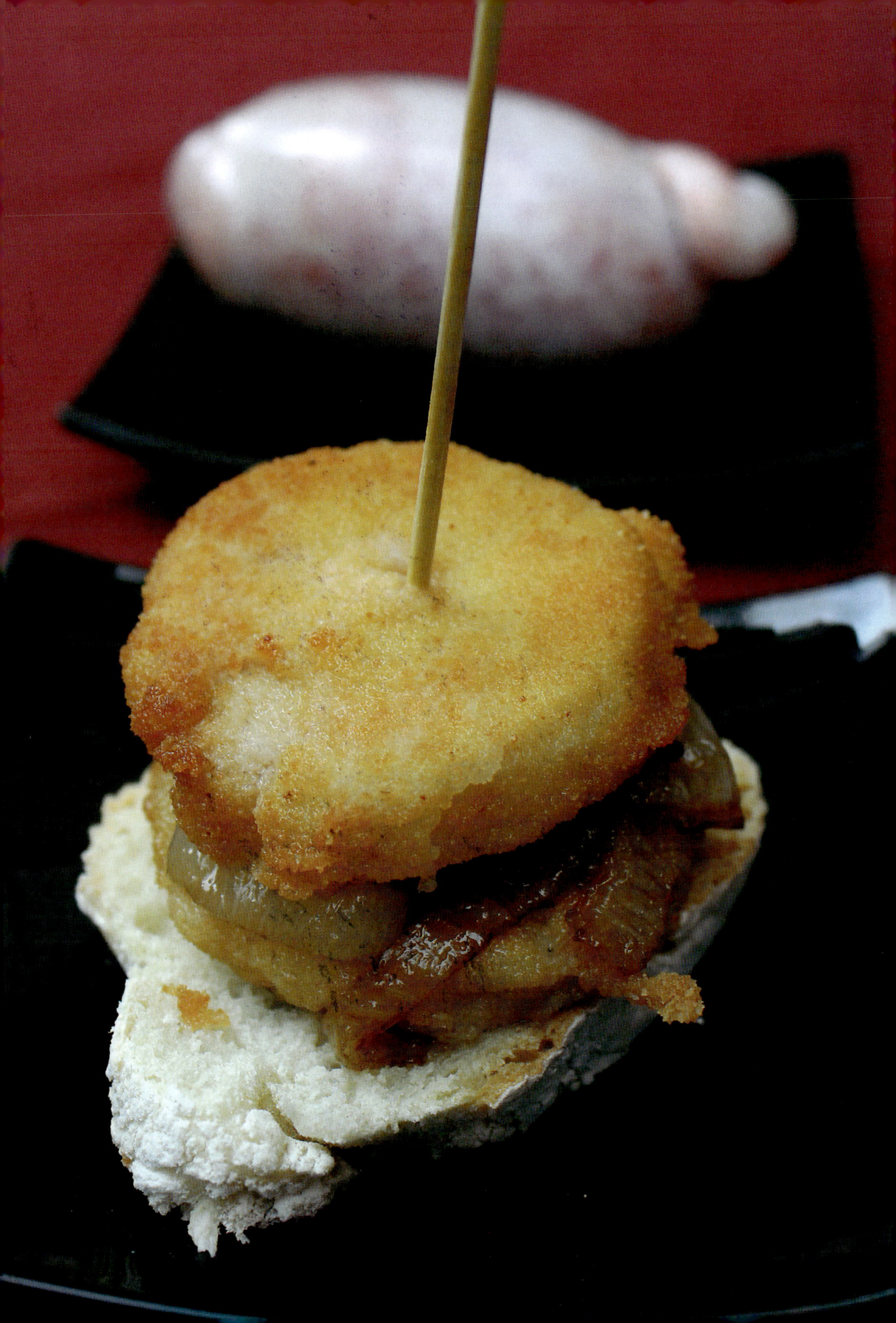

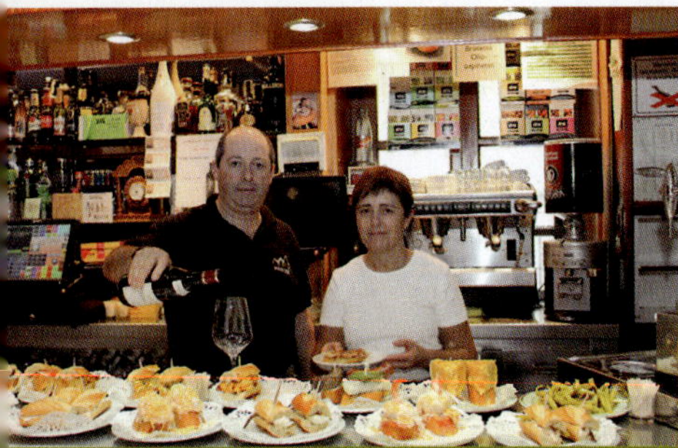

ARALAR

Zapa kalea, 8
HERNANI
943 33 15 06

Los hermanos Tolosa, Arantxa, Mikel y Miren, llevan desde 1982 al cargo de este céntrico bar, antes conocido como Baldo y al que los actuales propietarios rebautizaron en homenaje a su padre, natural de Azkarate. En cualquier caso, **la de los Tolosa es una vida dedicada a la hostelería.** Sus padres regentaron en su día el Joxe Mari en el barrio Lizeaga y ellos ya se habían estrenado llevando anteriormente el Americano de Kardaberaz. Aralar abre todos los días a las 10:30 de la mañana y cuenta con **una vistosa barra de pintxos en la que no sabremos qué elegir**, además de una amplia variedad de **ensaladas, sandwiches, bocadillos, hamburguesas, platos combinados y raciones** entre las que sobresalen los Txipirones frescos, simplemente pasados por harina, que gozan de gran éxito, al igual que las croquetas caseras. También tiene gran éxito el **campeonato de mus** que se juega en el Aralar todos los años entre abril y junio, una tradición a conservar.

Otros pintxos:

- *Croquetas caseras (De jamón, hongos, espinaca, gamba, queso y nueces, bacalao...)*
- *Tortilla de patata*
- *Tortilla de bacalao*
- *Champis*
- *Bacalao frito*
- *Chorizo cocido*
- *Morcilla*
- *Carrilleras en salsa de Oporto*
- *Foie a la plancha con manzana*

Brocheta de gambas y bacon

Ingredientes:

4 gambas
4 trozos de bacon
Pan

- **Para el aceite de ajo:**
Aceite de oliva virgen extra
Ajos

- **Para el aceite de perejil:**
Aceite de oliva virgen extra
Perejil

Elaboración:

Para el aceite de ajo: En una cazuela o cazo colocamos aceite de oliva y varios dientes de ajo pelados, la proporción en función a nuestros gustos o a la intensidad que le queramos dar. Llevamos a ebullición, pero sin dejar que hierva el aceite y se doren los ajos, bajamos a fuego lento y dejamos que se "cuezan" los ajos en el aceite durante 10-15 minutos. Dejamos enfriar el aceite y ya estará listo para ser utilizado.

Para el aceite de perejil: Picamos muy finamente perejil fresco y lo ponemos a macerar con aceite de oliva durante varias horas. Pasamos la batidora y lo conservamos en un recipiente hermético.

Insertamos en un palito de brocheta, intercalados, cuatro trozos de bacon y cuatro gambas peladas. Ponemos la plancha bien caliente y hacemos la brocheta por ambos lados con aceite de ajo.

Final y presentación: Sobre una rebanada de pan colocamos la brocheta recién hecha y la rociamos con aceite de perejil.

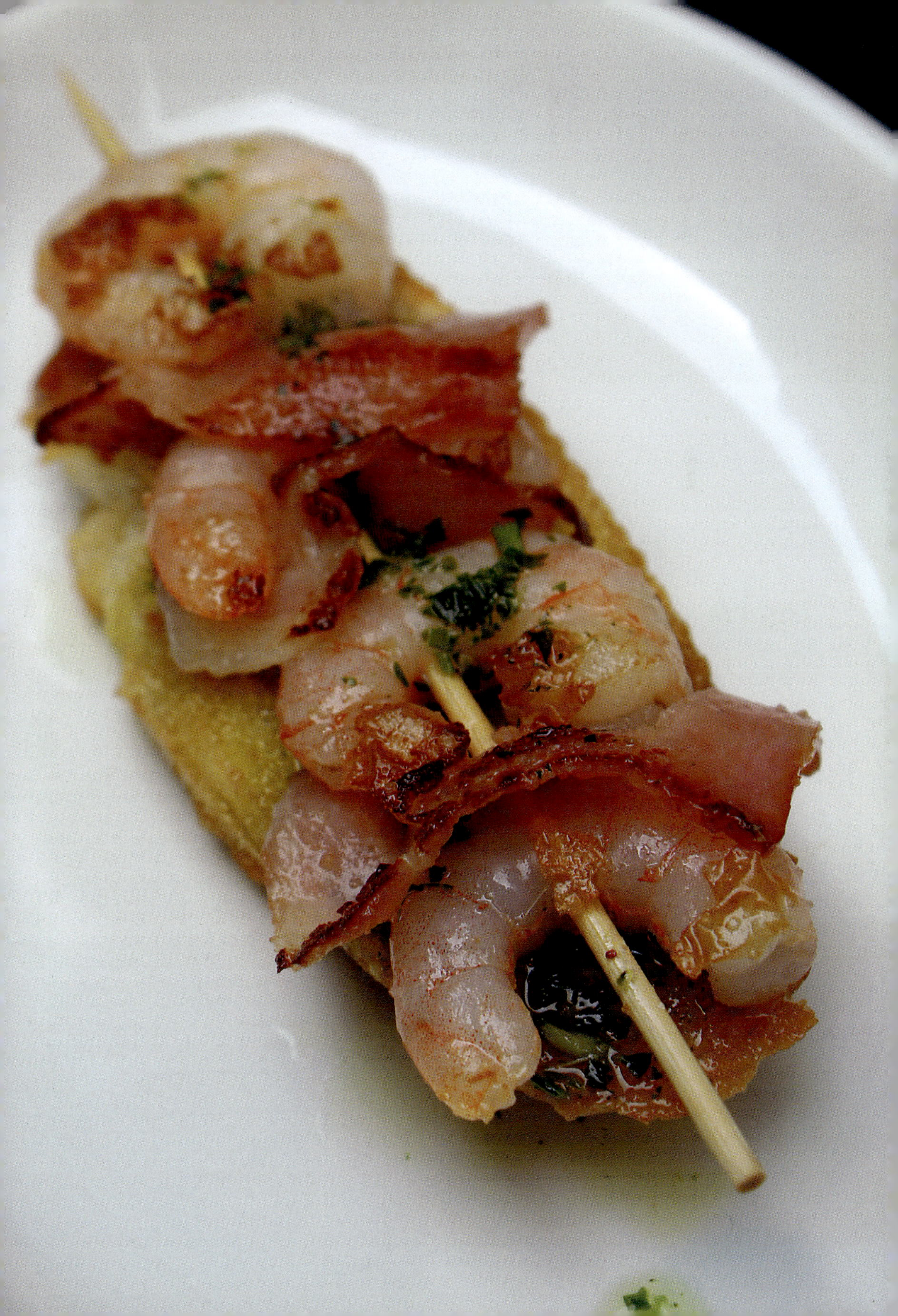

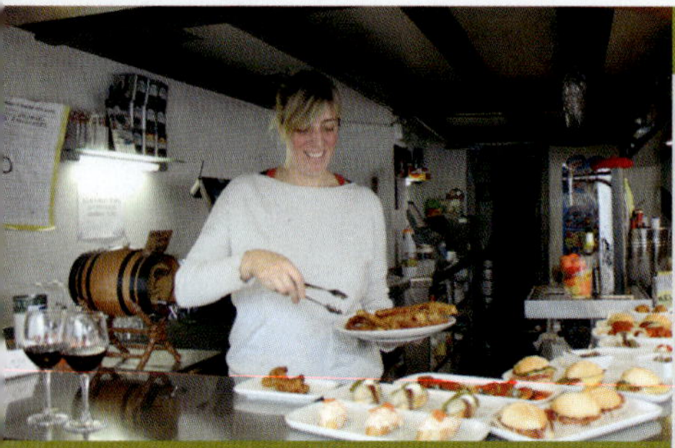

ARKUPE

Tras la jubilación de sus antiguos propietarios, que llevaban unos 20 años encargándose de él, la lasartearra **Jenni García**, que cuenta con más de 15 años de experiencia en hostelería, se hizo con este céntrico y veterano bar en abril de 2012. Jenni ha mantenido algunas de las especialidades del local, como los **Torreznos**, que tuvo que conservarlos "por votación popular", y ha añadido algunos nuevos productos como los Huevos rotos con jamón ibérico o las Tostas, destacando la de Jijas que se muestra a continuación y la que más éxito tiene: la Tosta de ibérico, txanpis y salsa de Roquefort. Arkupe abre todos los días a las 8:30 de la mañana y cuenta con una vistosa barra de pintxos desde primera hora. Por la tarde, los pintxos se ofrecen a precio popular, y los jueves a partir de las 7 hay pintxo-pote. Destacan también en Arkupe su terraza, su vermouth casero de Reus, su variedad en infusiones naturales, y el hecho de ser **punto de venta oficial de entradas para los partidos de la Real Sociedad.**

Largoenea, 1
LASARTE - ORIA
943 37 17 42

Otros pintxos:

- *Torreznos*
- *Champiñones en salsa*
- *Bola de carne*
- *Bola de marisco*
- *Callos caseros*
- *Albóndigas en salsa*
- *Croqueta de jamón*
- *Bacalao con piperrada*
- *Vieira gratinada*
- *Kokotxa de bacalao rebozada*

Tosta de jijas con huevo

Ingredientes:

Pan de pueblo
Jijas
Aceite de oliva
Huevo
Sal

Elaboración:

Cortamos una rodaja hermosa de pan de pueblo y la tostamos en la plancha o en el horno

Salteamos las jijas en aceite de oliva por espacio de unos minutos, sin dejar que se sequen en exceso.

Ponemos una sartén al fuego con aceite de oliva y freímos el huevo, añadiéndole una pizca de sal.

Final y presentación: Sobre la rodaja tostada de pan de pueblo extendemos las jijas y, sobre éstas, depositamos el huevo frito. Finalmente damos a la tosta un último golpe de calor en la salamandra antes de servirla.

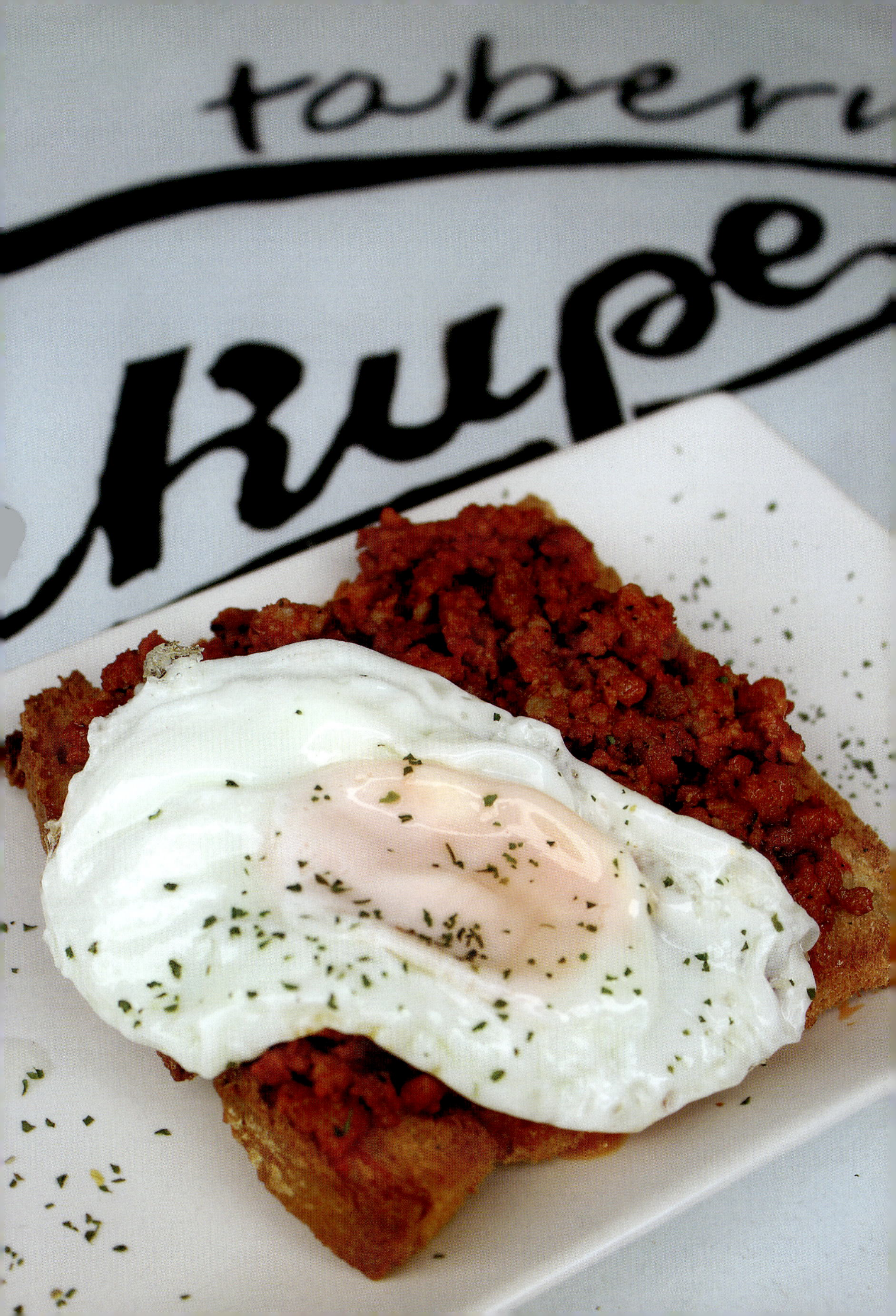

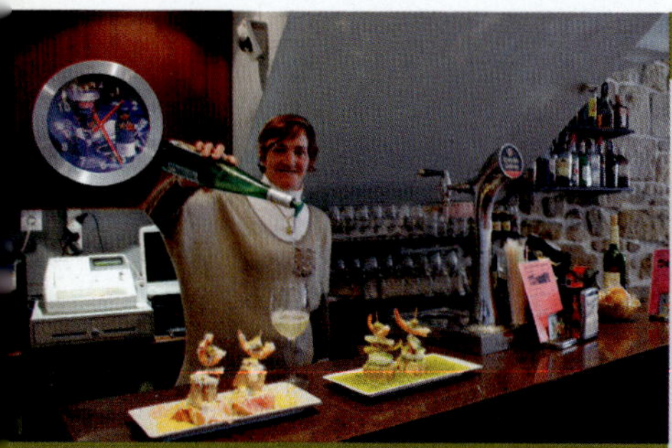

ARKUPEBERRI

Donibane 110-B
PASAI DONIBANE
943 34 15 48

Aunque lekeitiarra de origen, **Mª Carmen Mugika** lleva 25 años residiendo en Pasaia, donde contaba con una amplia experiencia en hostelería, traducida en 20 años tras la barra del Txulotxo y 2 años al frente del Bahía, en Pasai Antxo. En 2007, esta animosa hostelera se animó a coger las riendas del Arkupeberri, situado en plena plaza del Ayuntamiento. Con **Eduardo Benito** como jefe de cocina, Mª Carmen ofrece, los fines de semana, una gran cantidad de pintxos, así como platos de **cocina tradicional** como Merluza a la plancha con almejas y gambas, Ensaladas, Callos, Manitas de cerdo, Chuleta, Entrecot... Entre semana, además, cuenta con una carta de **Platos combinados, Bocatas, Hamburguesas y Raciones** como Calamares, Croquetas, Confit con patatas, Costilla... Arkupeberri abre todos los días a las 9:30 de la mañana.

Otros pintxos:

- *Ensaladilla*
- *Txaka*
- *Pulpo a la vinagreta*
- *Jamón*
- *Taco de bonito con jamón York y huevo*
- *Huevas de merluza*
- *Tortilla de patata*
- *Gildas*
- *Bola de carne*
- *Croquetas*

Taco de atún escabechado, jamón serrano, huevo y langostinos

Ingredientes:

1 taco de atún escabechado
1/2 huevo duro
1 filete de antxoa en salazón
2 langostinos cocidos
1/2 espárrago
1 aceituna rellena
1 rodaja de jamón serrano o ibérico
Mayonesa
Pan
Huevo rallado

Elaboración:

En la base de un platillo colocamos una rodaja de pan tostado al horno o a la plancha. Seguidamente, y con la ayuda de un palillo de brocheta, colocamos, primeramente, una rodaja de jamón serrano o ibérico. A continuación, medio huevo duro y el taco de atún en escabeche, de la mejor calidad posible.

Sobre el atún, disponemos una cucharada de mayonesa y una antxoa en salazón, a poder ser casera.

Sobre el atún y la mayonesa, seguimos dando altura al pintxo con dos langostinos cocidos, entre los cuales colocaremos un pedazo de espárrago de Navarra, y coronamos la "torre" con una aceituna rellena.

Terminamos el pintxo espolvoreando el conjunto con huevo duro rallado.

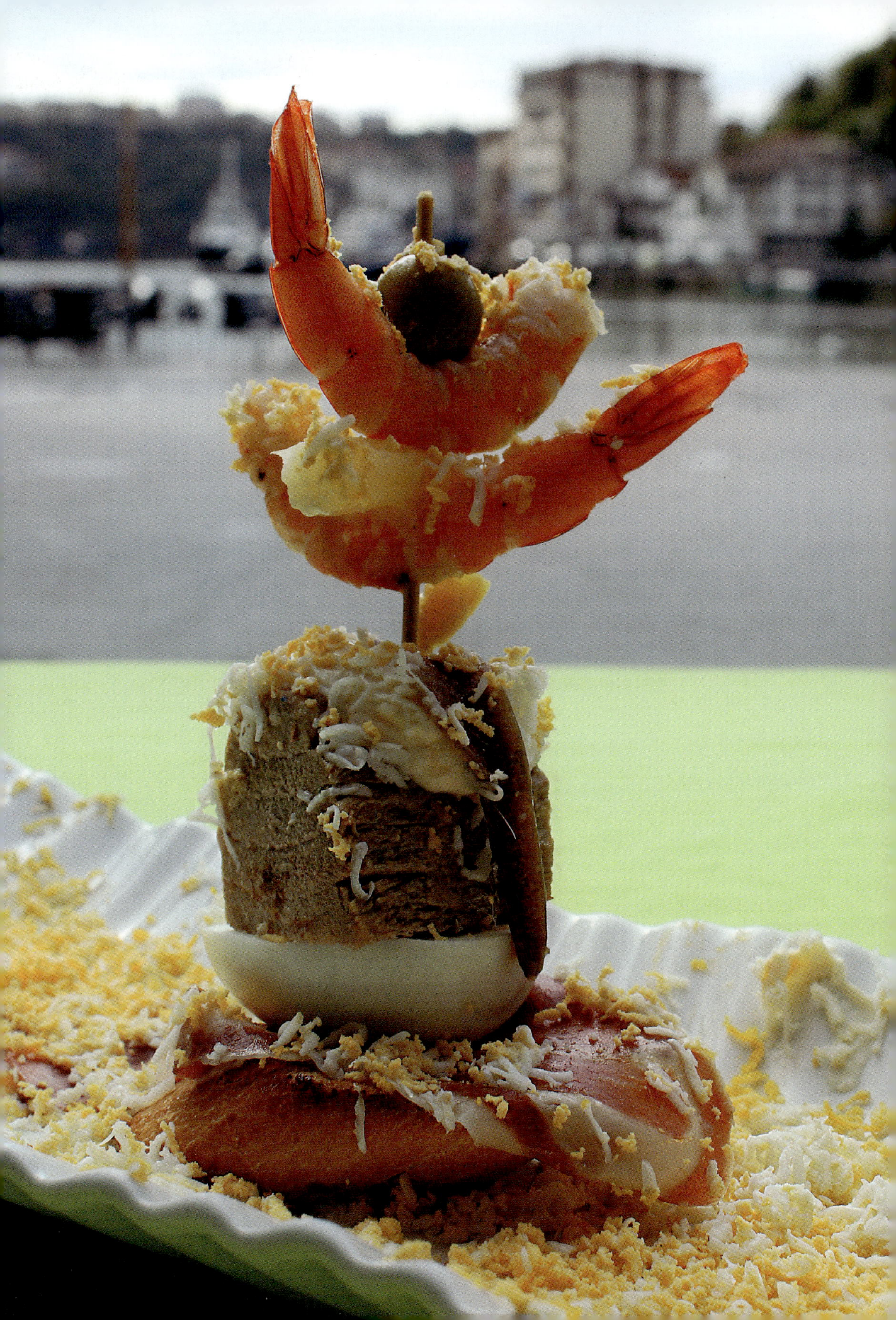

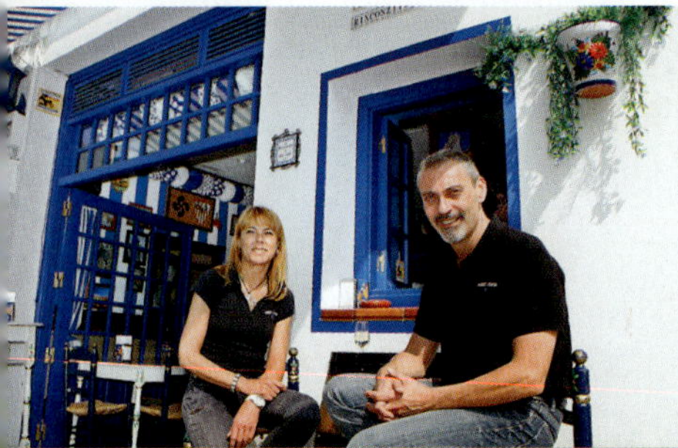

ARRIKITAUN

Igara bidea, 19 (Ibaeta)
DONOSTIA
843 98 31 41

Aunque llevaban más de 10 años residiendo en Donostia, no fue hasta junio de 2012 que los sevillanos **Mayca Madroñal y Ángel de la Chica** se animaron a abrir Arrikitaun, un txokito andaluz en pleno barrio de Igara, en el local ocupado durante décadas por el bar Lanperna. **Todo es andaluz en Arrikitaun, desde los propietarios y el personal hasta la gastronomía, pasando por los colores, la decoración y, como no, la alegría imperante en el local**. En este establecimiento encontraremos una amplia selección de tapas de marcado carácter andaluz donde no falta el excelente Jamón de Jabugo, las extraordinarias Puntillitas o productos menos conocidos como la "Pringá", una masa que contiene, bien picaditos, los sacramentos del cocido de garbanzos (chorizo, carne, tocino ibérico...). Los precios de Arrikitaun, al igual que los de las tascas andaluzas, son ajustados.

Otros pintxos:

- *Pringá*
- *Aliño del día*
- *Croqueta de chuletón de buey*
- *Carne mechá*
- *Langostino abrigao*
- *Carne al Pedro Ximénez*
- *Salmorejo cordobés*
- *Sopa de picadillo*
- *Flamenquín*
- *Croqueta de rabo de toro*

Tortita de camarón

Ingredientes:

Camarones
Harina de trigo
Harina de garbanzos
Agua
Sal
1 cebolleta
Perejil fresco
Aceite de oliva

Elaboración:

Picamos finamente la cebolleta y el perejil. Por otra parte, cogemos un vaso mediano, de aproximadamente 250 cl. de capacidad, y llenamos 3/4 con harina de trigo y 1/4 con harina de garbanzos.

Pasamos la harina a un bol más grande. Añadimos la cebolleta y el perejil picados, la sal, un puñado de camarones y un vaso y medio de agua, de manera que quede un poco líquido.

Trabajamos la masa hasta que ésta coja una consistencia algo uniforme.

Ponemos una sartén al fuego con aceite de oliva y cuando esté caliente, pero todavía no humeante, con la ayuda de un cucharón, vamos vertiendo porciones de masa de camarón en el aceite. Al contacto con el aceite la masa se expandirá y formará la tortita, a la que daremos la vuelta a la de un minuto para que se haga también por el otro lado. Una vez hecha, la dejamos sobre un papel absorbente para que suelte el aceite sobrante y la servimos rápidamente para que no se enfríe, pues calentitas están más ricas.

Final y presentación: No es un pintxo que requiera de grandes presentaciones, aunque una copa de buen fino siempre le sienta bien.

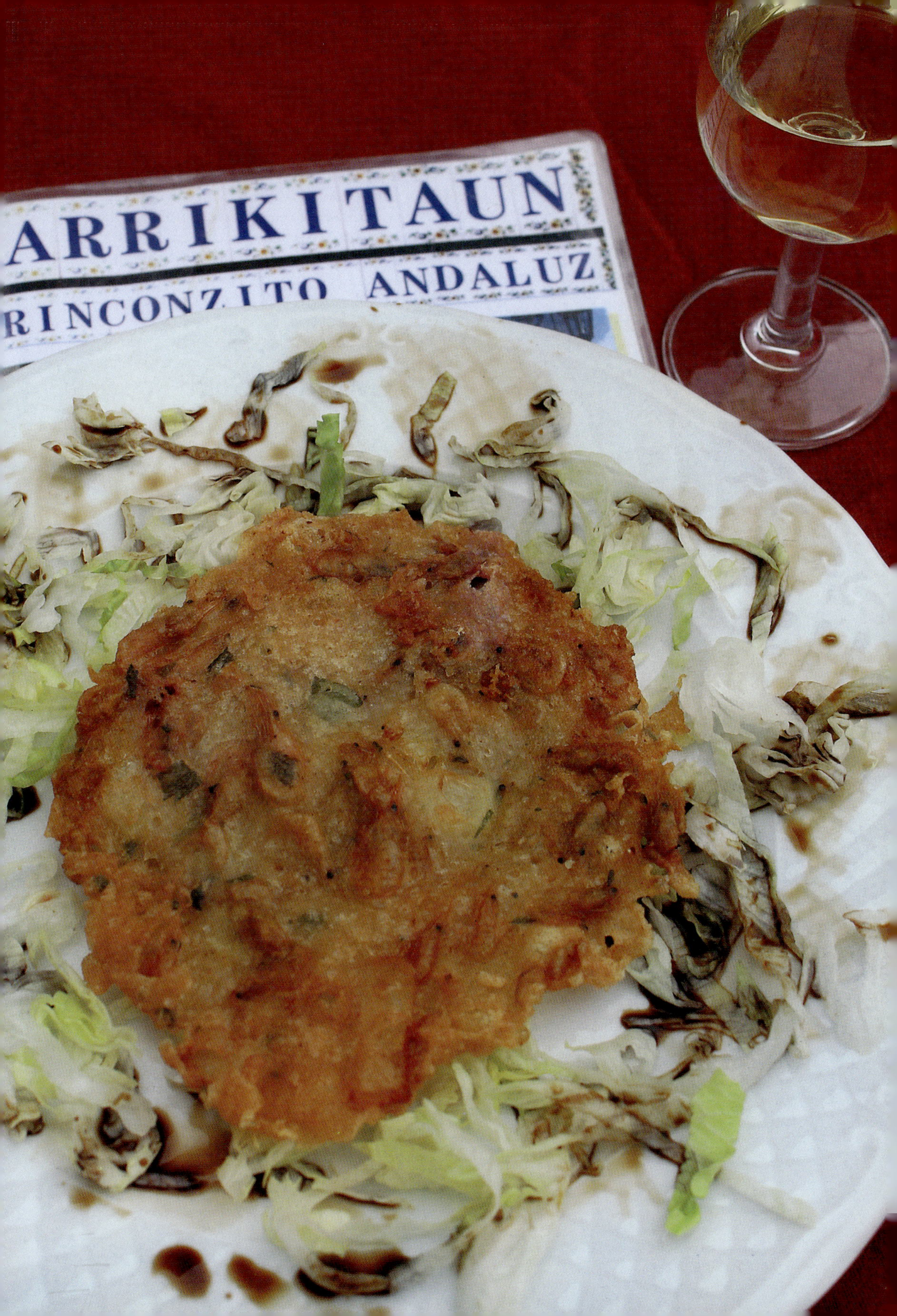
ARRIKITAUN
RINCONZITO ANDALUZ

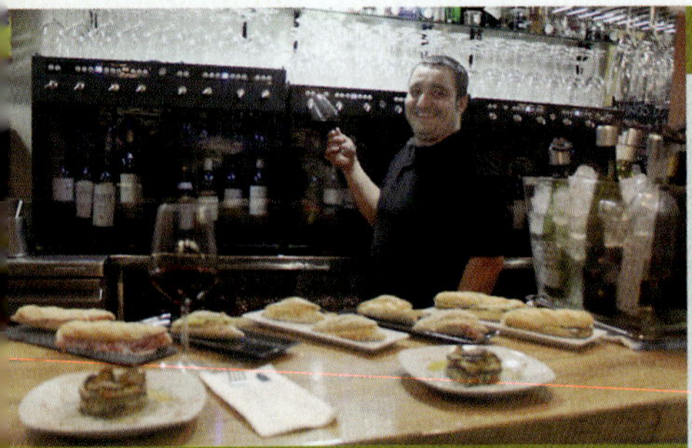

ASTELENA GASTROTEKA

Estaziño, 7
EIBAR
943 20 70 32
facebook: astelena.gastroteka.7

Aunque estudió cocina, **David Vallejo** se había mantenido aparte del sector hasta que en diciembre de 2013 se animó a abrir esta gastroteca en la que todo el año podemos disfrutar de **pintxos, raciones y medias raciones de caza** (ciervo, jabalí, gamo, liebre...), un producto que a David le encanta cocinar y que tiene gran aceptación. También encontraremos aquí una gran variedad de **Platos combinados, Cazuelitas, Ibéricos, Pintxos...** y sobre todo, **Txuletas a la brasa, tanto de vaca vieja como de buey.** Aparte de la comida, el fuerte de Astelena son **los vinos.** David empezó con 100 y a día de hoy cuenta con 150, 50 de los cuales se ofrecen por copas, gracias a **su dispensador de 20 grifos que conserva los vinos en perfectas condiciones durante 20 días.** Este eibartarra trata de trabajar con diferentes bodegas y ofrecer a sus clientes vinos especiales, que no vayan a encontrar en otros lugares. Cada semana recomienda un vino diferente y, además, organiza **actividades en torno al vino.**

Otros pintxos:

- *Brocheta de entrecot*
- *Morcilla de Olano*
- *Caza estofada (Ciervo, Jabalí, Liebre...)*
- *Carrilleras con hongos*
- *Callos*
- *Chipirones encebollados*
- *Tomate, queso de cabra y pimiento verde*
- *Champiñones a la plancha*
- *Ensalada de pulpo*
- *Calabacín, ibérico y queso Brie*

Milhojas de berenjena, bacalao y pisto

Ingredientes:

Berenjena
Bacalao
Cebolla
Pimiento rojo
Pimiento verde
Ajo
Aceite de oliva virgen extra Eusko Label Arrolan (Variedad Arroniz)
Aceite de trufa blanca
Perejil
Pimentón

Elaboración:

Cocemos el bacalao, a poder ser al vapor, lo desespinamos y lo desmigamos. Le añadimos un chorrito de aceite de oliva virgen extra y lo reservamos.

Picamos la cebolla, los pimientos y el ajo y los pochamos con el mismo aceite. Una vez pochadas las verduras, las escurrimos, las mezclamos con el bacalao y les añadimos un toque final de aceite de trufa blanca.

Cortamos la berenjena en rodajas muy finas y las freímos en aceite de oliva.

Final y presentación: Montamos el milhojas disponiendo una capa de berenjena, una de pisto, otra de berenjena, otra de pisto, y una capa final de berenjena formando una flor con los pedazos más pequeños. Terminamos decorando con perejil picado y pimentón dulce.

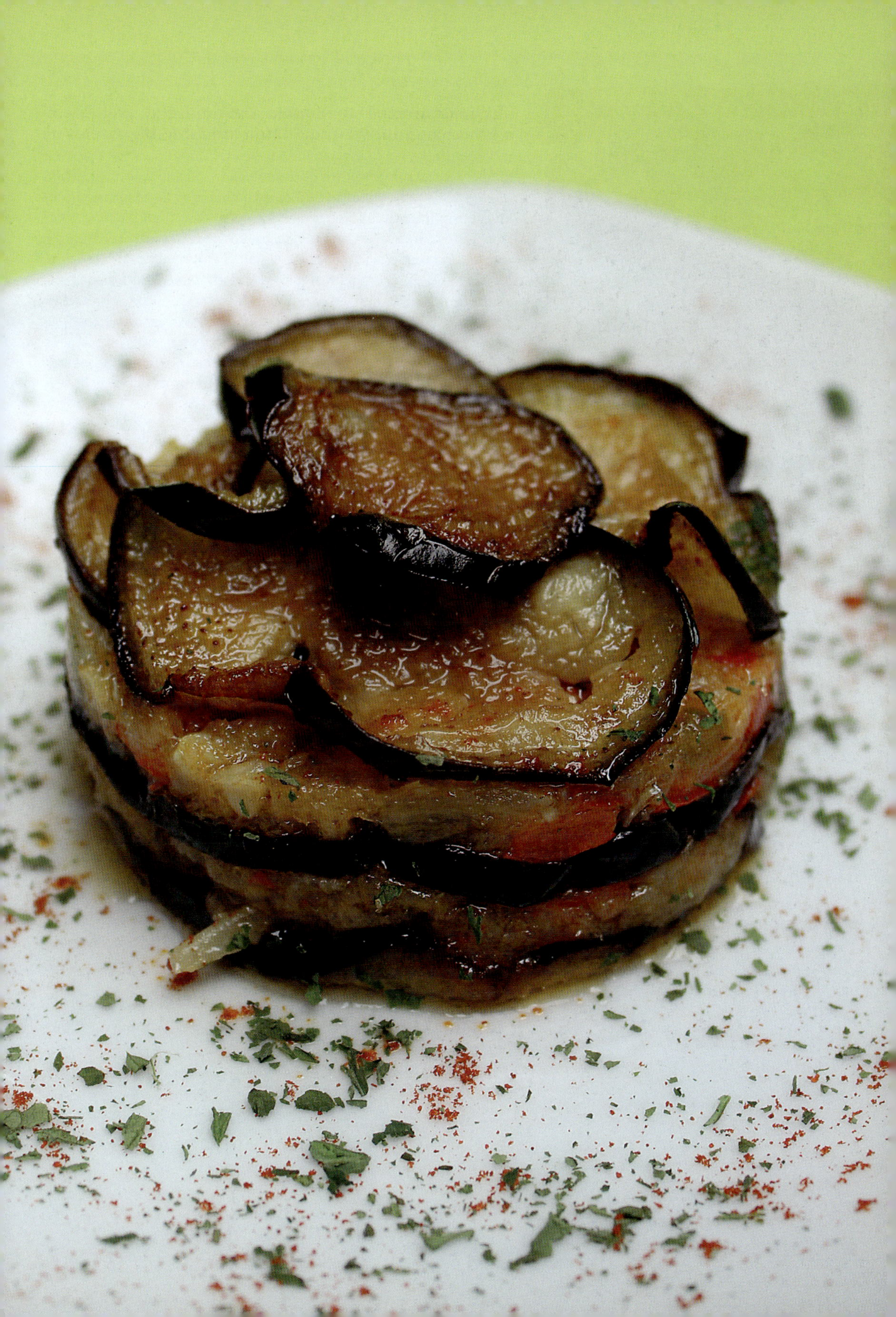

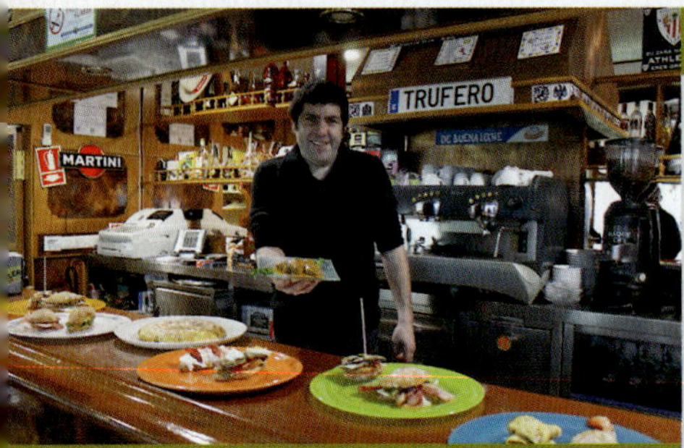

AURRERA

Egaña kalea, 13
ZARAUTZ
943 02 16 38

La **cocina casera** es la seña de identidad de este bar de toda la vida, dirigido desde octubre de 2011 por el zumaiatarra **Iñigo Trufero Pavo**, que anteriormente había dirigido el Kaia de Zumaia y había trabajado en diferentes establecimientos de Zestoa, Oikia, etc... En el Aurrera, Iñigo ofrece una **amplia variedad de Platos combinados, Sandwiches, Hamburguesas, Pintxos...** cómo él dice: "Lo que pida la clientela". En las **cazuelitas** es donde más patente queda el carácter casero de la cocina del Aurrera, con especialidades como Callos, Oreja, Manitas de cerdo... sin olvidar las Rabas y Croquetas. Es destacable también la Ensalada templada de txipirones servida con pan crujiente, que tiene una gran aceptación. Aurrera abre todos los días, salvo los martes, a las 10 de la mañana, y desde el primer momento cuenta con pintxos en barra. Es especialmente remarcable el pintxo-pote de los miércoles en el que en el Aurrera se ofrecen 9 tortillas de patata diferentes.

Otros pintxos:

- *Tortilla de patata*
- *Pavo con queso y pimientos*
- *Bacon, queso y pimiento*
- *Chaka*
- *Oreja con tomate*
- *Morros en salsa*
- *Callos caseros*
- *Albóndigas caseras*
- *Pimientos rellenos de bacalao*
- *Tortilla de jamón*

Manita de cerdo en salsa

Ingredientes:

1 manita de cerdo
Agua
Sal
Pan

- **Para la salsa:**

Zanahoria
Cebolla
Ajo
Un poco de tomate frito
Un poco de pimiento verde

Elaboración:

Para la salsa: Hacemos un sofrito con la cebolla, la zanahoria, el ajo y el pimiento verde. Una vez las verduras estén fritas, añadimos agua y llevamos a ebullición. Antes de que el agua empiece a hervir, añadimos un poco de miga de pan para que la salsa espese. Finalmente, añadimos el tomate frito y dejamos que hierva un rato. Pasamos por la batidora y la reservamos.

Cocemos las manitas unos 30 minutos en olla express con agua y sal, hasta que estén bien blandas. Incorporamos las manitas a la salsa que teníamos reservada y le damos un hervor.

Final y presentación: Servimos en el plato una manita de cerdo y la napamos con la salsa.

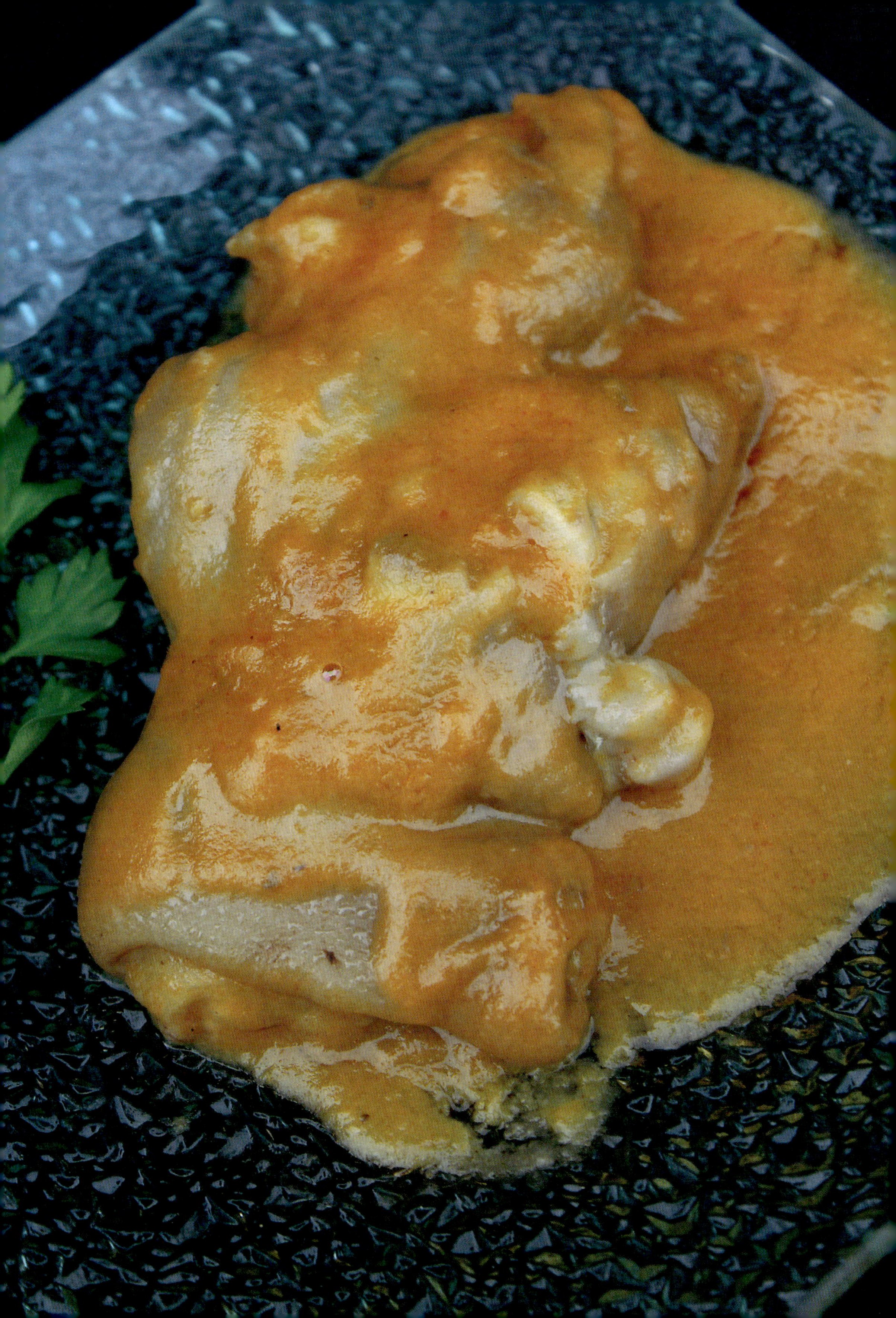

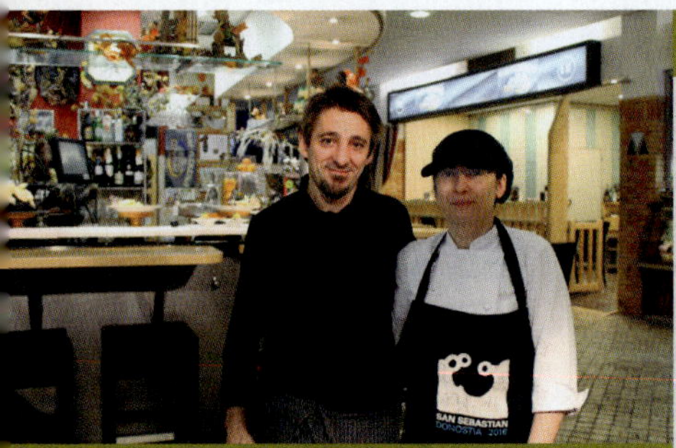

AZKENA

Mercado de la Bretxa, 36
(Parte Vieja)
DONOSTIA
615 79 26 55

Escondido entre los puestos del Mercado de la Bretxa se encuentra el bar Azkena, una agradable sorpresa en un lugar inesperado. Dirigido por **Iñigo Mas y Mertxe Bengoetxea**, en Azkena encontraremos una **cocina tradicional** elaborada en función de los productos de temporada disponibles en el mercado y una surtida barra con una gran variedad de pintxos fríos y calientes, siendo la mayoría de ellos, incluido este "Peine del viento", **elaborados sin gluten**, es decir, **aptos para celíacos**. Destacan asimismo en Azkena sus **desayunos especiales** con tostadas y tortillas variadas, y un café recién molido para llevar. En este bar también podremos adquirir exquisitos **tés naturales** que impregnan el establecimiento con sus sugerentes aromas a Ikebana, Marimba, Gyokuro... y que Iñigo se encarga de distribuir en hostelería.

Otros pintxos:

- *Paleta ibérica con tomate del país y virutas de pan de sésamo al aroma de hongos*
- *AZKENA: Berenjena frita, tortilla de champis, queso y fideos crujientes de arroz*
- *Bacalao confitado con salsa de cebolla y tinta*
- *Tronquito verde relleno de morcillo de ternera*
- *Ensalada templada de verduritas y pulpo*
- *Morcilla de cebolla, berza y salsa de alubia*
- *Rabo de ternera con champiñón y piña*
- *Flor de alcachofas y manitas de cordero*

Peine del viento (Carrilleras de ternera con pasta retorcida, fresas al vino tinto y aire de vainilla)

Ingredientes:

4 carrilleras de ternera
2 cebollas
1 puerro
1 zanahoria
1 copa de brandy
1/4 l. de Oporto
1 l. de vino tinto
1 l. de caldo de carne

• Para las fresas al vino tinto:
1/2 k. de fresas
6 cucharadas de azúcar
1/2 l. de vino tinto
la piel de una naranja
1 rama de canela

• Para el aire de vainilla
400 ml. de agua
100 ml. de leche
2 vainas de vainilla
1,5 g. de lecitina de soja

Elaboración:

Para las carrilleras: Pochar las verduras a fuego lento. Sazonar y dorar a fuego vivo las carrilleras, retirarles el aceite y flambearlas con el brandy. Agregar el Oporto y el tinto, juntar con las verduras, rehogar bien y agregar el caldo, cociendo suavemente hasta que estén tiernas. A continuación, reducir la salsa hasta que quede un cuarto del volumen inicial, introducir las carrilleras en lonchas en la salsa y hacerlas lentamente hasta que estén glaseadas.

Para las fresas: Cortar las fresas por la mitad. Calentar en un cazo el tinto con el azucar, la canela y la naranja. Cocinar 20 minutos, añadir las fresas y dejar 5 minutos más. Dejar templar.

Para el aire de vainilla: Hervir los ingredientes, colar y emulsionar.

Para la pasta retorcida: Poner un cazo al fuego con abundante agua. Cuando hierva, introducir los tallarines y cocerlos al dente. Refrescarlos, escurrirlos, reservarlos y freírlos dándoles la forma deseada.

Final y presentación: Ponemos una base de patata. Encima, unos trozos de carrillera con su salsa y fresas al tinto. Decoramos con la pasta retorcida que recuerda al peine, el aire de vainilla simulando el mar y las tortitas de maíz crujiente dándoles la forma de los adoquines.

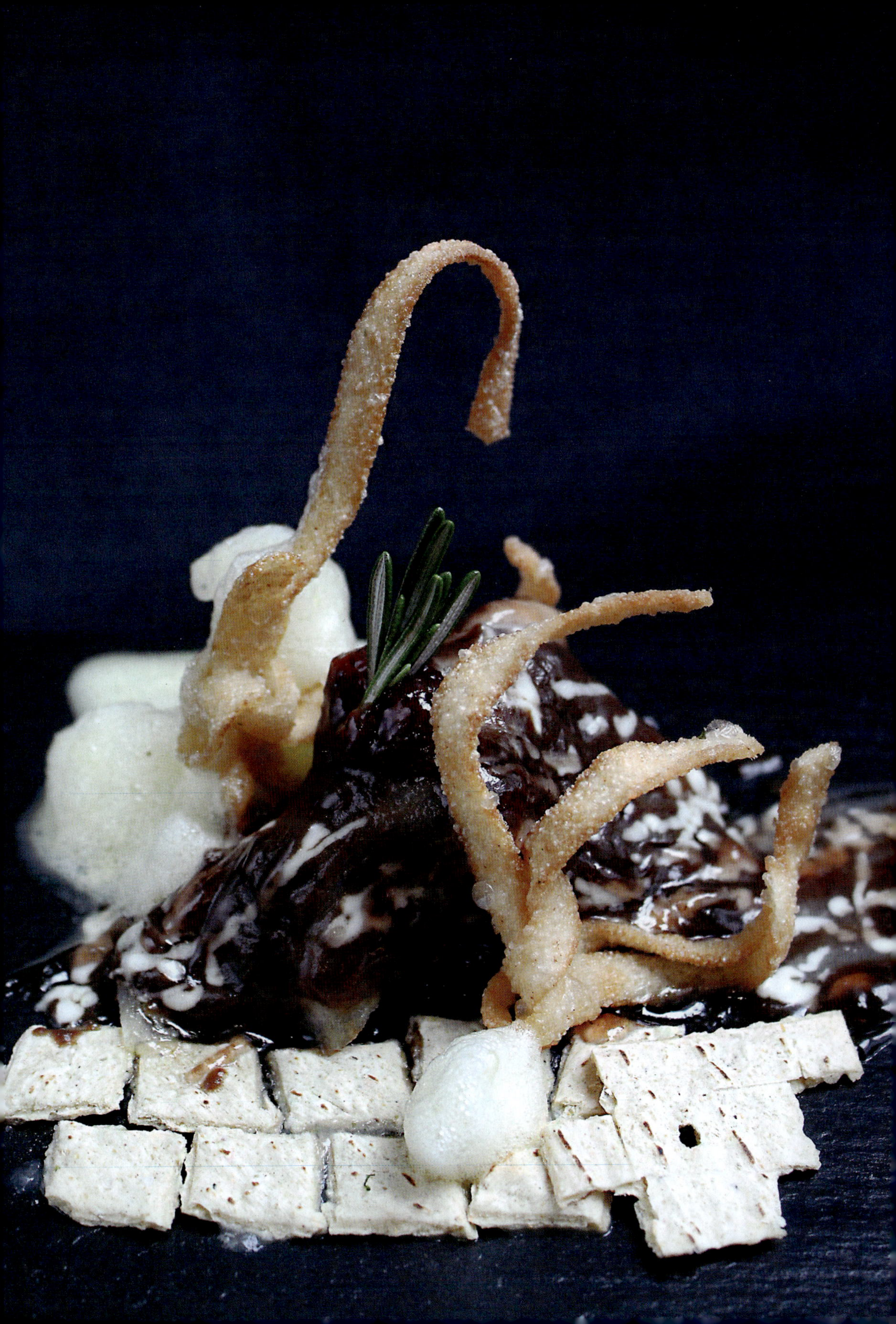

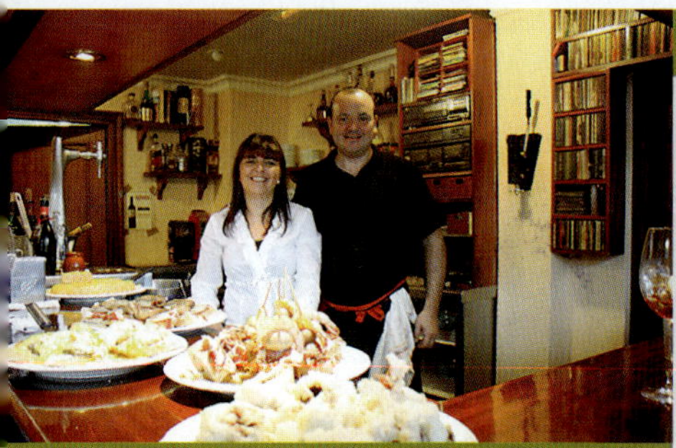

AZPIKOETXEA

Azpikoetxea, 1
LEGAZPI
943 73 13 87

La del Azpikoetxea es una de las barras de pintxos más tentadoras del sur de Gipuzkoa. A 45 minutos en coche de la Parte Vieja, **el mostrador que Juanjo Intxausti llena con su saber culinario rivaliza, superando en muchos casos, con las más reputadas barras donostiarras**, sin necesidad de buscar la cuadratura (o la esferificación) del círculo. Y es que la cocina de Intxausti no requiere de conocimientos de química ni alquimia, se basa en el **producto de calidad y las elaboraciones tradicionales** a las que aporta un gran gusto a la hora de presentar sus creaciones. Compruébenlo dejándose caer cualquier día (salvo los lunes) a mediodía por este local de ambiente familiar y disfrutando de su completísima barra, siempre bien aprovisionada de clásicos como su excelente Tortilla de patata o el imprescindible Bacalao al pil-pil con hongos. En su comedor, además, Juanjo ofrece una cuidada cocina tradicional, un solicitado **menú del día** y un interesante **menú de fin de semana**.

Otros pintxos:

- *Tortilla de patata*
- *Tortilla "campesana"*
- *Carrilleras al Rioja alavesa*
- *Alcachofas con foie*
- *Cochinillo crujiente*
- *Bacalao al pil-pil con hongos*
- *Bacalao de sidrería*
- *Oreja asada*
- *Crêpe de puerros, hongos y gambas*
- *Manos de ministro rellenas de foie*

Morritos "Jagger"

Ingredientes:

1 morro de ternera
2 pimientos morrones
2 pimientos verdes
1 cabeza de ajo
1 tomate natural
1 cebolla
Agua
Sal
Reducción de Módena
Aceite de perejil
Patatas

Elaboración:

Limpiamos y despepitamos los pimientos, pelamos la cebolla y los ajos y limpiamos y cuarteamos el tomate. Limpiamos asimismo a conciencia el morro de ternera y lo cocemos durante una hora en olla express con sal y todas las verduras mencionadas.

Una vez cocido, sacamos el morro y lo dejamos atemperar para que se solidifique. Mientras el morro se atempera, trituramos toda la verdura con el caldo obtenido de la cocción, colamos por el chino y dejamos que reduzca hasta la mitad.

Hacemos un tubo con el morro envolviéndolo en papel film, de manera que quede como un redondo, y lo metemos en la cámara hasta que se enfríe.

Una vez frío, lo cortamos en rodajas que haremos a la plancha o al horno.

Final y presentación: Montaremos en cada ración dos rodajas de morro, acompañándolas de la salsa que hemos obtenido con las verduras y el caldo. Terminaremos el plato con unas patatas paja o panadera y podemos adornarlo con unos hilos de reducción de vinagre de Módena y aceite de perejil.

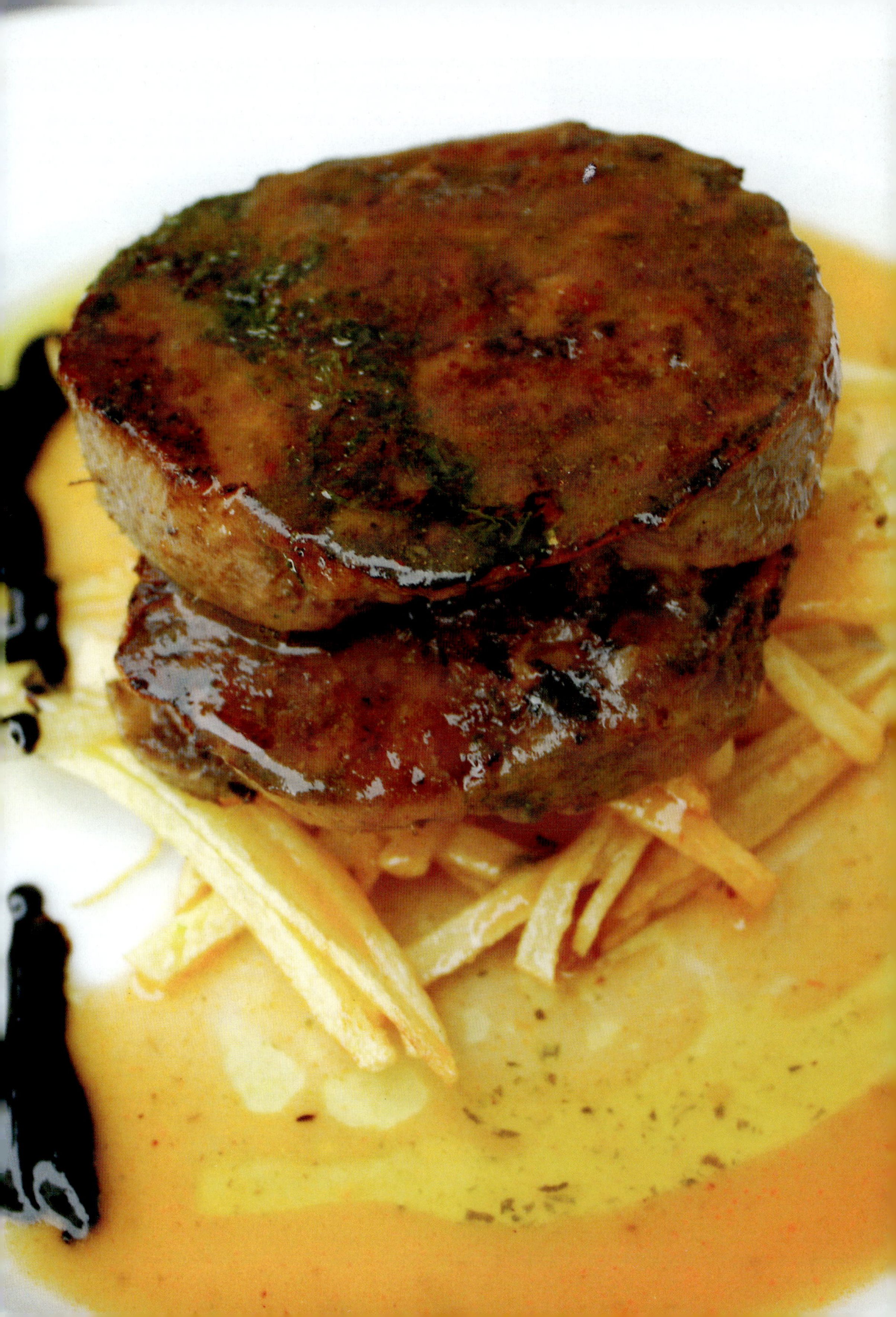

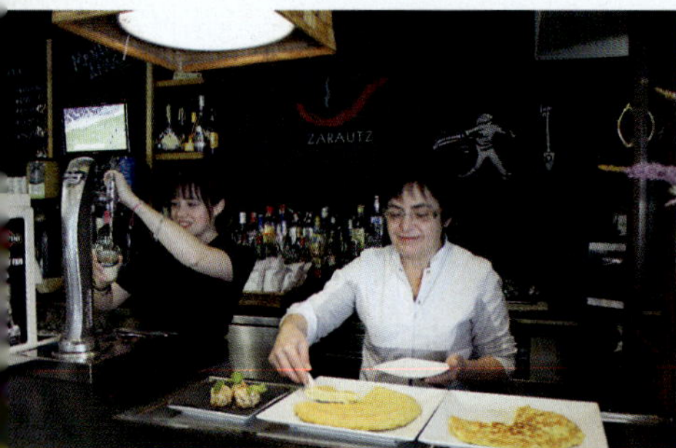

BAI BATZOKIA

Balea, 1 - ZARAUTZ
943 00 20 49
www.baibatzokiazarautz.eus
Fcb: Bai Batzokia Zarautz

Situado en pleno centro de Zarautz, a un paso de la playa, este local está dirigido desde mayo de 2010 por **Mª Jose de la Granja Alustiza**, cocinera con más de 35 años de experiencia, curtida en el Zumardi de Bidebieta. Además de las tortillas y sardinas marinadas, siempre presentes en la barra, **los fines de semana, Mª Jose prepara una gran variedad de pintxos** entre los que siempre encontraremos alguna novedad. Son también remarcables sus **rabas de begihaundi**, elaboradas siguiendo una vieja receta familiar, y los **callos caseros**, que cuentan con admiradores incondicionales. También se ofrece **Plato del día, Menú del día y de fin de semana y carta con platos tradicionales** como Arroz con almejas, Kokotxas de bacalao, Merluza al horno con verduras, Rabo de buey... Este establecimiento, dotado de una atractiva terraza cubierta, abre sus puertas a las 9 de la mañana, cerrando lunes noche y martes por descanso semanal (de julio a septiembre no cierra).

Otros pintxos:

- *Txiki - burguer*
- *Marisco crujiente en brick*
- *Pato confitado con mango*
- *Bacalao ajoarriero*
- *Croquetas de jamón*
- *Croquetas de txipirón*
- *Sardinas marinadas*

Raciones:

- *Rabas de begihaundi*
- *Callos caseros*

Bola de queso fresco y salmón

Ingredientes:

Queso fresco (de untar)
Cebolleta picada
Salmón marinado casero
Pimienta negra
Almendra tostada en grano

- **Para marinar el salmón:**

Sal Gorda
Azúcar
Pimientas variadas
Eneldo

Elaboración:

Para marinar el salmón: Desespinamos un trozo de salmón fresco de unos 500 gr. Mezclamos 300 g. de sal gorda y 300 g. de azúcar con un puñado de pimientas variadas y un manojo de eneldo. Colocamos una cama de esta mezcla en una fuente y, sobre ella, el salmón con la piel hacia arriba. Cubrimos el salmón con el resto de la mezcla y lo guardamos en el frigorífico entre 12 horas y un día. Una vez marinado, lo secamos con papel de cocina y lo cortamos en daditos muy finos para elaborar los pintxos.

Para la almendra tostada: Adquirimos la almendra en grano o la trituramos nosotros mismos en un mortero. Una vez triturada, la introducimos 5 minutos al horno a 180°, dándole vueltas constantemente.

Final y presentación: Mezclamos el queso con la cebolleta picada, el salmón marinado en daditos y la pimienta negra. Hacemos una bola y la "rebozamos" con las almendras tostadas. Optativamente, podemos decorar este pintxo con un crujiente de verdura (apio, albahaca o lo que tengamos a mano).

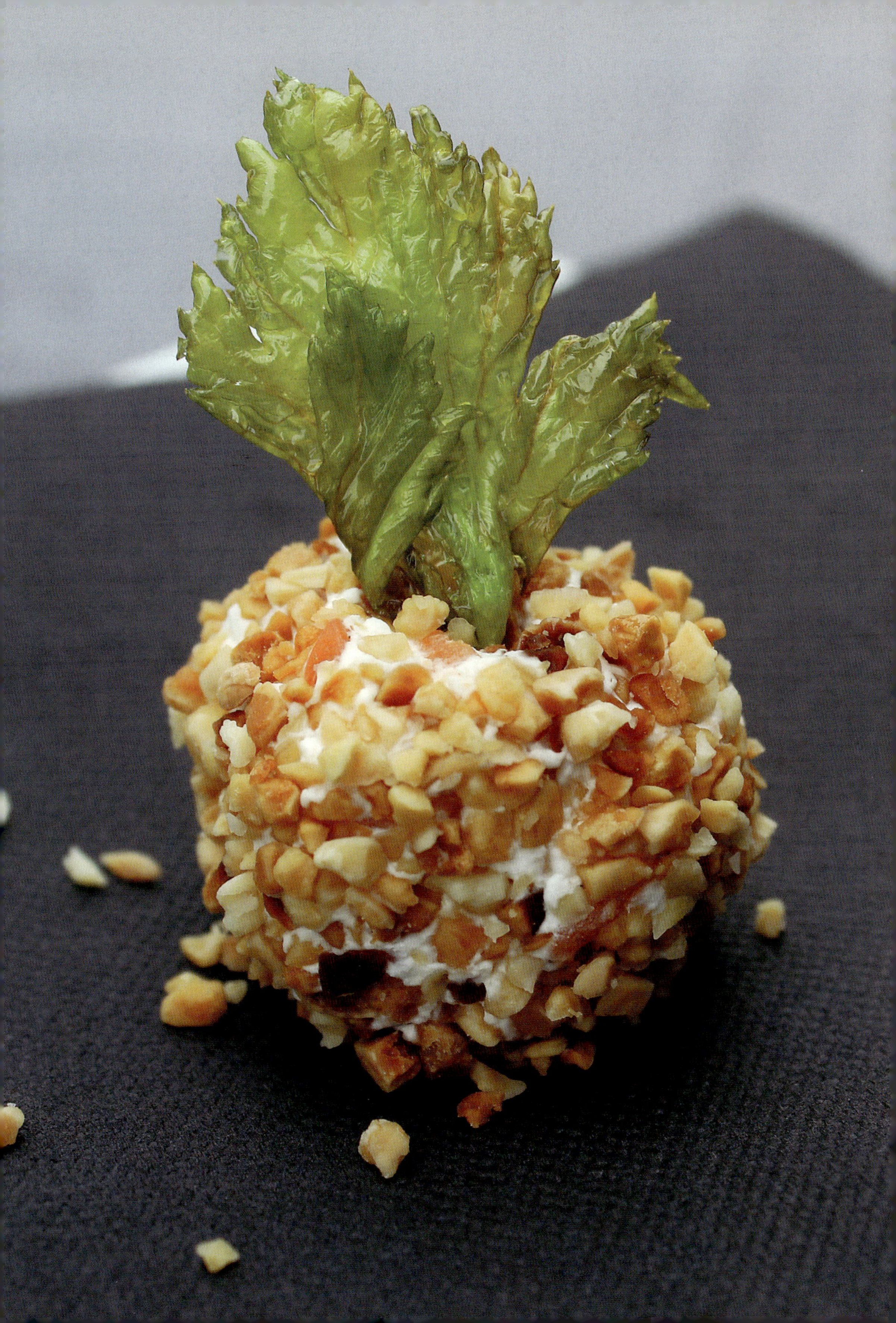

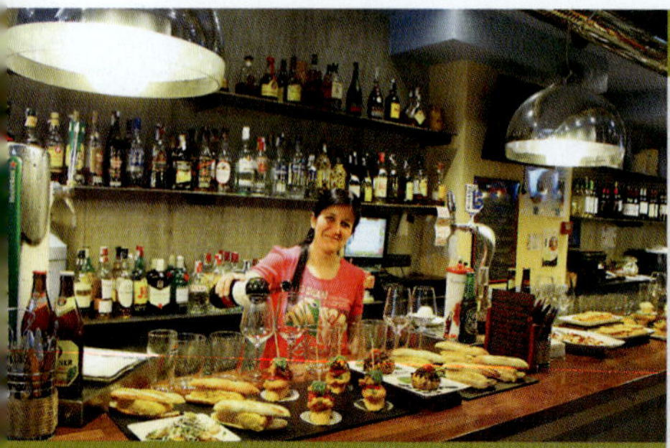

Patxiku, 10
ZARAUTZ
943 02 12 75

BASARRI

El Basarri es un bar con más de 3 décadas de existencia que **ha sido renovado de arriba a abajo por Nerea Artetxe** tras hacerse cargo de él en septiembre de 2013. Nerea ha cambiado de sitio la barra, ha dejado a la vista el comedor y ha convertido este veterano bar en un espacio más diáfano y moderno. La cocina también va a tono con el local con una **base tradicional acompañada de evidentes toques de autor**. Así encontramos platos como el Carpaccio de ternera, el Risotto de hongos con queso parmesano, la Ensalada "Basarri" templada con hongos... Asimismo, Nerea ofrece curiosidades como el **Perrito gigante** (el doble de una salchicha normal), la **Hamburguesa casera "Arrona" de tamaño gigante** o la **Hamburguesa "Lekeitio"**, de pescado. Todo se elabora en casa en este establecimiento que también ofrece **Menú del día, Menú de fin de semana, Bocadillos con pan recién horneado** y cenas todos los días de la semana. Todas las especialidades se preparan también para llevar.

Otros pintxos:

- *Brocheta de solomillo con salsa de hongos*
- *Solomillo al foie*
- *Risotto de hongos con queso parmesano*
- *Carrillera en salsa*
- *Brocheta de langostino*
- *Brocheta de ancas de rana*
- *Foie a la plancha*
- *Calabacín relleno de gulas con gambas*
- *"Nido de huevo"*
- *Vieira rellena de txangurro*

Espárrago con marisco

Ingredientes:

Espárrago de Navarra en conserva
Harina
Huevo
Calabacín
Gulas
Gambas

- **Para la salsa:**

Ajo
Perejil
Aceite de oliva virgen extra

Elaboración:

Para la salsa: En un bol o en una botella mezclamos ajo muy picado, perejil muy picado y aceite de oliva virgen extra. Removemos bien y dejamos que repose unas horas o de un día para otro.

Rebozamos el espárrago con harina y huevo y lo freímos en aceite de oliva hasta que adquiera un bonito color dorado.

Cortamos una rodaja de calabacín a lo largo y la freímos en aceite de oliva hasta que se dore.

Salteamos las gulas y las gambas con una gota de aceite.

Final y presentación: Hacemos una cruz con el espárrago rebozado y la rodaja de calabacín frito. En el centro de la cruz disponemos el salteado de gulas y gambas. Finalmente, rociamos el conjunto con la salsa o aceite de perejil que hemos preparado con antelación.

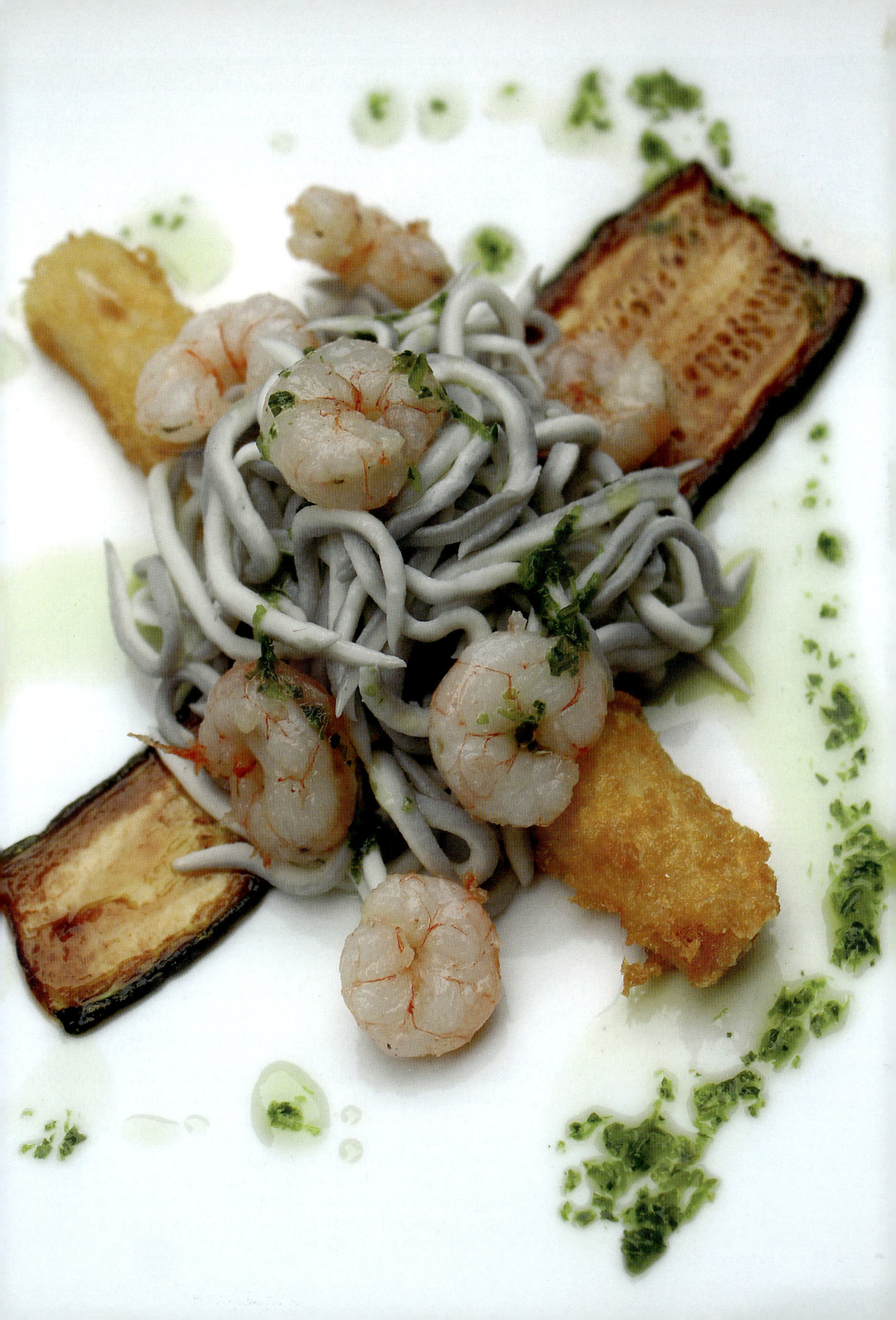

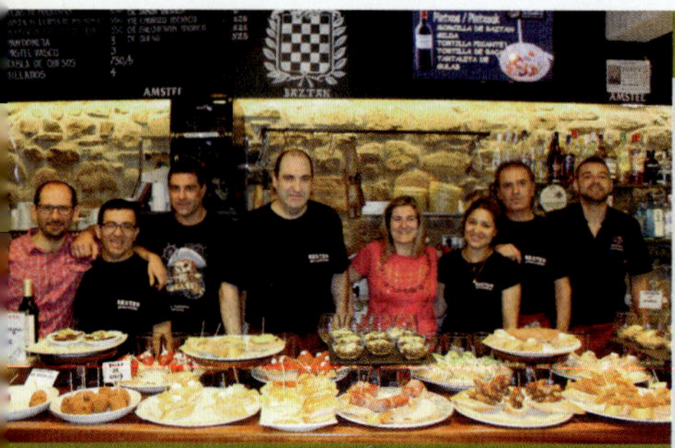

C/ Puerto, 8 (Parte Vieja)
DONOSTIA
943 42 42 72
www.barbaztan.com

BAZTAN PINTXOS & BAR

El local ocupado hasta finales de 2011 por el Portaletas, ha sido retomado por **Arantxa Ciaurriz Iraizoz, de Elizondo**, junto a sus hermanos **Joseba y Oskar**, y con la colaboración de su primo, **Eki Iraizoz**, del cercano bar Casa Alcalde (Ver página 68). En su amplia barra se ofrece una **gran variedad de pintxos fríos y calientes**, aunque en sus mesas puede disfrutarse también de una gran cantidad de **raciones, procedentes de una cocina que permanece abierta sin interrupción desde las 11:30 de la mañana hasta la medianoche.** No se puede dejar de probar la Koka estilo Baztan o los hojaldres, todo elaborado por la centenaria **pastelería Malkorra**, de Elizondo, con la que les une una gran relación que va más allá de lo estrictamente profesional.

Otros pintxos:

- *Pimiento relleno de morcilla de Baztan*
- *Solomillo a la plancha*
- *Ajoarriero con gambas*
- *Calabacín relleno con jamón y queso gratinado*
- *Foie a la plancha con cebolla caramelizada*
- *Txistorra de Baztan*
- *Albóndigas*
- *Bacalao rebozado*
- *Txanpiñones con crema de Idiazabal*
- *Revuelto de hongos de Baztan*

Bacalao de primavera

Ingredientes:

1 medallón de bacalao
3 lonchas finas de calabacín
1 gamba
1 rodaja fina de zanahoria
Pan

· Para el rebozado de la gabardina:
Harina
Cerveza
Agua
Sal

· Para la salsa de piquillos:
Cebolla
Pimientos del piquillo
Nata
Sal

Elaboración:

Para la salsa de piquillo: Picamos finamente la cebolla y la ponemos a pochar en una sartén con aceite de oliva. Una vez pochada, añadimos los pimientos del piquillo y los confitamos un rato a fuego muy lento. Cuando estén blanditos, retiramos el aceite y añadimos un poco de nata. Dejamos hervir un rato, lo trituramos todo con la batidora y lo pasamos por el chino.

Preparamos el rebozado de la gabardina mezclando en frío la harina con la cerveza, el agua y la sal.

Envolvemos el bacalao en la gabardina y lo freímos en abundante aceite de oliva a fuego suave hasta que adquiera un atractivo color dorado.

Freímos la rodaja de zanahoria y dos de las rodajas de calabacín en aceite muy caliente para que queden crujientes.

Final y presentación: Sobre una base decorada con mayonesa y salsa de piquillos colocamos una rodaja de pan. Sobre ella, una rodaja de calabacín frito, el medallón de bacalao en gabardina, otra rodaja de calabacín frito y la rodaja de zanahoria frita. Coronamos el pintxo con una rodaja cruda de calabacín y una gamba a la plancha.

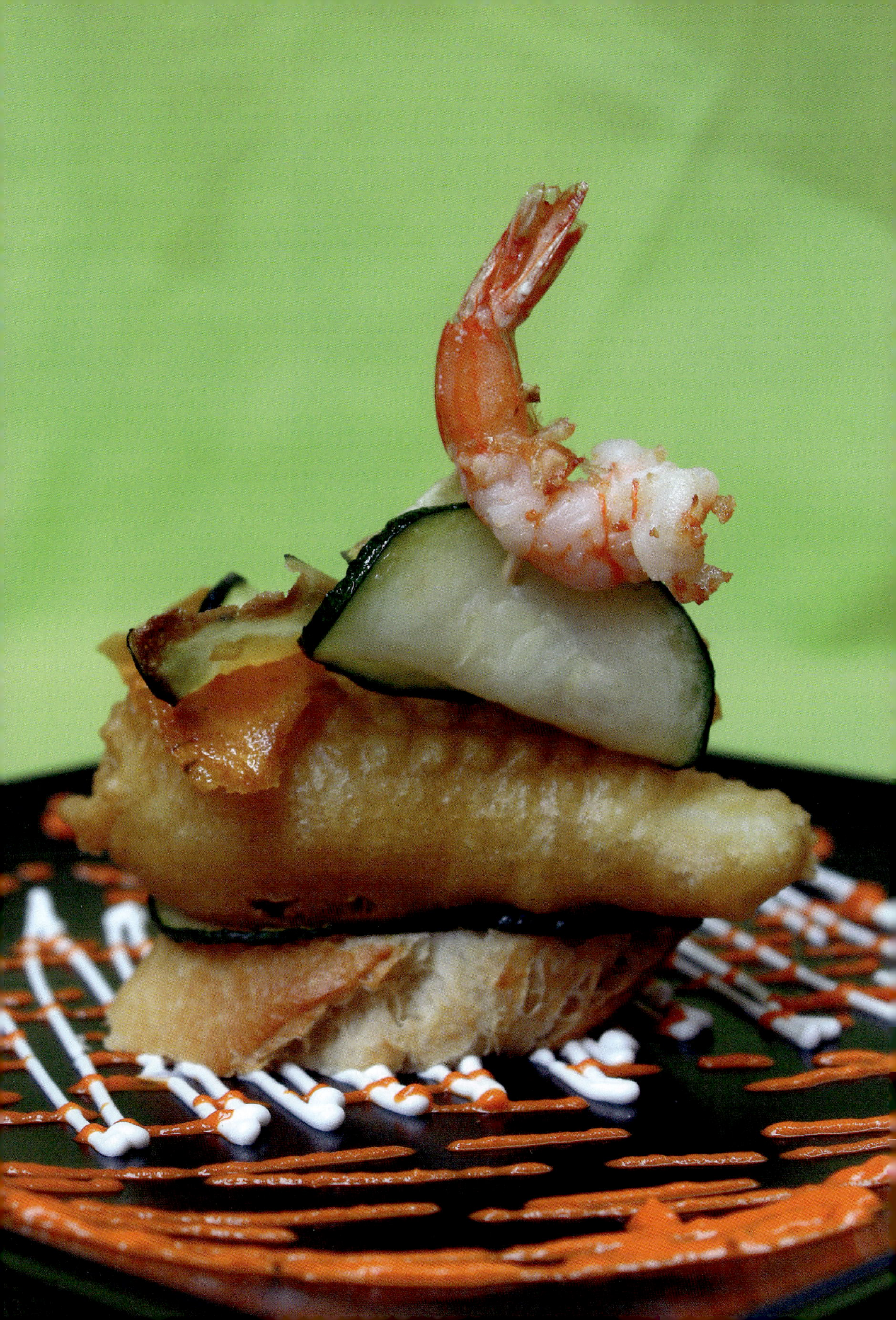

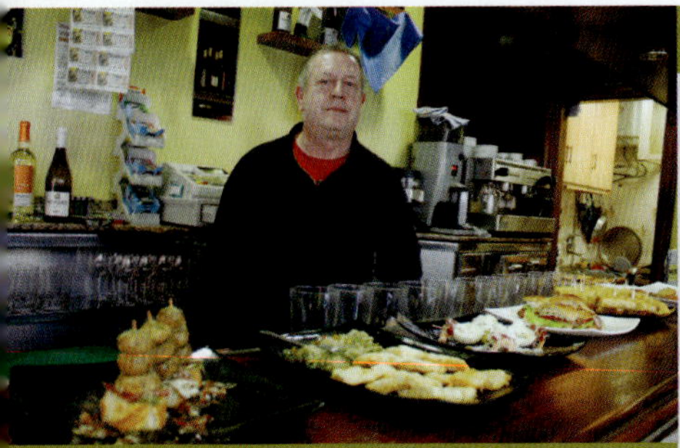

BAZTARRE

Virgen del Carmen, 25 (Egia)
DONOSTIA
943 11 63 50

A la hora en que empiezan a poner las calles en Egia, es decir, a las 6 de la madrugada, **Iñaki Asurmendi**, hijo del barrio, ya ha levantado la persiana para ofrecer a sus clientes buen café y bollería. Este experimentado hostelero trabajó más de 17 años en una conocida cafetería de Gros antes de animarse a coger, en agosto de 2007, este estratégico **bar con más de 3 décadas de historia** en el que la barra empieza a decorarse con toda clase de pintxos a partir de las 9 de la mañana. Txikito pero cálido y acogedor, Baztarre cuenta, además, con una **pequeña terracita** dotada de un práctico toldo, que cuando hace buen tiempo nos permite tomarle el pulso al barrio. Los domingos, Baztarre abre a las 9 de la mañana y cierra después del vermut por descanso semanal.

Otros pintxos:

- *Pulpo con txaka y gamba*
- *Torre de champiñón*
- *Tortilla de patata*
- *Merluza frita*
- *Bacalao encebollado*
- *Revuelto de morcilla*
- *Salmón ahumado*
- *Boquerón en vinagre*
- *Mejillón rebozado*
- *Gambas rebozadas*

Brocheta de alcachofa con gamba y jamón ibérico

Ingredientes:

2 alcachofas en conserva
1 trozo de espárrago de Navarra
1 aceituna rellena de antxoa
1 gamba cocida
1 loncha de jamón ibérico

- **Para la vinagreta**

Pimiento verde
Cebolla
Zanahoria
Aceite de oliva virgen extra
Vinagre
Sal

Elaboración:

Para la vinagreta: Picamos muy finamente la cebolla, el pimiento verde y la zanahoria. Una vez picadas las pasamos a un bol y las cubrimos de aceite de oliva virgen extra, vinagre y sal, removiendo bien. Reservamos.

En un palillo de brocheta ensartamos la loncha de jamón ibérico seguida de la gamba cocida, una alcachofa, el trozo de espárrago, la segunda alcachofa y la aceituna rellena.

Final y presentación: Disponemos en un platillo la brocheta y la cubrimos con la vinagreta.

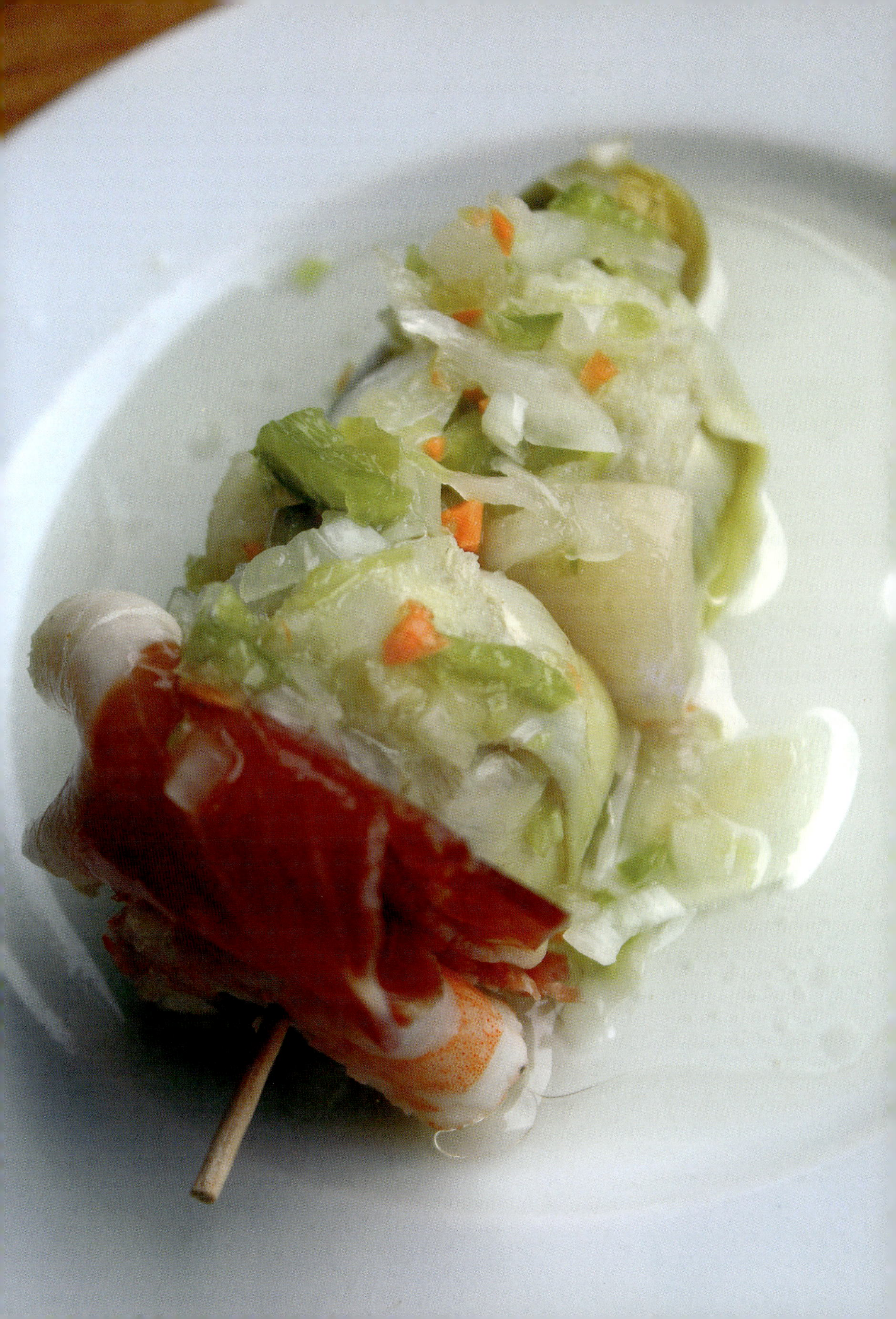

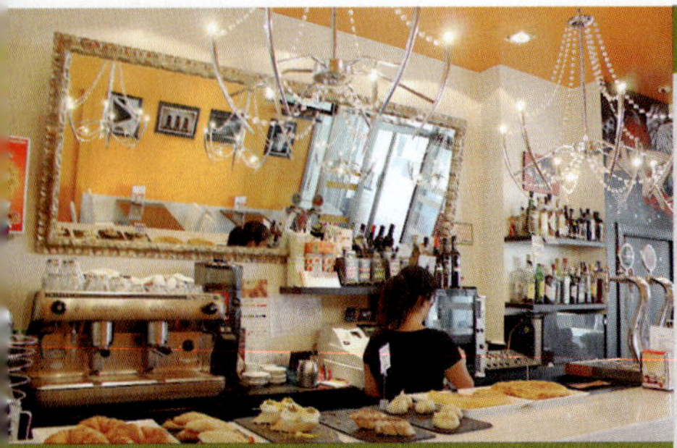

BCN

El BCN, cuyo nombre hace honor a la Avenida de Barcelona, en la que se encuentra, fue **el primer bar que abrió en el nuevo barrio de Riberas de Loiola.** Dotado de una atractiva **terraza aporticada**, este coqueto local cuenta con una amplia variedad de **Pintxos, Raciones, Bocadillos, Hamburguesas caseras y Platos combinados,** así como otras originales opciones como el **Plato Especial para dos personas**, una atractiva y económica propuesta compuesta de Chuleta de buey de 1 kilo, Ensalada verde, Patatas fritas y Botella de sidra o vino de la casa, que puede también ser solicitado con costilla de ternera en vez de chuleta. BCN abre todos los días a las 9:30 de la mañana y desde primera hora cuenta con pintxos en la barra. Destacan también sus rabas y sus solicitadas **Patatas BCN**, caseras y elaboradas al momento con bacon, queso y huevo frito. Los jueves por la tarde se ofrece servicio de **pintxo-pote** a partir de las 7.

Avda. Barcelona, 38
(Riberas de Loiola)
DONOSTIA
943 47 42 65

Otros pintxos:

- *Croquetas (de hongo, de carne con piquillos, de txipirón, de bacalao, de jamón...)*
- *Tortilla de patata*
- *Montadito de jamón ibérico*
- *Seta, bacon y pimiento verde*
- *Bola de carne o queso*

Raciones:

- *Patatas (BCN, Bravas o Ali-oli)*
- *Rabas*
- *Albóndigas caseras*

Bacalao estilo sidrería con vinagreta de perejil

Ingredientes:

Taco de bacalao
Harina
Aceite de oliva

▪ Para la guarnición:
Pimiento verde
Cebolla

▪ Para la vinagreta de perejil
Aceite de oliva
Vinagre
Sal
Perejil

Elaboración:

Para la vinagreta de perejil: Picamos el perejil muy fino, lo mezclamos con el aceite de olvia, el vinagre y la sal, y lo trituramos todo con la batidora.

Para la guarnición: Cortamos la cebolla y el pimiento verde en tiras alargadas y muy finas y lo freímos rápidamente (meter y sacar) en aceite muy caliente.

Para el bacalao: Pasamos el taco de bacalao por harina y lo freímos suavemente en aceite de oliva.

Final y presentación: Disponemos en un platillo el taco de bacalao, acompañado de la guarnición de cebolla y pimiento verde, y lo completamos con la vinagreta de perejil.

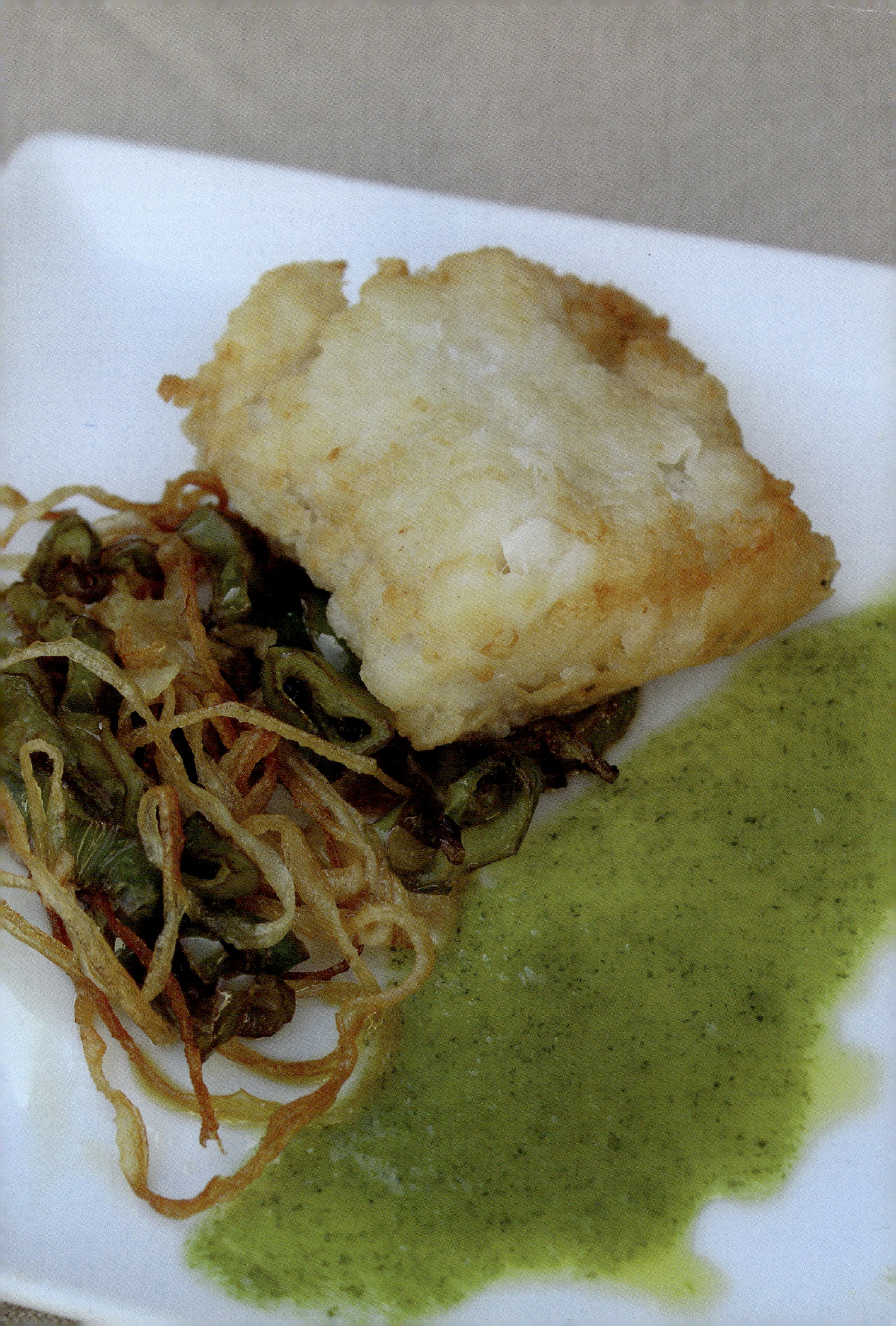

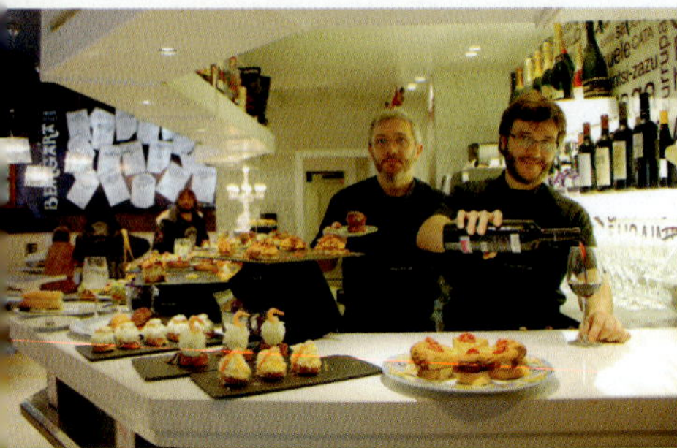

BERGARA

El Bergara de Gros sigue manteniéndose fiel al espíritu inicial del pintxo donostiarra: aquí los pintxos se siguen cogiendo con la mano y se ventilan, sin miramientos, en dos o tres bocados. Además, siguen dando una importancia primordial a la barra, una de las más elegantes y cuidadas de la ciudad, que les hizo ganar el premio a la **Mejor barra de pintxos del Estado** en el Congreso Lo Mejor de la Gastronomía. Fue en 1982 cuando **Patxi Bergara** se hizo cargo del mismo para convertirlo en uno de los más laureados bares de pintxos donostiarras. En 1989 ganó el **primer premio del Campeonato de Donostia de Pintxos** con el Cocktail Bergara. Desde 2008 Patxi ha pasado la dirección del bar a sus sobrinos **Monty y Esteban**, que junto a sus mujeres, **Katixa y Susana**, mantienen las estrellas de la casa y han añadido regularmente novedades dignas de mención como este Fideuá, que era parte del menú del personal del bar hasta que Elena Arzak les animó a sacarlo a la barra. Todo un acierto.

General Artetxe, 8 (Gros)
DONOSTIA
943 27 50 26
www.pinchosbergara.com

Otros pintxos:

- *Falsa lasagna de antxoas*
- *Gratinado de pisto con hongos e ibérico*
- *Revuelto individual de antxoas*
- *Delicias de pato al Calvados*
- *Hamburguesa de tomate raf con dátil y bacalao*
- *Itxaso (Rape y gambas con crema de puerros)*
- *Txalupa (Seta, langostinos, nata y cava)*
- *Udaberri (Calabacín a la crema con cigalitas)*
- *Cuchara de hongos*
- *Cocktail Bergara*

Fideuá en lata con langostino y txipirón

Ingredientes:

Fideo cabello de ángel
Langostinos
Calamares
Pimiento morrón
Pimiento verde
Cebolla
Ajo
Guindilla cayena
Aceite de oliva

• Para el fumet de pescado:
Espinas
Cáscaras de langostino
Agua

• Para el ali-oli:
Aceite de oliva virgen extra
Ajo
Leche

Elaboración:

Para el fumet de pescado: En una cazuela ponemos a cocer espinas de pescado con cáscaras y cabezas de langostinos, a fuego muy suave, durante unas dos horas como mínimo.

Para el ali-oli ligero: Mezclamos en un bol o batimos ajo muy picado, aceite de oliva virgen extra y una pizca de leche para aportarle suavidad.

Para el fideuá: En una sartén, freímos los fideos en crudo con un poco de aceite de oliva. Cuando cogen color, colamos el aceite con un escurridor y los reservamos. Por otra parte, picamos finamente los pimientos, la cebolla y el ajo y los rehogamos en una cazuela con aceite de oliva. Añadimos un poco de pimienta cayena, los langostinos y los txipirones troceados, y rehogamos todo junto un rato. Añadimos finalmente los fideos y el fumet de pescado y llevamos a ebullición. Cuando los fideos se ponen tiesos hacia arriba, quiere decir que ya están hechos.

Final y presentación: Llenamos una lata con una generosa porción de fideuá y lo decoramos con dos cucharaditas de ali-oli.

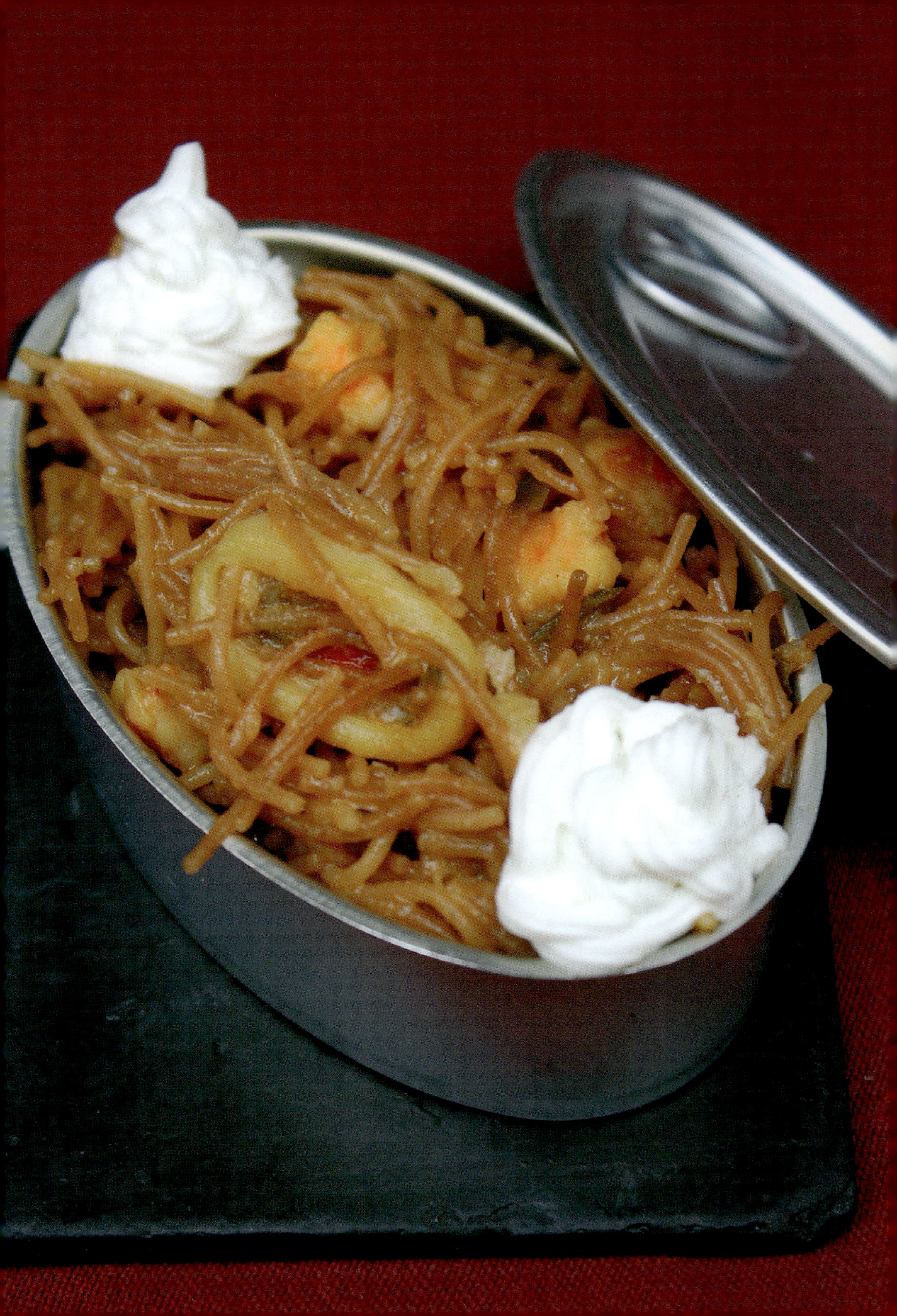

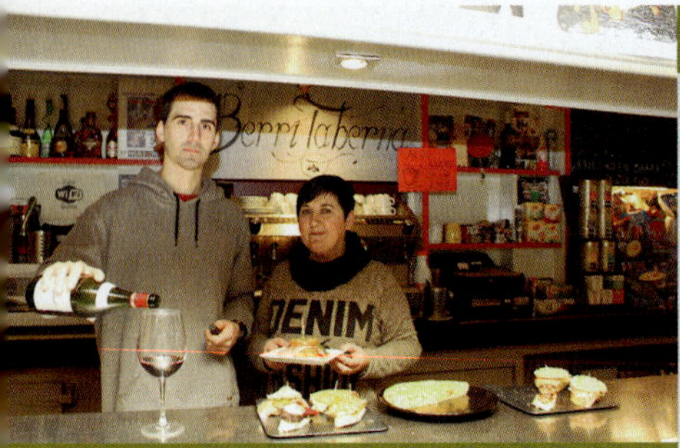

Soraluze, 3
ZUMARRAGA
943 25 29 06

BERRI

Mª Sol Bidarte se hizo en 2012 con este céntrico bar de Zumarraga. Desde enero de 2014 es su hijo, **Ander García de Albeniz**, conocido por su experiencia en bares como el Goiko Kale o el Denak de Urretxu, quien lleva las riendas del negocio. La tortilla de patata es la reina del mostrador del Berri, que abre todos los días (salvo los lunes) a las 10 de la mañana con una amplia variedad de pintxos en barra y raciones como Rabas, Croquetas, Alitas, Gambas a la gabardina o sus Bravas "de luxe". También está siempre disponible el caldito "de la amatxo", así como los exitosos **bokatas, perritos calientes y hamburguesas caseras.** El fin de semana es cuando más ambiente encontraremos en el Berri, empezando el viernes por la tarde con el **pintxo-pote** y principalmente el sábado por la mañana, debido a su proximidad con la plaza del mercado. Además Ángel, aficionado a la música, organiza de cuando en cuando alguna fiesta de DJ´s.

Otros pintxos:

- *Pimiento verde relleno de champi y bacon*
- *Txistorra picante o normal*
- *Tortillas variadas*
- *Morcilla con pimiento del piquillo y huevo de codorniz*
- *Pimiento relleno de morcilla y carne*
- *Croquetas de jamón*
- *Champiñones a la plancha con jamón*
- *Calabacín con queso de cabra y huevo cocido*
- *Bacon con queso y setas*
- *Beniz (bacon con queso y setas, en bocadillo)*

Tomate empanado sobre jamón serrano

Ingredientes:

Tomate
Huevo
Panko
Queso de fundir
Jamón serrano
Seta de cardo
Pimiento verde
Pan
Aceite
Perejil
Cebolla (opcional)

Elaboración:

Cortamos una rodaja de pimiento verde, y lo freímos en aceite de oliva bien caliente.

Hacemos una seta de cardo a la plancha.

Cortamos una hermosa rodaja de tomate, la rebozamos en huevo y panko y la freímos en aceite de oliva

Final y presentación: Sobre una rodaja de pan, disponemos la loncha de queso para fundir, y sobre ella y en este orden, la loncha de jamón serrano, la seta a la plancha, la rodaja de pimiento verde frito y la rodaja de tomate rebozado. Espolvoreamos el conjunto con perejil recién picado y ensartamos el pintxo con un palillo.
En el momento de ser servido este pintxo, se le da un golpe de calor al horno para que el queso se funda y el jamón se haga un poco.

Nota: Hay ocasiones en que este pintxo es coronado con un poco de cebolla pochada.

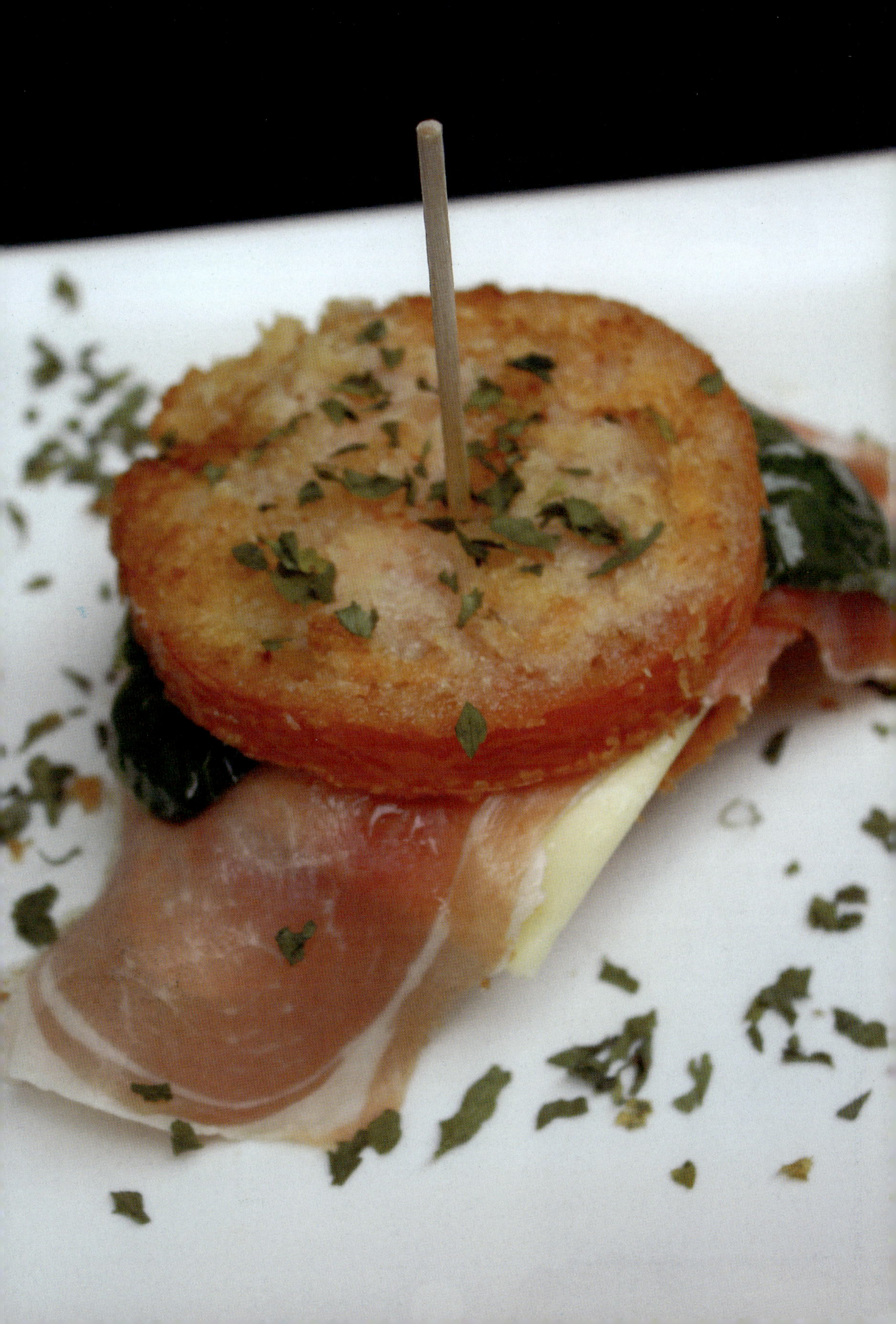

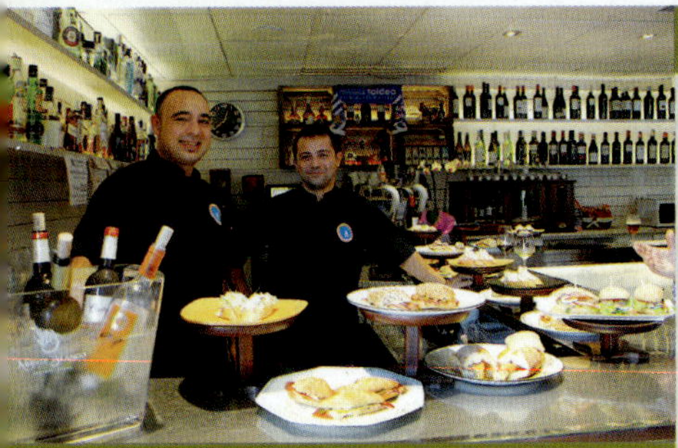

BIDEZAR

Bidezar, 17
ZUMARRAGA
943 25 38 56

En pleno centro de Zumarraga, dirigido por **Roger Hidalgo y Koldo Ruiz**, con **Elixabete García** al mando de la cocina, Bidezar cuenta con una carta asequible y atractiva con **gran variedad de bocadillos, tostas, ensaladas, sandwiches, hamburguesas, pintxos y platos combinados.** Las tostas, en concreto, se elaboran sobre una generosa rodaja de pan y se hornean al modo de las pizzas, resultando un plato idal tanto para comer de forma individual como para compartir. Se ofrecen, además, **2 menús infantiles y una gran variedad en ensaladas**, destacando la de Langostinos y cigalas, así como sus **raciones de picoteo** (Cecina, Callos y morros, Nachos, Codillo con patatas...) **y los espectaculares Huevos Rotos** (con jamón, con setas, etc...). **La oferta de vinos es remarcable** con una gran cantidad de denominaciones de origen y referencias continuamente renovadas. Bidezar cuenta además con una carta con **más de 40 ginebras** para quien quiera disfrutar de un buen gin-tonic.

Otros pintxos:

- *Cazuelita de bacalao*
- *Brocheta de champis, langostino y bacon crujiente*
- *Montadito de bacon, queso, pimiento verde y huevo frito*
- *Montadito de pechuga empanada queso, bacon y ali-oli*
- *Sandwich vegetal*
- *Tortillas variadas*
- *Ensaladilla rusa*
- *Calabacín rebozado con carne picada o gulas y gambas*
- *Croqueta de jamón*
- *Hojaldres rellenos variados (puerro, marisco...)*

Queso de cabra caramelizado sobre tomate y jamón a la plancha

Ingredientes:

1 rodaja de queso de cabra
1 rodaja de tomate
1 loncha de jamon
Cebolla
Pimiento del piquillo
Setas de cardo
Aceite de oliva
Pan
Perejil

Elaboración:

Hacemos el queso de cabra a la plancha hasta que los bordes se caramelicen, cuidando de que no se nos seque el interior.

Hacemos la rodaja de tomate igualmente a la plancha, al igual que la loncha de jamón.

Cortamos en Juliana la cebolla y la pochamos a fuego muy lento en aceite de oliva.

Salteamos en aceite de oliva las setas troceadas y el pimiento del piquillo en tiras.

Final y presentación: Sobre una base de pan tostado al horno o en la plancha colocamos la rodaja de tomate a la plancha. Encima de ella el jamón. Encima del jamón hacemos una cama con la cebolla pochada, los pimientos y las setas y sobre ella depositamos la rodaja de queso de cabra. Espolvoreamos el conjunto con un poco de perejil fresco recién picado.

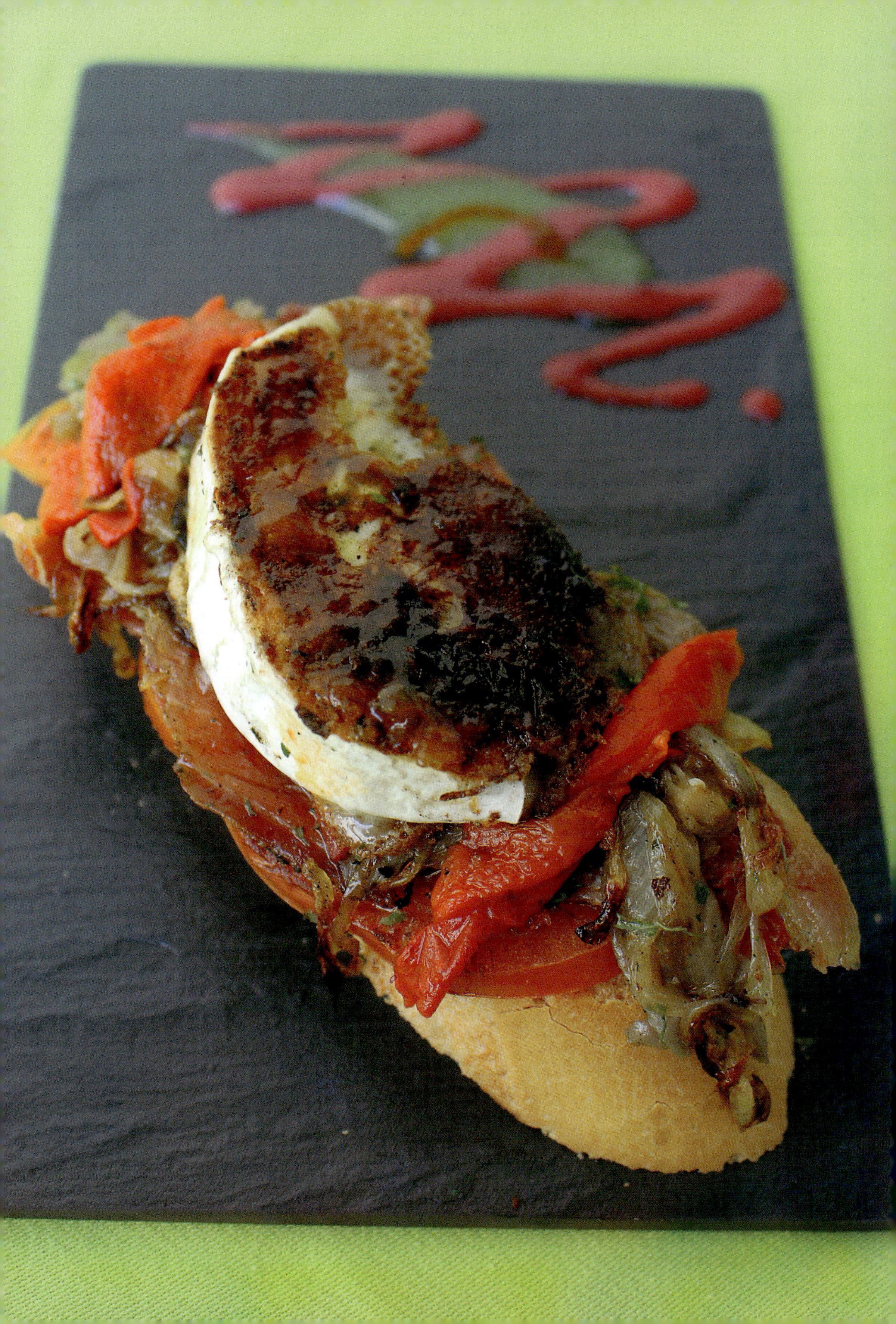

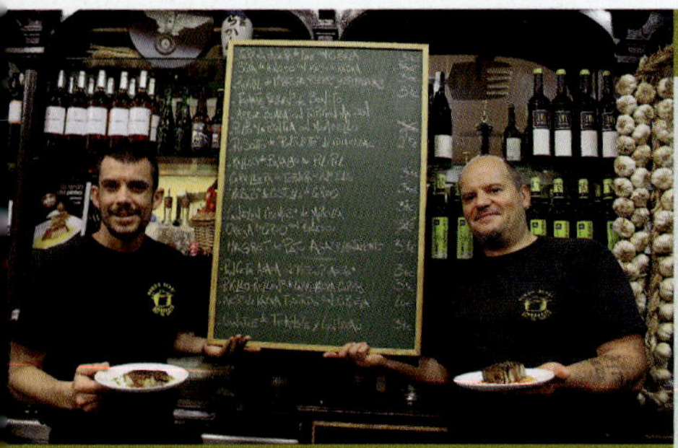

BORDA BERRI

El donostiarra **Iñaki Gulin** y el catalán **Marc Clua** se hicieron cargo en 2007 de este veterano local tras trabajar varios años en La Cuchara de San Telmo, bar del que Iñaki fue miembro fundador. Desde entonces, esta creativa pareja no deja de sorprendernos con ocurrencias como sus extraordinarios Callos de bacalao, imitados sin disimulo en cocinas cercanas, o el original Kebab de kostilla ibérika, que refleja su vena más viajera e internacional. Pregunten también por el Mar y Montaña, que cambia en función de la temporada. Otras tentaciones ineludibles en **su pizarra, en continua evolución**, son la Oreja de cerdo crujiente con tximitxurri, el Arroz bomba con txipirón-maiden, el Tomate relleno... Como reza el original rótulo que preside la entrada del local: **"Akí se guisa".**

Fermín Calbetón, 12
(Parte Vieja)
DONOSTIA
943 43 03 42

Otros pintxos:

- *Foie plantxa con un golpe de pimienta*
- *Tomate relleno de bonito*
- *Terrina casera de foie con ciruela*
- *Kallos de bacalao al pil-pil*
- *Guiso de pollo y txipirón*
- *Pikillo relleno de karri-kabra*
- *Ravioli a la plantxa de molleja, puerro y lemon-grass*
- *Morro de ternera en salsa bizkaína*
- *"Kebab" de kostilla ibérika*
- *Arroz "bomba" con txipiron-maiden*

Panceta de basatxerri asada con ketchup casero

Ingredientes:

Panceta de Basatxerri

- **Para el caldo de cocción de la panceta:**

Caldo de carne
Pimienta
Jengibre
Soja

- **Para el Ketchup casero:**

1 cebolla roja
½ hinojo
2 ramas de apio
100gr genjibre
2 dientes de ajo
2 clavos
Granos de pimienta
500gr. Tomate pera
500gr. Salsa de tomate

Elaboración:

Para elaborar este pintxo, en Borda Berri utilizan pancetas enteras de Basatxerri, que alcanzan los 7 kilos de peso. Partimos la panceta por la mitad y la cocemos en caldo de carne con pimienta, jengibre y soja. No la coceremos en exceso para que quede jugosa.

Para el Ketchup casero: Se sofríen todos los ingredientes menos el tomate durante unos 15 minutos. Se añade el tomate y se deja cocer hasta esté todo bien hecho. Se tritura, se pasa por el chino y se coloca al fuego otra vez, añadiendo una reduccion de 200ml de vinagre de vino con 70 g. de azúcar. Se deja espesar y se reserva.

Dejamos enfriar la panceta, la cortamos al tamaño deseado, la marcamos en la plancha y la lacamos con el ketchup casero.

Final y presentación: Servimos en un platillo una porción de panceta lacada con ketchup. La podemos acompañar con un puré de coliflor o con un Trinchat de la Cerdanya, que se elabora cociendo col y patata troceadas y añadiendo unas rodajitas de panceta frita.

Nota: La receta de Ketchup casero está basada en una receta de Jamie Oliver.

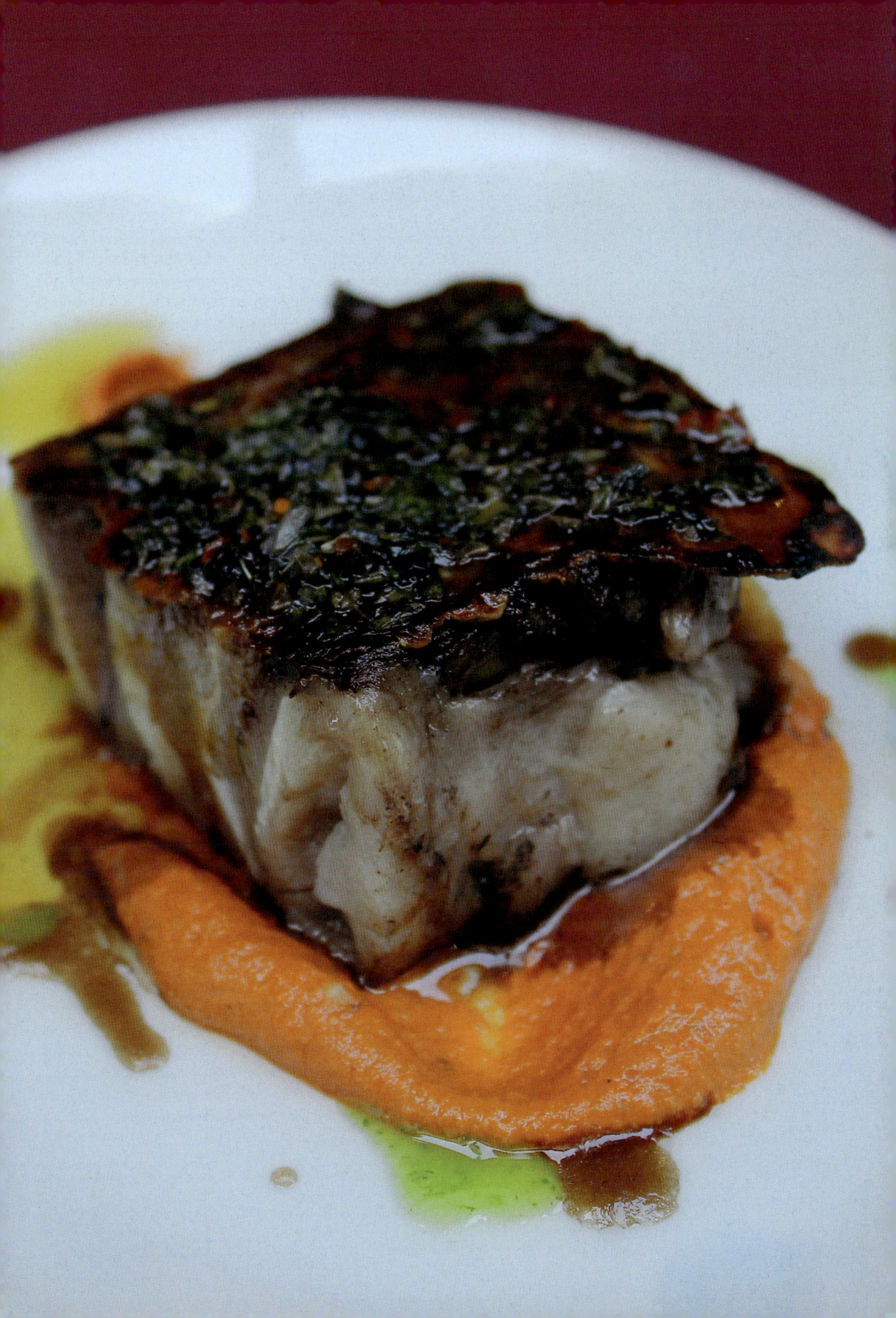

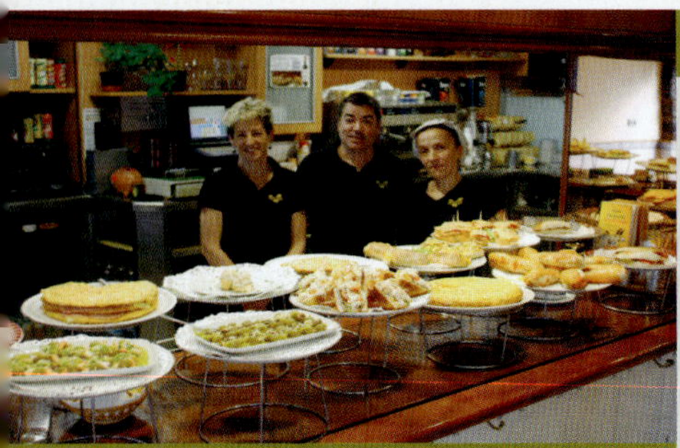

BOSSA

Los eibarreses **Castor García y Gari Luengo**, que arrastran a sus espaldas más de 30 años de experiencia en hostelería, dirigen desde el año 2001 este bar, principalmente especializado en bocadillos, con una carta en la que encontramos **casi 50 referencias entre bocadillos fríos, bocadillos calientes, sandwiches y hamburguesas**. Además, los clientes pueden pedir variantes de los bocadillos añadiendo uno o varios ingredientes de la lista que se propone, con lo que la variedad es casi infinita. Tanto los bocatas como los pintxos se sirven en **pan recién horneado** y el producto se cuida al máximo, como lo atestigua la carne de las hamburguesas caseras, adquirida en la carnicería de Ramón Albizu. Bossa abre todos los días a las 7 de la mañana ofreciendo buen café, bollería y tartas, y los pintxos hacen su aparición a partir de las 8:30. Los jueves, se ofrece **pintxo-pote**, regalando un pintxo incluso a los que entran a tomar un café.

Ego-Gain, 7
EIBAR
943 20 67 53

Otros pintxos:

- *Torreta de huevo*
- *Revuelto de setas*
- *Tortillas variadas*
- *Sandwich*
- *Gilda*
- *Champiñones a la plancha o en salsa*
- *Albóndigas en salsa*
- *Atún en vinagreta*
- *Verduras en tempura*
- *Tomates verdes fritos rebozados*

Tosta de seta de temporada

Ingredientes:

Pan de hogaza o de pueblo
Setas de cardo
1 loncha de jamón ibérico
Aceite de oliva virgen extra

· Para el refrito:
Jamón
Ajo
Guindillas
Aceite de oliva

· Para la sal de tomate seco:
Salsa de tomate casera

Elaboración:

Para el refrito: Picamos muy finamente una loncha de jamón serrano, ajo y guindillas, y lo freímos todo en aceite de oliva.

Para la sal de tomate seco: Partimos de una salsa de tomate casera, que dejamos secar al horno a baja temperatura durante toda la noche. Una vez bien seca, la pasamos por el molinillo para que quede picada con consistencia de sal.

Hacemos las setas a la plancha

Final y presentación: Tostamos al horno una rodaja de pan de hogaza y la regamos con aceite de oliva virgen extra. Sobre ella colocamos una loncha de jamón ibérico en crudo y, sobre ella, las setas a la plancha. Terminamos vertiendo el refrito de jamón, ajo y guindilla y espolvoreando el conjunto con la sal de tomate seco.

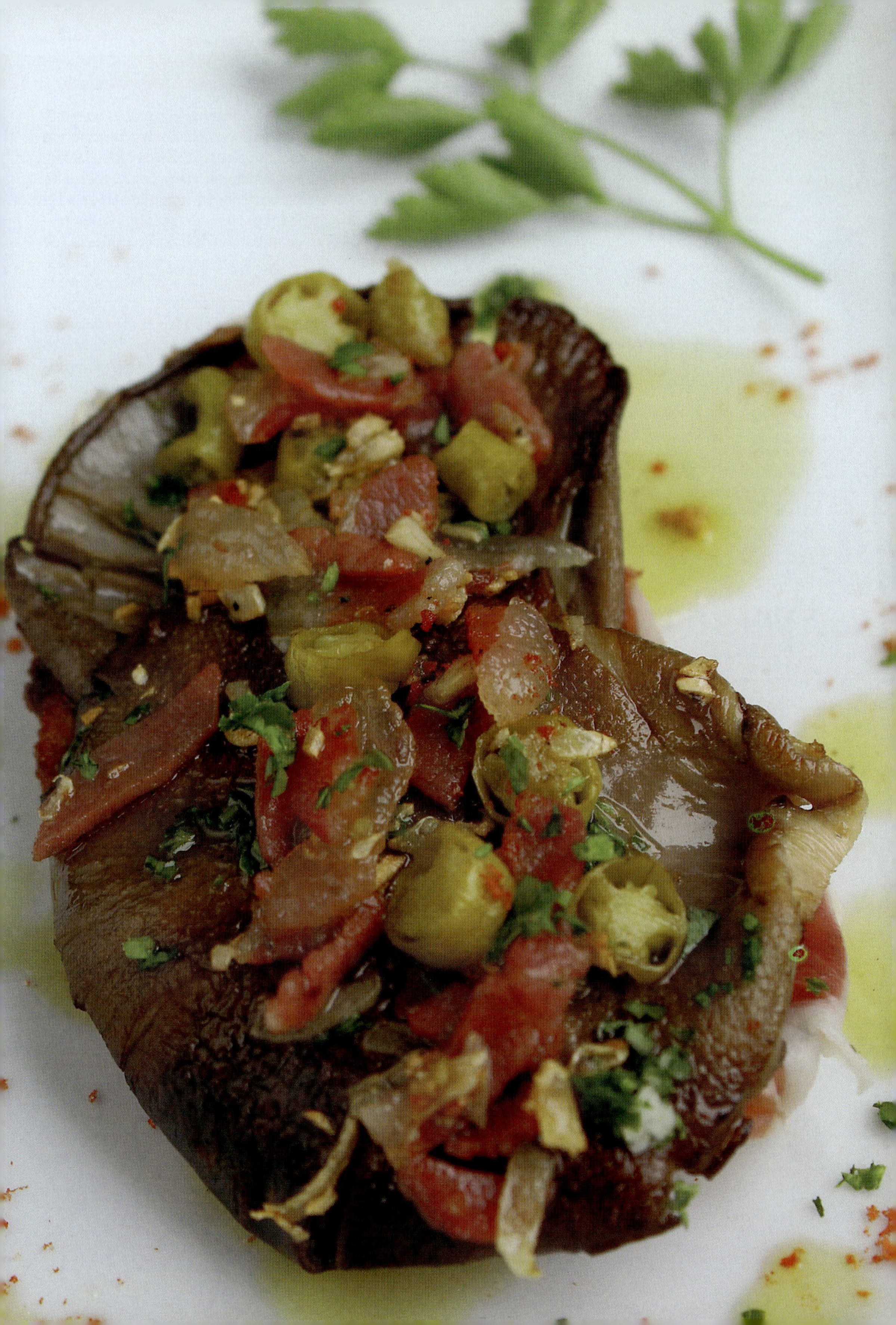

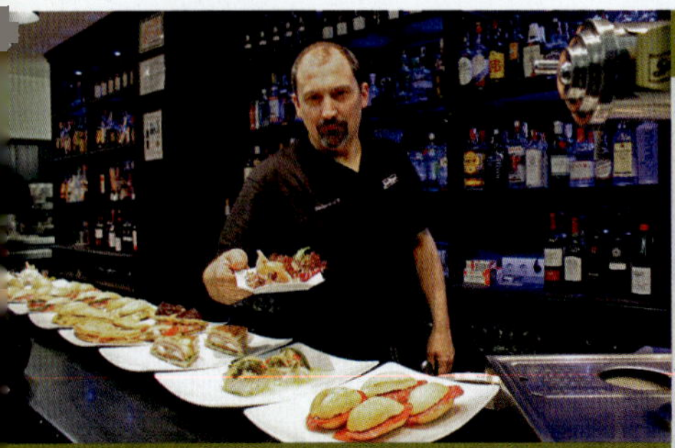

BOULEVARD 9

Alda. del Boulevard, 9 (Centro)
DONOSTIA
943 42 21 14
www.boulevard-9.com

El Jueves Santo de 2009 este local dirigido por el donostiarra **Mikel Díaz**, y hasta entonces conocido como Koquis, sufrió una profunda renovación que lo ha convertido en un lugar todavía más exitoso, si cabe, que el anterior. Además de mejorar y ampliar su oferta de pintxos de cocina, Boulevard 9 ofrece desde su fundación una variada y atractiva oferta gastronómica con una completa **carta tradicional** que incluye una **gran variedad de Ensaladas templadas** (de Gula del norte, de cabra, de pulpo y gambas...), **Risottos** y platos como Bacalao asado con piperrada, Txipirones a la plancha, Entrecot con piquillos y patatas, Muerte por chocolate... así como una amplia oferta de menús (Menú del día, Especial de fin de semana y Menús especiales para grupos) Boulevard 9 abre a las 6 de la mañana y sirve la **carta de cafetería durante todo el día sin interrupción** (pintxos, bocadillos, sandwiches...).

Otros pintxos:

- *Foie a la plancha*
- *Solomillo de cerdo a la plancha con queso de cabra*
- *Brocheta de gambas*
- *Bakalao asado con piperrada*
- *Morros guisados en salsa*
- *Queso de cabra con cebolla caramelizada*
- *Carrillera ibérica al vino tinto*
- *Txipirón a la plancha*
- *Crustáceo crujiente*
- *Brocheta de pulpo a la gallega*

Mini ensalada de gulas y gambas

Ingredientes:

Un pequeño bouquet de ensalada (Lechuga, lollo rojo, lombarda...)
4 gambas
Un puñado de gulas
2 tomatitos cherry
Ajo
Aceite de oliva

- **Para la vinagreta:**

Aceite de oliva virgen extra
Aceite de vino
Sal

Elaboración:

Para la vinagreta: En un bol, mezclamos cuidando de emulsionar bien el aceite de oliva virgen extra, el vinagre de vino y la sal. Reservamos.

Pelamos los ajos, los laminamos y los ponemos a freír en una sartén con un poco de aceite de oliva a fuego vivo. Cuando empiecen a coger color añadimos las gambas previamente peladas, las salteamos y cuando estén casi hechas incorporamos las gulas y les damos un par de golpes a fuego vivo.

Cortamos los tomatitos cherry por la mitad y los reservamos.

Final y presentación: En un pequeño bol disponemos el bouquet de lechuga. Sobre él, los tomatitos cherry y, finalmente, el salteado de gulas y gambas. Aliñamos el conjunto con la vinagreta .

Nota: Con un precio similar al de un pintxo, estas miniensaladas (en Boulevard 9 también las hay de pulpo y langostinos o de queso de cabra y nueces) son la alternativa ideal y sana al pikoteo tradicional.

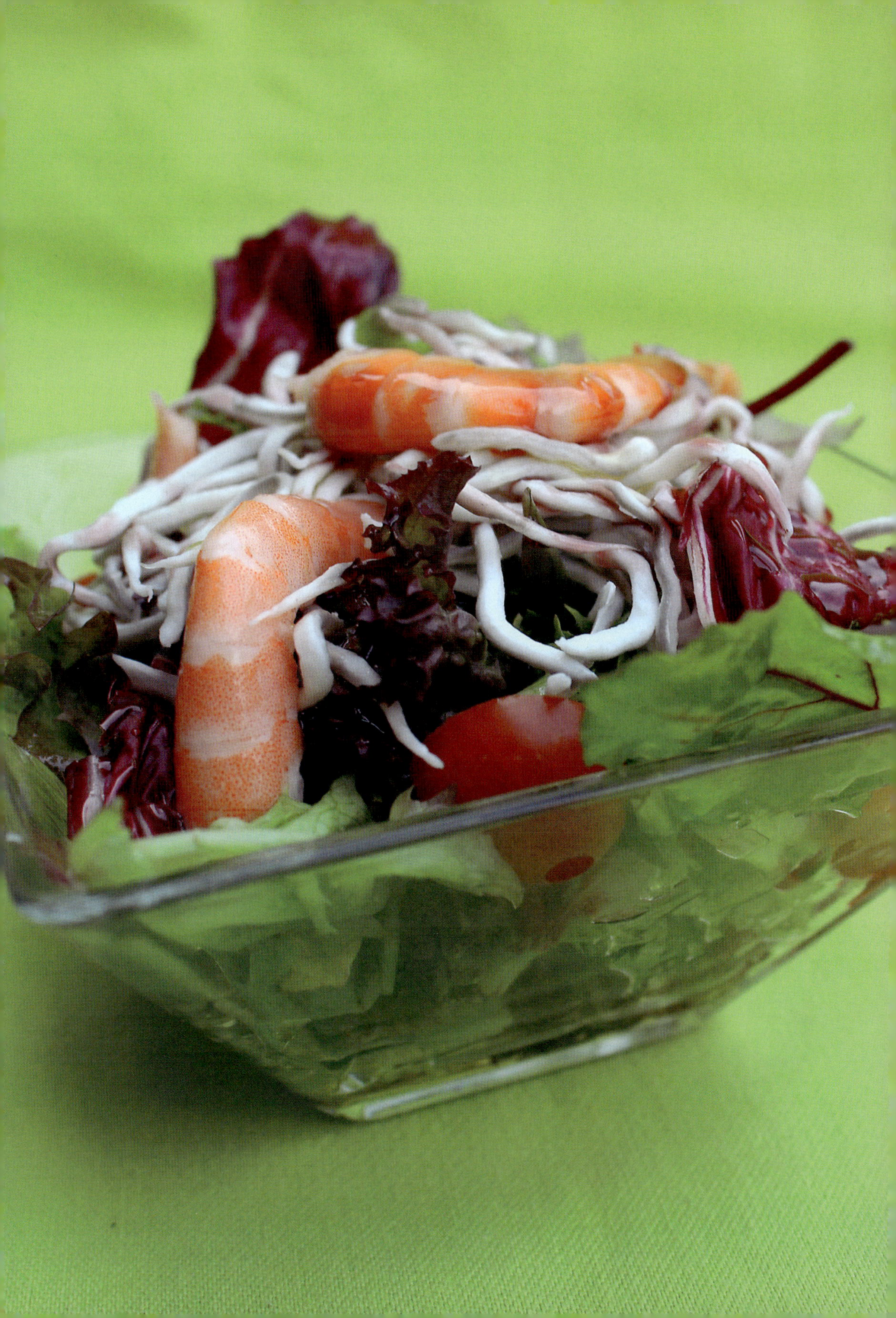

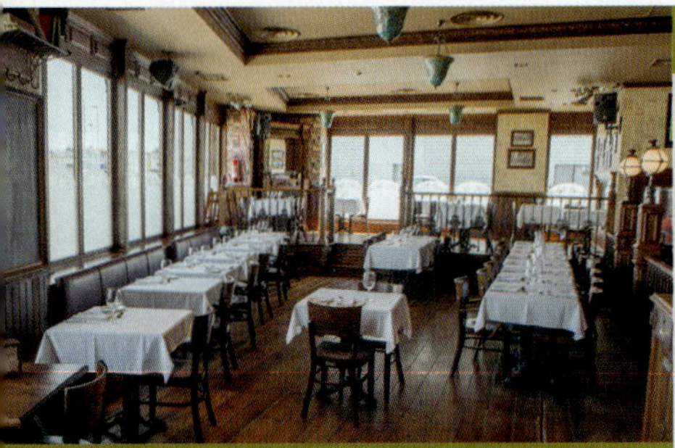

CAFÉ IRUN

Inaugurado en julio de 2008, Café Irun es un espacio **especialmente indicado para celebrar todo tipo de eventos** (Comidas de empresa, celebraciones familiares, bodas, post-bodas...) debido a la versatilidad de sus salones, discoteca incluida, su cómodo y amplio parking y su gran capacidad, pudiendo acoger **hasta 240 personas sentadas** entre sus tres plantas. En su restaurante podemos optar por el solicitado menú con 10 primeros, 10 segundos y 10 postres a elegir, su menú especial o su carta con **carnes y pescados a la parrilla** y platos entre los que destacan sus ensaladas o sus cuidados postres. En su barra podemos encontrar desde primera hora de la mañana una **esmerada selección de pintxos y un café especialmente mimado**, tanto en su calidad como en su servicio. Café Irun cuenta, además, con un **Club de fumadores** en su planta de sótano.

Avda. Letxunborro, 91
IRUN
943 63 73 77
www.cafeirun.com

Otros pintxos:

- *Croqueta de jamón, hongos o bacalao*
- *"Champis" en salsa*
- *Langostino crujiente*
- *Ravioli crujiente de alcachofa con jamón ibérico de Bellota*
- *Pan de cristal con tomate y aceite de oliva virgen extra*
- *Vieira gratinada*
- *Chorizo a la sidra*
- *Txipirón a la plancha*
- *Foie Gras fresco a la plancha*

Lata de micuit sobre cama de manzana y cebolla

Ingredientes:

Foie micuit
Manzana Granny Smith
Cebolla
Azúcar moreno
Mantequilla
Pan

Elaboración:

Cortar la manzana y la cebolla en Juliana y caramelizarla en una sartén con mantequilla a fuego muy suave.

Disponer en el fondo de la lata la cebolla y la manzana caramelizada. Colocar encima una rodaja de foie micuit y espolvorear con el azúcar moreno.

Con la ayuda de un soplete, quemar la superficie del micuit para que el azúcar se tueste.

Presentar sobre plato de pizarra negra acompañado de unas rodajas de pan tostado al horno o a la plancha.

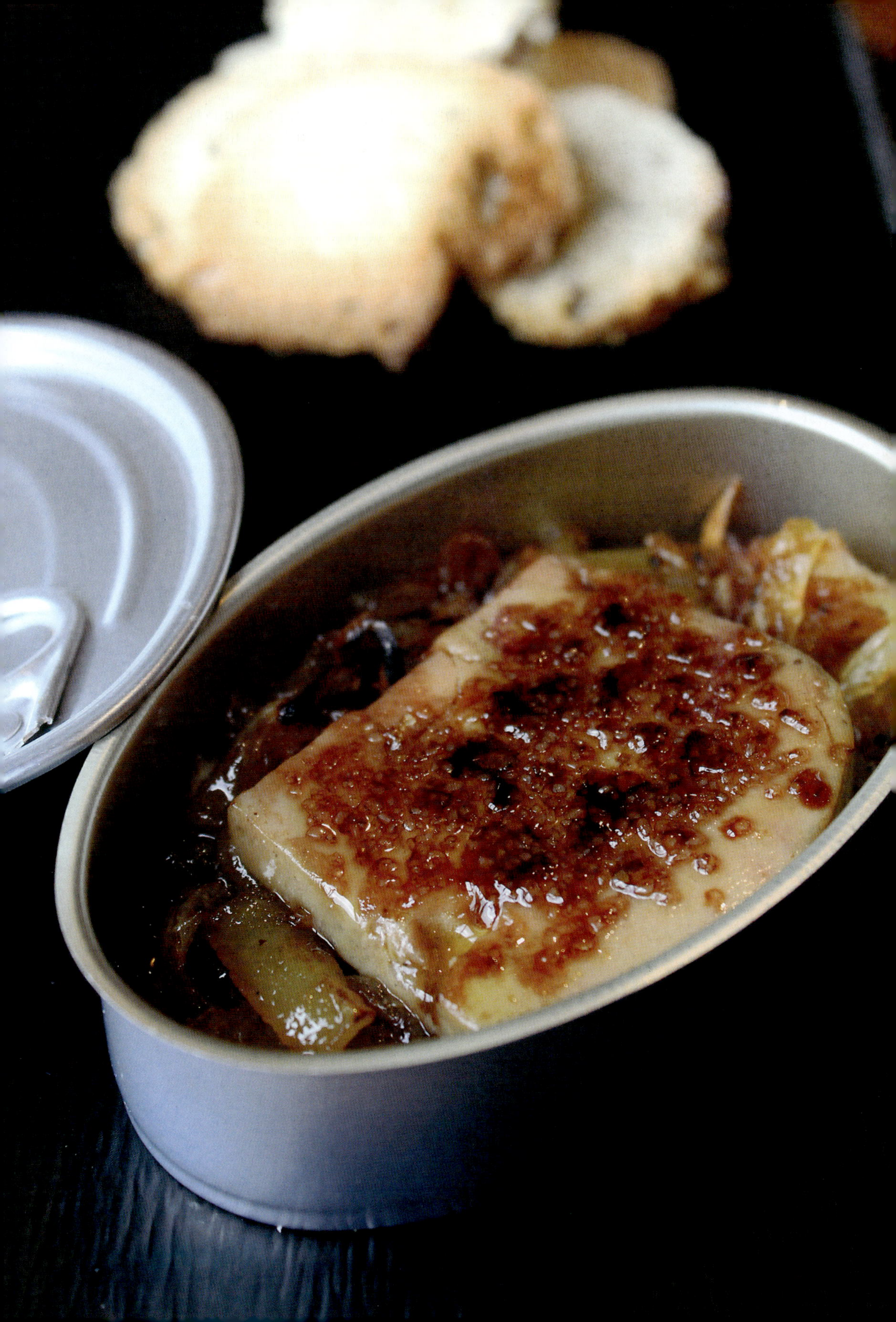

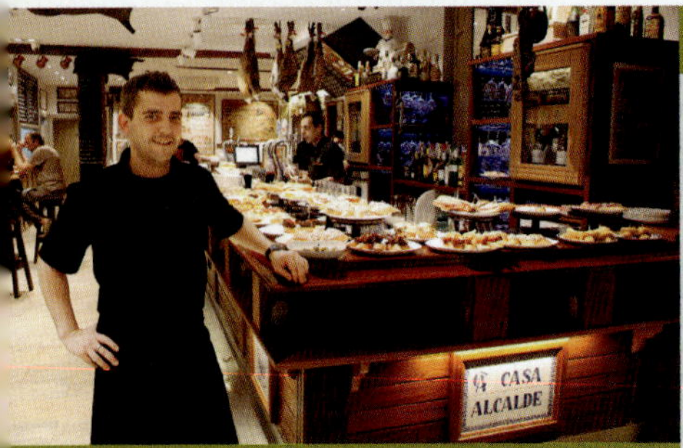

CASA ALCALDE

Casa Alcalde es el legado de **Joseba Iraizoz**, cocinero de Baztan fallecido en 2011 que, tras haber trabajado como jefe de cocina siendo muy joven y de la mano de Luis Irizar en lugares como el Hilton de Londres y los mejores establecimientos de dicha cadena en Oriente Medio, recaló en 1980 en la Parte Vieja donostiarra para adquirir el hoy centenario establecimiento **(Restaurante fundado en 1897)** y poder atender mejor a su familia. Entonces acababa de nacer su hijo **Eki**, que es hoy en día el responsable del bar tras haber aprendido el oficio de la mano de su padre. Eki lleva desde 1997 trabajando en Casa Alcalde y conoce todos los entresijos del negocio a los que poquito a poco va introduciendo pequeñas novedades, como la reforma a la que sometió al bar a inicios de 2014 y que ha cambiado sensiblemente su fisonomía, manteniendo, eso sí, su estilo y su espíritu.

Mayor, 19 (Parte Vieja)
DONOSTIA
943 42 62 16
www.casaalcalde.com

Otros pintxos:

- *"Txapela"*
- *Remix (Jamón, queso, pimiento)*
- *Queso de cabra con membrillo, nueces y miel*
- *Alcachofa albardada con bacon y vinagreta*
- *Jamón con pimiento verde, rojo y antxoa*
- *Bonito con tomate, cebolla pochada y vinagreta*
- *Albóndiga caliente con patata panadera*
- *Antxoa rebozada*
- *Crema de Roquefort con caramelo y nuez*
- *Tartaleta de txangurro*

Lazo de antxoa y boquerón

Ingredientes:

Antxoa en salazón
Boquerón marinado
Jamón ibérico
Tomate cherry del Baztan
Perejil
Cebolla
Aceite de oliva
Semillas de amapola
Pan
Reducción de Módena

Elaboración:

Cortamos la cebolla en juliana y la pochamos lentamente, a fuego suave, en aceite de oliva hasta que quede bien blandita.

Hacemos el tomate cherry del Baztan al horno durante unos 10minutos, a 180°.

Freímos en aceite de oliva muy caliente el perejil para que quede crujiente.

Final y presentación: Tostamos una rodaja de pan al horno o a la plancha. Sobre ella disponemos la cebolla caramelizada, una rodaja de jamón ibérico en crudo y la antxoa y el boquerón formando un lazo como puede apreciarse en la imagen. Coronamos con el tomate cherry asado al horno e insertamos el conjunto con un palillo. Terminamos de decorar con el perejil crujiente, la reducción de Módena y las semillas de amapola.

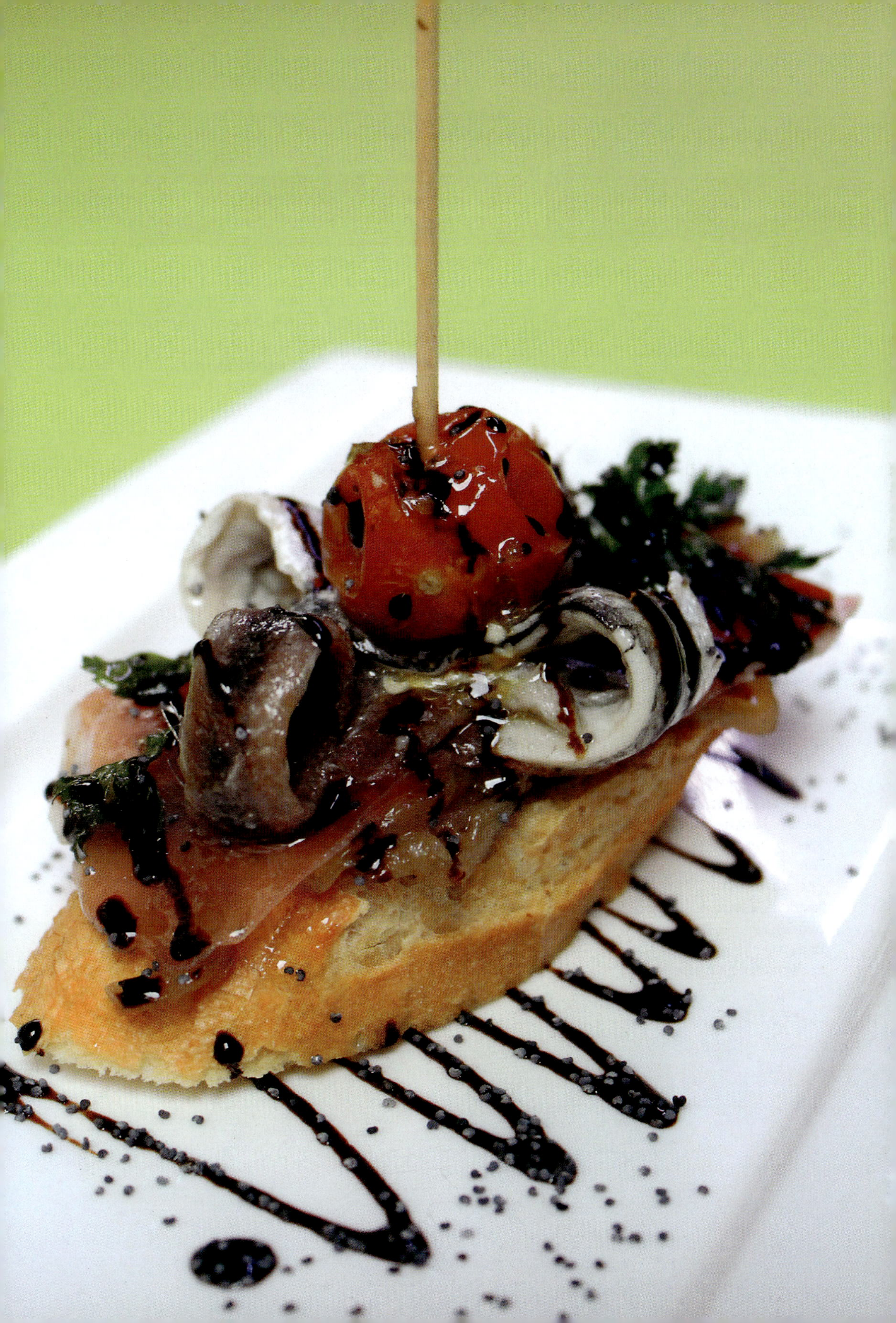

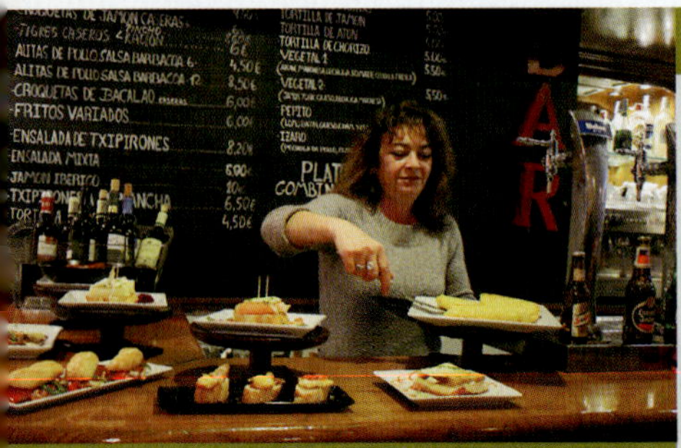

Azara, 4
ZARAUTZ
943 13 28 44
www.casa-izaro.com

CASA IZARO

Nathalie Rebichon, nacida en Dax y asentada desde 2010 en Zarautz dirige desde 2012 este emblemático y céntrico bar situado a un paso de la playa donde el cliente será perfectamente atendido en euskara, francés, castellano, inglés o incluso en brasileño. En su barra, se sirve una amplia variedad de pintxos, así como Croquetas caseras y unos recomendables calamares en tempura elaborados al momento. En Casa Izaro se ofrece una **cocina tradicional vasca con productos de calidad adquiridos en Iparralde** como el Confit de pato, el Magret o el Foie Gras, que goza de gran éxito tanto en pintxo como en ración. También están introduciendo algunos platos de inconfundible sabor francés como el Gratin Dauphinois, el Beauf Bourgignon o la Tarte Tatin. Son también remarcables sus **postres caseros** como el Tiramisú, el Arroz con leche, la Mamia o su exitosa Tarta de queso. Casa Izaro abre todos los días a las 9:00 de la mañana, salvo los lunes de invierno, y cuenta con servicio de menú del día.

Otros pintxos:

- *Tortillas variadas*
- *Boquerón con atún y pimiento*
- *Antxoas con atún*
- *Salmón con atún y mayonesa*
- *Jamón ibérico con pa amb tumaca*
- *Txipirón a la plancha*
- *Txistorra navarra*
- *Queso de cabra a la plancha con jamón serrano*
- *Tortilla de patatas*
- *Pan pita vegetal*

Pato con salsa de melocotón

Ingredientes:

Foie fresco
Magret de pato crudo
Jamón de pato ahumado
Pan

- **Para la salsa:**

Melocotón en conserva
Azúcar
Caldo de carne
Vinagre de Módena
Sal
Pimienta negra

Elaboración:

Para la salsa: Ponemos el azúcar al fuego en una sartén antiadherente y según se va fundiendo, añadimos un poco de vinagre balsámico. Echamos el melocotón en almíbar cortado en pequeños trozos y los rehogamos ligeramente. Añadimos el caldo de carne, un poco de agua y llevamos a ebullición, dejando que hierva durante un minuto. Trituramos la salsa con la batidora y la pasamos por el chino.

Cortamos una rodaja de foie fresco y la hacemos en la sartén, vuelta y vuelta. Procedemos de la misma manera con una rodaja de magret de pato.

Final y presentación: Tostamos una rodaja de pan en la plancha y colocamos sobre ella la rodaja de foie a la plancha. Sobre ella, disponemos la rodaja de magret y encima de ésta, una loncha de jamón de pato ahumado. Napamos el conjunto con la salsa de melocotón y servimos acompañado de unas hojitas de lechuga y unos hilitos de reducción de módena.

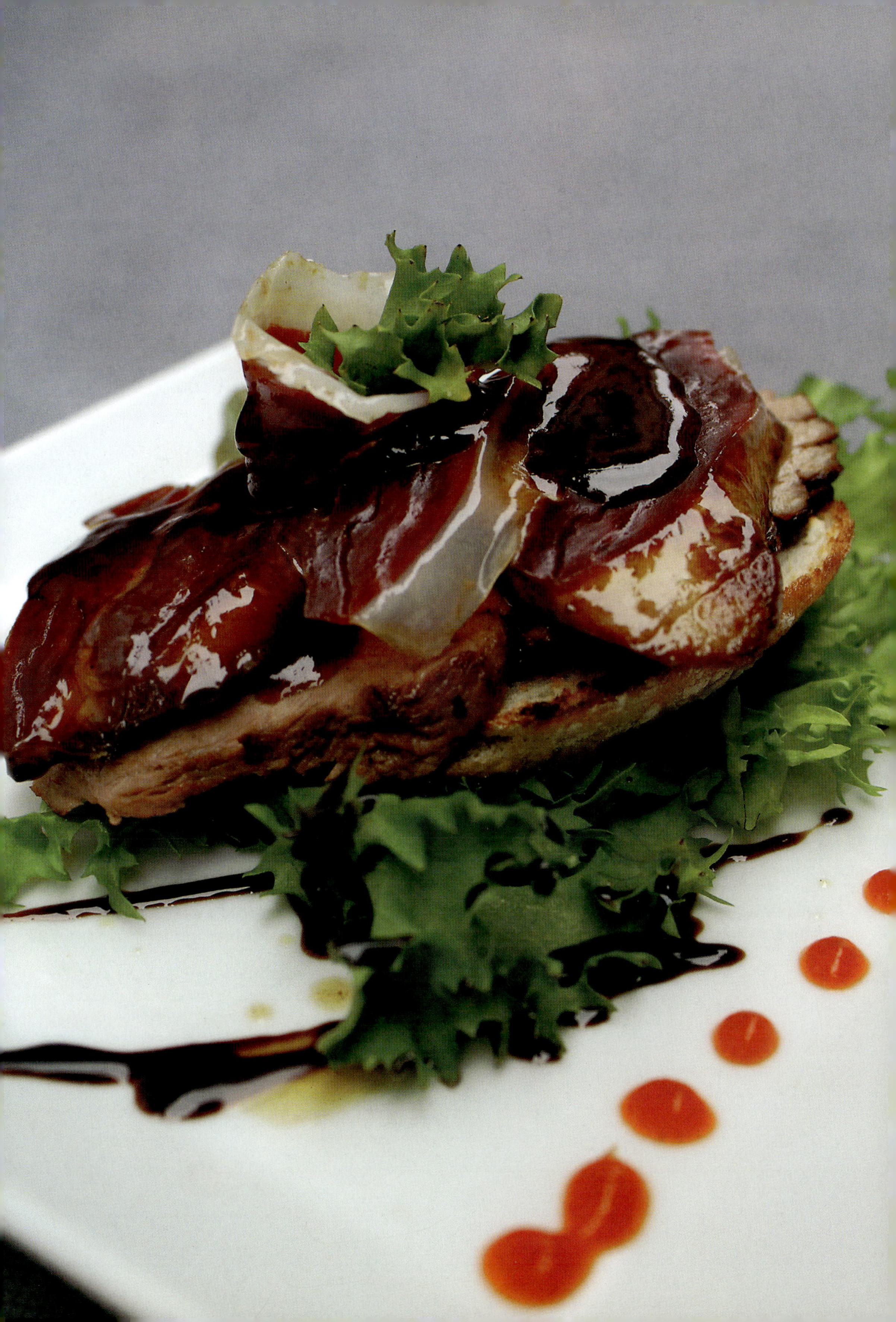

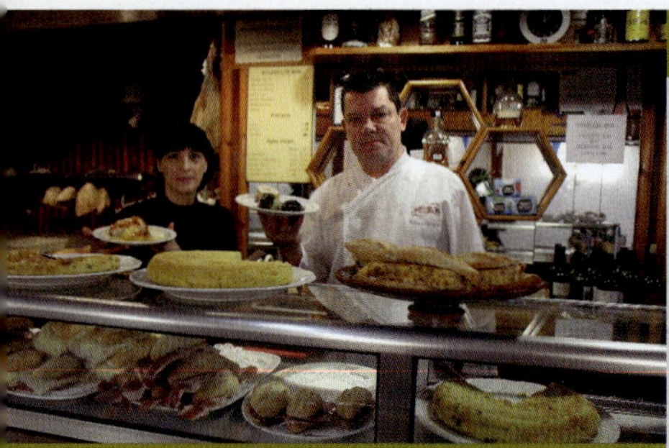

P° de Vizcaya, 14 (Amara)
DONOSTIA
943 46 10 62
www.casamaruxa.com

CASA MARUXA

"Un rincón de Galicia en Donosti" es el slogan que utiliza **Sebas Liñeiro** al referirse a su restaurante, y el lema del mismo, en sus propias palabras: **"Simpatía, precio, calidad, cantidad y buen ambiente"**. Sebas aprendió a cocinar compartiendo los fogones con su madre, **Maruxa Liñeiro**, que vino de A Coruña en 1967. Comenzó con una casa de comidas en Intxaurrondo para pasar a llevar la Casa de Galicia de la calle Zabaleta en 1980. En 1984 abrió el restaurante actual, que ha pasado a dirigir su hijo Sebas junto con su compañera **Ana Bermejo**, en 2010. Sebas sigue la tradición familiar cocinando como lo hacía su madre, en los mismos pucheros de los que salen las mejores especialidades gallegas: pulpos cocinados divinamente, caldos gallegos, caldeiradas y mariscos de primera categoría. En Maruxa se sirve también un gran jamón de Jabugo, hermosas mariscadas por encargo y una gran variedad de pintxos de cocina.

Otros pintxos:

- *Pimiento relleno de bacalao*
- *Bola de carne picante*
- *Bola de marisco*
- *Pintxo de lacón*
- *Croquetas caseras de jamón*
- *Tortillas variadas*

Raciones:

- *Pulpo*
- *Caldo gallego*
- *Pimientos de Padrón (En temporada)*

Pimiento relleno de calamar y gamba

Ingredientes:

Pimiento del piquillo
Calamar
Gambas
Cebolla
Aceite
Sal
Tomate frito
Tinta de calamar
Nata
Pan

Elaboración:

Picamos muy finamente la cebolla y la ponemos al fuego a pochar casi hasta que caramelice. Mientras se hace la cebolla, cortamos en porciones pequeñitas el calamar y las gambas y los salteamos. Una vez hecho, mezclamos todo con la cebolla y le damos el punto de sal.

Rellenamos los pimientos del piquillo con la farsa de calamar, gambas y cebolla.

En una cazuela ponemos el tomate frito a coger calor y le añadimos las tintas de calamar y un poco de nata. Removemos bien y cuando la salsa esté ligada, añadimos los pimientos ya rellenos. Dejamos hervir todo junto durante 10 minutos.

Final y presentación: Servimos en el plato un pimiento, lo napamos con la salsa y lo acompañamos de un trozo de pan. Podemos complementarlo con un cachelo o patata cocida.

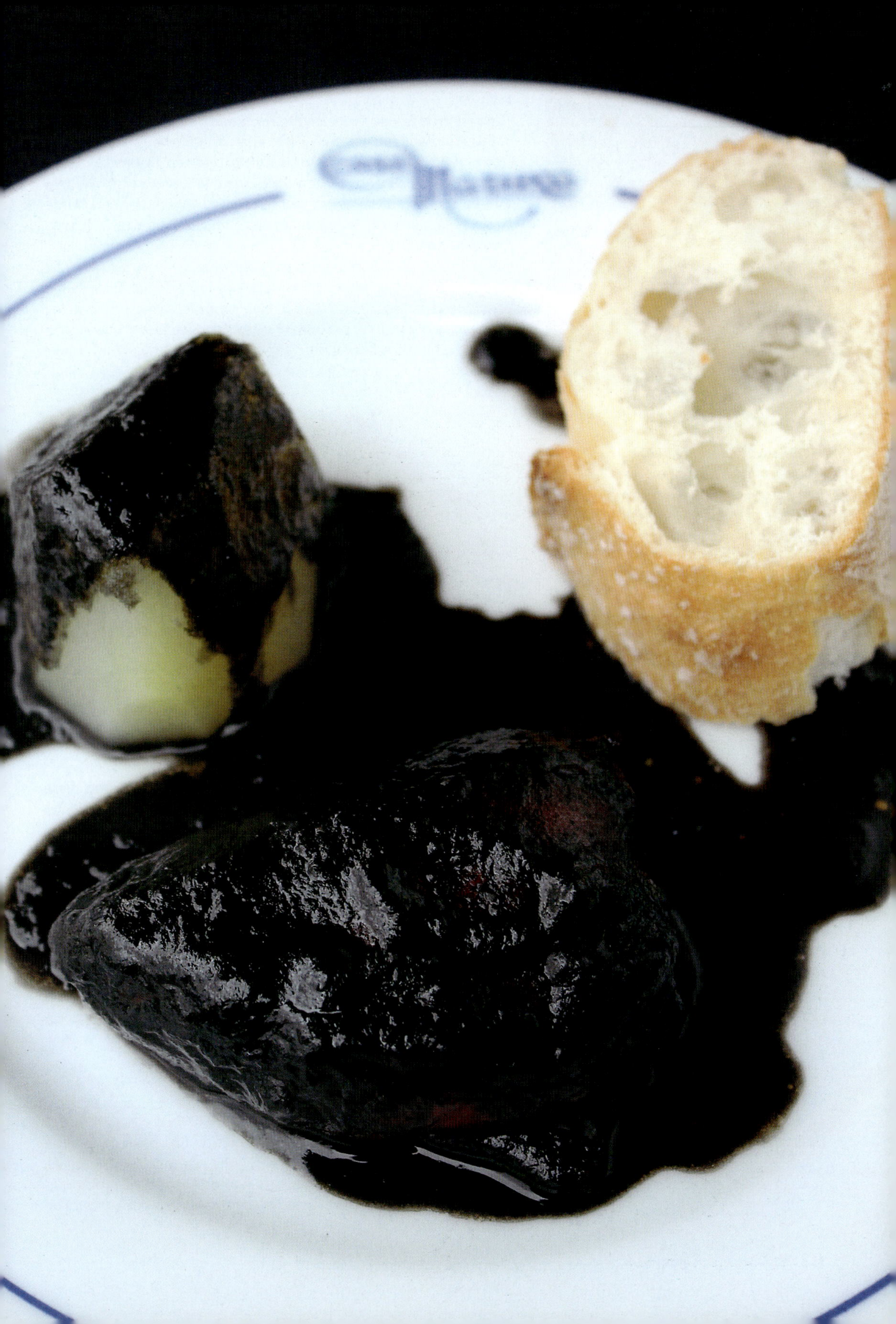

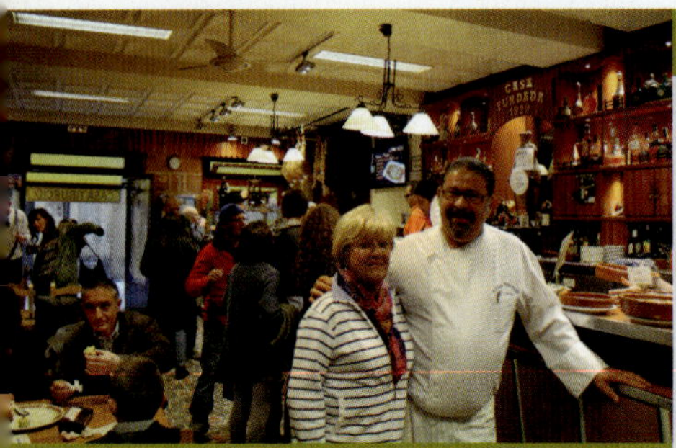

CASA TIBURCIO

Casa Tiburcio es uno de los bares en los que más fielmente ha perdurado la tradición familiar de la Parte Vieja. Dirigido hoy en día a los fogones por **Tibur Eskisabel,** fue su abuelo, también **Tiburcio**, quien lo inauguró en 1929 y sus padres, **José Luis y Mª Carmen**, todavía presentes en el local, quienes han mantenido viva la llama del restaurante hasta la actualidad en la que, además de Tibur, trabaja en el mismo su hermano **Jon**.
Casa Tiburcio es tradición en estado puro. Tradición de la buena. Su alto mostrador, sus mesas de madera, sus cazuelas llenas de callos, txipirones, ajoarriero y otros guisos elaborados en casa... son señas de una estética que, inexorablemente y por desgracia, está desapareciendo de nuestros bares para dar paso a un futuro más frío y estandarizado.

Fermín Calbetón 40 (Pte. Vieja)
DONOSTIA
943 42 31 30 - 943 42 06 80
www.casatiburcio.com

Otros pintxos:

- *Tartaleta de hongo y gambas*
- *Bouquet de setas con panceta*
- *Tomates variados (seco, fresco, mermelada)*
- *Bonito en escabeche con vinagreta*
- *Tartaleta de ajoarriero*
- *Callos*
- *Cucharilla de queso con caviar de Müjol*
- *Apurras de bacalao*
- *Kokotxas de bacalao con piperrada (Ración)*
- *Txipirones de anzuelo en su tinta (Ración)*

Hongo confitado con trancha de foie y patata trufada

Ingredientes:

Hongo
Una rodaja de foie fresco
Aceite de oliva
Ajo
Sal
Cebollino

· Para la patata trufada:
Patata
Agua
Sal
Leche
Mantequilla
Aceite de trufa

· Para el consomé:
Caldo de carne
Oporto

Elaboración:

Para la patata trufada: Elaborar un puré de patata tradicional. Para ello, ponemos agua a hervir, añadimos las patatas, y una vez cocidas retiramos el agua y añadimos un poco de leche y mantequilla. Antes de triturar, añadiremos un chorro generoso de aceite de trufa.

Para el consomé: Ponemos a calentar el caldo de carne y le añadimos una copa de Oporto. Llevamos a ebullición y dejamos reducir hasta obtener una textura cremosa.

Para los hongos: Confitamos el hongo con un poco de ajo, sal yl aceite de oliva en la Thermomix, por espacio de hora y media aproximadamente, a 70-80°

Para el foie: Cortamos una rodaja de foie fresco y la hacemos a la plancha, vuelta y vuelta.

Final y presentación: Hacemos en el platillo una base de puré de patata trufado. Colocamos encima el hongo confitado y, junto a él, la trancha de foie a la plancha. Terminamos napando el pintxo con la reducción de consomé al Oporto y decoramos con una ramita de cebollino fresco.

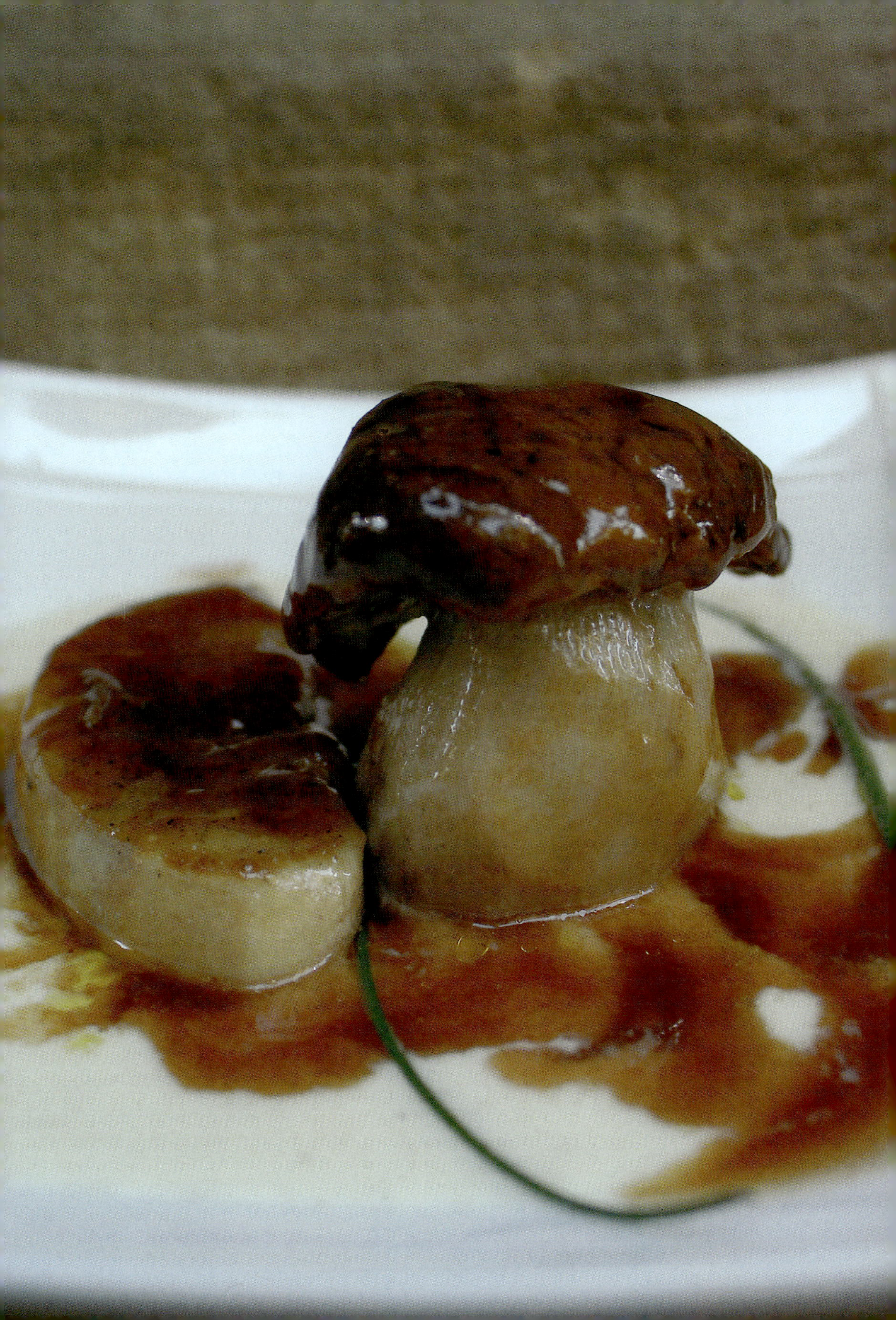

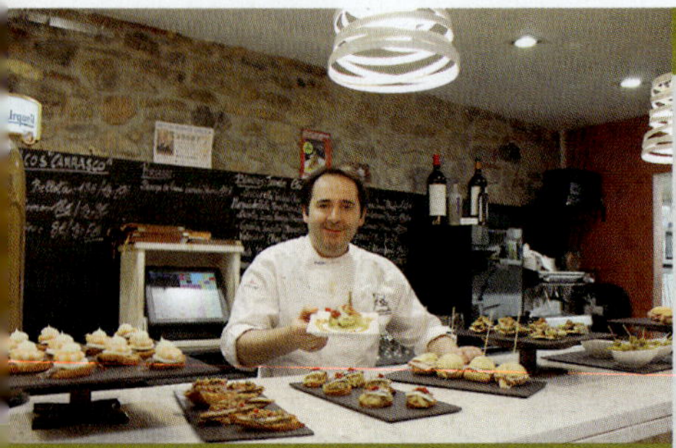

Fermín Calbetón, 20 (P. Vieja)
DONOSTIA
943 44 13 71
www.casaurolajatetxea.es

CASA UROLA

Los pintxos de temporada como éste de alcachofa y cardo a la plancha son el motor de la barra de este veterano restaurante de la Parte Vieja que ha adquirido un interesante rumbo desde que el chef donostiarra **Pablo Loureiro Rodil** se hiciera con sus riendas en 2012. Así, este pequeño pero bien abastecido mostrador se renueva con cada estación, ofreciéndonos pintxos de caza y cerdo ibérico fresco en invierno, guisantes de lágrima en primavera, hongos en verano y otoño y otras mil exquisiteces del tiempo. Pasando al comedor de la planta superior, podremos disfrutar de una carta en la que **Pablo ha renovado sin estridencias el clasicismo que siempre ha caracterizado a esta gran casa, manteniendo el carácter tradicional de su cocina y la elegancia de sus instalaciones, actualizando las cocciones y las presentaciones** y conservando algunos emblemas del restaurante como la imprescindible chuleta a la parrilla.

Otros pintxos:

- *"Urola" (Cuchara de salpicón de bogavante)*
- *Brocheta de pulpo y papada con sopa de patata*
- *Bacalao confitado, zurrukutuna y panaderas*
- *Vieira con crema de ajoblanco y vinagreta de café*
- *Carrillera guisada, verduritas y espuma de patata*
- *Foie a la plancha con puré de melocotón*
- *Taco de chuleta con piquillo*
- *Croqueta de jamón o bogavante*
- *Cazuelita de ajoarriero*
- *Txapela de hongo asado con piñones y yema de huevo*

Alcachofa y cardo a la plancha con praliné de almendras

Ingredientes:

Alcachofa
Cardo
Aceite de oliva
Almendras tostadas
Polvo de almendras tostadas
Jamón ibérico

• Para la crema de jamón:
Hojas y tallos sobrantes de la alcachofa
Aceite de jamón
Aceite de oliva
Puntas de jamón

• Para el praliné de almendras
Almendras tostadas
Aceite de girasol
Flor de sal

Elaboración:

Para la alcachofa: Quitarle todas las hojas de fuera dejando tan sólo el corazón ahuecado. Confitarla al vacío con aceite de oliva en la Thermomix 50 minutos a 95° y marcarla a la plancha.

Para el cardo: Pelar el cardo, trocearlo y cocerlo en agua con sal durante dos horas aproximadamente.

Para la crema de jamón: Cocemos las patas del tallo de la alcachofa y las hojas centrales que hemos quitado para dejarla ahuecada. Una vez cocidas les añadimos aceite de jamón, un poco de aceite de oliva y unas puntas de jamón. Trituramos el conjunto y lo confitamos al vacío en la Thermomix, por espacio de 20 minutos a 60°.

Para el praliné de almendra: Mezclamos almendras tostadas con un poco de aceite de girasol y flor de sal y lo trituramos en la Thermomix hasta alcanzar la textura deseada.

Final y presentación: Sobre una base de crema de jamón colocamos 2 alcachofas y dos pedazos de cardo. Rodeamos el pintxo con el praliné de almendras y lo terminamos añadiendo unas lascas de jamón ibérico al natural, unas almendras tostadas picadas y polvo de almendra tostada.

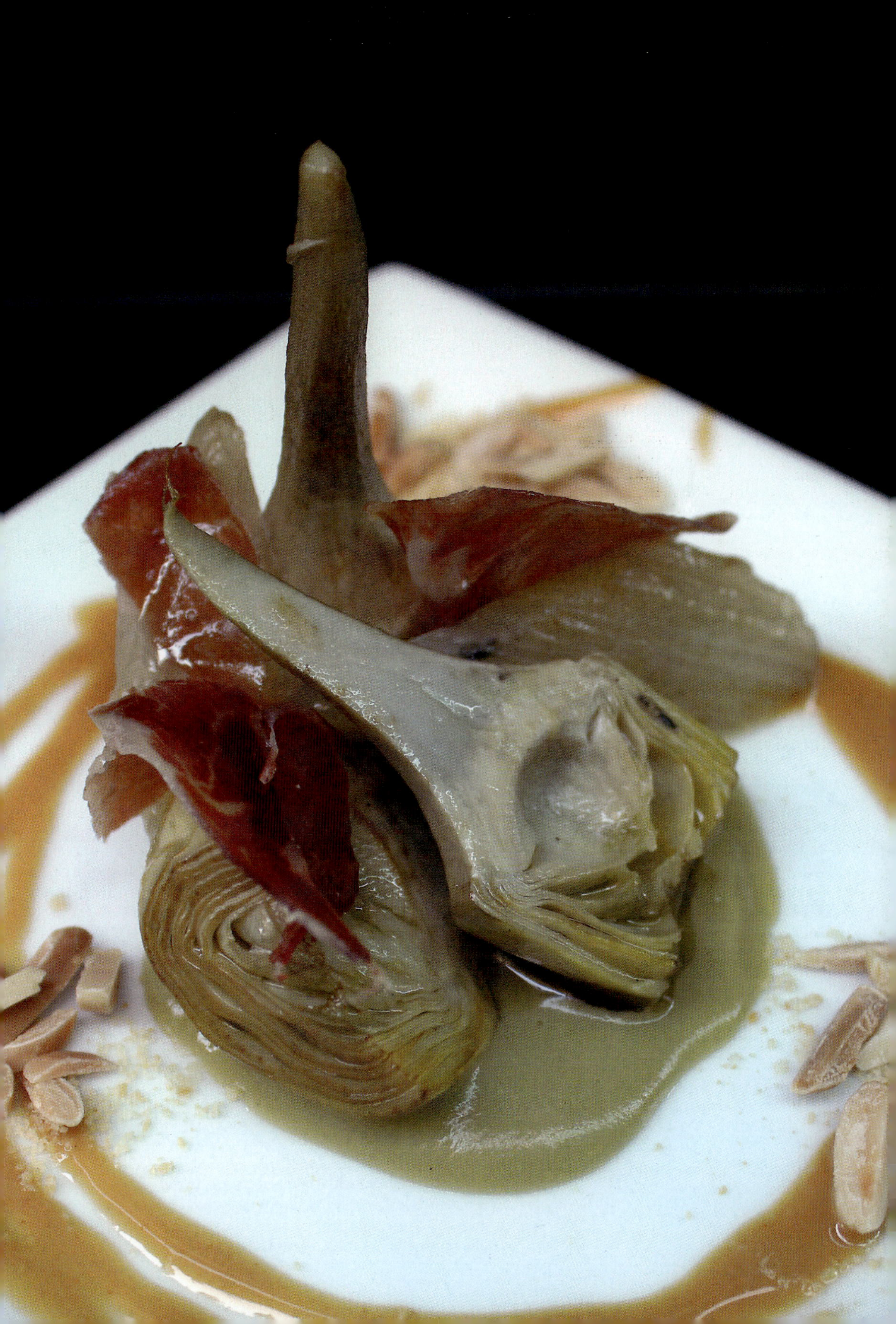

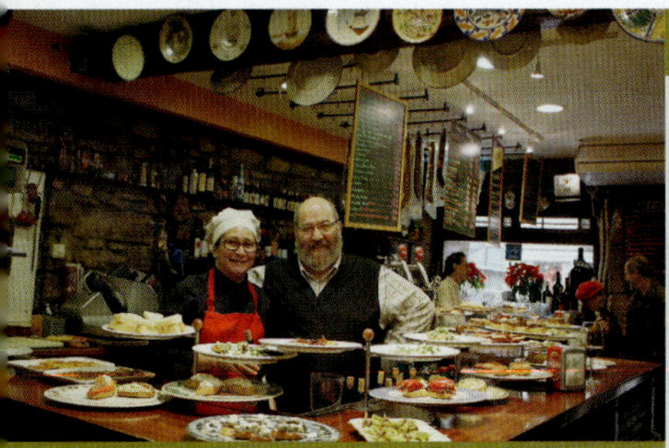

CASA VERGARA

La arrolladora personalidad de **Álvaro Manso** es la principal seña de identidad de este emblemático local de la Parte Vieja que **se ha alzado en tres ocasiones con el Premio al Label Vasco en el Campeonato de Pintxos de Gipuzkoa** gracias a sus pintxos "Manolo", "Mauri" y "Habanito", además del premio a la Originalidad por su pintxo "El incomprendido". Desde sus inicios, la cocina ha estado dirigida por la brasileña **Vera María Cruz da Silva**, esposa de Álvaro, que tras estudiar en la escuela de Luis Irizar ha alcanzado un dominio envidiable de la cocina tradicional vasca. La oferta de este local es abrumadora, con **más de 50 pintxos fijos en barra, una carta de vinos con más de 300 referencias** y una atractiva carta en la que destacan los pescados traídos directamente del puerto, la chuleta y el exquisito Arroz con bogavante.

Mayor, 21 (Pte. Vieja)
DONOSTIA
943 43 10 73
www.casavergara.com

Otros pintxos:

- *Habanito*
- *Manolo*
- *Incomprendido*
- *Colas de macaco*
- *Kali*
- *Txangurro al horno*
- *Pulpo asado*
- *Solomillo al Roquefort*
- *Bola de cabrón*
- *Crema de erizo*

Ternera agridulce

Ingredientes:

Carrilleras de ternera
Cebolla
Puerros
Zanahorias
Vino tinto
Aceite de oliva
Agua
Sal
Pimienta
Patata
Dulce de membrillo
Aceite de oliva
Vinagre de Módena
Cebollino

Elaboración:

En una cazuela, rehogamos y sellamos las carrilleras y las reservamos. En ese mismo aceite, pochamos bien la cebolla, la zanahoria y el puerro.

Una vez pochados, añadimos las carrilleras y el vino y un chorro generoso de vinagre de Módena. Hervimos a fuego fuerte 10 minutos y, cuando haya reducido bien, añadimos agua hasta que cubra sobradamente las carrilleras.

Cocemos las carrilleras unas dos horas a fuego lento y, si hiciera falta, añadimos algo de agua. Una vez se han ablandado, retiramos la cazuela del fuego y pasamos la salsa por la batidora.

Desmigamos las carrilleras y las mantenemos otros 10 minutos cociéndose en su salsa para que terminen de soltar su gelatina.

Cortamos una rodaja de patata panadera y la confitamos en aceite de oliva.

Final y presentación: Con la ayuda de un aro de cocina, colocaremos una capa de patata confitada. A continuación una rodaja de dulce de membrillo y, sobre ésta, la carrillera desmigada. Napamos con su salsa y espolvoreamos con cebollino recién picado.

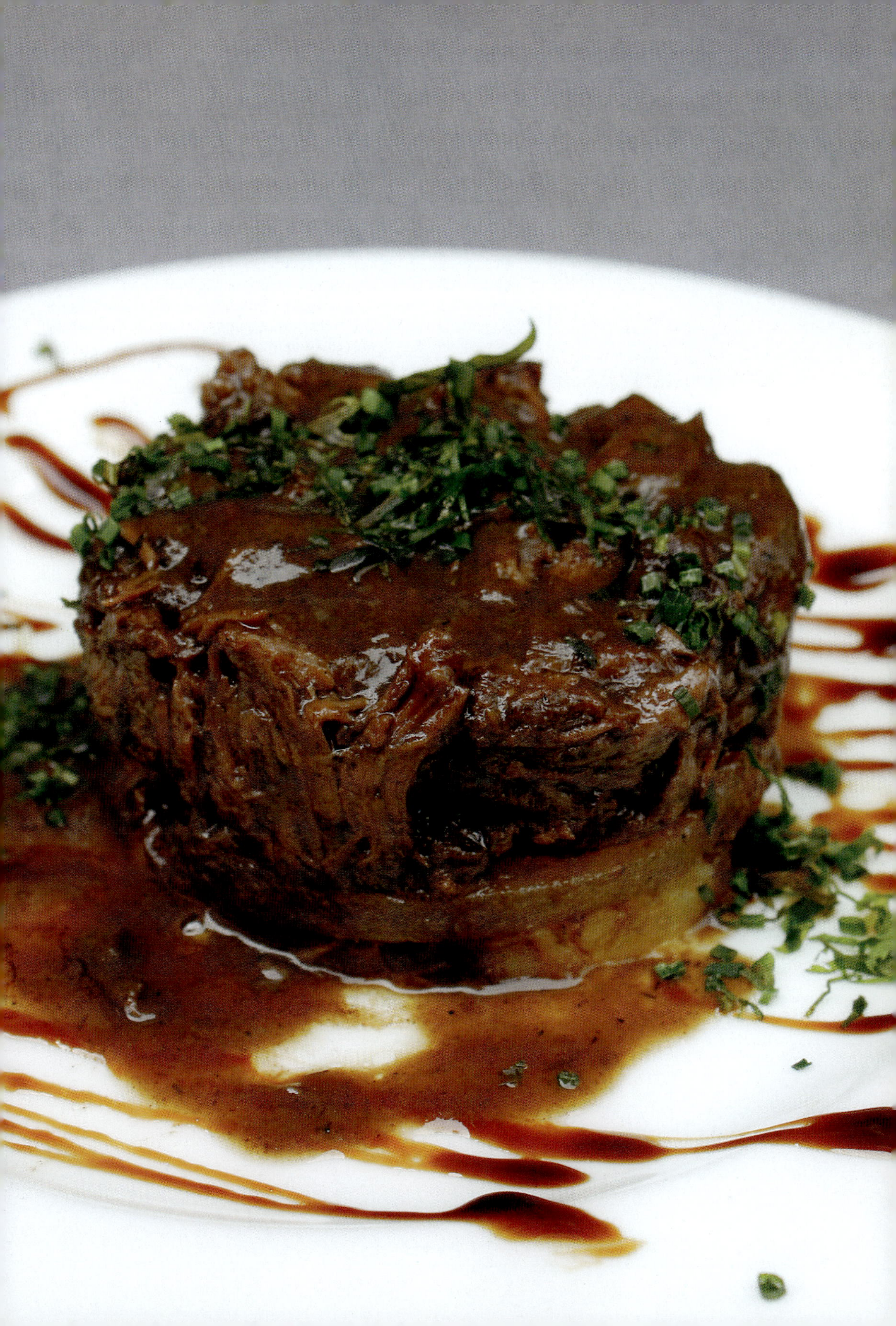

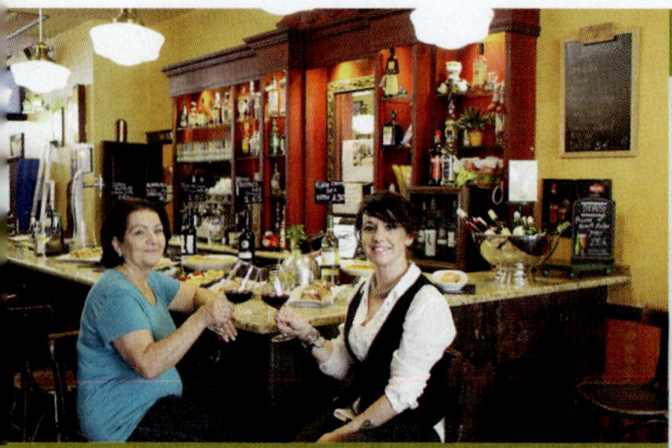

Av. Sancho el Sabio, 4 (Amara)
DONOSTIA
943 45 75 57

DERBY

La jovial y dinámica **Kriss Tarrio Barrocal** es la clave del éxito de esta cafetería en la que encontramos una variedad gastronómica no habitual en los locales de su género. Con la ayuda de su madre, **Mª Ángela Barrocal**, Kriss ofrece a su fiel clientela todo tipo de **Pintxos, Raciones, Bocadillos con pan recién horneado, buen jamón ibérico y montaditos con bonito y antxoas de Olasagasti**. Los lunes tarde, no hay que perderse la espectacular **Empanada de hojaldre de atún, elaborada al estilo gallego**, y aunque no cuenta exactamente con servicio de pintxo-pote, los sábados y domingos los pintxos se cobran al ajustado precio de 1 euro. Derby abre todos los días a las 8 de la mañana (fines de semana a las 9) ofreciendo muy buen café de Pantxito. A mediodía es recomendable degustar sus **vermouths preparados**, y al atardecer nada mejor que un buen Gin-tonic, pues no en vano Kriss obtuvo el **4° puesto en el Concurso de Gin-Tonics de Donostia** de 2013.

Otros pintxos:

- *Tortilla de patata*
- *Tortilla de champiñón*
- *Cojonudo*
- *Ibérico con queso de cabra y cebolla pochada*
- *Hojaldre de txistorra*
- *Hojaldre de bacon-queso*
- *Txipirones troceados en su tinta*
- *Gildas en vaso*
- *Rollito de pollo con bacon y queso*
- *Calabacín relleno*

Rollito de ibérico con Idiazabal

Ingredientes:

1 loncha de paletilla ibérica
1 loncha de jamón cocido
Queso Philladelphia
Queso de Idiazabal
Harina de tempura
Ajos frescos
Tomate natural
Aceite de oliva

Elaboración:

Juntamos la loncha de jamón de York con la de paletilla ibérica y las enrollamos untando el interior de queso Philladelphia. Pasamos el rollo por harina de tempura y lo freímos suavemente en abundante aceite de oliva.

Cortamos los ajos frescos en tiras largas y finas y las freímos dándoles un golpe en aceite de oliva muy caliente.

Final y presentación: Hacemos una camita con lascas de queso Idiazabal y, sobre ella, disponemos unas cucharaditas de tomate natural. Colocamos encima el rollo de jamón con tempura y coronamos el pintxo con el ajo tierno frito. Ensartamos todo con un palillo y espolvoreamos el conjunto con lascas de Idiazabal.

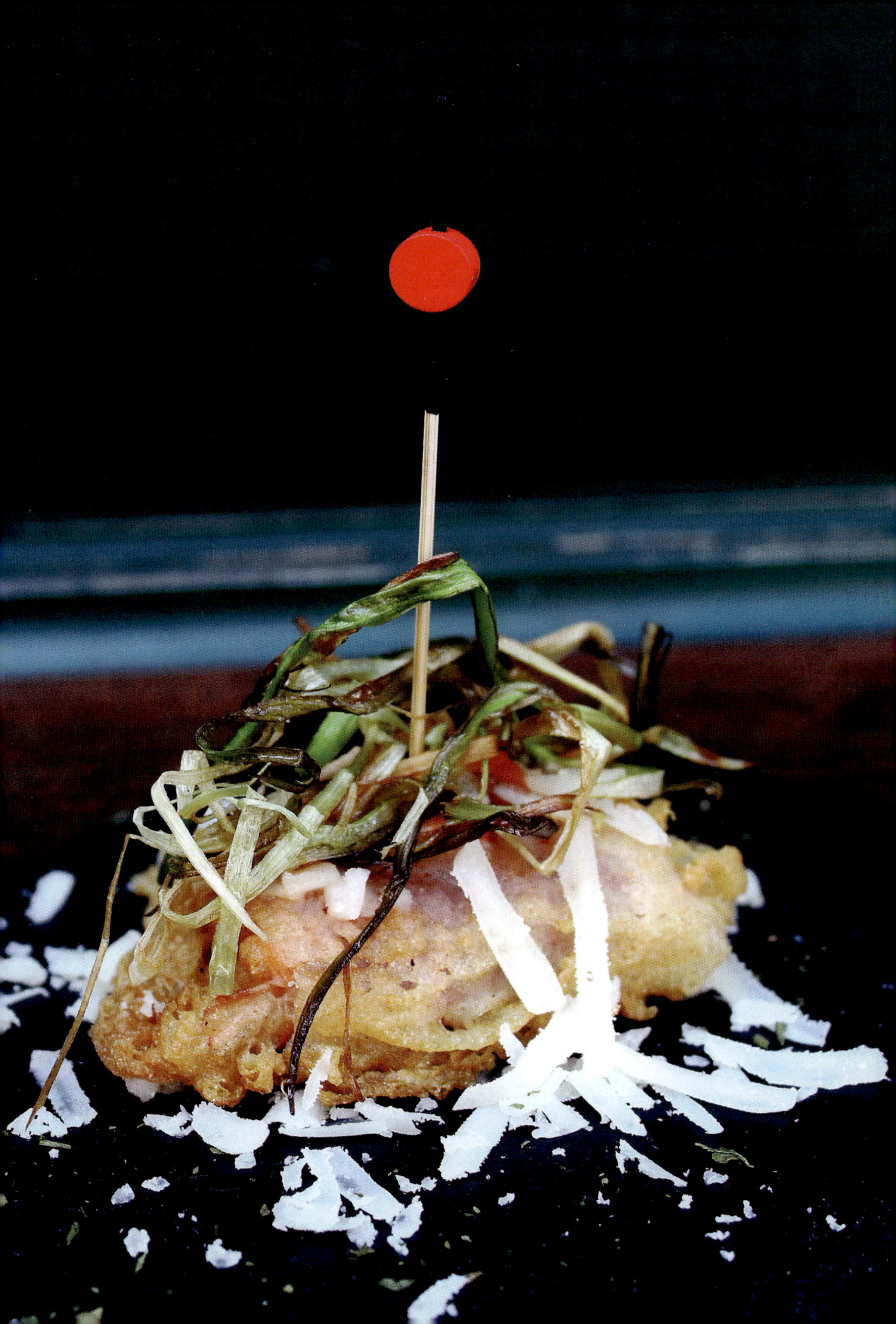

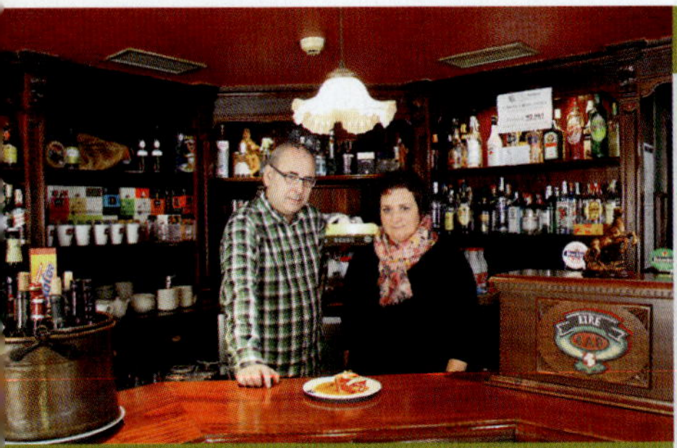

EIRE

Gernikako Arbola, 3
URRETXU
943 72 64 66
www.eiretaberna.com

Fue en mayo de 1999 cuando **Txema Iriberri** abrió este local en lo más céntrico de Urretxu, tras haber regentado durante 14 años el bar de la Estación de Renfe en Zumarraga. Eire no es un bar de pintxos, aunque su inclusión en este libro está plenamente justificada, pues de un tiempo a esta parte, **todos los jueves se pone de bote en bote durante el pintxo-pote**, momento al que se encarga de sacar chispas la media naranja de Txema, la donostiarra **Karmele Graña**, que cada jueves idea un pintxo diferente: Pulpo a feira, Brocheta de champis, bacon y gamba, Croqueta de hongos... Por otra parte, desde que abrió, Eire ofrece los sábados y domingos a mediodía Tigres y Rabas y los fines de semana al mediodía los clientes son obsequiados, además, con un frito casero. Eire es mundialmente conocido por acoger desde hace 15 años el **Torneo Eire-Bankoa de ajedrez**, declarado "de especial interés" por la Federación Vasca de Ajedrez.

Otros pintxos:

- *Pulpo a feira*
- *Brocheta de champiñones, bacon y gambas*
- *Croqueta de hongos*
- *Croqueta marinera*
- *Gamba a la gabardina*

Raciones

- *Tigres*
- *Rabas*

(Las raciones se sirven los sábados y los domingos al mediodía)

Timbal de ventresca y pimiento del piquillo

Ingredientes:

Patata
Pimiento del piquillo
Aceite de oliva
Ajo
Ventresca de bonito
Guindillas de Ibarra

- **Para la vinagreta:**

Aceite de oliva virgen extra
Vinagre de Módena
Sal

Elaboración:

Cocemos la patata durante media hora con piel. La dejamos enfriar, la pelamos y la cortamos en rodajas finas.

Cortamos los piquillos en tiras y los salteamos con un poquito de ajo picado en aceite de oliva.

Final y presentación: En un platillo, colocamos una capa de patata, sobre ella ponemos una capa de pimiento del piquillo. Repetimos la operación con una segunda capa de patata y una segunda capa de piquillo. Sobre ella, colocamos unas tiras de ventresca de bonito y coronamos el pintxo con unas guindillas de Ibarra picadas. Finalmente, aliñamos el pintxo con la vinagreta.

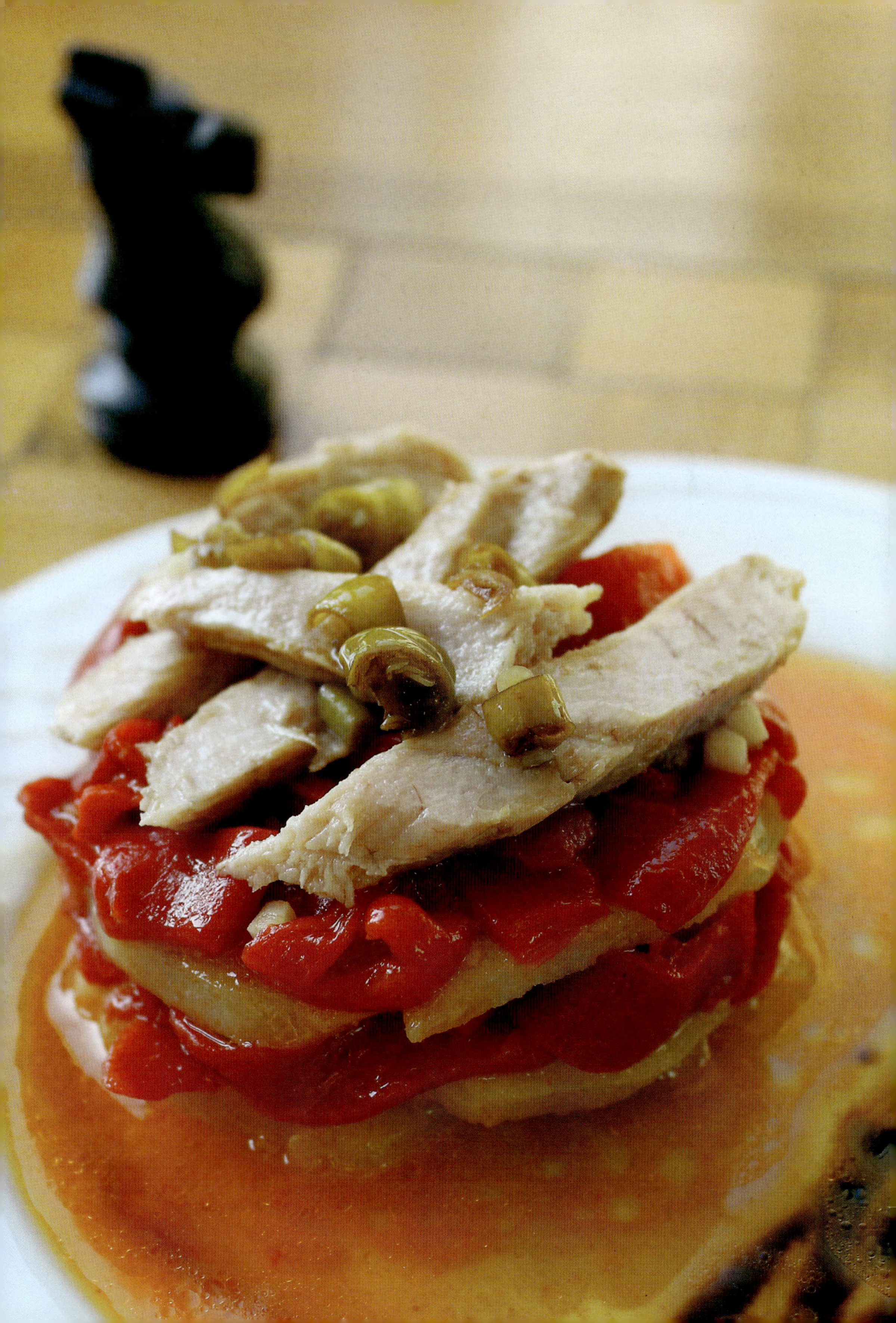

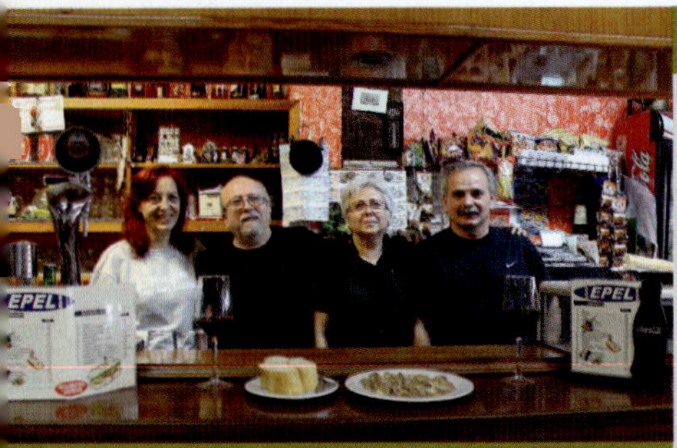

Goikale, 1
LASARTE - ORIA
943 36 27 01

EPEL

Fernando Carballés, natural de Zamora y **Paco Navarro,** granadino, llevan más de 25 años al frente de este céntrico bar de Lasarte, inaugurado a inicios de los años 60. Impulsados por el paro y la necesidad, estos cuñados apostaron por la hostelería con la indispensable ayura de sus mujeres, **Marisa y Charo. La oreja es el buque insignia de este bar, y puede ser solicitada en pintxo, en ración o en bocadillo.** De hecho, hasta cuentan con un plato combinado que incluye también la oreja entre sus ingredientes. No son pocos, además, los que la adquieren para llevar a casa. El motivo del éxito reside en su simpleza. La oreja se sirve bien cocida y acompañada de una salsita ligera como un caldo que no tiene (dicen) ningún secreto. Lo que cuenta, eso sí, es que esté bien limpia de pelo, algo de lo que se ocupan los propios responsables del bar, que queman las orejas manualmente, a base de soplete. El resultado es un bocado exquisito, de una ternura excepcional.

Otros pintxos:

- *Albóndigas*
- *Callos*
- *Champiñones*
- *Carne adobada*
- *Chorizo*

Raciones:

- *Pulpo a la gallega*
- *Carrilleras en salsa*
- *Manitas de cerdo*
- *Rabo guisado*

Oreja

Ingredientes:

Oreja de cerdo
Agua
Sal

• Para el sofrito:
Cebolla
Ajo
Guindilla
Aceite de girasol

Elaboración:

Cortamos las orejas y las depositamos en una cazuela. Las cubrimos con agua y las ponemos a cocer por espacio de una hora más o menos.

Mientras se están cociendo y va reduciendo el caldo, echamos el sofrito a la cazuela. Para ello calcularemos por cada 5 orejas, media cebolla, 2 dientes de ajo y guindilla al gusto. Picamos la cebolla, el ajo y la guindilla, lo freímos en una sartén con aceite de girasol, trituramos el sofrito y lo añadimos a la cazuela para que dé sabor al caldo de la cocción.

Terminamos de cocer las orejas y le damos el punto de sal

Final y presentación: Serviremos la oreja acompañada simplemente del caldo de la cocción.

Nota: Para elaborar este pintxo partimos de una oreja inmaculada, completamente limpia de pelo. En el Epel se encargan de hacerlo manualmente, a soplete, una a una. Teniendo en cuenta que es un bar que algunas semanas vende más de 150 kilos de oreja, eche cuentas el lector del trabajo que ello supone.

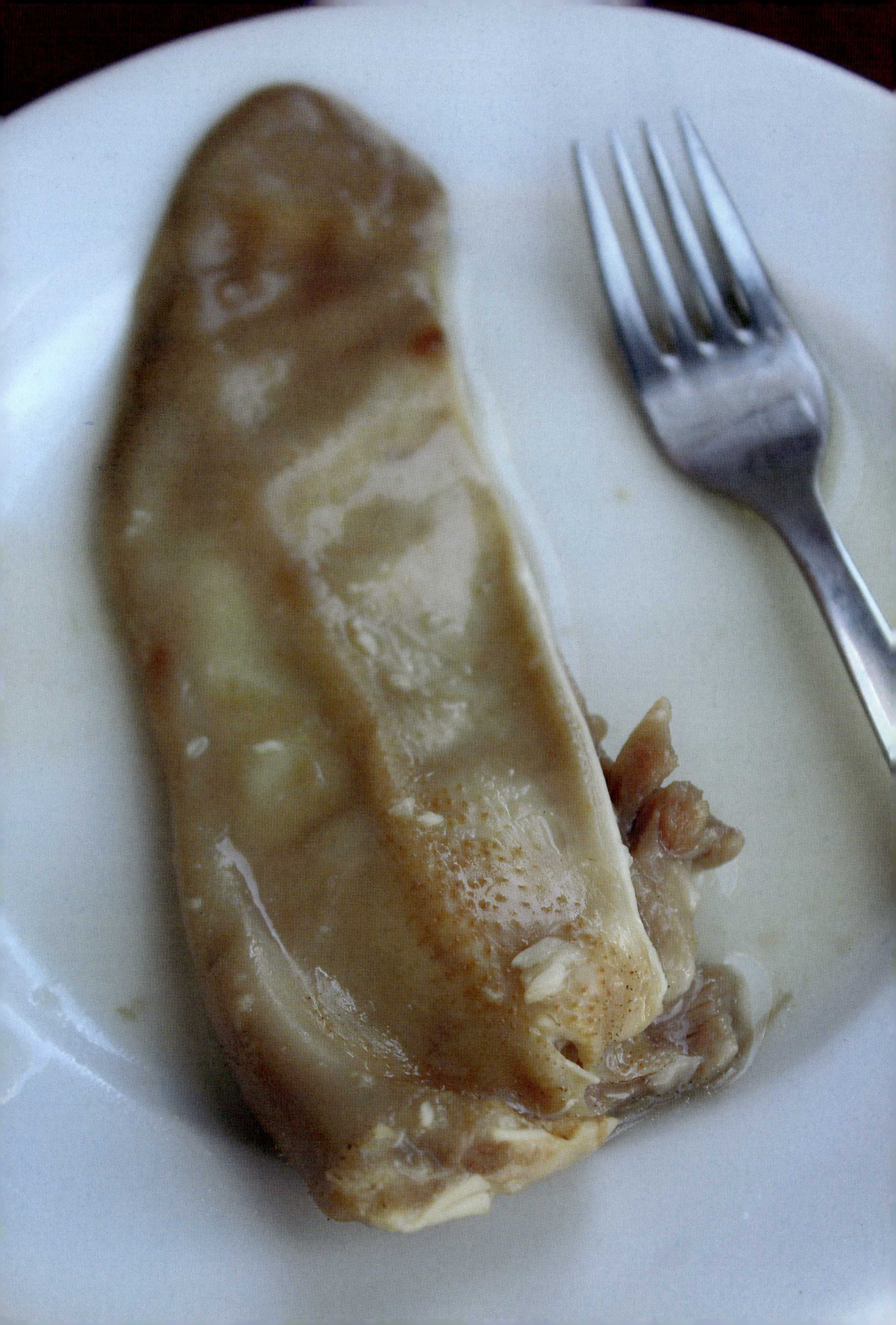

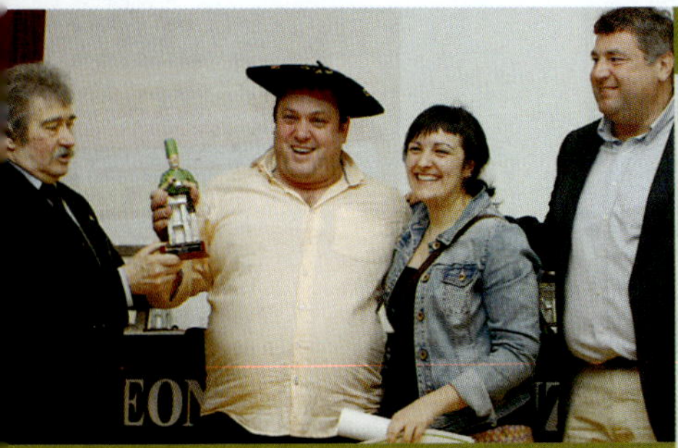

ERRENTERIAKO BATZOKIA

Iñaki Gezala es una eminencia en el mundo de la cocina en miniatura de Gipuzkoa. El pintxo cuya receta ofrecemos en este libro le valió el **Premio al Label Vasco en el Campeonato de Pintxos de Gipuzkoa de 2013** y, posteriormente, se hizo con el **Plato de Bronce en el Campeonato de 2014** con el pintxo 'Artalokume', un bocado consistente en un cuello de cordero asado a baja temperatura, al vino tinto de Rioja Alavesa y tomillo entre talos de maíz. Como se ve, la utilización de productos vascos (Txipirón, Huevo Eusko Label, Tinto de Rioja Alavesa...) es una constante en la trayectoria de este cocinero, como también lo atestigua la "Euskalburgertxerri", una hamburguesa de ternera vasca con crema de queso Idiazabal, jamón serrano y queso, que se sirve en un pan decorado con un lauburu y puede ser degustada en el bar del Batzoki de Errenteria, dirigido por Iñaki desde 2007 y donde podemos disfrutar de sus mejores pintxos así como de una excelente cocina tradicional y buenos menús.

Pza. Koldo Mitxelena, 4
ERRENTERIA
943 00 24 68

Otros pintxos:

- *Tortillas variadas*
- *Ensalada landesa de pato*
- *Arroz cremoso de hongos y foie*
- *Rulo de cordero a baja temperatura*
- *Torrija caramelizada con helado*

Raciones:

- *Morros de basatxerri*
- *Calamares*
- *Croquetas caseras*
- *Carrilleras*

No hay huevos... y el txipirón dijo "Sí !"

Ingredientes:

Txipirón
Huevo Eusko Label
Cebolla
Pan negro
Aceite de oliva
Fideos chinos

Elaboración:

Limpiamos el txipirón y le introducimos la yema de huevo y la cebolla previamente pochada en aceite de oliva.

Tapamos el txipirón con la clara de huevo montada. Freímos los tentáculos. A continuación freímos el txipirón rebozado en la clara de huevo en aceite durante 20-30 segundos. Lo reservamos en el horno o sobre una fuente de calor.

Final y presentación: Pasamos una brocha con aceite de oliva por la base del plato. Colocamos encima el txipirón con sus tentáculos y lo espolvoreamos con pan negro rallado. Terminamos de decorar con unos fideos chinos fritos.

Nota: Este pintxo le valió a Iñagi Gezala el Premio Eusko Label en el Campeonato de Pintxos de Gipuzkoa de 2013, y está incluido en el Menú de pintxos que todos los días se ofrece en el local.

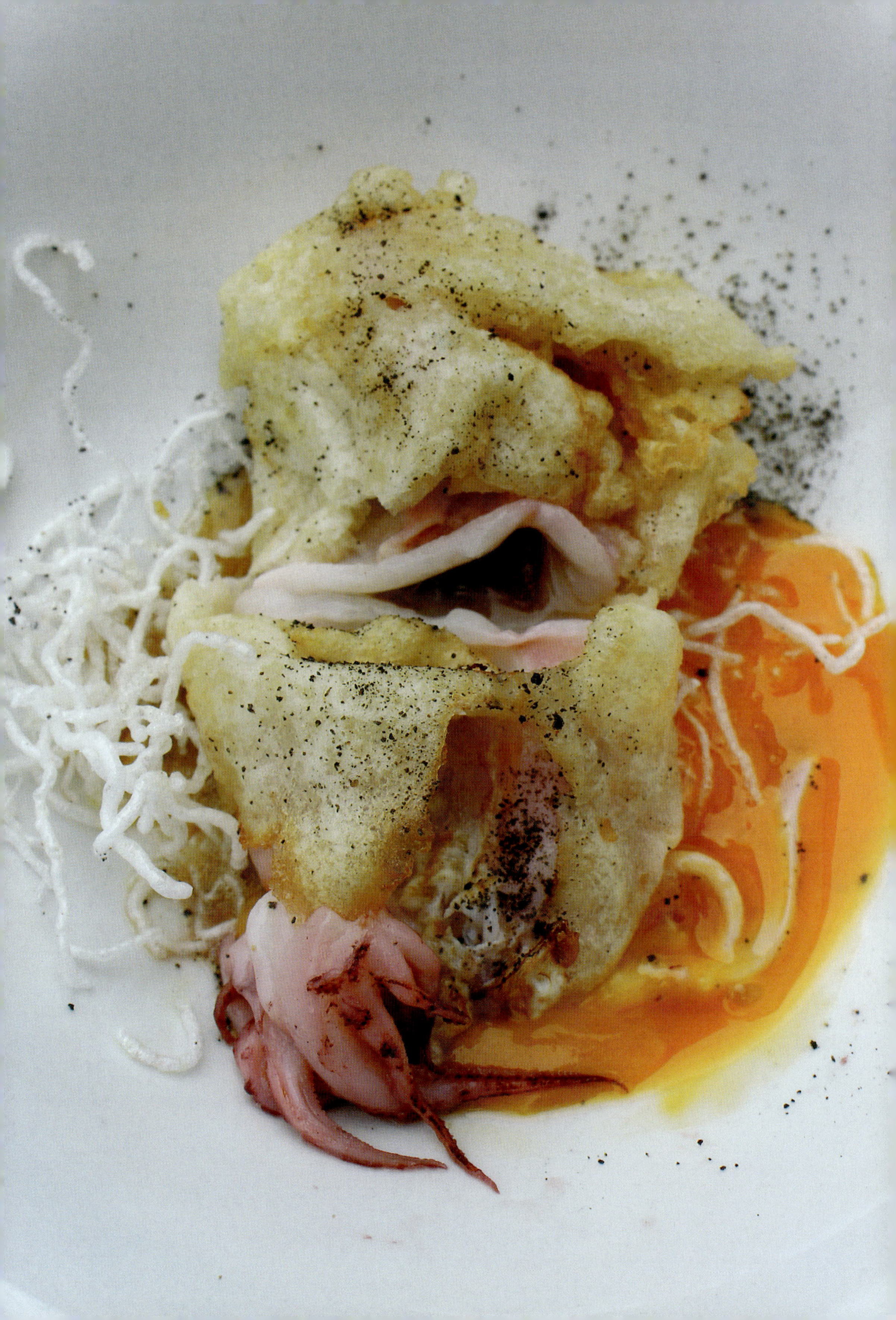

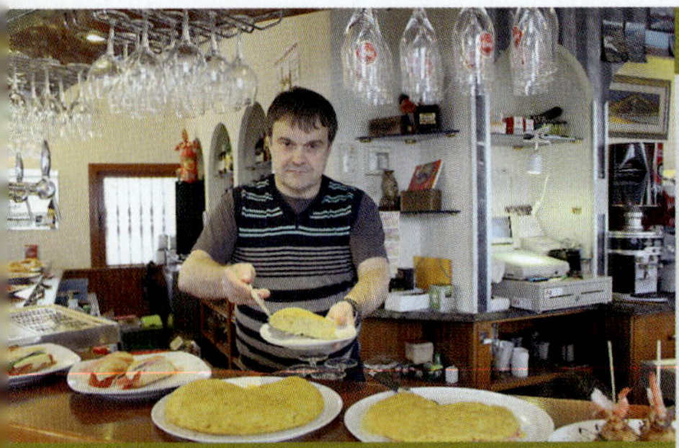

ETXAIZ

Gipuzkoa kalea, 57 (San Pelayo)
ZARAUTZ
843 98 27 31

Este amplio local, situado en la República independiente de San Pelayo, "a kilómetro y medio de Zarautz" como rezan los mojones locales, está dirigido desde febrero de 2011 por **Joseba Elorza Enbil,** que atesora **más de 30 años en hostelería**, habiendo recorrido las barras de algunos de los establecimientos más emblemáticos de la zona. En Etxaiz, además de una **amplia variedad de pintxos**, encontraremos **cazuelitas tradicionales** (Callos, Txipirones en su tinta, Albóndigas, Rabo de buey...), **bocadillos, sandwiches y hamburguesas**, brillando con luz propia la "Caprichosa", compuesta de hamburguesa, cebolla caramelizada, lechuga, tomate, bacon, jamón de york, queso, huevo frito y patatas fritas. En su comedor, Etxaiz cuenta con una **carta tradicional** con platos como Ensalada templada de bacalao, Merluza a la plancha con pimientos verdes, Costilla con ensalada... y una **gran oferta de vinos.** Una amplia y concurrida terraza complementa el local los días de buen tiempo.

Otros pintxos:

- *Jamón ibérico, queso y pimiento*
- *Tortilla de patata con cebolla*
- *Tortillas variadas*
- *Carne cocida*
- *Croquetas caseras*
- *Chorizo de Extremadura picante*
- *Txipirón a la plancha*
- *Tigre*
- *Txipirón con pimiento verde, ibérico y langostino*
- *Tosta de ibérico con tumaca*

Pan de pita con vegetal

Ingredientes:

Pan de pita
Lechuga
Tomate
Jamón de York
Queso para fundir
Huevo
Aceite de oliva
Sal

Elaboración:

Lavamos unas hojas de lechuga y las escurrimos. Lavamos el tomate y lo cortamos en rodajas.

Freímos el huevo en aceite de oliva y le damos el punto de sal.

Pasamos el pan de pita por la plancha hasta que se tueste ligeramente.

Final y presentación: Abrimos el pan de pita y sobre la base colocamos, en este orden, las hojas de lechuga, tres o cuatro rodajas de tomate, la loncha de jamón de York, el queso para fundir y el huevo frito. Cerramos el conjunto con el pan de pita.

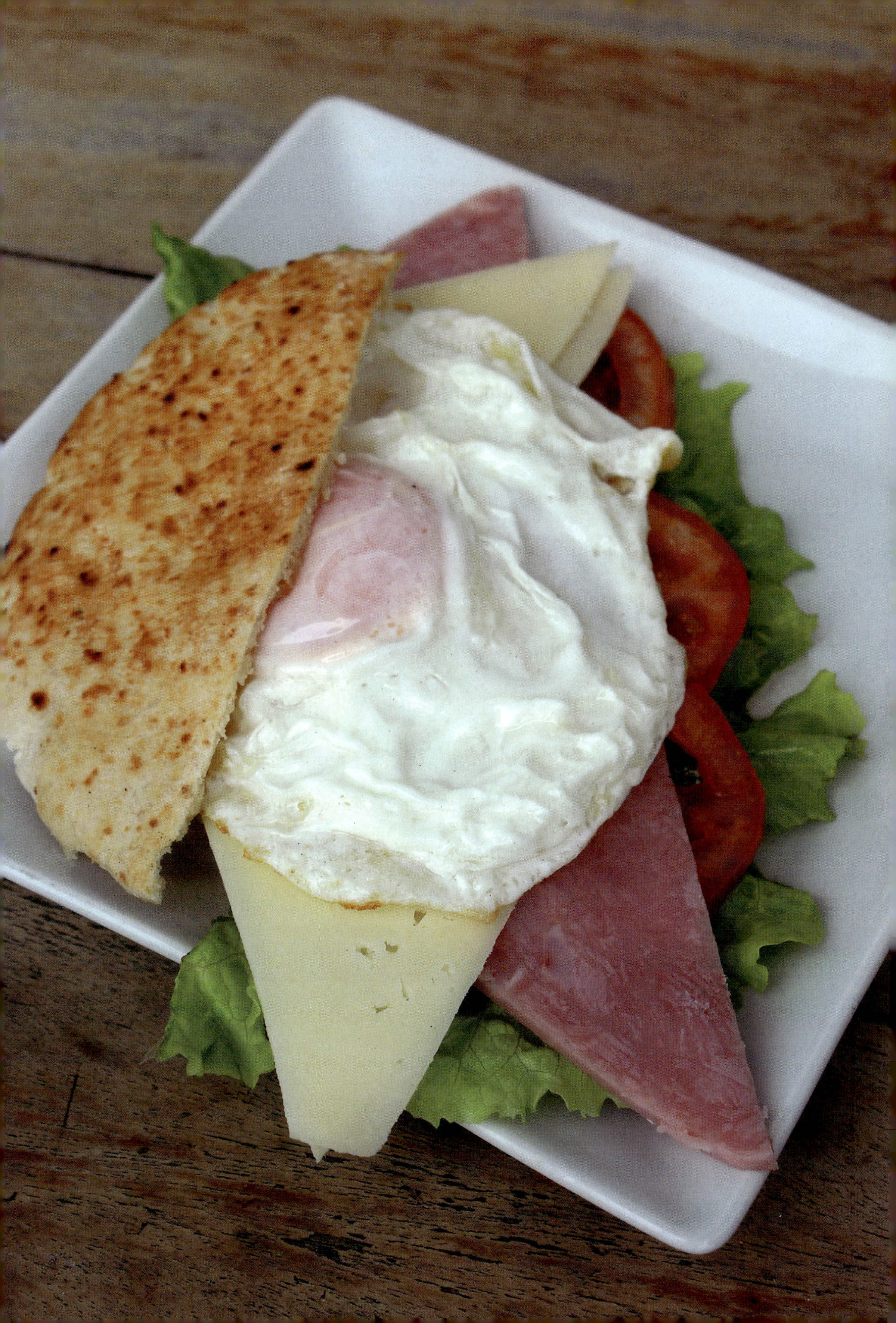

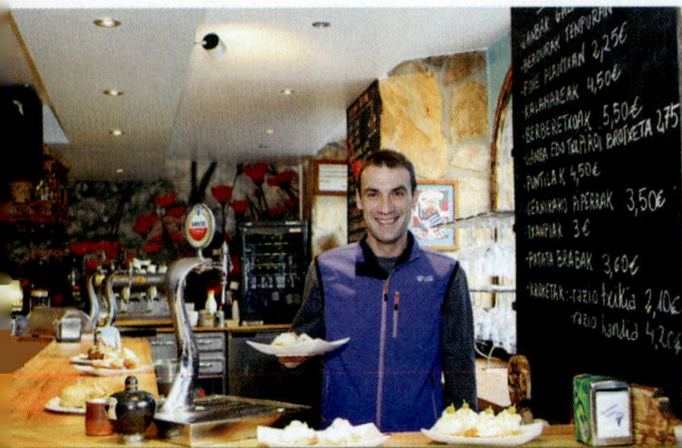

ETXE - ZURI

Pérez Arregi, 19
AZPEITIA
943 02 68 56

El Etxe-Zuri, bar de toda la vida, ya se llamaba así cuando **Iñaki Areizaga** pasó a dirigirlo allá por 1997. (De hecho, esta zona situada en un rincón de la parte vieja de Azpeitia es conocida por el nombre de Etxe-Zuri). Por aquel entonces era un local viejo y este azpeitiarra lo sometió a una profunda reforma que le dotó de su agradable aspecto actual. A día de hoy, con la ayuda de **Dahbia** en la cocina, Iñaki ofrece una **amplia variedad de pintxos, raciones, platos combinados... aunque son los bocadillos los que gozan de más éxito** en este bar: De berenjena, bacon, queso y pimiento; de perretxiko, queso, pimiento y jamón; de lomo, txampi, queso y patatas... y un largo etcétera. Etxe-Zuri abre sus puertas todos los días a las 10 de la mañana y los pintxos hacen su aparición en barra a primera hora. Los jueves, además, ofrece **pintxo-pote** de 7 a 9 de la tarde.

Otros pintxos:

- *Pulpo a la gallega*
- *Brocheta de gamba o de txipirón*
- *Ensalada rusa, atún, cebolla y mayonesa*
- *Bacon con txanpi*
- *Huevo, gamba, mayonesa y huevo rallado*
- *Tortillas variadas*
- *Ensalada de puerro y jamón york*
- *Chaka con gamba*
- *Albóndigas (Ración)*
- *Bacalao al pil-pil (Ración)*

Champiñones en salsa

Ingredientes:

Champiñones
Ajo
Aceite de oliva
Sal
Perejil

Elaboración:

Picamos finamente el ajo y lo ponemos a dorar en una cazuela con aceite de oliva. Lavamos los champiñones, les quitamos los rabos y los añadimos a la cazuela, donde no dejamos de remover afuego alto hasta que empiecen a soltar su agua. A partir de ese momento, bajamos el fuego, les damos el punto de sal y los dejamos que se vayan haciendo de media hora a una hora, removiéndolos de vez en cuando.

Final y presentación: Servimos los champiñones en cazuelita de barro, espolvoreándolos con perejil fresco recién picado.

Nota: A pesar de no ser un pintxo, el precio popular de esta ración de champis, por debajo del de muchos pintxos donostiarras, hace que sea uno de los productos con más aceptación del bar. De hecho, en Etxe-Zuri los champis se elaboran en grandes cantidades, preparando cada vez un mínimo de 8 kilos.

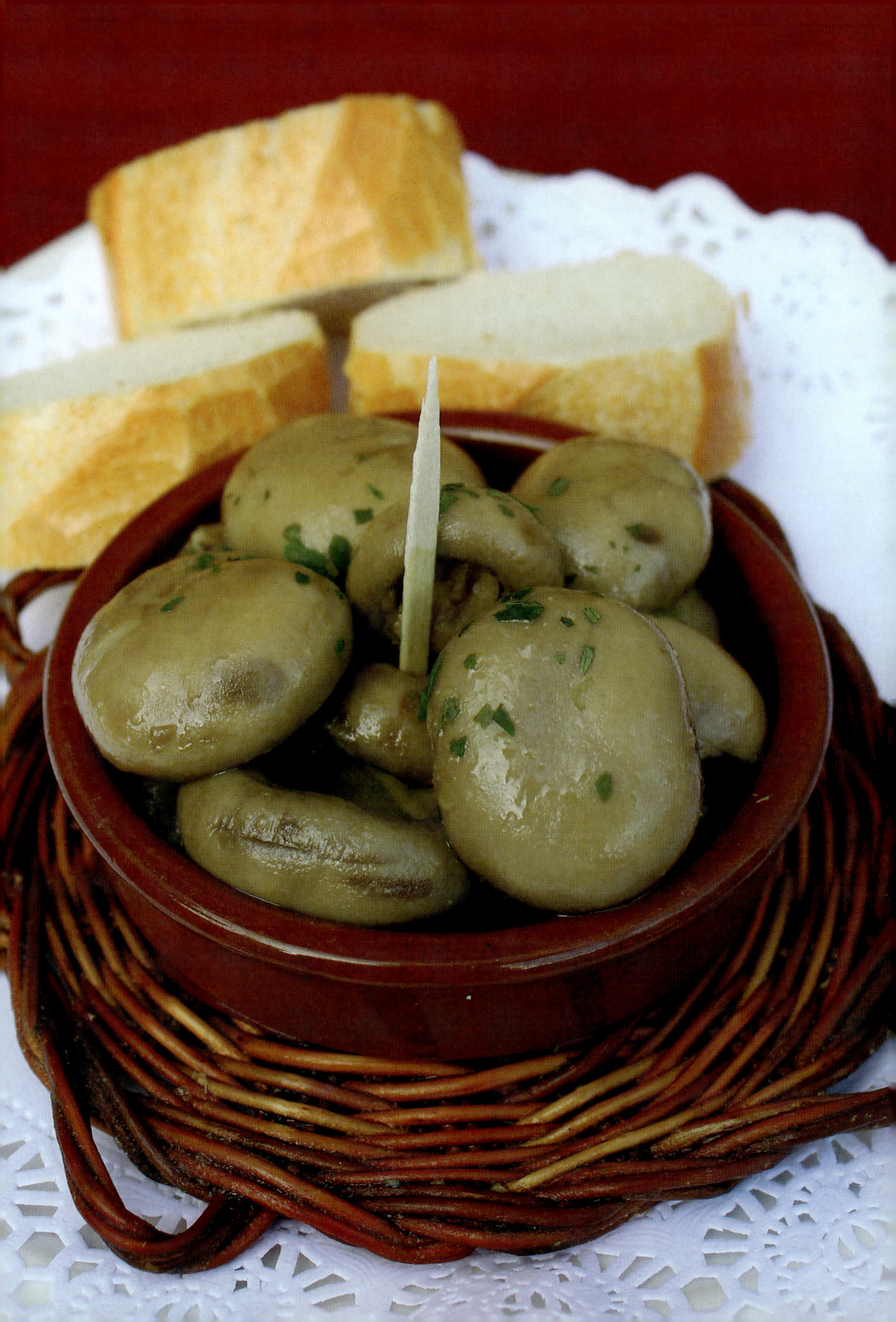

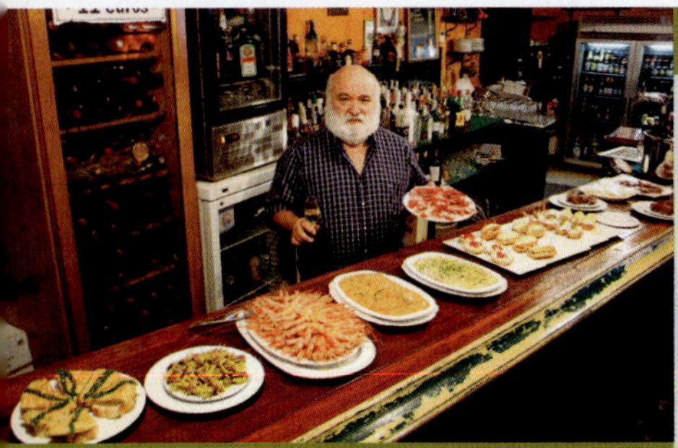

Iñigo, 6 (Parte Vieja)
DONOSTIA
943 42 13 90

ETXEBE

Helio Cano Jiménez nació en Sevilla y lleva aquí, según cuenta, "3 fines de semana". Tras un periplo que incluyó Ergobia, Astigarraga y Hernani, este inquieto hostelero recayó en Donostia donde se hizo con las riendas del entonces Restaurante Etxeberria en 1983. Durante 3 años lo mantuvo como restaurante, pero finalmente optó por la fórmula actual de bar y barra de picoteo que hoy en día es atendida por la cocinera **Arantxa Agirre,** de Mutiloa. Para acompañar los pintxos, Helio cuenta con una **amplia variedad de vinos de gran cantidad de denominaciones de origen, así como 34 marcas diferentes de cervezas.** En su día llegó a tener hasta 194 cervezas, pero con el tiempo ha decidido reducir la variedad ante la evidencia, en sus palabras, de que "los chavales están sin un chavo". El Etxebe abre todos los días, salvo los domingos, de 12 a 15:30 y de 18:30 hasta que el cuerpo aguante.

Otros pintxos:

- *Gildas "de verdad" (hechas con aceituna con hueso)*
- *Tortilla de patata*
- *Mixto (jamón ibérico con quesito)*
- *Bonito con pimiento del piquillo*
- *Antxoa con guindilla*
- *Tartaleta de queso de cabra con mermelada de tomate*

Raciones:

- *Gambas a la plancha*
- *Antxoas en vinagreta*
- *Embutidos ibéricos del valle de Los Pedroches*

Cazuelita de callos

Ingredientes:

Callos
Cebolla
Puerro
Sal

· Para la salsa:
Cebolla
Zanahoria
Pimiento verde
Ajo
Salsa de tomate casera
Pimiento choricero
Guindilla
Aceite de oliva

Elaboración:

Limpiamos concienzudamente los callos y los cocemos en olla a presión durante una hora con sal, una cebolla y un puerro.

Mientras se cuecen, hacemos la salsa. Para ello, picamos muy finamente y pochamos en aceite de oliva la cebolla, la zanahoria, el pimiento verde y el ajo. Una vez bien pochado todo, añadimos la salsa de tomate casera y la carne de un par de pimientos choriceros. Emulsionamos todo bien y añadimos guindilla al gusto.

Una vez los callos se hayan cocido, los cortamos en cuadritos con la ayuda de unas tijeras y los añadimos a la salsa. Dejamos que hiervan unos 10 minutos y los dejamos reposar. Mejor de un día para otro.

Final y presentación: Servimos los callos en una cazuelita de barro y los acompañamos, como no, de un buen tinto.

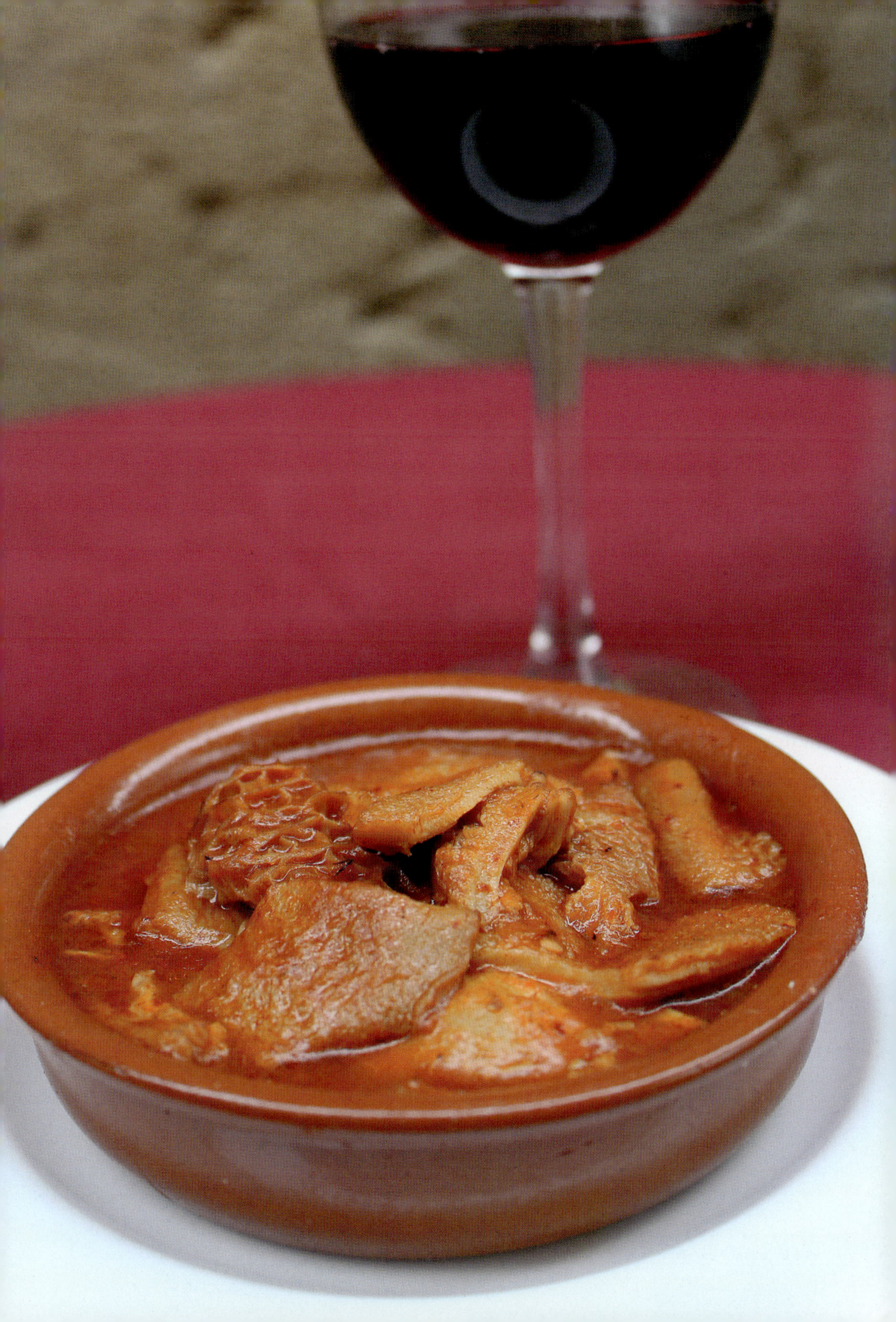

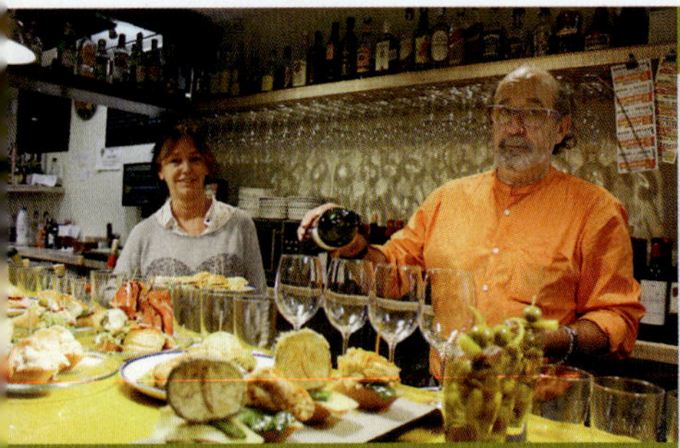

EUSKALDUNA

Nagusia, 37
ZARAUTZ
943 13 03 73

Son curiosas las efemérides del Euskalduna, **uno de los bares más emblemáticos de Zarautz**: Se inauguró en el aciago año en que empezó la Guerra Civil, y fue el día de la República del 2000 cuando se hicieron cargo de él sus actuales gestores: **Félix Borda, Marian Dulanto y Jesús Otazua.** Este inquieto trío ha convertido a este establecimiento en un agente cultural más de la villa costera, acogiendo en sus paredes **más de 100 exposiciones de fotografía** coordinadas por **Ramón Serra** de Photomuseum, u organizando, el último jueves de cada mes, el interesante **"Kafé Torero"**, una excusa para ofrecer actividades en torno al euskara (actuaciones, poesía...) que han atraído a gente como **Niko Etxart, Jesús Mari Lopetegi, Mikel Markez...** En cuanto a su oferta culinaria, Euskalduna ofrece una **cocina tradicional de temporada** (no podía ser menos estando junto al mercado) y una amplia variedad de **Ensaladas, Cazuelitas, Platos combinados, Bocadillos, Brochetas de solomillo...**

Otros pintxos:

- *Txipirón "Euskalduna"*
- *Tosta de jamón*
- *Huevo roto con txitxikis*
- *Solomillo de cerdo con salsa de Roquefort*
- *Solomillo con foie*
- *Secreto ibérico en salsa con viruta de puerros*
- *Croquetas caseras*
- *Tortillas variadas*
- *Txipirón con berenjena*
- *Pimiento relleno de bacalao*

Txipirón "Xirita"

Ingredientes:

1 Txipirón
Arroz
Pan
Aceite de oliva

- **Para la salsa del txipirón:**

Cebolla
Puerro
Tinta de txipirón
Sal

- **Para la salsa de piquillo:**

Cebolla
Pimiento del piquillo

Elaboración:

Para la salsa del txipirón: Picamos finamente la cebolla y el puerro y los ponemos a rehogar en una cazuela de barro. Cuando esté la verdura bien pochadita, añadimos la tinta del txipirón, agua y sal y la llevamos a ebullición.

Limpiamos el txipirón, salteamos sus patitas y las introducimos dentro del cuerpo de éste. Introducimos el txipirón en la salsa negra y le damos un hervor dejándolo que se cueza unos minutos.

Para la salsa de piquillo: Pochamos muy lentamente cebolla y pimiento del piquillo bien picaditos y los trituramos con la batidora.

Final y presentación: En una cazuelita disponemos el txipirón cubierto por su salsa y con una cucharadita de salsa de piquillo, acompañado de una rodaja de pan frito en aceite de oliva. Junto a la cazuelita, en una cucharita, servimos un arroz blanco mezclado con ajilimójilis (aceite con ajo picado y perejil)

Nota: Este pintxo se sirve en homenaje a "Xirita" (Cecilia), la cocinera de casa de Marian, natural de Oñati, que estuvo durante 6 generaciones al servicio de la familia y elaboraba así los txipirones. "Xirita" era, según Marian, como una abuela para ella.

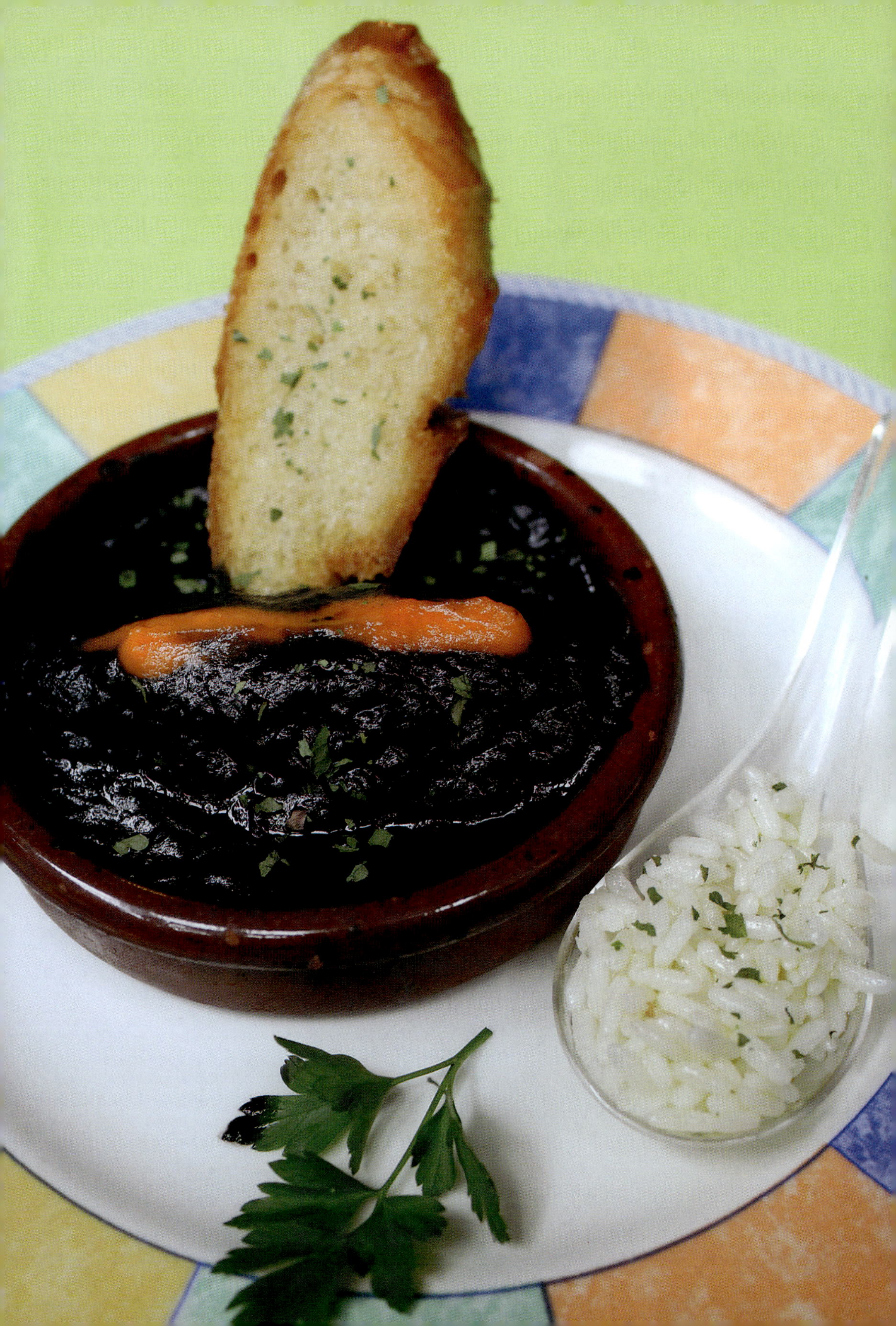

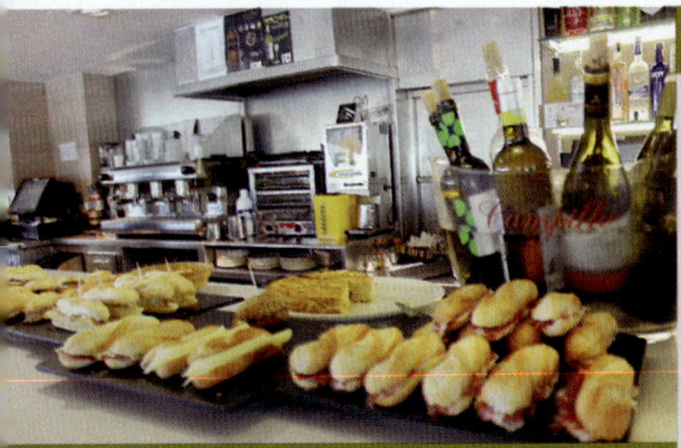

EZEIZA

El hotel Ezeiza es un **establecimiento centenario que que desde 1904 ha sido dirigido por la familia Ezeiza**, que se trasladó de Igeldo a Ondarreta, lugar en el que sigue el negocio, aunque en 1994 sufrió una amplia transformación que le dotó del aspecto actual y convirtió también en hotel lo que hasta entonces sólo había sido restaurante. La cocina está en las manos del donostiarra **Iñaki Etxenike**, miembro de la familia, que se curtió en la Euskal Etxea de Madrid de la mano de Luis Irizar y ha trabajado en lugares tan dispares como México o el desaparecido Clery de la plaza de la Trinidad. Iñaki practica una **cocina tradicional con toques personales** en la que se cuidan especialmente los postres. En Ezeiza se ofrece un cuidado menú del día y los fines de semana cuentan con un **menú especial que incluye Cochinillo asado.** La cafetería de Ezeiza abre todos los días a las 8 de la mañana y su terraza cubierta goza de gran aceptación, especialmente los domingos a la hora del aperitivo.

Avda. Satrustegi, 13
DONOSTIA
943 21 43 11
www.hotelezeiza.com

Otros pintxos:

- *Brocheta de champiñón*
- *Croqueta casera de jamón*
- *Hojaldre de puerros con gambas*
- *Frito de jamón y queso*
- *Talo de txistorra y queso*
- *Taco de marisco*

Raciones:

- *Calamares*
- *Gambas*
- *Jamón ibérico*

Tostada de gulas, setas y langostino con crema de ajos frescos

Ingredientes:

1 langostino
Setas de cardo
Ajo
Pan
Perejil picado
Aceite de oliva

· Para las gulas al ajillo:
Gulas
Ajo
Guindilla
Aceite de oliva

· Para la crema de ajos frescos:
Ajos frescos
Ajos
Aceite de oliva

Elaboración:

Para la crema de ajos frescos: Confitamos los ajos frescos junto a cuatro ajos pelados a fuego lento en aceite de oliva. Colamos los ajos y hacemos un puré que pondremos a punto de crema.

Para las gulas al ajillo: En una sartén doramos los ajos con aceite de oliva y una rodaja de guindilla y añadimos las gulas, salteándolas un momento. Salteamos las setas, finamente picadas en juliana, en aceite de oliva con un poco de ajo. Finalmente, juntamos las gulas y las setas.

Cocemos el langostino 30 segundos, lo pelamos, le hacemos un corte en la espalda y lo pasamos por la plancha.

Final y presentación: Tostamos una rodaja hermosa de pan al horno, y sobre ella montamos con cuidado la mezcla de gulas y setas de cardo. Colocamos encima de todo el langostino a la plancha y espolvoreamos el conjunto con perejil fresco recién picado. Finalmente, acompañamos el pintxo con la crema de ajos frescos como decoración.

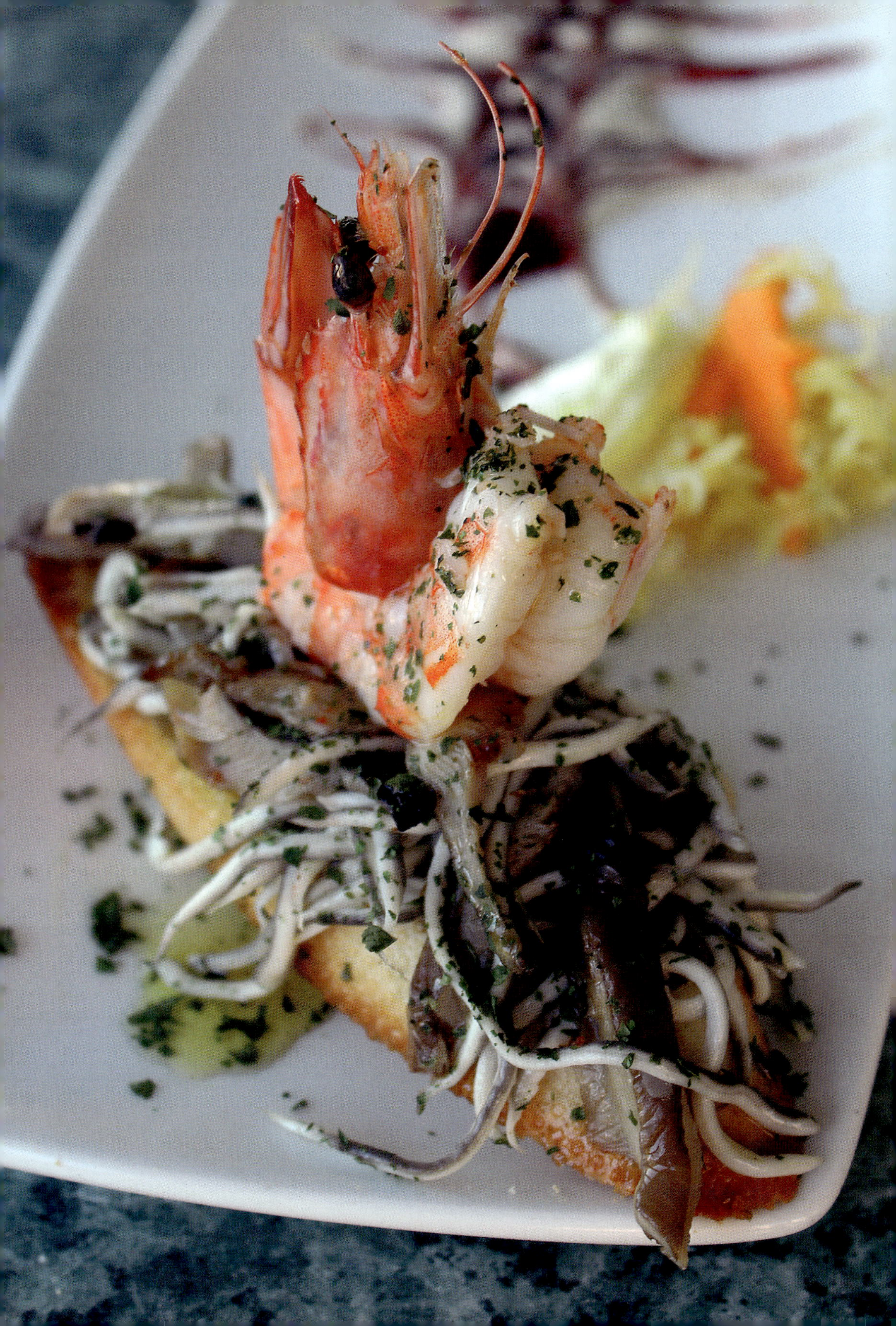

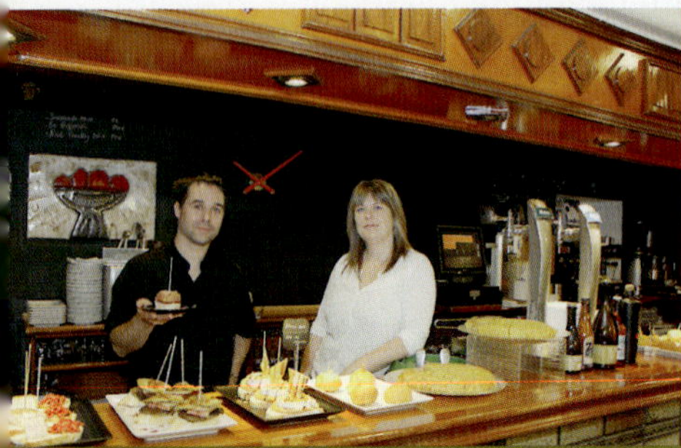

Olarte, 25
ARRASATE
943 04 43 88
facebook-ezkiña taberna

EZKIÑA

Tras pasar varios años cerrado, este acogedor bar situado frente al Palacio de Monterroi, a las puertas del centro histórico de Arrasate, ha adquirido nueva vida desde 2003 de la mano de **Asier Antia y Gurutze Villar**, que llevan décadas trabajando en el mundo de la hostelería local. Esta joven pareja ha dotado al Ezkiña de una variada oferta gastronómica en la que **además de sus pintxos destacan las Hamburguesas caseras**, principalmente la exitosa Hamburguesa de buey y la hamburguesa 100% vegetal, aunque **cada semana ofrecen una hamburguesa diferente** que puede ser de ciervo, de cordero... También tienen gran demanda los **bocadillos**, entre los que sobresale el "Ezkiña" (Pechuga a la plancha, tomate a la plancha, bacon, cebolla pochada y salsa Roquefort). Y para los valientes, nada como la **"Eusko Pizza"**, una monumental pizza para 6-7 personas, elaborada con pan casero de Aretxabaleta, que debe ser solicitada por encargo.

Otros pintxos:

- *Tortilla de patata con puerro y cebolla*
- *Tortilla de patata rellena de jamón y queso*
- *Bola de carne*
- *Bola de queso*
- *Bola de marisco*
- *Berenjena, seta, bacon, queso y cebolla pochada*
- *Calabacín, queso, bacon y pimiento verde*
- *"Ander" (Calabacín, rulo de cabra y espárrago triguero)*
- *Rulo de cabra con tomate y galleta de queso*
- *Montadito de patata*

"Villar"

Ingredientes:

Tronco de bonito
Pimiento del piquillo rojo
Pimiento del piquillo verde
Antxoa
Pan de caserío
Reducción de Pedro Ximénez

· Para la vinagreta:
Pimiento rojo
Pimiento verde
Zanahoria
Cebolla
Pepinillo
Aceite de oliva virgen extra
Vinagre
Sal

Elaboración:

Para la vinagreta: Picamos muy finamente el pimiento rojo, el pimiento verde, la zanahoria, la cebolla y el pepinillo, Disponemos todo en un bol y cubrimos las verduras con aceite de oliva virgen extra, vinagre y sal. Mezclamos bien y dejamos reposar.

Cortamos una rodaja de pan de caserío y, sobre ella, disponemos un pimiento verde y un pimiento rojo, ambos del piquillo. Sobre ambos pimientos, colocamos el tronco de bonito en conserva, y sobre este conjunto vertemos la vinagreta que hemos dejado reposando.

Finalmente, sobre la vinagreta colocamos una buena antxoa en conserva, y ensartamos todo con un palillo.

Terminamos decorando el pintxo con unos hilitos de reducción de Pedro Ximénez.

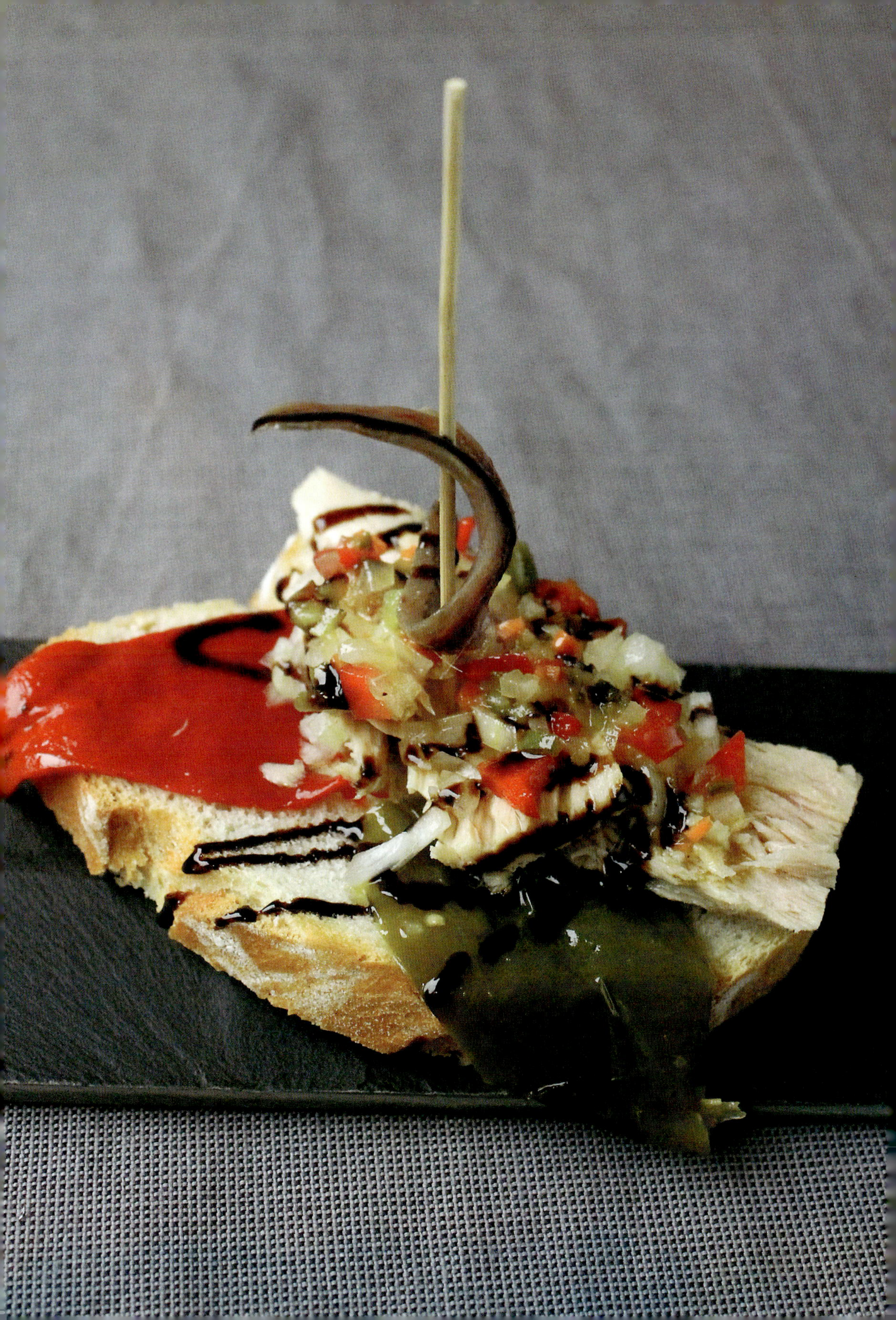

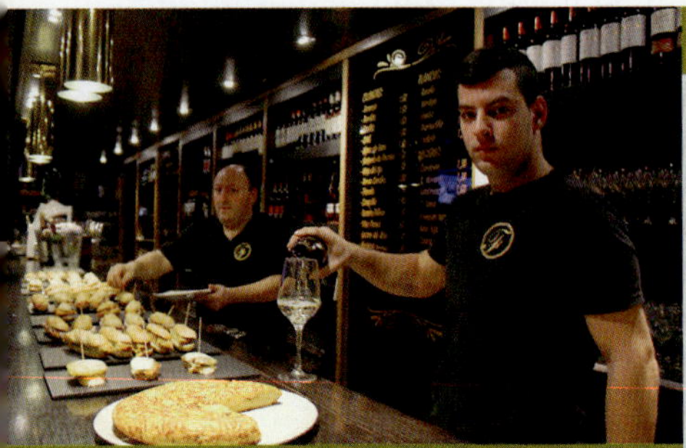

Plaza Barria, 6
EIBAR
943 12 12 55
www.foxtterbar.com

FOXTTER

El Foxtter es el ejemplo perfecto de cómo la vida le puede encauzar a uno por donde menos se lo pensaba. Los hermanos **David y Alberto Morcillo**, trabajadores con su vida enfocada hacia la construcción y la automoción, sufrieron como tantos otros los embates de la crisis, pero tuvieron la oportunidad de hacerse en 2012 con este céntrico bar que en su día fue la cafetería Niza, una de las mejores de Eibar. Con la ayuda en barra de su padre, **Juan José**, y en cocina de su madre, **Mª Pilar**, estos hermanos han dotado al Foxtter de **un ambiente más familiar y casero, manteniendo la elegancia del local y la calidad de su oferta**. En Foxtter, además de una gran variedad de vinos, encontraremos una carta de **más de 18 bocadillos**, destacando el de Foie fresco, excelentes **Hamburguesas** entre las que sobresale la de Wagyu y contundentes **Sandwiches** como el de Pechuga de pollo. Como novedad destacan las **Fajitas mexicanas** que poco a poco van logrando su hueco entre la clientela.

Otros pintxos:

- *Foie con manzana a la plancha*
- *Rulo de tortilla con gulas y langostino*
- *Tortilla de espinacas con langostino*
- *Paleta ibérica y queso de cabra sobre cebolla pochada*
- *Brocheta de rape, langostino y bacon*

Raciones:

- *Fritos variados*
- *Rabas*
- *Patatas bravas*
- *Chopitos*

Dulce de foie

Ingredientes:

1 rodaja de sobao pasiego
Hongos
Chalota
1 chorrito de Oporto
Sal
Agua
1 huevo de codorniz

Elaboración:

PIcamos finamente la chalota y la rehogamos con aceite de oliva. Añadimos un chorrito de vino de Oporto y dejamos que éste se evapore. Adjuntamos los hongos previamente picados y los hacemos junto con la chalota por espacio de una hora a fuego lento, añadiendo agua según vayan pidiendo.

Antes de terminar de hacer los hongos, añadimos la sal y les damos varias vueltas a fuego vivo durante los últimos 10 minutos para que el hongo pierda su mucosidad.

Marcamos ligeramente en la plancha una rodaja de sobao pasiego. (Justo marcarla, puesto que si se deja mucho tiempo, ésta se amarga) y hacemos el huevo de codorniz también en la plancha.

Final y presentación: Sobre la rodaja de sobao pasiego disponemos los hongos rehogados con la chalota y, sobre estos, el huevo de codorniz. Adornamos el conjunto con un poco de reducción de Módena.

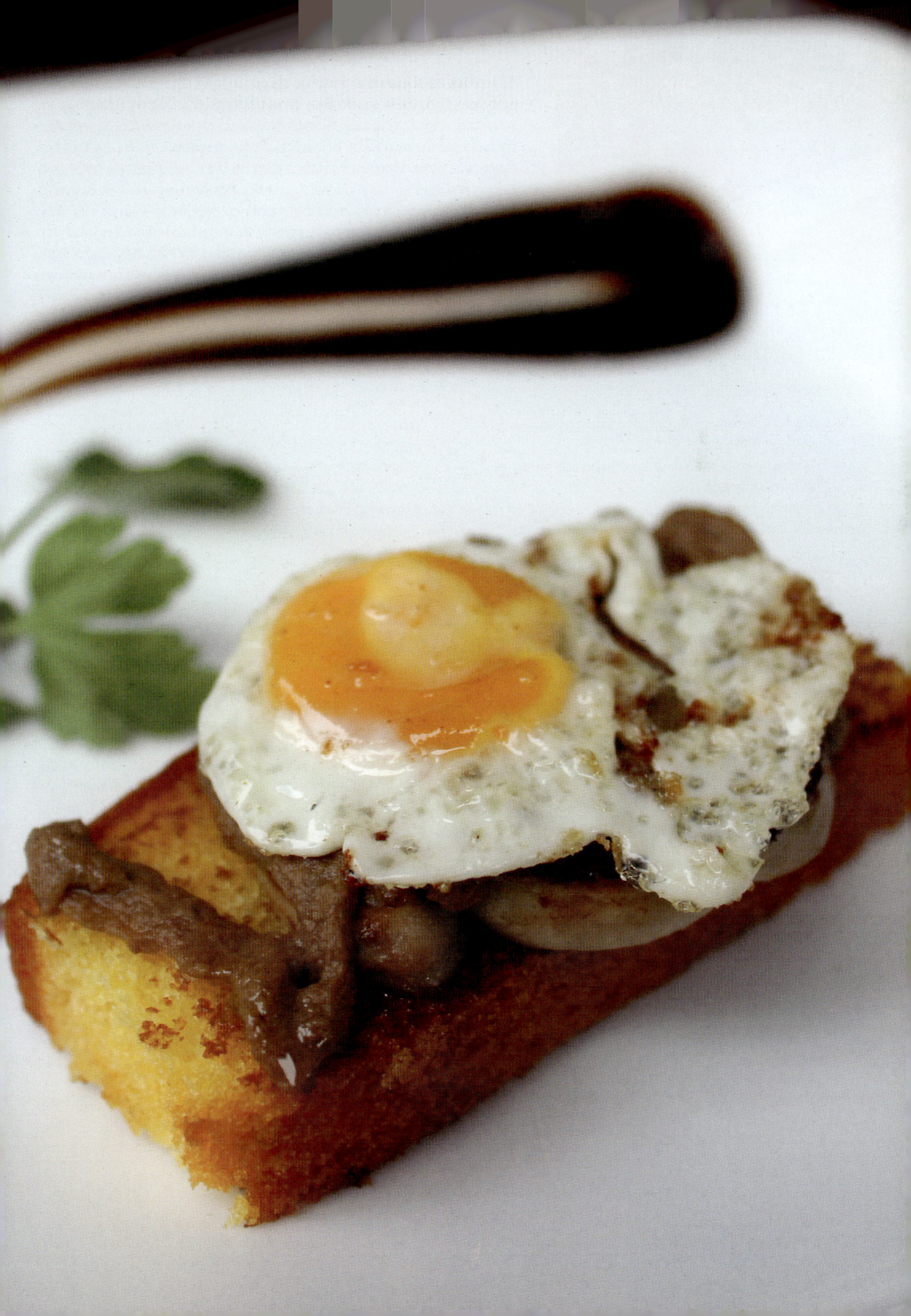

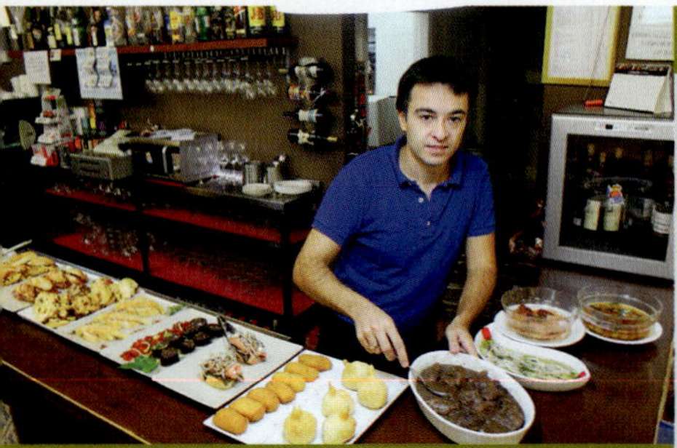

Serapio Mujika, 21
DONOSTIA
943 39 05 66

GUARDAPLATA

José Miguel Alcaraz, vecino de Bidebieta de toda la vida, empezó siendo un chaval en el mundo de la hostelería, echando una mano a su padre, José Luis, en el Osinaga de Amara, y **desde 2005 lleva la dirección del Guardaplata, el bar del Hogar del Jubilado de Bidebieta,** un local con una vida terrible y una clientela fiel y exigente como pocas. Con la indispensable ayuda de su mujer, **Naiara Segura** y el cocinero, **Garikoitz Barandiaran**, José Miguel ofrece desde las 9 de la mañana una barra que llama la atención por la variedad de croquetas, pintxos y cazuelitas que en ella se ofrecen. Asimismo, en Guardaplata se trabaja mucho con el **menú del día, que es totalmente casero, muy económico, y se cambia todos los días.** Los viernes, la afluencia de público se duplica con el **pintxo-pote** que se ofrece de 7 a 9, y en el que se cobra la consumición al precio habitual, regalándose un pintxo a elegir.

Otros pintxos:

- *Croquetas variadas (jamón, bacalao, hongos...)*
- *Carrilleras en salsa*
- *Tortilla de piquillo con base de morcilla de verdura*
- *Buñuelo de bacalao*
- *Champi con jamón*
- *Flamenquín*
- *Crujiente de langostino*
- *Bola de carne o de marisco*
- *Morcilla con piquillos*
- *Espárrago rebozado*

Bacalao en tempura con piperrada y tosta de ali-oli

Ingredientes:

1 taco de bacalao
Pan
Aceite de oliva

· Para la piperrada:
Cebolla
Pimiento verde
Pimiento rojo

· Para la masa de gabardina:
Harina
Cerveza
Sal

· Para el ali-oli
Mayonesa
Ajo
Perejil

Elaboración:

Para la piperrada: Picamos finamente la cebolla, el pimiento verde y el pimiento rojo y los dejamos pochar un buen rato a fuego muy lento.

Para la masa de gabardina: Ponemos en un bol la harina, añadimos la cerveza y mezclamos muy bien. Añadimos la sal y batimos enérgicamente hasta que adquiera el espesor deseado. Una vez lo tenemos, dejamos la masa 10 minutos en una zona caliente para que se levante.

Para el ali-oli: Batimos mayonesa, ajo picado y perejil picado.

Para el bacalao: Rebozamos el bacalao con la masa de gabardina, y lo freímos en abundante aceite de oliva, cuidando de que quede jugoso.

Final y presentación: Cortamos una rodaja de pan, la untamos de ali-oli y la horneamos hassta que se haga una costra. Sobre ella colocamos el taco de bacalao frito con la masa de gabardina, y coronamos el pintxo con una cucharada de piperrada.

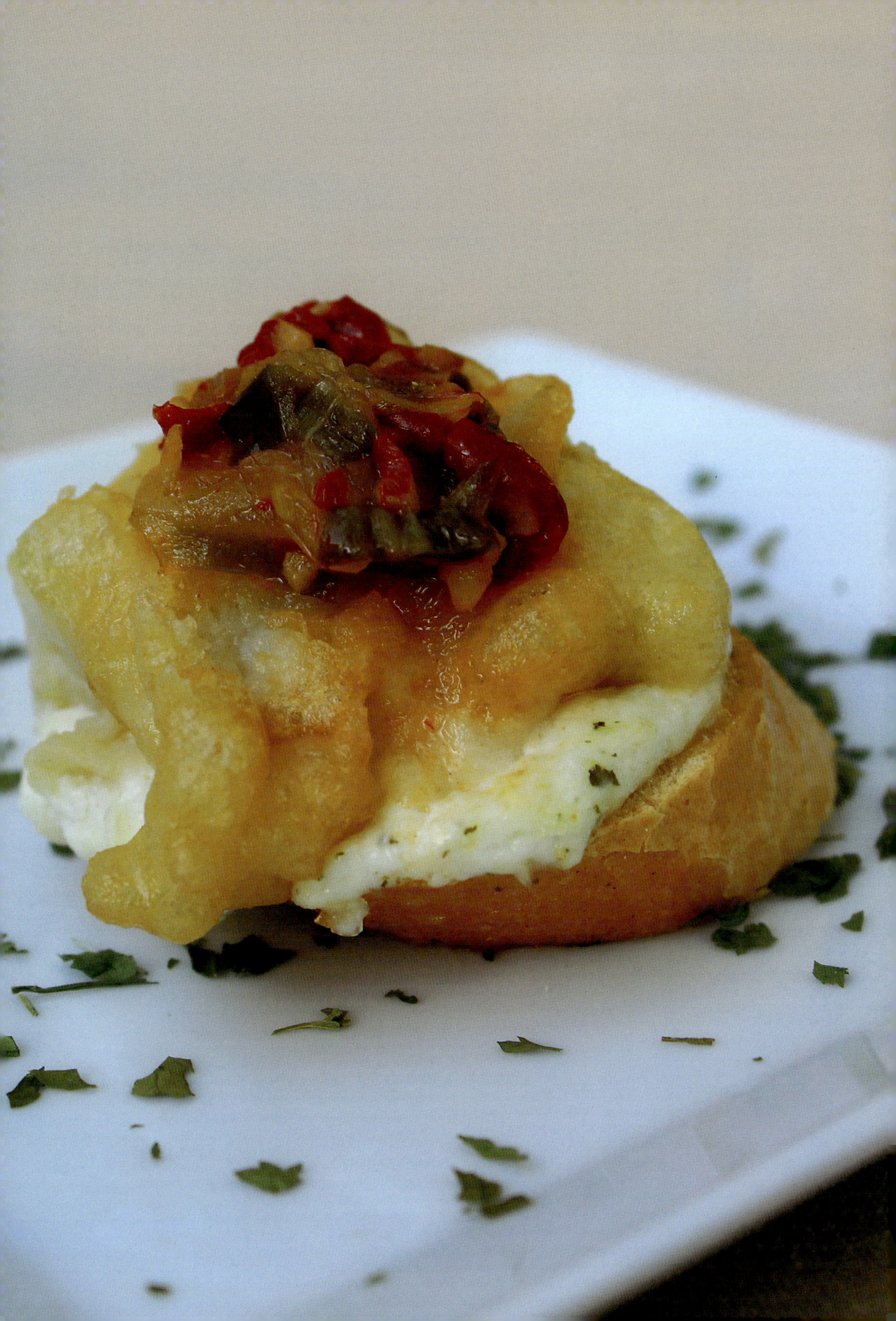

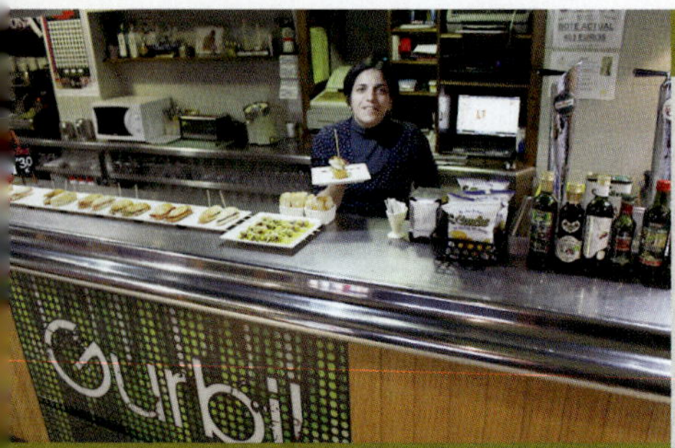

GURBIL

Este pequeño y céntrico establecimiento, situado casi en plena Plaza de Unzaga, ofrece bastante más de lo que parece a simple vista. Dirigido por **Roberto Póveda y Marga Gómez**, Gurbil abre todos los días a las 7 de la mañana y, además de la selección habitual de pintxos ofrece raciones, platos combinados y especialidades como Codillo, Rabo guisado o Cochinillo y cordero al horno (estos últimos, por encargo). En Gurbil también podemos disfrutar de un menú diario con postres caseros o de una original curiosidad como es el **Menú de bodega**, que por el precio que cuesta habitualmente un menú del día ofrece el siguiente festín, elaborado con productos de Salamanca adobados artesanalmente: Morcilla picante, pintxo moruno, chorizo, panceta, patatas fritas y ensalada. En Gurbil, además, se organizan **fiestas de cumpleaños con cuentacuentos**. Los viernes y sábados, además, se ofrece pintxo-pote a partir de las 7 de la tarde.

Isasi, 1
EIBAR
943 20 11 52

Otros pintxos:

- *Embutidos ibéricos de Bellota*
- *Queso de Idiazabal*
- *Tortillas variadas*
- *Chorizo a la sidra*
- *Croquetas caseras*
- *Champiñones en salsa*
- *Gildas*

Raciones:

- *Caracoles en salsa vizcaína*
- *Muslitos de codorniz*
- *Albóndigas en salsa*

Pimiento verde del piquillo relleno de merluza

Ingredientes:

Pimiento verde del piquillo
Merluza
Jamón serrano
Cebolla
Pimiento verde
Leche entera
Tomate frito
Harina
Huevo
Aceite de oliva
Pan
Reducción de Módena

Elaboración:

Picamos la cebolla y el pimiento verde y los ponemos a pochar. A medio hacer, añadimos la cebolla previamente desmigada. Sofreímos todo a fuego bajo y, cuando esté hecho, añadimos un poco de leche entera y dejamos que vaya a ebullición, dejándolo hervir un minuto. Añadimos una cucharada de tomate frito, dejamos hervir otro poco y retiramos del fuego.

Cuando la farsa esté templada, la pasamos por la batidora y rellenamos el pimiento verde.

Rebozamos el pimiento en harina y huevo y lo freimos en aceite de oliva.

Final y presentación: Envolvemos el pimiento relleno con una loncha de jamón serrano, lo ensartamos en un palillo de brocheta y lo servimos sobre una rodaja de pan, adornando el conjunto con un poco de reducción de Módena. También podemos, optativamente, acompañar este pintxo de una salsa de pimiento elaborada con cebolla, zanahoria, pimiento verde, piquillo verde, vino blanco, tomate frito, harina y sal.

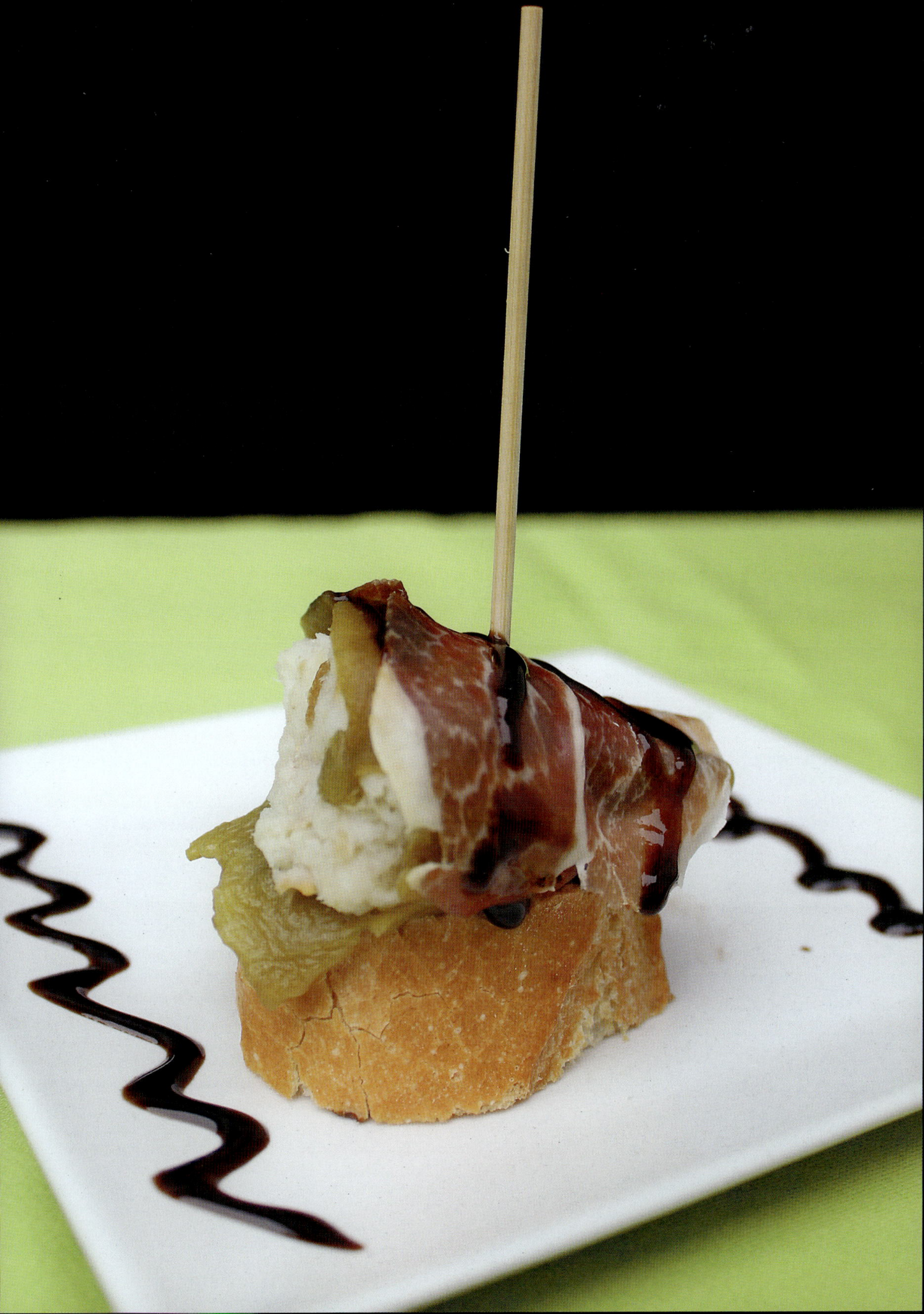

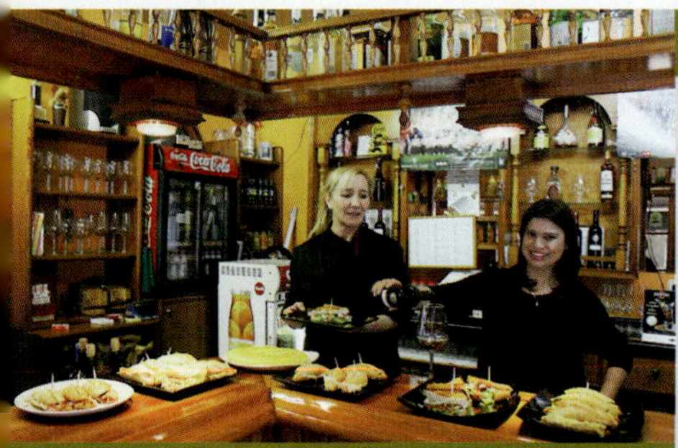

Gurmendi kalea, 10
ZARAUTZ

HARITZA

En la zona de Azken Portu, **Idoia Aristi** dirige este bar abierto por sus padres, **Joxe y Mª Paz**, en 1982, y en el que han trabajado desde sus hermanos **Ana, Sergio y Pakea**, hasta su sobrino **Ibai.** En solitario desde finales de la década pasada, Idoia ofrece, con la ayuda de **Paula** en barra, **desayunos desde las 6:30 de la mañana con repostería casera y pintxos a partir de las 8**, destacando la tortilla de patata, siguiendo la receta de su madre, que le ha hecho ganar el concurso veraniego popular de tortilla organizado por el Zast (Club Deportivo de Zarautz) en 2014. Idoia no ha dotado de novedades al bar, de hecho, trata de mantener los mismos proveedores que tenían sus padres y que tan buenos productos le proporcionan, como los cafés de Aitona o los huevos, traídos directamente del mercado de Zarautz. La patata también sigue siendo la misma patata alavesa que su madre usaba en las tortillas.

Otros pintxos:

- *Tortilla de patata*
- *Tortilla de jamón*
- *Tortilla de chorizo*
- *Atún con mayonesa*
- *Chaka*
- *Sardinillas*
- *Jamón*
- *Antxoas con guindillas*
- *Tortilla francesa, jamón, antxoa, pimiento verde y mayonesa*

Sandwich vegetal

Ingredientes:

Pan de molde
Mayonesa
Lechuga
Tomate
Aceite
Huevo
Atún en aceite
Antxoas (opcional)
Pimiento verde (opcional)

Elaboración:

Cocemos el huevo y lo partimos en rodajas.

Limpiamos la lechuga y la cortamos en Julliana. Limpiamos asimismo el tomate y lo cortamos en daditos pequeños.

Cortamos por la mitad una rodaja de pan de molde y la tostamos ligeramente en la sartén con un poco de aceite.

Untamos uno de los trozos de pan de molde con mayonesa por la parte sin tostar, y disponemos sobre él y en este orden la lechuga en Juliana, los daditos de tomate y unas rodajas de huevo duro. Finalmente, añadimos una cantidad generosa de atún o bonito en aceite.

Nota: En función de quien lo pida, hay ocasiones en las que Idoia añade a este sandwich un par de antxoas o unos trozos de pimiento verde frito.

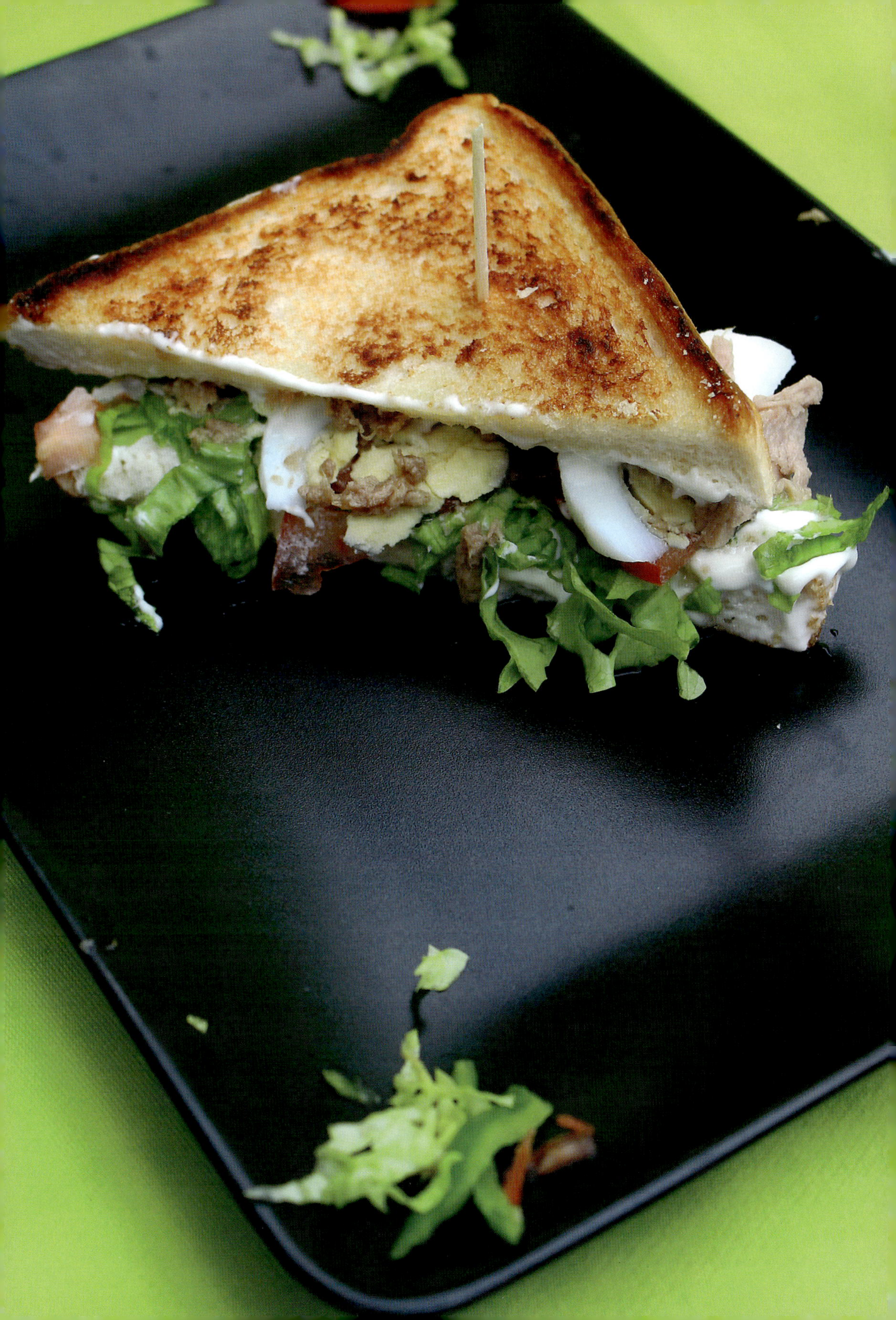

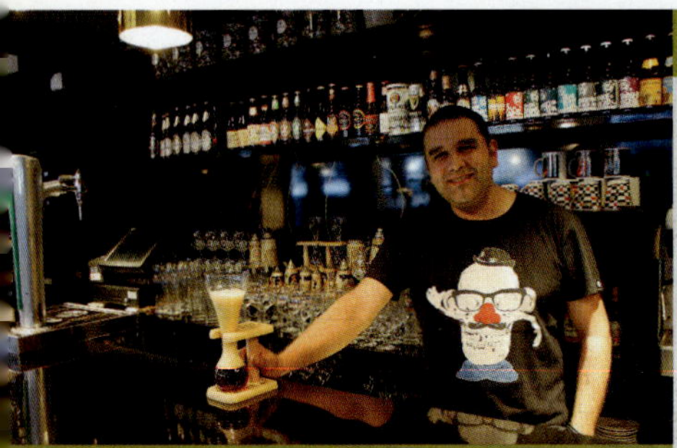

Areizaga, 18
URRETXU
647 96 33 76

HOKABA

Antonio Fernández dirige desde diciembre de 2013 este moderno local al que ha **especializado en cervezas, con una carta con más de 43 referencias en botella**. Todos los meses, se ofrece la "cerveza del mes" y quien quiera puede adquirir cualquier cerveza de la carta para llevar a casa, a un precio más ventajoso que el del local. Además, en breve, se pondrá en marcha un "menú cervecero". Por lo demás, en Hokaba se sigue ofreciendo una **cuidada variedad gastronómica con los platos clásicos del local y nuevas incorporaciones** como el suculento Bocadillo de estofado de ternera, o nuevos platos como Ensalada de bacalao, Txipirones rellenos de langostinos, Lomo relleno de jamón y queso... Además, todos los fines de semana se ofrecerán uno o dos platos nuevos fuera de carta para que la gente tenga una mayor variedad para elegir. Antonio, además, quiere dotar de vida al local organizando regularmente diversas **actuaciones, monólogos, conciertos, etc...**

Otros pintxos:

- *Brocheta de pulpo*
- *Callos caseros*
- *Tortilla de morcilla (en temporada)*
- *Tosta de bacon*
- *Tosta de jamón*
- *Montadito de lomo con pimiento rojo y queso*
- *Brocheta de tempura de verduras*
- *Gildas*
- *Albóndigas*
- *Estofado de ternera*

Txapela de bacon y patata

Ingredientes:

Bacon
Patata
Huevo
Sal
Aceite de oliva
Pimiento verde
Pimiento rojo
Queso

Elaboración:

Cortamos la patata y la confitamos en aceite de oliva de la misma manera que si fuéramos a hacer una tortilla de patata. Una vez confitada, la escurrimos bien de aceite y la echamos al huevo batido.

Colocamos unas tiras de bacon en un molde semicircular. Vertemos en él la mezcla de huevo y patata sin cuajar y cerramos con las tiras de bacon, formando una especie de paquete.

Metemos el molde al horno previamente calentado y lo tenemos unos 20 minutos a 170° aproximadamente.

Una vez cocido, se espera 10 minutos para desmoldarlo.

Final y presentación: Presentamos la txapela en el centro de un platillo, decorada con dos rodajas de piquillo, verde y rojo, un poco de queso de barra y unos hilillos de reducción de Módena.

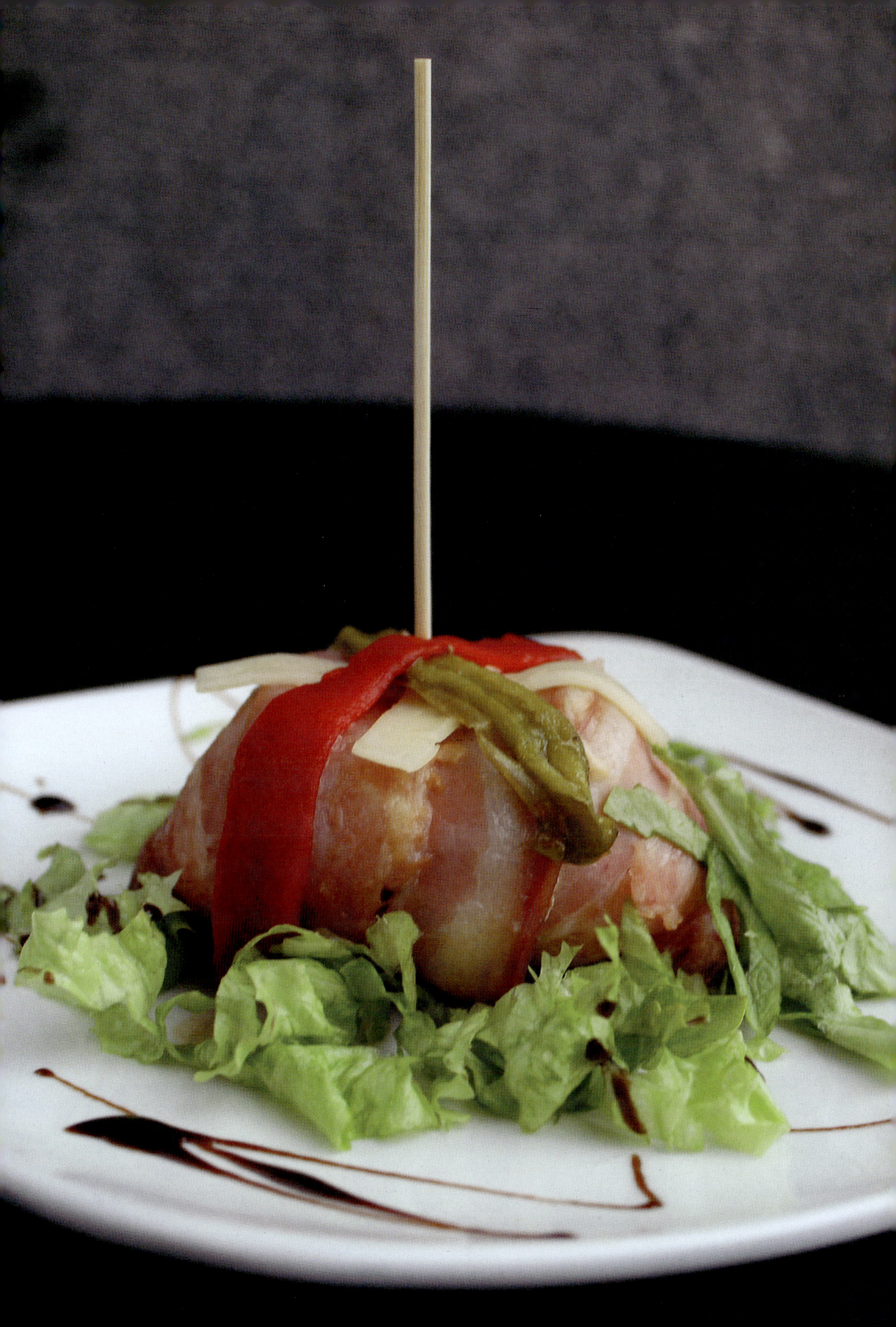

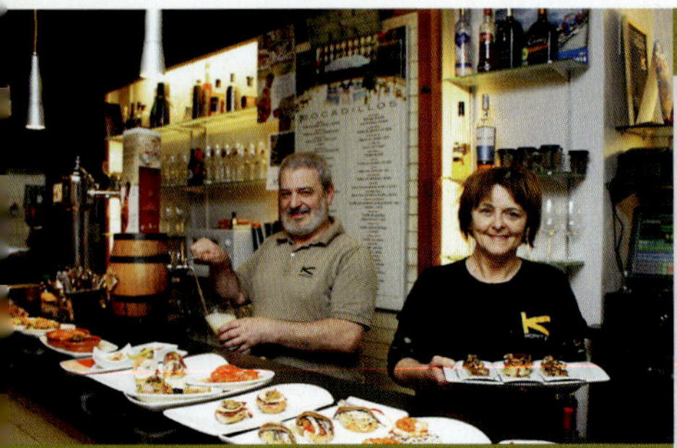

IKATZA

Plaza Berria, 6
TOLOSA
943 67 49 13

Kontxi Dorronsoro y **Jesus Mari Artutxa**, con más de 30 años de experiencia en hostelería, dirigen desde 2003 este **estratégico bar con entrada tanto desde Plaza Berria como desde la calle Rondilla.** En Ikatza, además de los pintxos, se ofrece **Menú del día**, **Raciones**, **Platos combinados** y su gran especialidad, sus casi 30 **Bocadillos**, bautizados con los nombres de los más importantes lugares naturales de Euskal Herria, como **Abodi** (Tortilla de patata, lechuga y tomate), **Zurriola** (Calamares), **Hondarribi** (Gambas, champis y tortilla de algas), **Deba** (Antxoas rebozadas), **Uzturre** (Bacon, queso, lechuga y tomate)... Los clientes, además, pueden "fabricarse" el bocata a su gusto. Ikatza abre todos los días de 9 de la mañana a 12 de la noche y los jueves ofrece pintxo-pote. **Los txipirones son el producto estrella** de este bar donde se sirven como pintxo, como ración, en bokata, a la plancha, encebollados, en su tinta... habiendo fines de semana en que han sido servidos más de 60 kilos de ellos

Otros pintxos:

- *Pimientos rellenos de txipirón*
- *Pimientos rellenos de bacalao*
- *Carrillera rellena con hongos*
- *Berenjenas rellenas con hongos*
- *Callos*
- *Champiñones*
- *Pasta brick rellena de pisto y pato*
- *Tortilla de bacalao*
- *Bacalao con tomate*
- *Puding de verdura*

Calabacín relleno de carne con hongos y frutos secos

Ingredientes:

Calabacín
Cebolla
Hongos
Carne picada
Queso Mascarpone
Piñones
Nueces
Un chorrito de Moscatel
Huevo

- **Para la menestra:**

Zanahoria
Guisantes
Vainas
Calabacín
Puerro...

- **Para el acompañamiento:**

Hongos
Cebolla
Aceite de oliva

Elaboración:

Para el relleno: Picamos finamente la cebolla y los hongos y los pochamos en una sartén con aceite de oliva. Una vez pochado, añadimos la carne picada y rehogamos todo junto. Cuando todo se ha rehogado, añadimos los frutos secos (piñones y nueces) previamente pelados y machacados en el mortero, y un chorrito de Moscatel. Lo mezclamos todo bien y añadimos un poco de queso Mascarpone.

Con el cortafiambres, cortamos dos lonchas largas de calabacín y las cruzamos formando una cruz. Colocamos la farsa en el centro de la cruz y la cerramos, la rebozamos con huevo y la freímos con aceite de oliva.

Para la menestra: Picamos finamente las verduras que se indican, pudiendo añadir alguna verdura más de temporada y las cocemos en agua con sal hasta que queden al dente.

Para el acompañamiento: Salteamos unos hongos picados con un poco de cebolla.

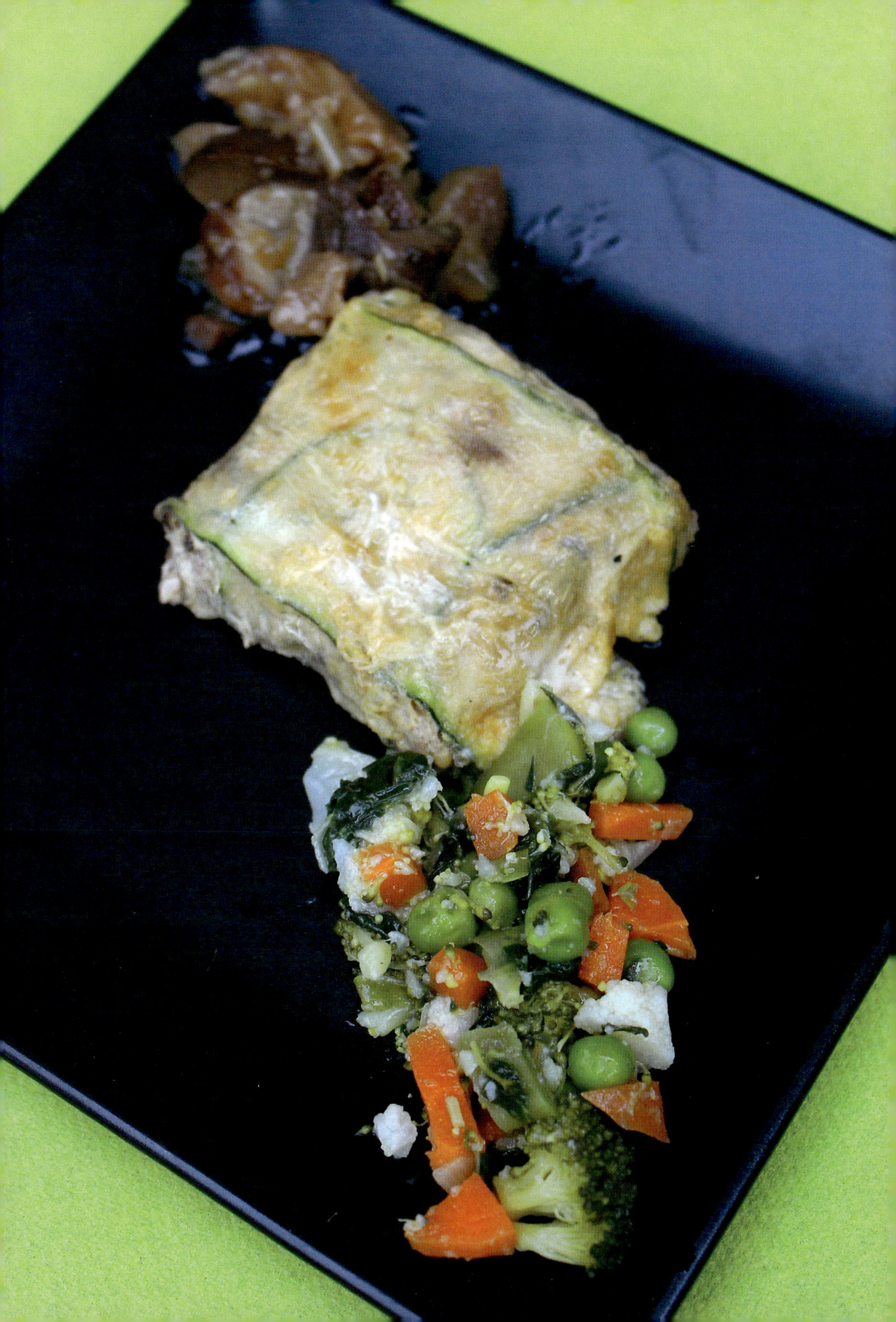

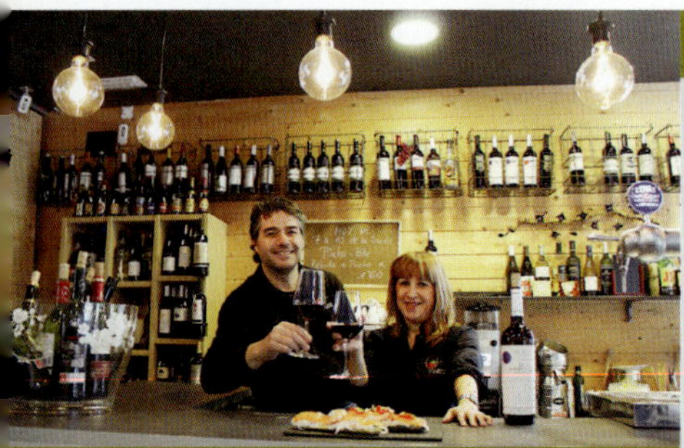

Zelai-Ondo, 23
ZARAUTZ
636 41 71 99
663 34 30 55

ILUNTZE

Tras trabajar 5 veranos seguidos llevando los merenderos de Asti, **Javier Benítez y Eli Cano** se animaron, en junio de 2014, a abrir Iluntze, un **establecimiento especializado en el mundo del vino**, un tema que apasiona a ambos y para el que se han preparado a conciencia visitando bodegas, asistiendo a catas y acudiendo a diversos eventos relacionados con el vino. Así, en este gastrobar situado frente al Polideportivo de Zarautz, encontraremos **unas 100 referencias de vinos, de los que unos 30 pueden consumirse por copas** y el resto por botellas, a precio de comercio, pagando 3 euros por el descorche. Para acompañar al vino, en Iluntze podemos optar por una **gran variedad de pintxos y raciones de cocina fría elaborados con productos de calidad comprobada y muy bien presentados.** Son altamente recomendables, sobre todo de cara al verano, sus **dos terrazas**, una al sol y otra a la sombra, para todos los gustos.

Otros pintxos:

- *Bonito con antxoa y boquerón*
- *Ibérico con pa amb tumaca*
- *Pulpo en vinagreta*
- *Pulpo a la gallega*
- *Tortilla de patata con pimiento*
- *Gildas variadas*

Raciones:

- *Jamón ibérico de Guijuelo*
- *Antxoas de Getaria*
- *Salmón ahumado*

Chaka con salmón y langostino sobre pan de amapolas

Ingredientes:

Pan con semillas de amapola
Chaka
Gambas
Mayonesa
1 rodaja de salmón ahumado
1 langostino

- **Para la vinagreta:**

PImiento rojo
Pimiento verde
Cebolleta
Aceite de oliva virgen extra
Vinagre de manzana
Sal

Elaboración:

Picamos la chaka y las gambas y las mezclamos con la mayonesa. Reservamos.

Cocemos el langostino y lo pelamos.

Para la vinagreta: Picamos finamente el pimiento rojo, el pimiento verde y la cebolleta y los mezclamos con aceite de oliva virgen, sal y vinagre de manzana. Dejamos que repose.

Horneamos el pan con semillas de amapola.

Final y presentación: Sobre la rodaja de pan con semillas de amapola, disponemos la base de chaka, gambas y mayonesa. Sobre ella, una hermosa rodaja de salmón ahumado que regaremos con la vinagreta. Finalmente, coronaremos el pintxo con un langostino cocido.

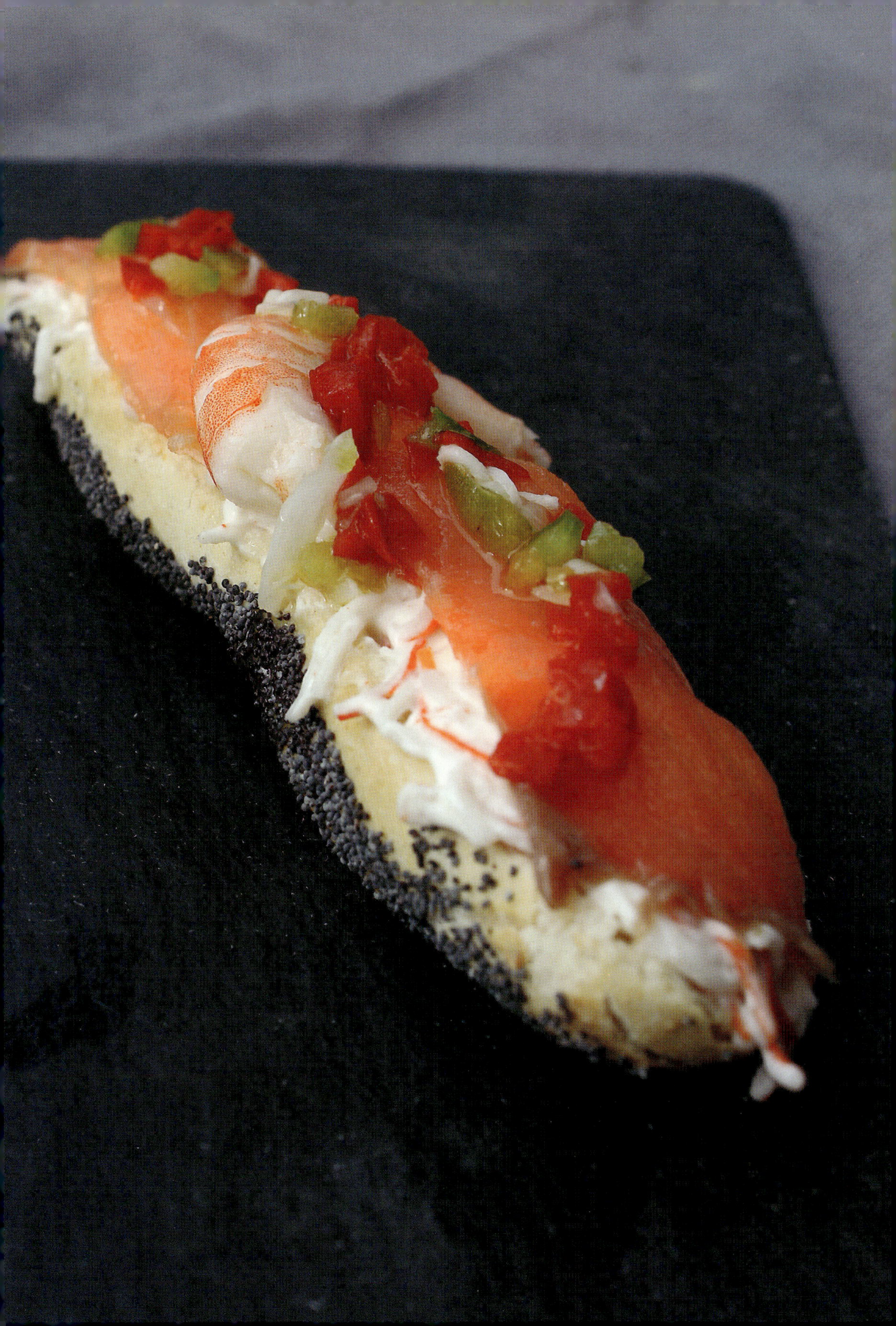

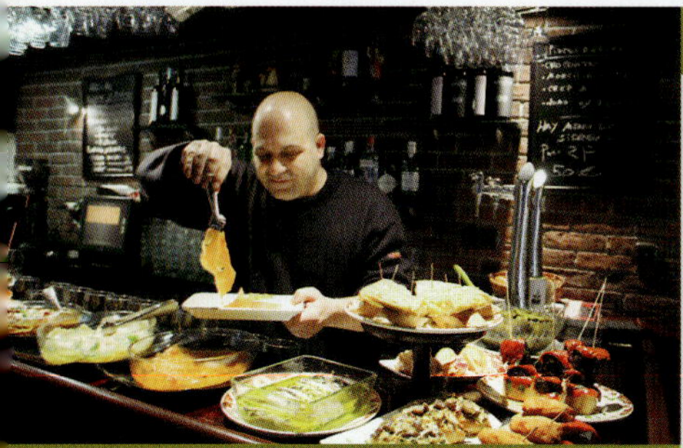

INFERNUKOA

Mahastarreka, 23
BERGARA
943 76 18 49
www.infernukua.com

Pocos establecimientos pueden presumir de haberse abierto en el siglo XIX y haber llegado a nuestros días. Es el caso del Infernukua, abierto como **Restaurante Matilde Alkarain** hacia 1890 por la tatarabuela del actual regente, **Alex González**, y que en un momento de su trayectoria cambió su nombre a Infernukua, pero sin dejar de ser regentado, salvo en un corto periodo a mediados del siglo XX, por la misma familia. Reformado en 2011 pero con un comedor que guarda el sabor de antaño, Infernukua ofrece hoy una **exquisita variedad de pintxos, carnes y pescados a la brasa y especialidades de cocina tradicional** como Txipirones en su tinta o a la plancha, Bacalao en varias formas (con piperrada, a la bizkaina, al pil-pil...), Ensaladas, Fritos caseros... La txuleta a la brasa es la reina del local, y puede ser consumida sola o dentro del Menú de sidrería, eso sí, solicitándose siempre con antelación.

Otros pintxos:

- *Tortilla de patata*
- *Tortilla de bacalao*
- *Bonito con mayonesa, guindilla y antxoa*
- *Revuelto de hongos*
- *Champiñón en vinagreta con bacon*
- *Morcilla con piquillos*

Ahumados caseros:

- *Salmón ahumado*
- *Bacalao ahumado*
- *Antxoas y boquerones*

"Rolling Stone"

Ingredientes:

Lomo adobado cocido
Harina
Huevo
Pan rallado
Pimiento del piquillo asado
Pan
Sal
Aceite de oliva

- **Para la bechamel:**

Mantequilla
Harina
Nuez moscada
Ajo
Leche

Elaboración:

Para la bechamel: Fundimos la mantequilla a fuego lento, hacemos en ella el ajo y añadimos la harina cocinándola un rato sin dejar de remover. Añadimos la leche y la nuez moscada, removiendo constantemente, y lo terminamos de cocinar durante 10-15 minutos a fuego lento.

Final y presentación: Pasamos el lomo por harina, huevo y pan rallado y lo freímos en aceite de oliva. Sobre una rodaja de pan disponemos un pimiento del piquillo asado y, sobre él, el lomo rebozado, haciendo que el pimiento sobresalga, recordando la lengua que le da nombre al pintxo. Terminamos ensartando el conjunto con un palillo.

Nota: Este pintxo, conocido también como "Lomo especial", se sirve también como bocadillo, cosechando un gran éxito, y también puede elaborarse con pechuga de pollo.
Es un pintxo que puede ser congelado, aunque se recomienda hacerlo después de freír, para evitar así que al freír se rompa.

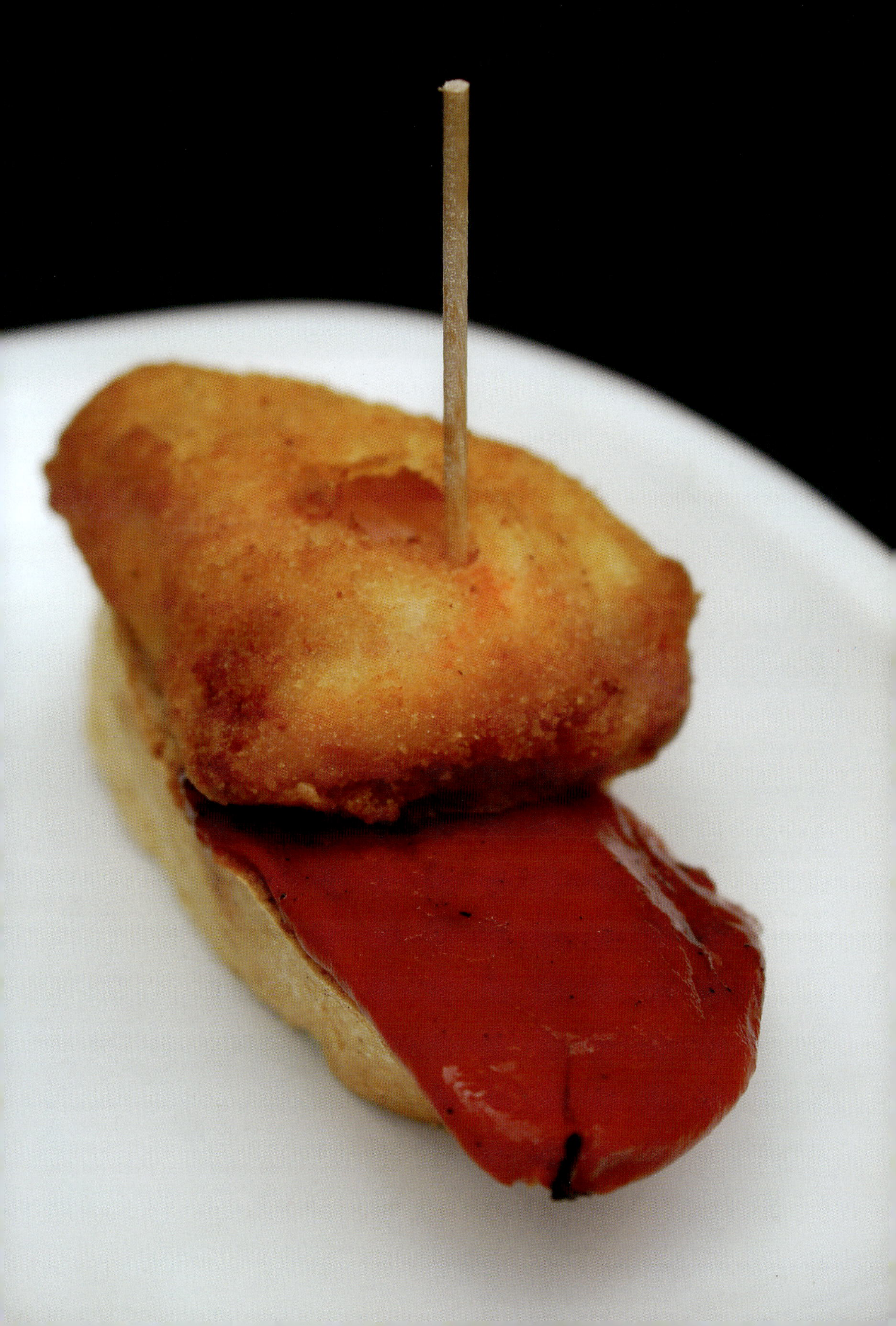

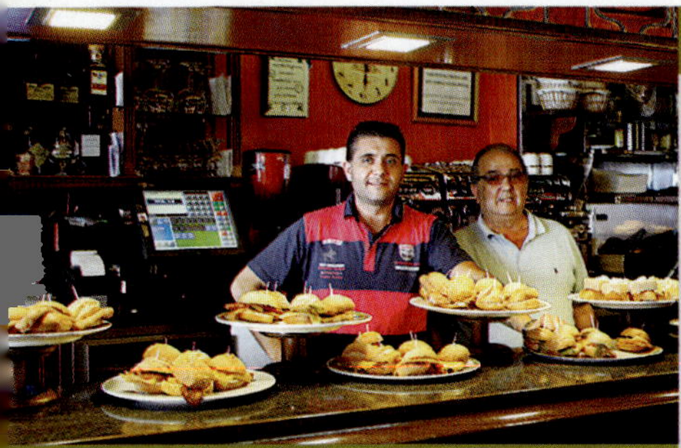

Gabiria kalea 3 (Políg. Ventas)
IRUN
943 63 52 17

IÑAKI

El Iñaki está estratégicamente situado a la entrada del Polígono Industrial de Ventas, uno de los más grandes de Irun. Al cargo del mismo se encuentra desde 1996 **Iñaki Cid** con la inestimable ayuda de su hermano **Mikel** en la cocina. **Los pintxos y los menús del día son la especialidad indiscutible de este bar restaurante** que abre todos los días (salvo domingos) a las 7 de la mañana y que desde las 8 presenta una barra llena de tentaciones como sus **múltiples tortillas de patatas rellenas y sus montaditos variados**, todo ello sin olvidar sus callos caseros. Destacan también en el Iñaki sus **platos combinados**, así como sus **bocadillos**, con nombres tan curiosos como Iñakito, Mikelito o Pantxito. También son muy solicitados los bocadillos vegetales o el de Solomillo con pimiento verde. Iñaki ofrece todos los días servicio de comidas y cenas salvo los sábados que cierra por las tardes.

Otros pintxos:

- *Callos caseros*
- *Tortilla de patata tradicional*
- *Tortilla de patata rellena de jamón y queso*
- *Tortilla de patata rellena de mayonesa, tomate y bacon*
- *Tortilla de patata rellena de chaka*
- *Montadito de lomo*
- *Montadito de bacon*
- *Montadito vegetal*
- *Montadito "tradicional" (Tomate, jamón y huevo frito)*
- *Pimientos rellenos de carne (ración)*

Montadito de berenjena rellena de bacon con salteado de pimientos

Ingredientes:

Berenjena
Bacon
Queso de cabra
Huevo de codorniz
Harina
Huevo
Aceite de oliva
Sal Maldon negra
Un bollito de pan
Reducción de Módena
Ajilimójilis

- **Para el salteado de pimientos:**

Pimiento rojo
Pimiento verde
Cebolla
Perejil
Aceite de oliva

Elaboración:

Para el salteado de pimientos: Picamos muy finamente el pimiento rojo, el pimiento verde y la cebolla y lo rehogamos en aceite de oliva a fuego vivo hasta que se dore bien, incluso que quede ligeramente tostado.

Cortamos dos rodajas finas de berenjena, las pasamos por harina y huevo y las freímos en aceite de oliva. Pasamos el bacon por la plancha.

Freímos en aceite de oliva el huevo de codorniz y lo sazonamos con sal Maldon negra.

Cortamos una rodaja fina de queso de cabra y la pasamos por la plancha por los dos lados.

Final y presentación: Abrimos un bollito de montadito y colocamos, en este orden, el queso de cabra, una rodaja rebozada de berenjena, el bacon, otra rodaja de berenjena y el huevo de codorniz. Cerramos el montadito y lo atravesamos con un palillo de brocheta para que no se desparrame. Lo servimos acompañado del salteado de pimientos, unos hilos de reducción de Módena y unas gotas de ajilimójilis.

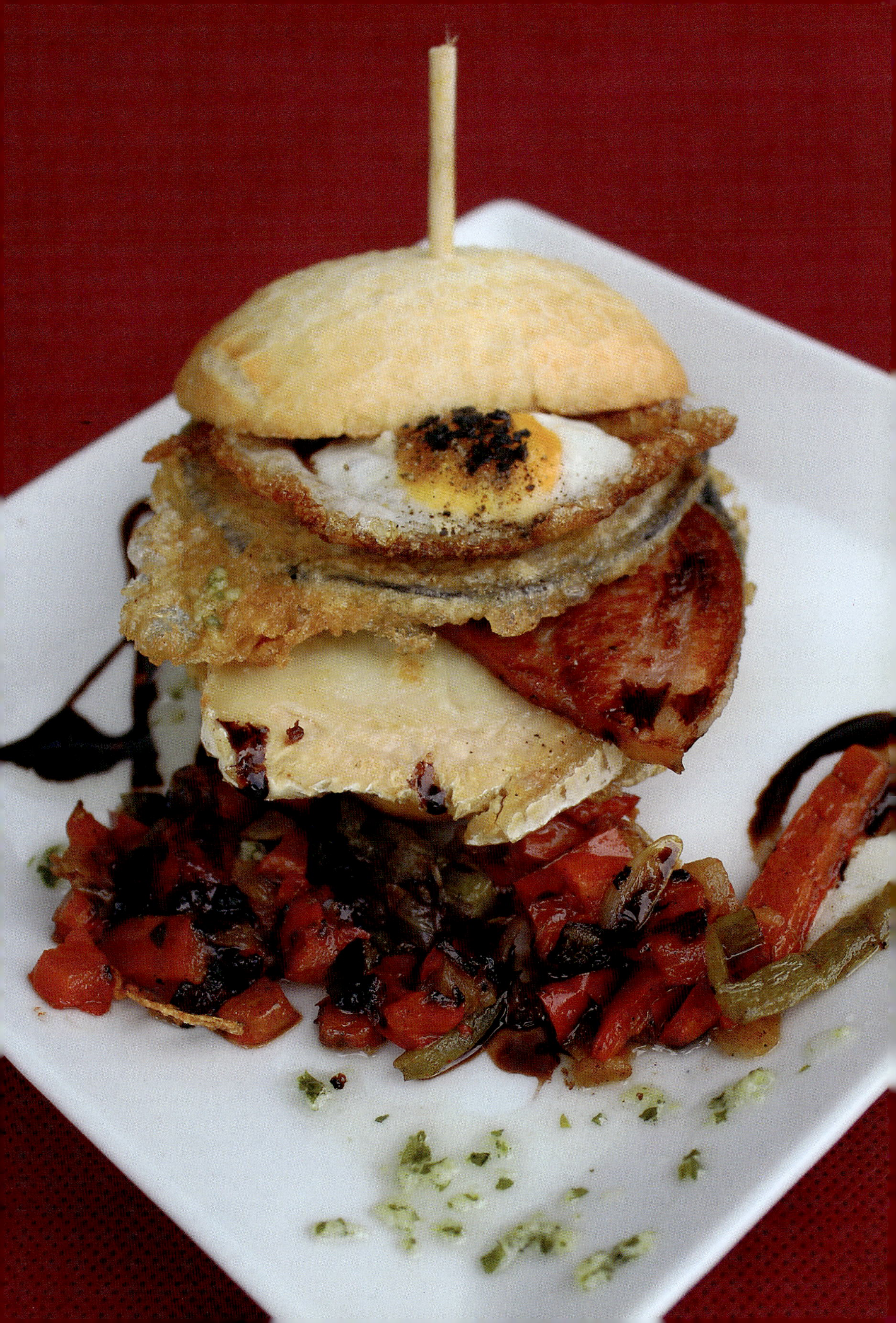

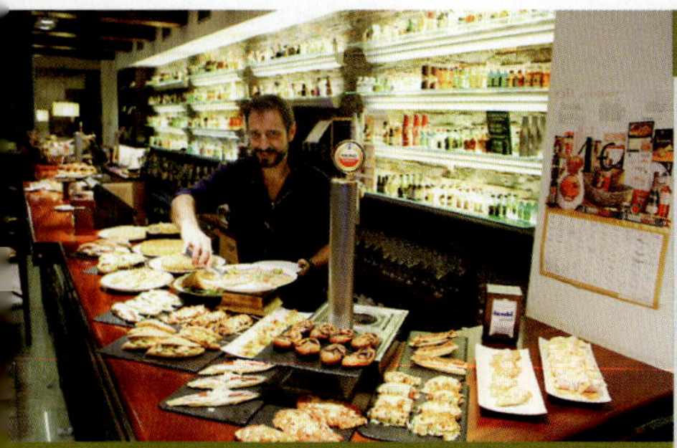

Gipuzkoa plaza, 15 (Centro)
DONOSTIA
943 42 84 23
www.iombi.com

IOMBI

El bar Iombi fue inaugurado por el tolosarra **Joxe Mari Zunzunegi** en marzo de 1983, aunque en sus inicios fue la primera tienda de caramelos a granel de Donostia. Para 1988 ya era bar y hoy son los hijos de **Joxe Mari, Ion, Cristina y Elena**, junto a su yerno **Uri**, quienes lo gestionan, al frente de un excelente equipo bien asentado. Estratégicamente situado en el corazón del área romántica de la ciudad y dotado de una atractiva terraza aporticada, Iombi abre todos los días de lunes a sábado a las 8:30 de la mañana para ofrecer **desayunos y pintxos** y a lo largo de todo el día permanece abierto con una vasta oferta que incluye **Menú del día, Raciones, Ensaladas, Bocadillos, Platos de carta, Platos de huevos, Hamburguesas, Sandwiches...** es destacable su jamón ibérico de bellota de gran calidad así como el hecho de que todo el pan se hornea en el día.

Otros pintxos:

- *Rollito de calabacín relleno de Philladelphia con jamón dulce y queso italiano*
- *Barquita*
- *Tosta de berenjena con tomate troceado y queso*
- *Rollito de lomo adobado con queso*
- *Croqueta de jamón*
- *Rollito de salmón*
- *Brick relleno de hongos y gambas*
- *Flor de jamón con revuelto de ajo confitado*
- *Pintxo de pastel de merluza fresca*

Pintxo "Iombi"

Ingredientes:

Yema de huevo de codorniz
Foie fresco
Sal Maldon

- **Para la salsa de caramelo:**

Azúcar
Agua
Vinagre
Pasas de corinto

Elaboración:

Para la salsa de caramelo: Poner una sartén al fuego con azúcar y, cuando empiece a fundirse, añadir un poco de agua, vinagre y unas pasas de corinto, tratando de que la salsa no quede sólida.

Cortar una pequeña rodaja de foie fresco y hacerla a la plancha, vuelta y vuelta.

Separar la yema de la clara del huevo de codorniz.

Final y presentación: En una cucharita de cerámica, disponer la yema de huevo y cubrirla con la salsa de caramelo intentando que incluya una o dos pasas de corinto. Depositar encima la rodajita de foie a la plancha y coronar con unas escamas de sal Maldon. Este pintxo debe servirse inmediatamente para que al ser degustado el comensal perciba el contraste entre las temperaturas de la yema (fría), la salsa de caramelo (templada) y el foie (caliente).

Nota: Este pintxo obtuvo el Plato de Bronce en el Campeonato de Pintxos de Gipuzkoa de 2002.

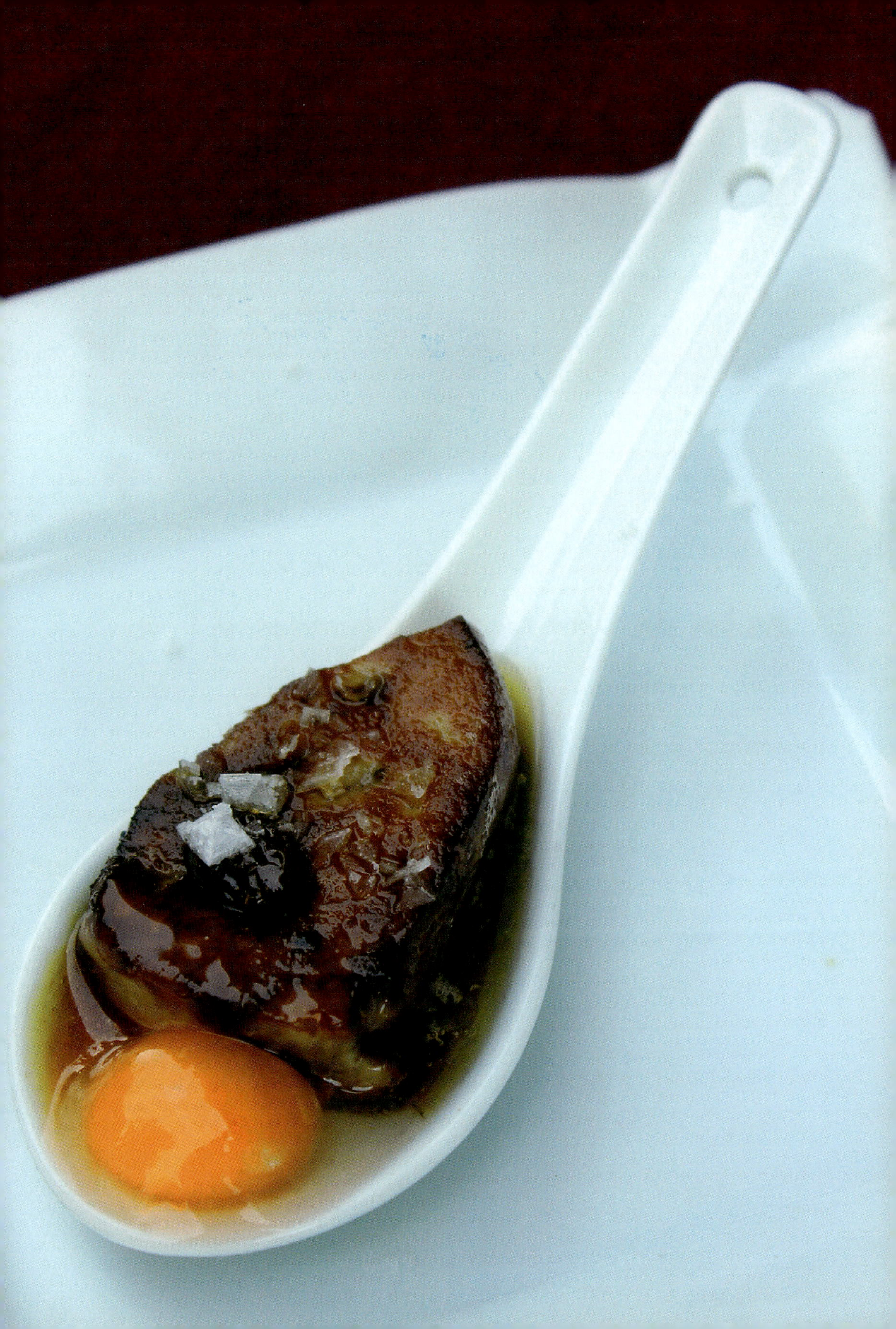

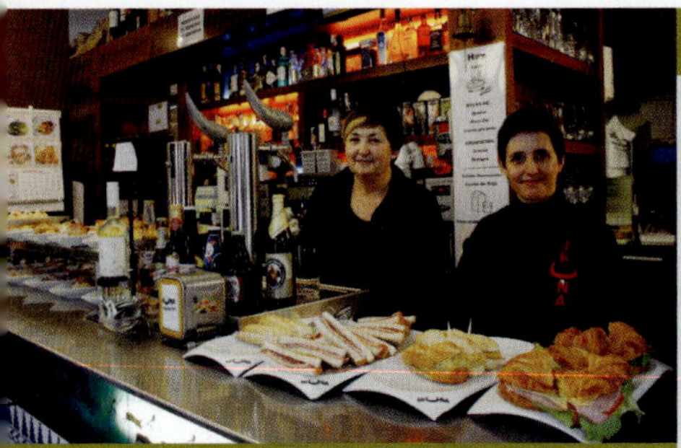

Easo, 73 (Centro)
DONOSTIA
943 45 69 17

IRUÑA

Puy Ustaroz, natural de Urbiola (Tierra Estella) abrió el Iruña en la plaza Easo en junio de 2004, pero anteriormente había regentado tres emblemáticos bares en la Parte Vieja de Pamplona: La Granja, Café Roch y La Bodeguita de en medio. Como buena navarra, a Donostia se trajo los **pintxos de verdura** que hacía en Iruña, aunque no todos tuvieron el mismo éxito, perdurando el de acelga y el de berenjena. Iruña abre todos los días a las 7 de la mañana y desde primera hora ofrece diversos pintxos. **La cocina permanece abierta todo el día con una gran variedad de bocadillos, sandwiches, platos combinados, raciones, tostas** (como su afamada Tosta de jamón con rulo de cabra) **y ensaladas**, destacando la Ensalada Iruña (Lechuga, cebolla, pollo a la plancha, pasas, queso de cabra y vinagre de Módena). Los ibéricos también son destacables en este establecimiento que sólo cierra en Navidad y Año Nuevo.

Otros pintxos:

- *Acelga con bechamel de espinacas*
- *Berenjena con bechamel de jamón y jamón ibérico*
- *Pimiento relleno de bacalao*
- *Revuelto de hongos y gambas*
- *Revuelto de morcilla (en invierno)*
- *Foie con salsa agridulce o al Oporto*
- *Vieira rellena de txangurro*
- *Hojaldre de foie y manzana*
- *Brick de setas y gambas*
- *Hojaldre de chorizo*

Cesta de patata con hongos y foie

Ingredientes:

1 patata
Agua
Aceite de oliva
Sal
Hongos
Foie fresco
Harina
Reducción de Módena
Sal Maldon

Elaboración:

Cocemos la patata sin quitarle la piel durante tres cuartos de hora en agua con sal a la que añadimos también un chorrito de aceite de oliva para que se pele mejor.

Una vez cocida, la dejamos enfriar, la pelamos, le hacemos un hueco y la reservamos.

Limpiamos los hongos, los picamos finamente y los salteamos en aceite de oliva.

Cortamos una rodaja de foie fresco, la enharinamos y la hacemos en la plancha vuelta y vuelta.

Final y presentación: Rellenamos el hueco de la patata con los hongos salteados. Colocamos encima la rodaja de foie. Añadimos unas escamas de sal Maldon y decoramos el pintxo con unos hilitos de reducción de Módena.

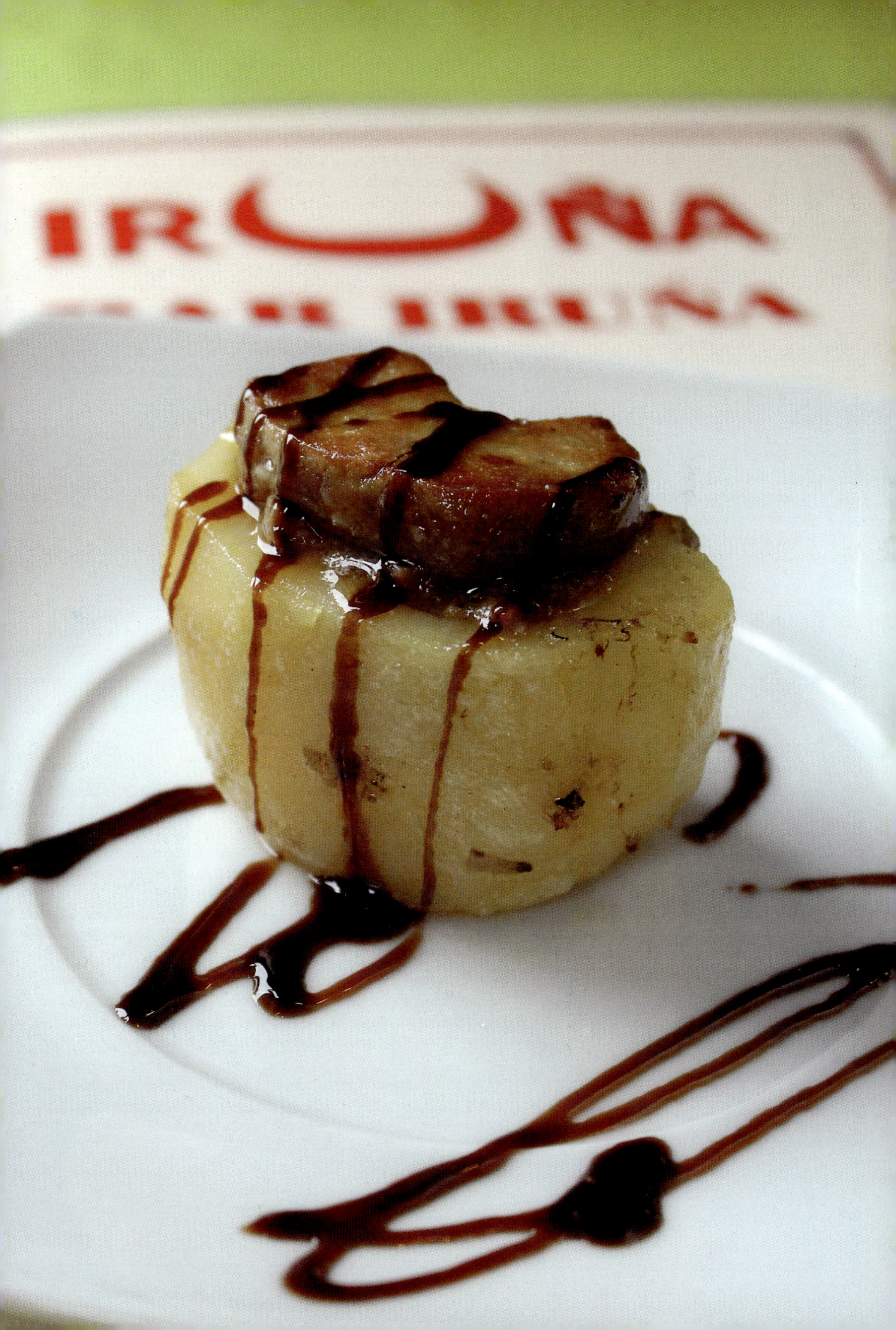
IRUÑA

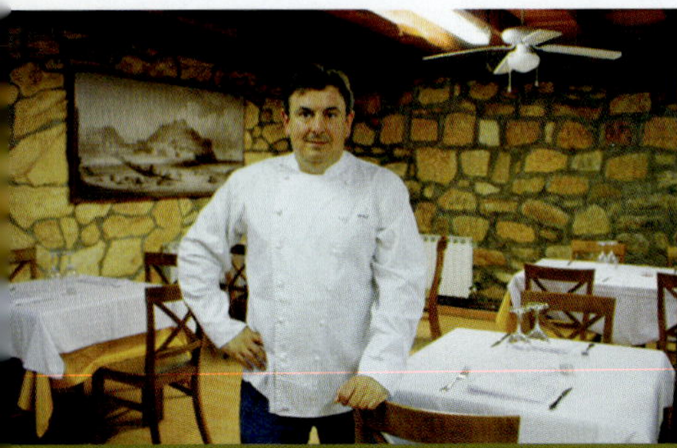

ITURRIETA - BERRI

Camping de Igeldo
DONOSTIA
943 22 65 83
www.iturrietaberri.com

Quienes se acerquen a Iturrieta Berri, el restaurante del camping de Igeldo, se llevarán una agradable sorpresa gastronómica de la mano del donostiarra **Mikel Mayán**, que **fue campeón estatal de cocina hacia 1995 y representó a España en el prestigioso certamen Bocusse de Oro**. Mikel comenzó en Arzak hace más de 20 años y pasó cinco años como jefe de cocina en el restaurante de Karlos Arguiñano antes de ponerse por su cuenta. En Igeldo, **Mayán ofrece una carta tradicional con evidentes toques de autor, en la que lo más interesante resulta el original Menú degustación de Gastroparrilla**, una muestra de que la parrilla no está reñida con la modernidad. Por supuesto, los pescados frescos a la parrilla, acarreados a diario de Getaria, son otro de los fuertes del local, así como las **carnes, generalmente procedentes de la zona** (Aia, Oiartzun...) adquiridas en la carnicería Mikel de El Antiguo. Destacan también sus **hamburguesas, 100% de ternera**, servidas en pan "de verdad".

Otros pintxos:

- *Morcilla de arroz asada*
- *Champi guisado*
- *Zancarrón con tomate*
- *Croquetas caseras*
- *Pintxo Moruno*

Raciones:

- *Rabas "de verdad"*
- *Calamares frescos*
- *Pimientos verdes fritos*
- *Patatas bravas con salsa picante casera*

Cogollo a la parrilla con vinagreta de frutos secos

Ingredientes:

½ cogollo de Tudela
Antxoa en salazón
Lascas de Idiazabal
Cebollino

· Para la vinagreta de frutos secos:
Pipas de girasol
Pipas de calabaza
Nueces
Pasas
Pistacho
Aceite de oliva virgen extra
Vinagre de Módena
Sal

Elaboración:

Para la vinagreta de frutos secos: Picar la nuez y el pistacho en un mortero. Añadir las pipas de girasol y calabaza y las pasas, y hornear 5 minutos a 180°. Una vez horneados los frutos secos, añadir aceite de oliva virgen extra, vinagre de Módena y sal y dejar macerar un mínimo de dos horas.

Hacer el cogollo de Tudela 5 minutos a la parrilla y terminarlo con 2 minutos de horno a 180°.

Final y presentación: Servir en un platillo el cogollo y verter encima la vinagreta de frutos secos. Sobre la vinagreta, disponer una buena antxoa en salazón y coronar con unas lascas de queso Idiazabal. Finalmente, decorar con un poco de cebollino fresco.

Nota: Es recomendable no preparar más vinagreta de frutos secos que la estrictamente necesaria, y no guardar la que sobre.

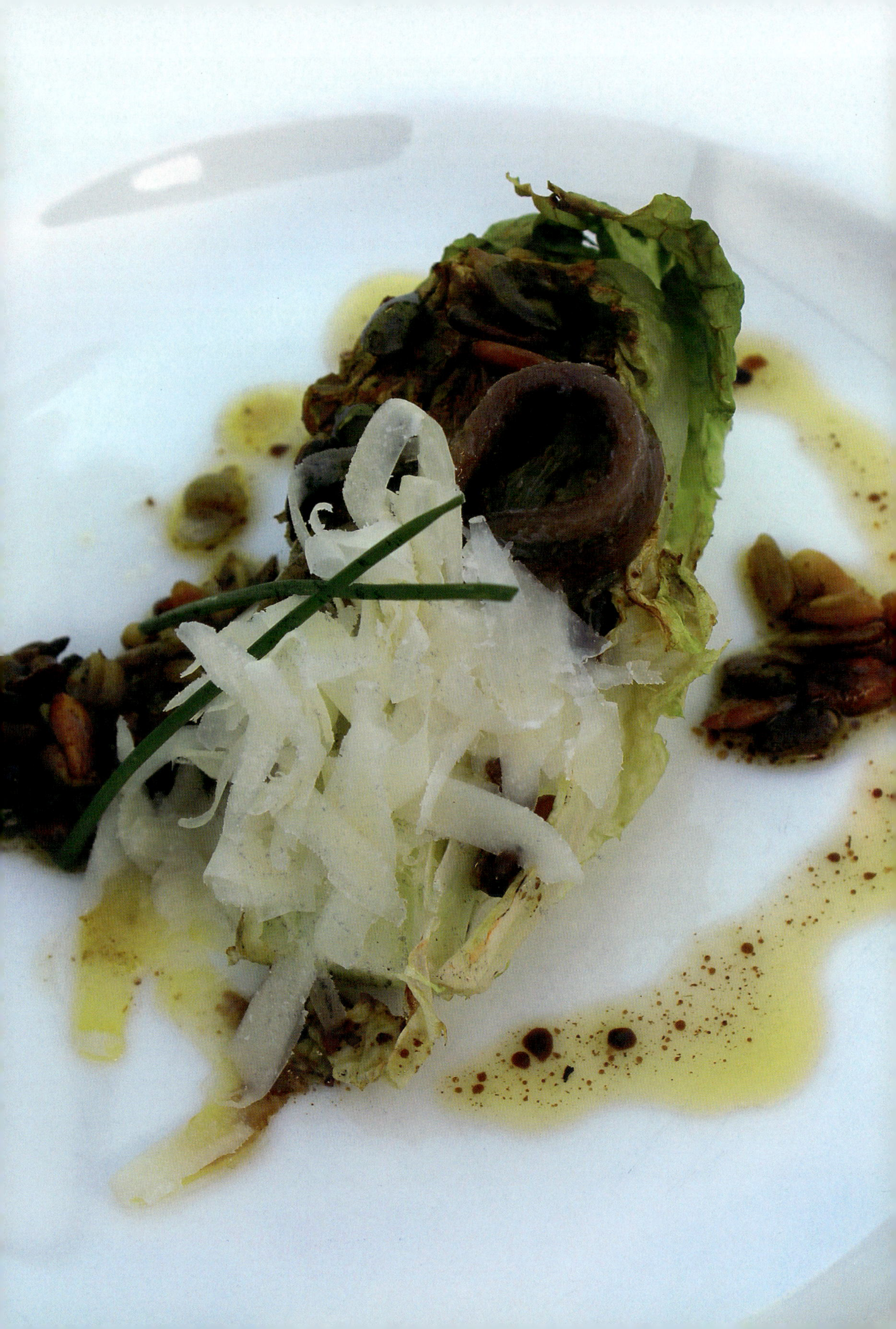

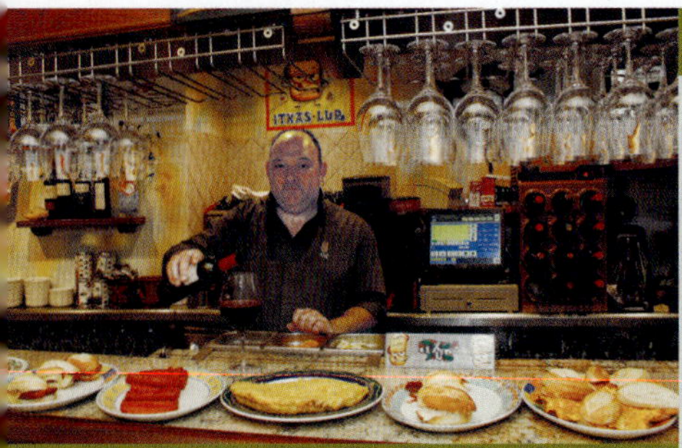

ITXAS-LUR

Plaza Santuiturri, 3
ZARAUTZ
943 89 01 38
www.itxaslur.com

Los **bocadillos elaborados con pan horneado al momento** son sin duda el buque insignia de este establecimiento inaugurado por **Pascu Expósito y Gurutze Gorostidi** en junio de 1999, con una impresionante carta con más de 60 referencias de bokatas entre las que destaca el Itxas-Lur (Bacon, queso, pimientos y setas) o los Vegetales (con pollo, con bacon, con jamón de York...). También llama la atención la variedad de **Platos combinados**, con más de 12 a elegir, sin incluir el **Plato infantil**, y las 7 **Hamburguesas caseras**, cuyo top ocupa la Santuiturri, servida en pan de bocadillo con doble de carne a lo ancho, lechuga, tomate, queso, cebolla, jamón York, mahonesa y un huevo. Itxas-Lur abre todos los días a las 10 de la mañana y ofrece servicio de **Menú del día y Menú especial de fin de semana**, así como cenas todos los días. Su terraza en una plaza peatonal equipada con columpios la convierten en un lugar ideal para acudir en familia.

Otros pintxos:

- *Chorizo cocido*
- *Txistorra frita*
- *Champiñón al ajillo con langostino*
- *Tortilla de patata*
- *Pechuga empanada, queso y bacon*
- *Ensaladilla natural*

Raciones:

- *Patatas bravas y ali-oli*
- *Rabas naturales*
- *Txipirones a la plancha*

Brocheta de pulpo y langostinos

Ingredientes:

Pulpo
Langostinos
Pimentón picante
Pimentón dulce
Sal gorda
Aceite de olliva virgen extra

Elaboración:

Cocemos el pulpo a la manera tradicional, en una cazuela con agua hirviendo en la que habremos introducido una patata sin pelar. Cuando el agua está hirviendo, sumergimos en ella el pulpo y lo dejamos medio minuto dentro, repitiendo el proceso 7 veces. La séptima vez, dejamos que se siga cociendo hasta que la patata se abra.

Mezclamos en una salsera o en un bol pimentón dulce, pimentón picante, sal gorda y aceite de oliva virgen extra. Reservamos.

Final y presentación: Cortamos tres rodajas de una de las patas del pulpo y las ensartamos en un palillo de brocheta junto a dos langostinos crudos. Hacemos la brocheta a la plancha, la colocamos en un plato y vertemos encima la mezcla de pimentones, aceite y sal gorda.

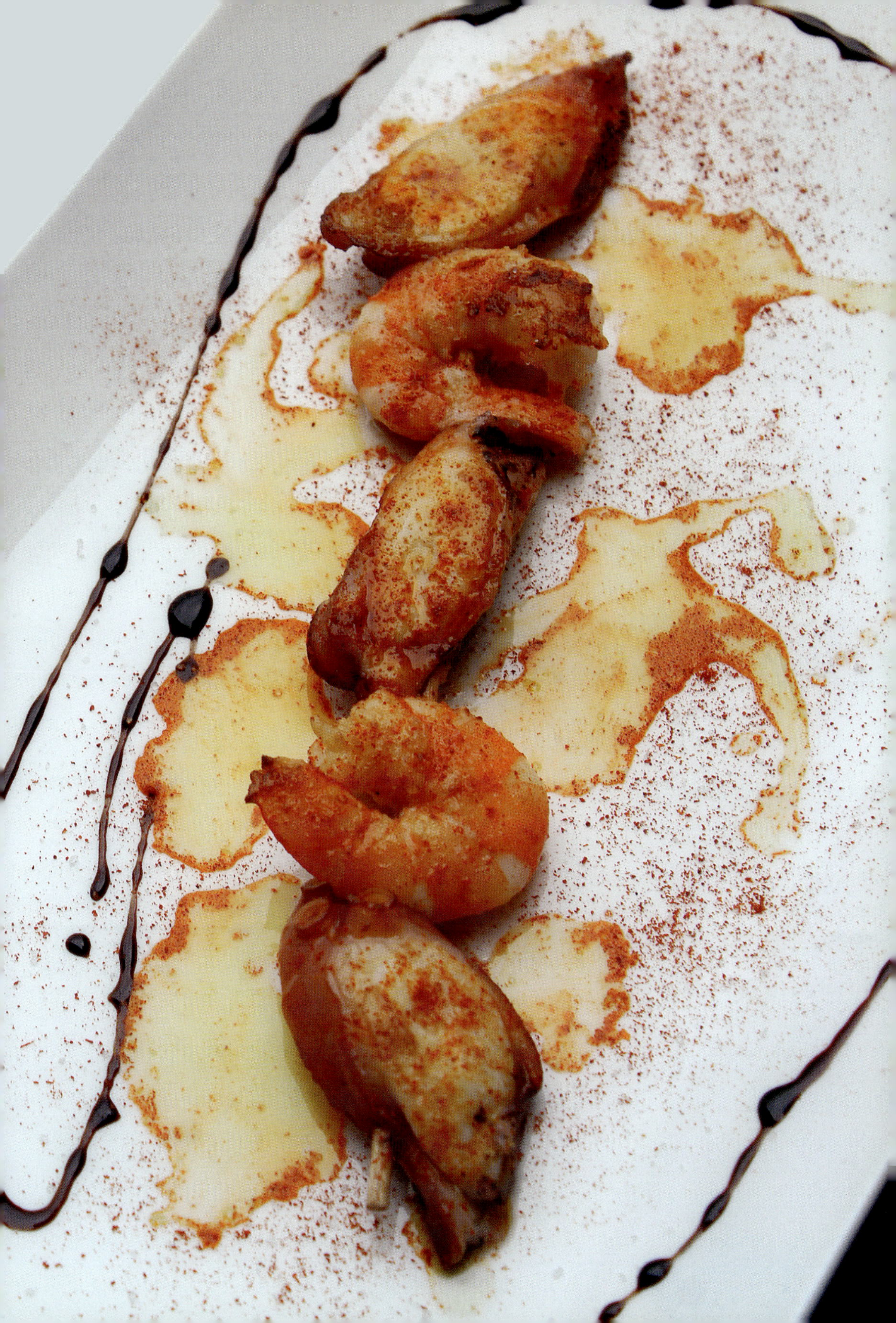

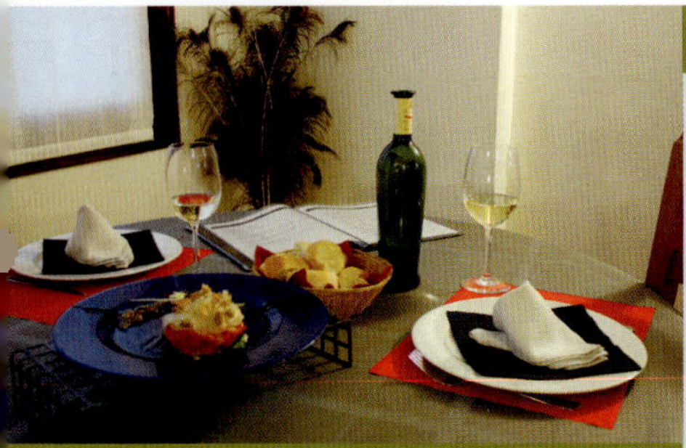

JAI - ALAI

La urretxuarra **Aloña Bosque**, curtida en los fogones del Etxeberri de Zumarraga y el Ostatu de Gabiria, dirige desde marzo de 2012 este bar-restaurante en el que ofrece una cocina colorista y divertida. En el Jai podremos optar entre **dos niveles de carta: una informal con raciones, bocadillos y platos combinados y otra con platos más elaborados**, además de un completo menú del día y un menú de fin de semana en el que encontraremos platos de la carta. Todo ello sin olvidar su completa barra de pintxos. En Jai-Alai, además, podemos disfrutar de diferentes **especialidades vegetarianas**, como el Ravioli relleno de espinaca y gorgonzola o la exitosa Hamburguesa de avena, que se ofrece como plato, como bocata o como pintxo. Y para los más pekes, hay 6 platos infantiles y una divertida zona de juegos para que puedan explayarse a gusto.

Iparragirre, 10
URRETXU
943 25 38 84

Otros pintxos:

- *Mini pizza*
- *Tosta de 4 quesos*
- *Jamón, queso y pimiento verde*
- *Revuelto de langostino con cebollino*
- *Tortilla de patata*
- *Brick relleno de calabacín, bacon y langostino*
- *Brick relleno de morcilla con manzana y salsa de piquillo*
- *Ventresca con pimiento asado*
- *Crema de hongos con jamón ibérico*
- *Hamburguesa de avena*

Brick relleno de hongos con salsa de foie

Ingredientes:

Pasta Brick
Cebollino fresco
Aceite de perejil

· Para el relleno del brick:
Cebolla
Hongos
Harina
Nata

· Para la salsa de foie:
Foie micuit
Cebolla
Un chorrito de Cognac
Nata

Elaboración:

Para la salsa de foie: Picamos finamente y rehogamos la cebolla. Añadimos un chorrito de Cognac y dejamos que reduzca. Añadimos un poco de nata y el foie micuit cortado en daditos. Ponemos a fuego bajo para que se derrita el foie y, en caso de que esté sobrado de aceite, se lo retiramos. Finalmente, trituramos todo con la batidora y pasamos la salsa por el chino.

Para el relleno del brick: Picamos finamente y pochamos la cebolla. Añadimos los hongos picaditos y dejamos que se rehoguen un poco. Añadimos una pizca de harina y un poquito de nata y lo llevamos a ebullición, dejando que hierva durante un minuto a fuego bajo.

Rellenamos una lámina de pasta brick con la farsa de cebolla y hongos. La cerramos dándole forma de saquito y la introducimos al horno dejándolo entre 3 y 4 minutos a 180ª

Final y presentación: Servimos el saquito de brick acompañado de la salsa de foie y unos hilitos de aceite de perejil. Podemos decorarlo con una ramita de cebollino fresco.

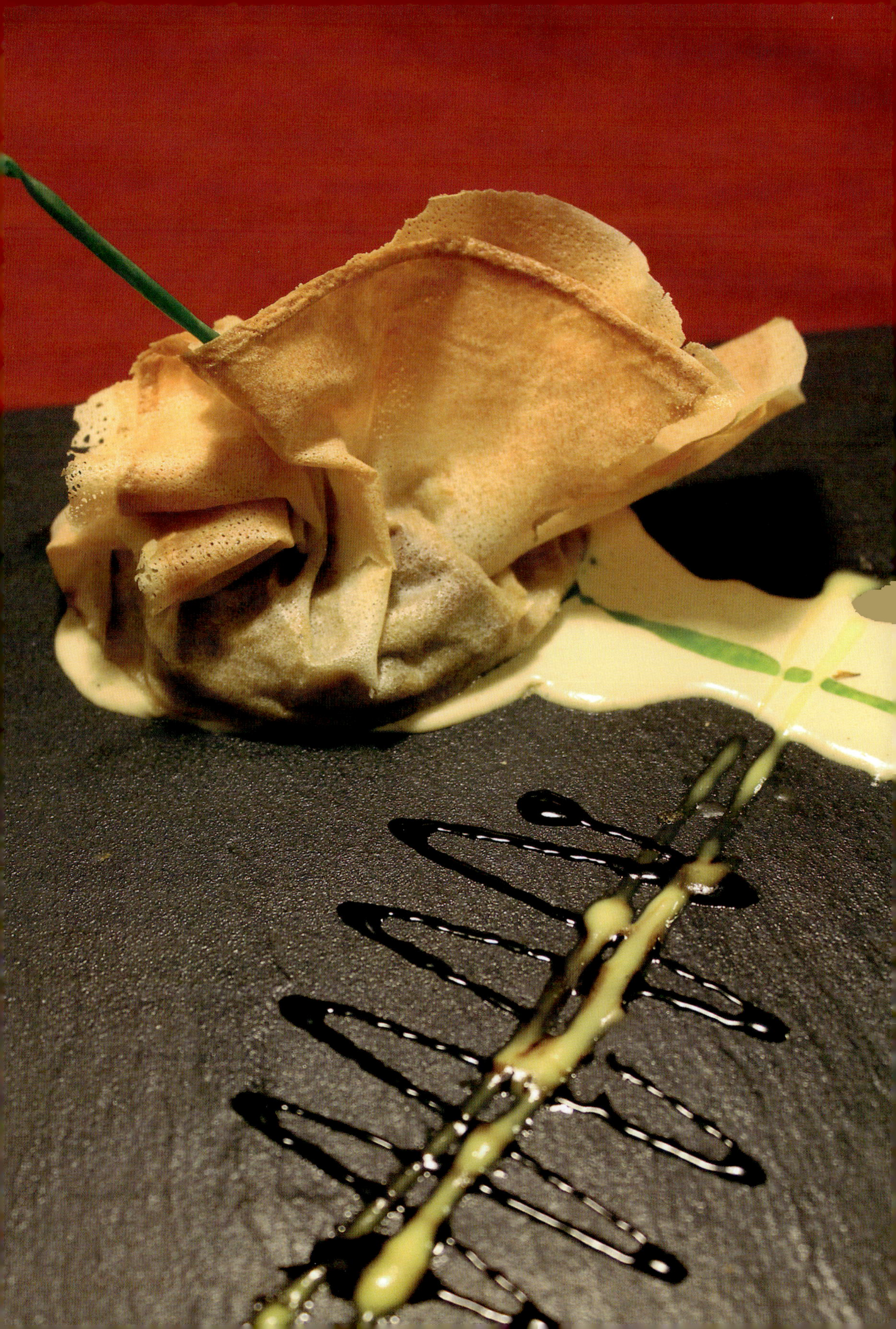

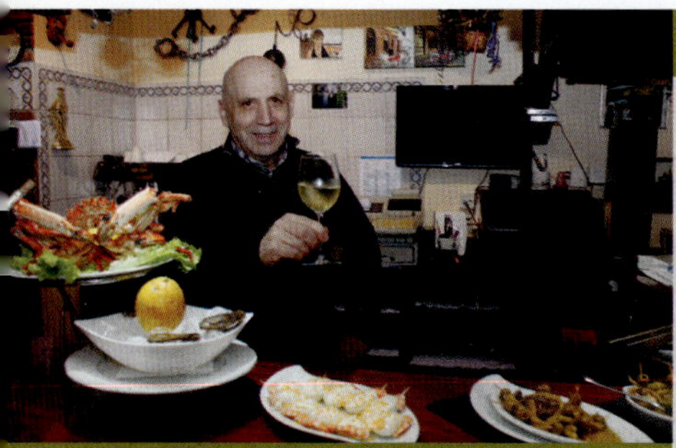

Iparkalea, 13
ZARAUTZ
943 31 42 36

JOE

Inmejorablemente situado entre el paseo marítimo y Musika Plaza, este bar abierto en 1991 por el arronatarra **José Luis Sánchez** ocupa el solar que en su día albergó al bar Bixkiak (también conocido como "El corderito"). José Luis contaba con una gran experiencia adquirida en La Cabaña del Tío Tom de Arrona y en el Alai de Zarautz, y con la ayuda en barra de su hija **Lorea**, ha convertido a su pequeño pero bien aprovechado bar en toda una institución del buen comer con **raciones de marisco fresco** (Camarón, Ostras, Centollo cocido, Ensalada de bogavante...) y **productos de temporada** (Antxoas, Bonito, Guisantes con huevo escalfado, Habitas con jamón...). Amante, y hasta en su día practicante, de los deportes más diversos, José Luis organiza los autobuses para acudir a Anoeta y **vende en su bar entradas para los partidos de la Real Sociedad**. Los miércoles, además, ofrece pintxo-pote a partir de las 7 de la tarde.

Otros pintxos:

- *Txipirón encebollado con cebolla caramelizada*
- *Trainera (huevo, antxoa y mayonesa sobre una rodaja de pan tostado)*
- *Tortilla de patata (especialidad)*
- *Gilda con taco de bonito del Norte*
- *"El clásico" (Pintxo de Gamba, huevo duro y mayonesa)*

Raciones:

- *Ostras*
- *Centollo cocido*
- *Antxoas (en temporada)*

Salpicón de marisco

Ingredientes:

Bogavante
Centollo
Buey de mar
Langostino

- **Para la vinagreta:**

Cebolleta
Pimiento rojo
Pimiento verde
Sal
Aceite de oliva virgen extra
Vinagre de Módena

Elaboración:

Para la vinagreta: Picamos muy finamente la cebolleta, el pimiento rojo y el pimiento verde y los disponemos en un bol, cubriéndolos con aceite de oliva virgen extra, sal y vinagre de manzana. Mezclamos bien y reservamos para que repose.

Cocemos el bogavante, el centollo, el buey de mar y el langostino. Salvo el langostino, que dejaremos entero, picamos muy finamente la carne del resto del marisco.

Mezclamos la carne picada del marisco con la vinagreta que hemos dejado reservada.

Final y presentación: Servimos en una cuchara la mezcla de la vinagreta con la carne picada de marisco y coronamos el pintxo con el langostino pelado.

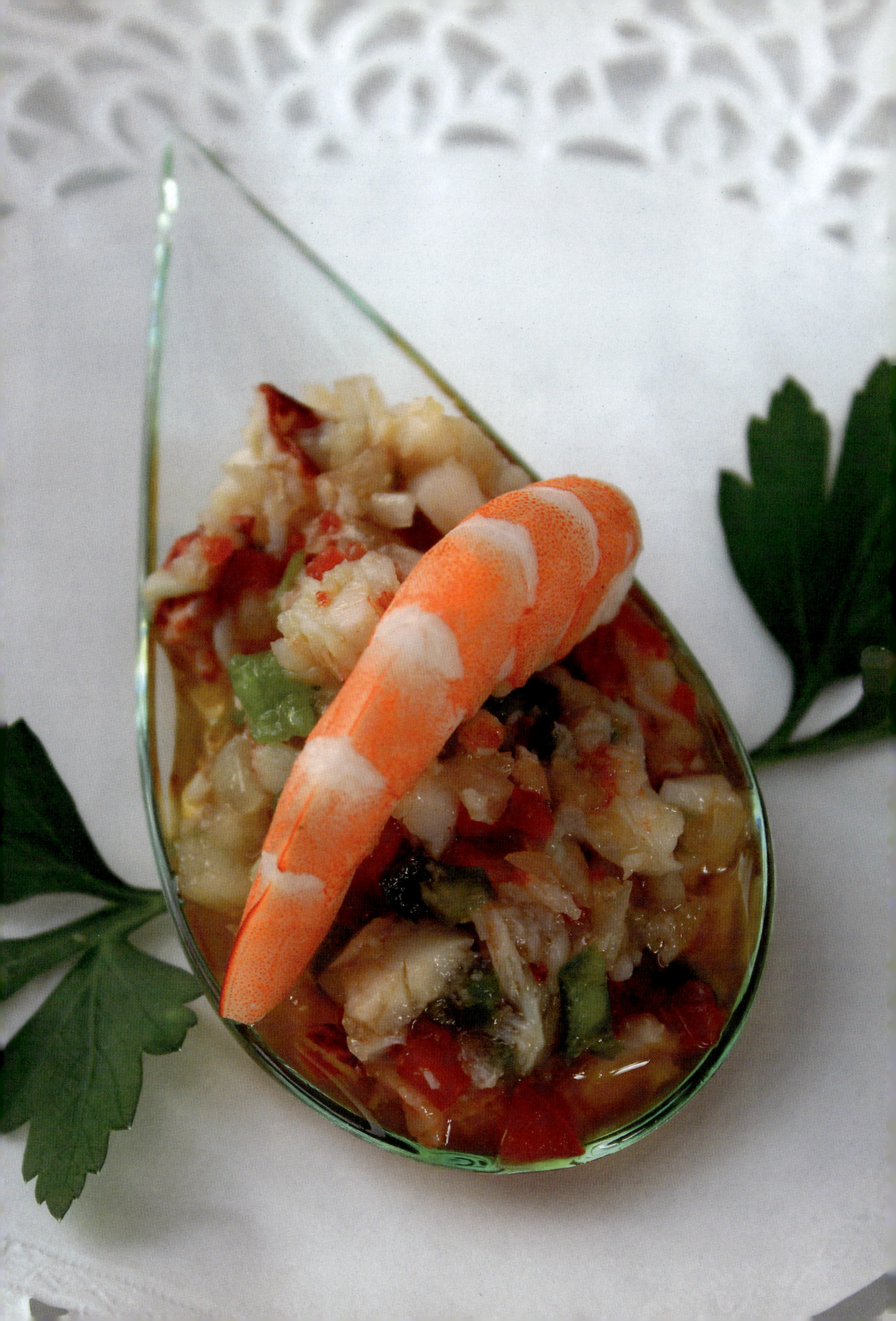

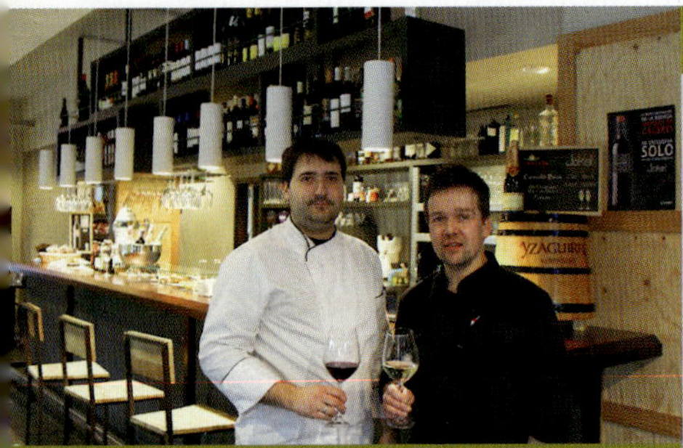

JOKEL

Martin Jose Iraola, 10
TOLOSA
943 11 60 17

Jose Ignacio Ferreras (Jo) y Mikel Moreno (Kel) dan nombre a su nuevo proyecto, Jokel, **un local que pretende huir del corsé de un restaurante, yendo más allá de un simple bar de pikoteo.** En Jokel encontraremos pintxos y raciones convencionales (Tortilla de patata, pastel de pescado...), pero también platos de indudable entidad gastronómica como Champiñones brasa-oli, Hongos a la parrilla con yema líquida, Ensalada templada de vieira y alcachofa... eso sí, **huyendo de la estructura primero-segundo-postre.** Lo que Jo y Kel quieren es que la gente venga a su casa, pique un pintxo, comparta un plato y termine con un gin-tonic, o que se limiten a picotear o, ¿por qué no? que se den un homenaje. Libertad sin condicionantes es la propuesta de esta **casa que trabaja con ahínco la parrilla** (Pulpo, verduras, pescados...), que **mima el producto de temporada** (espárragos en primavera, tomate en verano...) y que **cuida el detalle** (buenos hielos, bebidas frías, buena carta de vinos, rico vermouth de grifo...)

Otros pintxos:

- *Tortilla de patata*
- *Huevo a 60° con migas crujientes*
- *Chorizo encarbonado*
- *Langostino con panceta ibérica con mango*
- *Taco de solomillo de salmón noruego ahumado*
- *Txistorra con huevo roto*

Raciones:

- *Ibéricos variados*
- *Mejilloncitos bravos*
- *Kokotxas de bacalao*

Vieira a la plancha sobre crema de calabaza

Ingredientes:

1 vieira (la nuez, sin el coral)
Alga nori

· Para la crema de calabaza:
Calabaza
Cebolla
Cáscara de naranja
Fumet de pescado
Nata
Sal

· Para la salsa de soja y gengibre:
Salsa de soja
Gengibre rallado
Sésamo

Elaboración:

Para la crema de calabaza: Picamos finamente y pochamos la cebolla en aceite de oliva. Una vez sudada la cebolla, rehogamos los trozos de calabaza y rallamos un poco de peladura de naranja por encima. Mojamos el conjunto con un poco de fumet de pescado, añadimos un poco de nata y llevamos a ebullición. Damos un hervor al conjunto, rectificamos de sal y trituramos.

Para la salsa de soja y gengibre: Mezclamos en un bol u otro recipiente salsa de soja, gengibre rallado y sésamo. Trituramos todo ello en frío.

Freímos el alga nori en la freidora para que quede crujiente y lo troceamos.

Hacemos la vieira a la plancha cuidando que quede jugosa.

Final y presentación: Colocamos en el fondo de un bol o una copa unas cucharadas de crema de calabaza. Sobre ella, disponemos la vieira, que naparemos con la salsa de soja y gengibre. Finalmente, decoraremos el pintxo con alga nori frita.

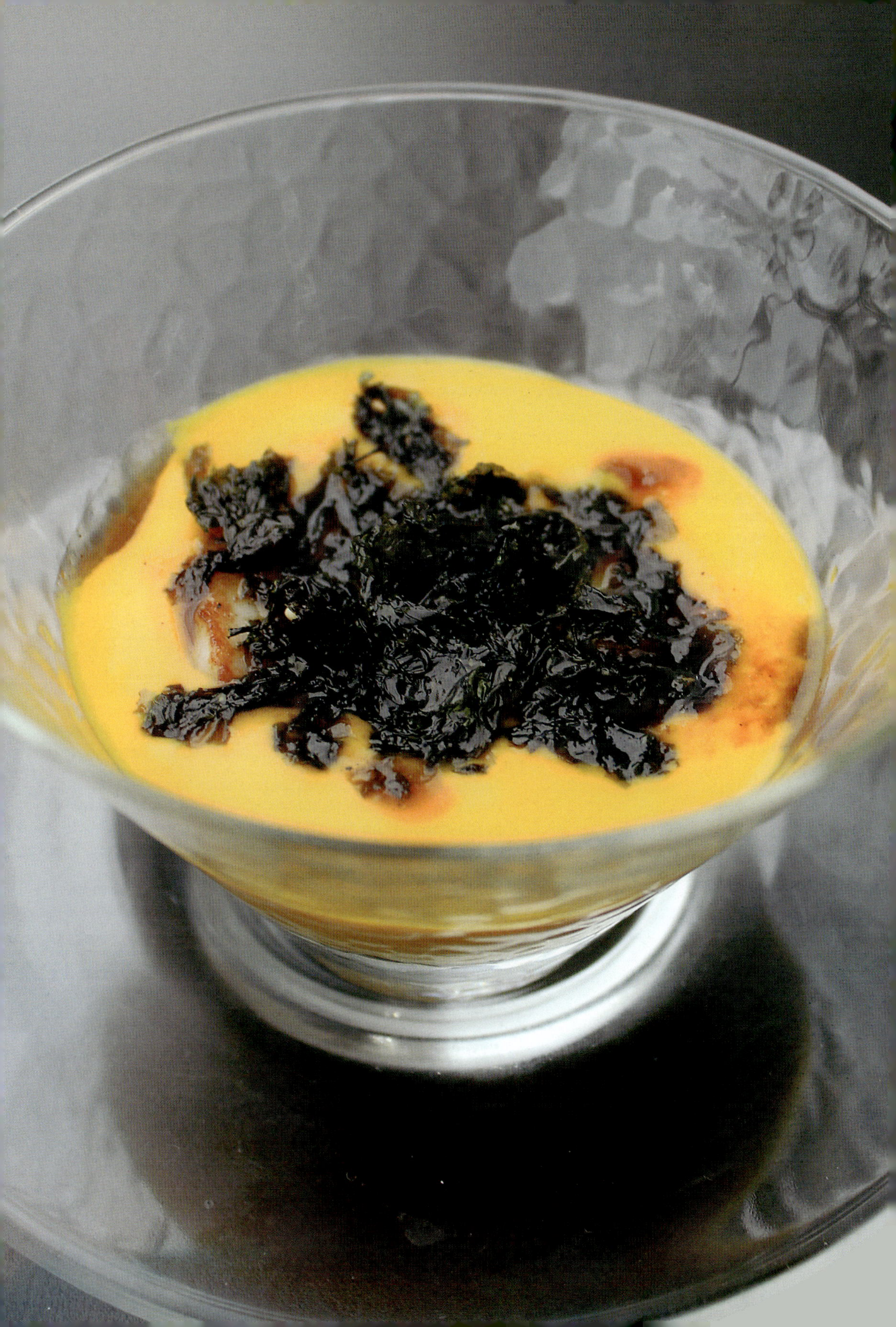

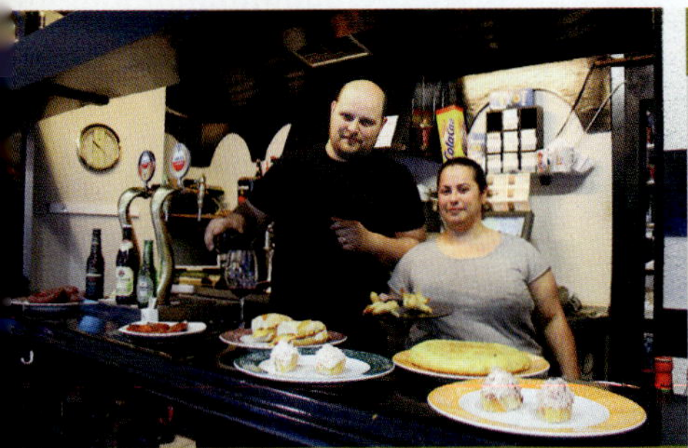

P° de los Olmos, 24
DONOSTIA
943 39 78 71

KAYAK

A pesar de estar alejado del centro de la ciudad, hay mucha vida en el Kayak y en la pequeña plaza en la que se encuentra, en la que se monta su concurrida terraza cuando el tiempo lo permite. El donostiarra **Gaizka Ruiz** y su mujer, **Izaskun Montero**, ambos con una larga trayectoria en hostelería, se hicieron con este local en diciembre de 2012, y lo han convertido en una de las paradas imprescindibles del barrio, principalmente por sus extraordinarios **calamares**, elaborados de manera artesanal y disponibles todos los días. También tienen gran aceptación sus **sandwiches "alargados"** y sus txipirones a la plancha, sin olvidar sus croquetas caseras, chiquititas y muy sabrosas. Kayak abre todos los días a las 8 de la mañana (excepto los lunes) y desde primera hora dispone de diferentes opciones de pikoteo en barra a las que a lo largo del día les siguen **las raciones, los bocadillos, las hamburguesas caseras...**

Otros pintxos:

- *Tortillas variadas*
- *Tigres*
- *Bonito con espárrago y gamba*
- *Serrano con huevo, chaka y gambón*
- *Huevo relleno de chaka con gamba gabardina*

Raciones:

- *Calamares fritos*
- *Croquetas caseras*
- *Patatas bravas y ali-oli*
- *Txipirones a la plancha*

Gambas a la gabardina

Ingredientes:

3 gambas
Aceite de girasol

· Para la gabardina:
Harina
Sal
Levadura
Cerveza, sifón o agua

Elaboración:

Para la gabardina: En un bol mezclaremos harina, sal, levadura y cerveza o, en su defecto, sifón o agua. De hecho, la gabardina se puede elaborar con cualquiera de los tres productos, siendo una cuestión de gusto personal el decantarse por uno u otro.

Mezclaremos bien los cuatro productos, batiendo sin cesar, teniendo en cuenta que lo más importante es que el líquido esté frío. Cuanto más frío, mejor sale la gabardina.

Elegimos tres buenas gambas, las pelamos, las pasamos por la gabardina y las freímos en abundante aceite de girasol hasta que adquieran un bonito color dorado.

Final y presentación: Ensartamos las tres gambas a la gabardina en un palillo de brocheta y las servimos en un platillo.

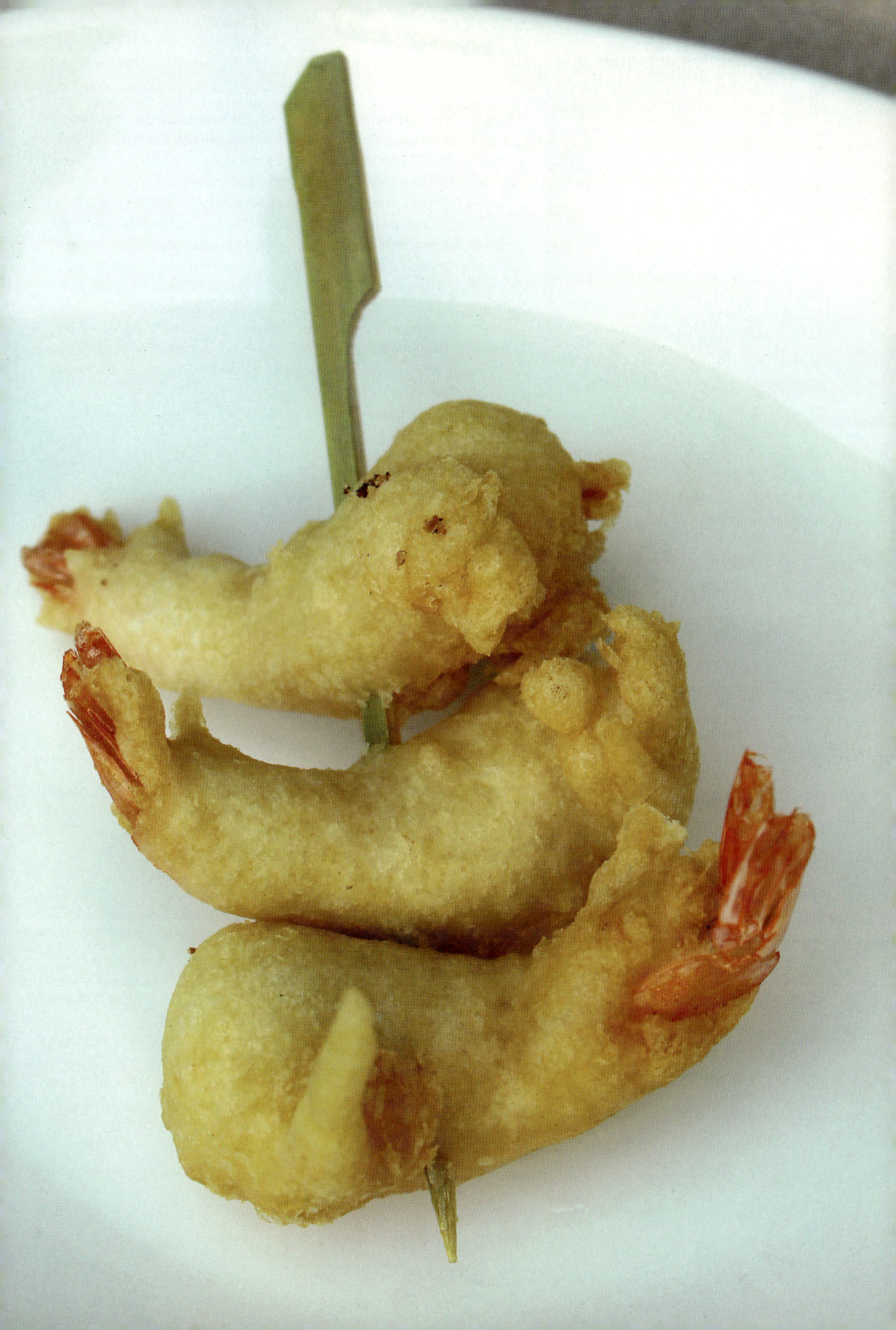

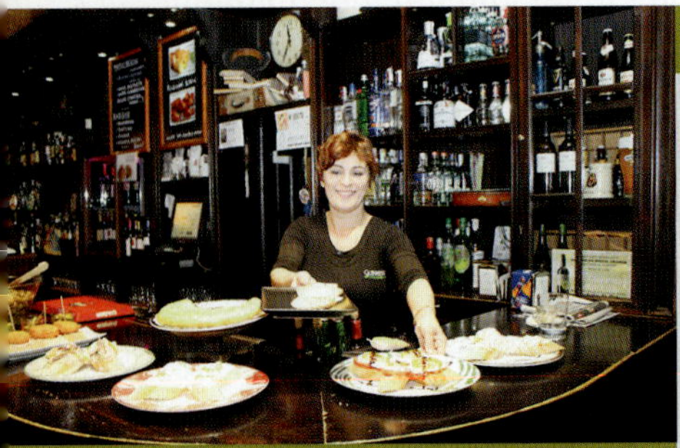

KIXKAL

Fue en 1998 cuando las hernaniarras **Jasone Astobiza y Jone Barrenetxea** comenzaron a dirigir este local que desde 2003 luce la placa de **Cervecería Oficial Guiness**. Por lo tanto, nunca falta la cerveza negra ni otro tipo de cervezas especiales en este dinámico establecimiento que **una vez a la semana ofrece monólogos, conciertos o algún tipo de actividad cultural**. Los vinos, con una selecta variedad de caldos de diferentes denominaciones, es otro de los fuertes del Kixkal. De hecho, siempre que tienen ocasión de hacerlo, Jasone y Jone organizan **catas de vinos con responsables de bodegas o enólogos**, que casi siempre son seguidas de su correspondiente degustación de pintxos. Kixkal abre todos los días a las 8:00 y para las 9 ya comienzan a hacer aparición los pintxos en barra. También trabajan mucho con **raciones** como Jamón ibérico, Pimientos del Padrón, Antxoas en salazón, Calamares, etc...

Nagusia, 15
HERNANI
943 33 66 99

Otros pintxos:

- *Croquetas (de jamón, de txipirón, de morcilla...)*
- *Tortillas variadas*
- *Brocheta de gambas*
- *Gamba a la gabardina*
- *Bola de marisco*
- *Bola de carne*
- *Foie a la plancha*
- *Tigres rellenos*
- *Milanesa*
- *Rollito de langostino con salsa agridulce*

Falsa vieira

Ingredientes:

Foie micuit
Cebolla
Bacalao desmigado
Queso Edam rallado

- **Para el puré de patata:**

Patata
Agua
Sal
Pimienta
Aceite de oliva virgen extra

Elaboración:

Para el puré de patata: Cocemos las patatas troceadas con agua y sal. Una vez cocidas, retiramos parte del agua y batimos las patatas, emulsionándolas con aceite de oliva virgen extra. Seguiremos batiendo hasta lograr la consistencia deseada.

Picamos finamente la cebolla y la ponemos a pochar. Cuando esté bien hecha, agregamos el bacalao desmigado y lo dejamos rehogar durante un rato.

Mezclamos la farsa de bacalao y cebolla con el puré de patata, obteniendo así una brandada de bacalao.

Final y presentación: Colocamos en mitad de la concha una bolita de foie micuit a modo de vieira. Cubrimos con la brandada de bacalao hasta ocupar la concha entera. Espolvoreamos la concha con queso Edam rallado y la introducimos a gratinar al horno a 250°. Cuando vemos que la concha está suficientemente dorada, la sacaremos del horno.

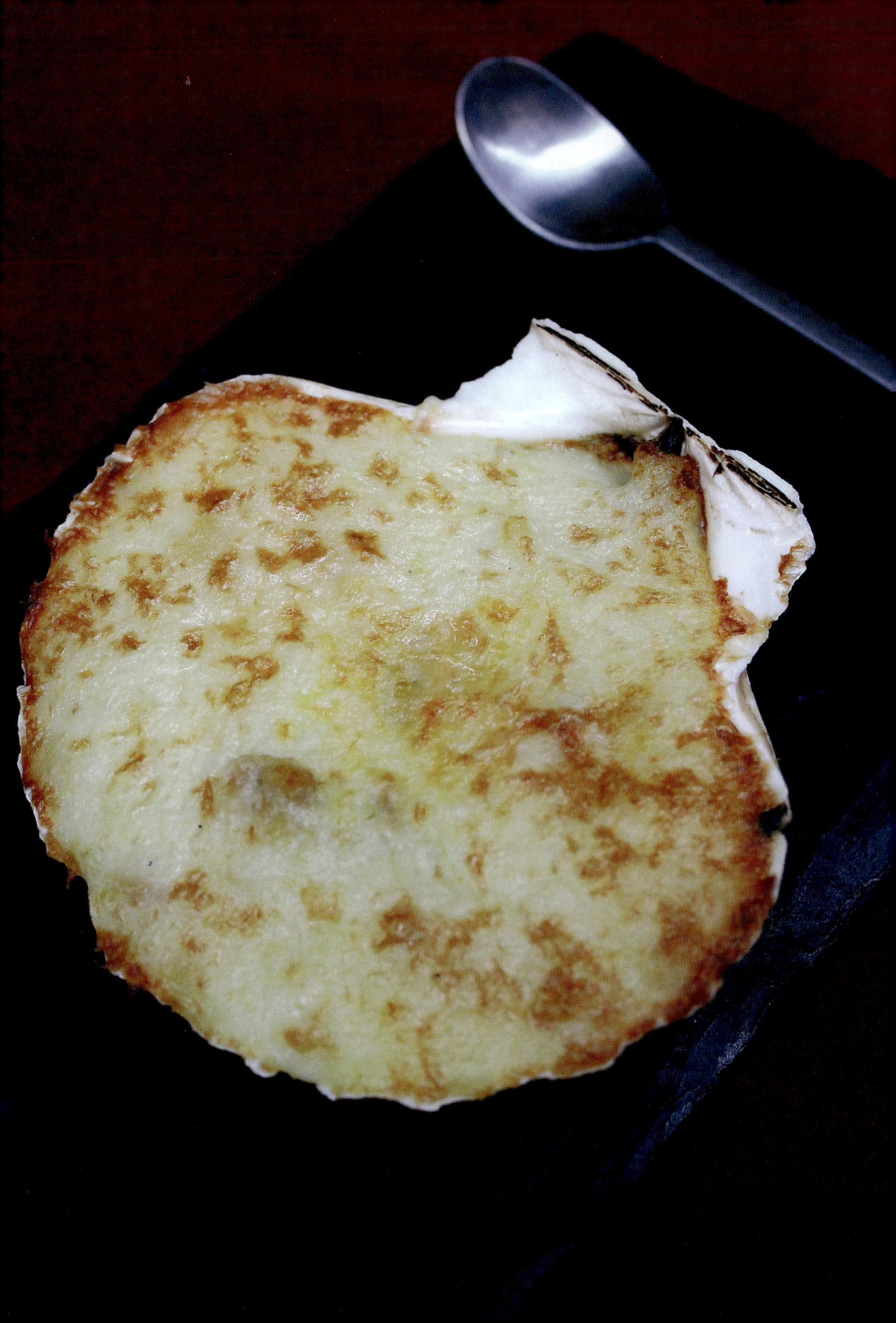

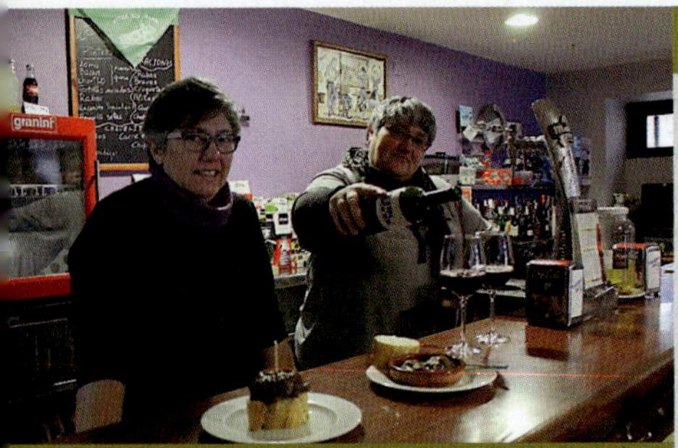

San Gregorio, 20 (Eitza)
ZUMARRAGA
943 72 27 86

KORTA TABERNA

Desde 2011, las hermanas **Mª Jose e Inés Rodrígue**z dan vida a este centenario bar, auténtico punto de encuentro de los vecinos del barrio de Eitza. **Inés y Marijo mantienen la línea de cocina tradicional y trato directo y cercano que se ha ofrecido siempre en este bar con platos de elaboración casera elaborados con mimo** como Jamón de paletilla, Espárragos rellenos, Bacalao ajoarriero, Bacalao con salsa de piquillos, Txipirones en su tinta, Rabo en salsa al vino tinto, Callos caseros, Albóndigas, Carrilleras... No deben dejarse sin probar las exitosas Croquetas ni los Tigres. Además del **menú del día, menú de fin de semana y carta**, en su bar podemos optar por una buena selección de **pintxos, bocadillos, cazuelitas y platos combinados.** También se preparan menús concertados para grupos según presupuesto.

Otros pintxos:

- *Tortillas variadas*
- *Callos*
- *Albóndigas en salsa*
- *Croquetas*
- *Txipirones en su tinta*
- *Tigres*
- *Carne en salsa*
- *Lomo con pimientos*
- *Chorizo cocido*
- *Revuelto de bacalao o de setas*

Carrilleras con salsa al vino tinto

Ingredientes (25-30 pintxos):

6-7 carrilleras
5 cebollas
2 puerros
3 zanahorias
2 botellas de vino
Aceite de oliva
Agua
Sal

Elaboración:

En una cazuela, rehogar y sellar las carrilleras y reservarlas. En ese mismo aceite, pochar bien la cebolla, la zanahoria y el puerro.

Una vez pochados, añadir las carrilleras y las dos botellas de vino. Hervir a fuego fuerte 10 minutos y, cuando haya reducido bien, añadir agua hasta que cubra sobradamente las carrilleras.

Cocer unas dos horas a fuego lento y, si hiciera falta, añadir algo de agua. Una vez se han ablandado, retirar la cazuela del fuego y pasar la salsa por la batidora.

Cortar las carrilleras en pedazos y volver a introducirlas en la salsa. Cocer aproximadamente una hora a fuego lengo para que las carrilleras terminen de soltar su gelatina.

Final y presentación: Aunque la imagen que acompaña a esta receta es la versión "pintxo tradicional" de la misma, sobre una rodaja de pan, en Korta Taberna el pintxo se sirve en una cazuelita de barro conteniendo una hermosa porción de carrillera acompañada de su correspondiente salsa y un pedazo de pan para disfrutar de la misma.

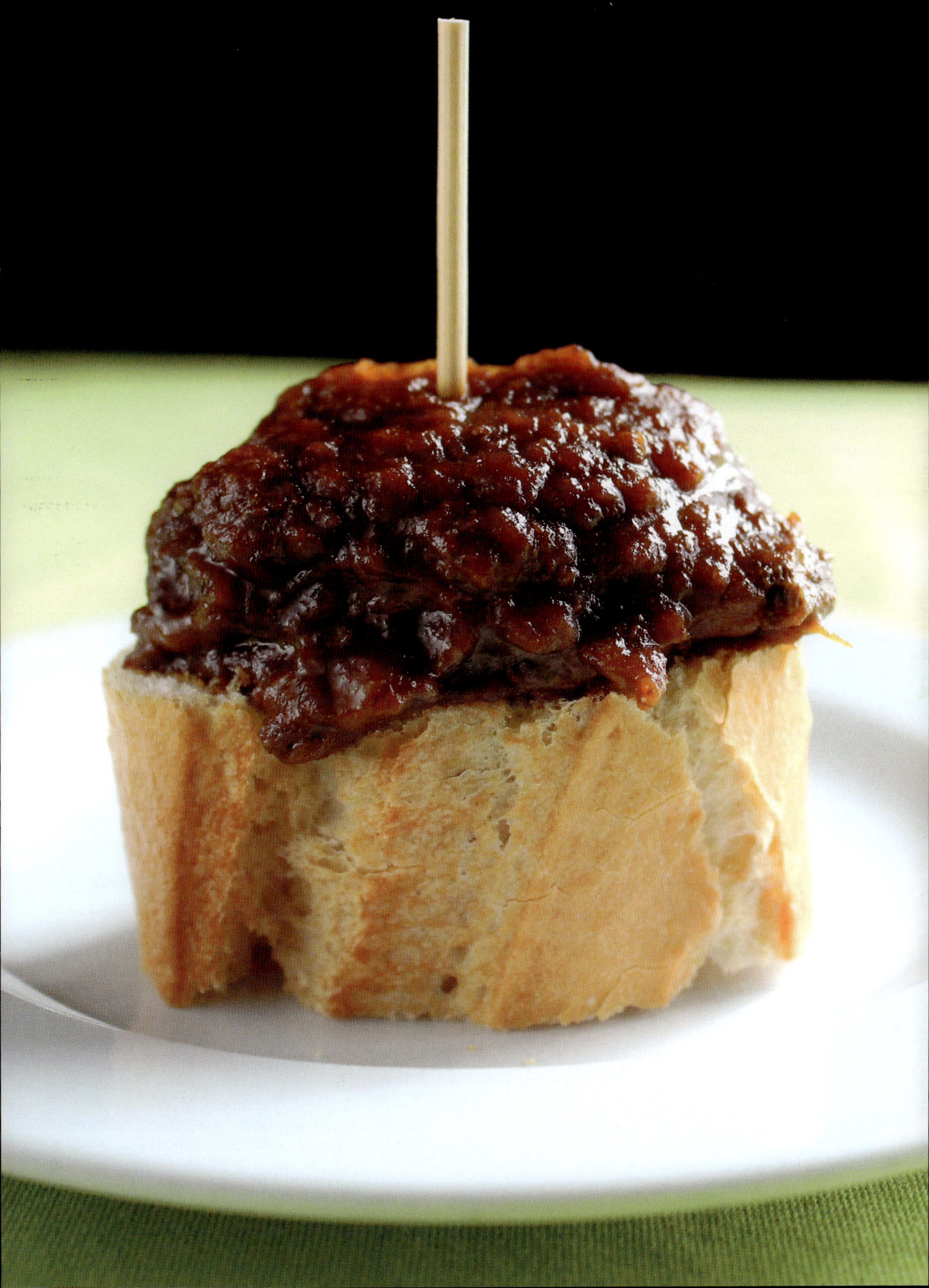

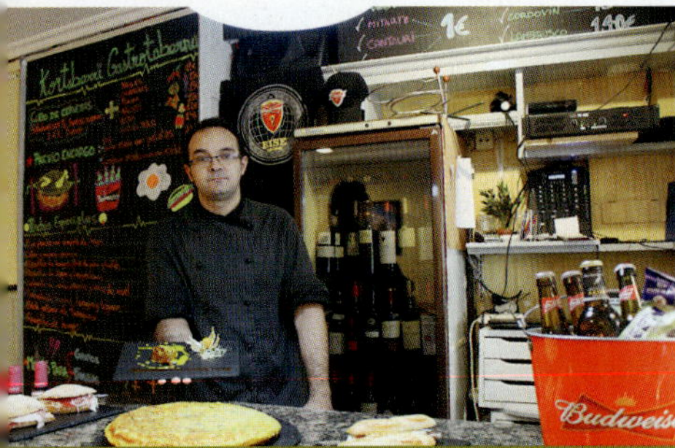

Kalebarren, 26
ZUMARRAGA
943 72 04 47

KORTABERRI

Jonathan Santamaría, zumarragatarra con más de 12 años de experiencia hostelera en locales como el Kabia, Santa Barbara, Zelaikoa, Hokaba... ha reabierto el Kortaberri convirtiéndolo en un **Gastrobar con cocina ininterrumpida de 10:00 a cierre.** Todos los platos se elaboran con productos frescos y de calidad, desde los **Pintxos especiales** (Solomillo de cerdo, Foie a la plancha...) hasta las **Tortillas de barra** (Tortilla de patata, Tortilla Riojana con chorizo y alegrías...) pasando por sus platos de **Carta** (Rape gratinado con hongos y parmesano, Terrina casera de foie...) hasta sus 10 **Ensaladas** (De bacalao, De queso de cabra, de Txipirones y langostinos...). Destacan sus **Ibéricos de Extremadura, que se sirven como pintxo, en bokata o como ración**, así como sus **Hamburguesas caseras**, especialmente la solicitada "Hamburguesa Pija", compuesta de carne de Wagyu con hongos, foie, jamón ibérico y queso de Idiazabal.

Otros pintxos:

- *Croquetas variadas caseras*
- *Foie plancha con compota de higos*
- *Callos y morros caseros*
- *Risotto de hongos, foie de pato y trufas*
- *Risotto de rape y langostinos*
- *Solomillo de ternera, hongos y trigueros*
- *Brick relleno de txangurro*
- *Revuelto de hongos*
- *Pulpo plancha con espuma de patata y pimentón (ración)*
- *Ibéricos de Extremadura (ración)*

Solomillo de cerdo, panceta y salsa de miel

Ingredientes:

1 medallón de solomillo de cerdo
1 loncha de panceta adobada
1 chorrito de nata
2 hebras de azafrán
1 cucharadita de mostaza de Dijon
1 cucharadita de miel
Escamas de sal
Pimienta negra

Elaboración:

Limpiamos y cortamos el solomillo en medallones del tamaño que vayamos a utilizar para el pintxo.

Envolvemos cada medallón en una loncha de panceta previemente frita y lo sellamos con un palillo.

Calentamos la nata y disolvemos en ella la miel, la mostaza y el azafrán. Llevamos a ebullición e introducimos en ella el medallón de solomillo. Dejamos que se haga durante un par de minutos.

Final y presentación: Servimos el medallón de solomillo y lo napamos con la salsa de mostaza. Lo espolvoreamos con unas escamas de sal y pimienta negra.

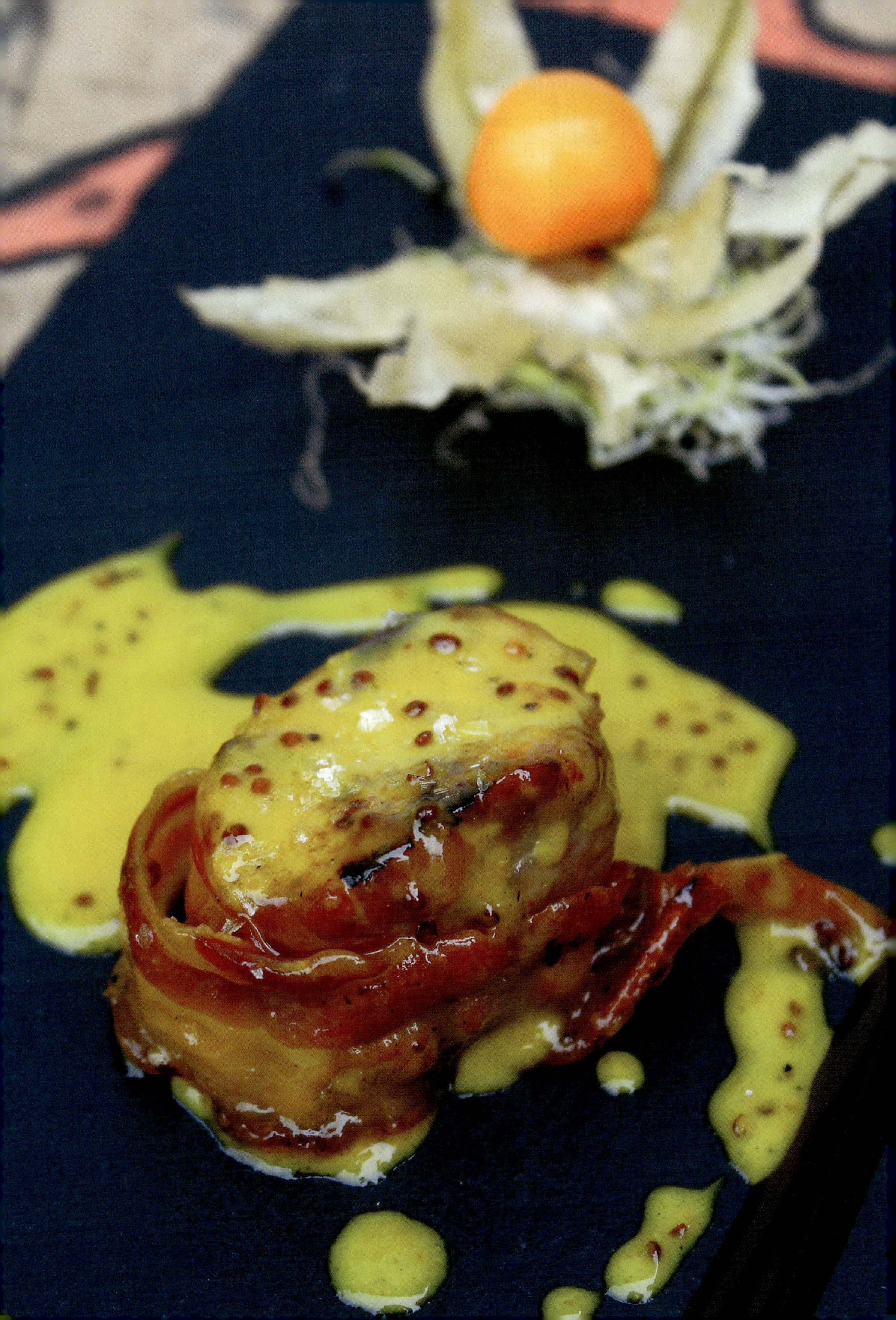

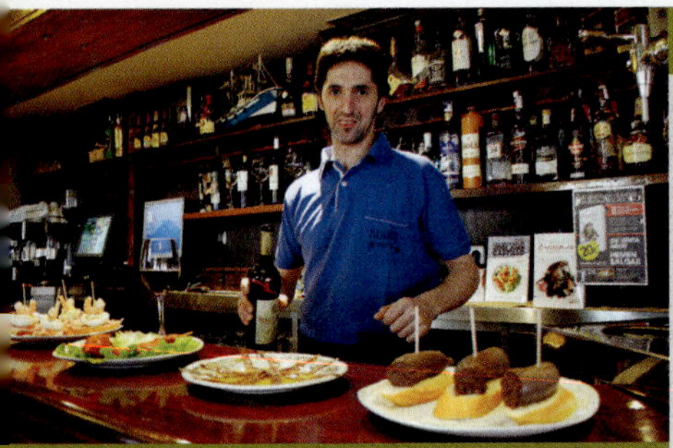

Larraitz Auzoa, 25
ALEGIA
634 61 17 46

KURPIL

Xabier Garmendia, conocido hostelero alegitarra de dilatada experiencia en el sector, se hizo con la dirección del bar Kurpil en 2008. Tras su prematuro fallecimiento en 2012, han sido dos de sus hermanos, **Luxio** y **Joseba**, quienes se han hecho cargo del establecimiento, manteniendo el estilo y el espíritu impuesto por su hermano. Kurpil abre todos los días (salvo los lunes) a las 11 de la mañana, ofreciendo **pintxos y cazuelitas** hasta las 11 de la noche, y alargando ligeramente el horario de cierre los fines de semana, momento en que Luxio y Joseba cuentan también con la ayuda de **Idoia Garmendia**, compañera de éste último. De viernes a domingo, también se ofrecen **bocadillos**. Además de estas opciones, en Kurpil se cuidan especialmente los Gin-tonics, con una carta de **más de 19 ginebras premium** de diferentes lugares del mundo.

Otros pintxos:

- *Bola de carne o marisco*
- *Antxoas de Santoña*
- *Morcilla*
- *Chorizo a la sidra*
- *Ensaladilla casera*
- *Atún encebollado*
- *Jalapeños con mozzarela*
- *Brocheta de cerdo*
- *Pintxo "Kurpil"*
- *Cazuelita de champiñones en salsa*

Pulpo a la gallega

Ingredientes:

Pulpo
Aceite de oliva virgen extra
Sal gorda marina
Pimentón dulce de La Vera
Pimentón picante de La Vera

Elaboración:

Cocemos el pulpo a la manera tradicional, en agua sin sal por espacio de hora y media aproximadamente, aunque puede variar en función de cada pulpo. Lo pincharemos con un palillo para comprobar el punto de cocción y lo sacaremos cuando consideremos que ha adquirido la textura deseada.

Con la ayuda de unas tijeras de cocina o un cuchillo bien afilado, cortaremos el pulpo en rodajas.

Final y presentación: En un platillo rectangular dispondremos 9 rodajas de pulpo que rociaremos con un buen aceite de oliva virgen extra. A continuación lo espolvorearemos con sal gorda marina, pimentón dulce de La Vera y pimentón picante de la misma denominación de origen.

Lo importante en este pintxo del Kurpil es la calidad del producto, empezando por un buen pulpo y terminando por un gran aceite de oliva, u "oro líquido" como acostumbraba a llamarlo Xabier.

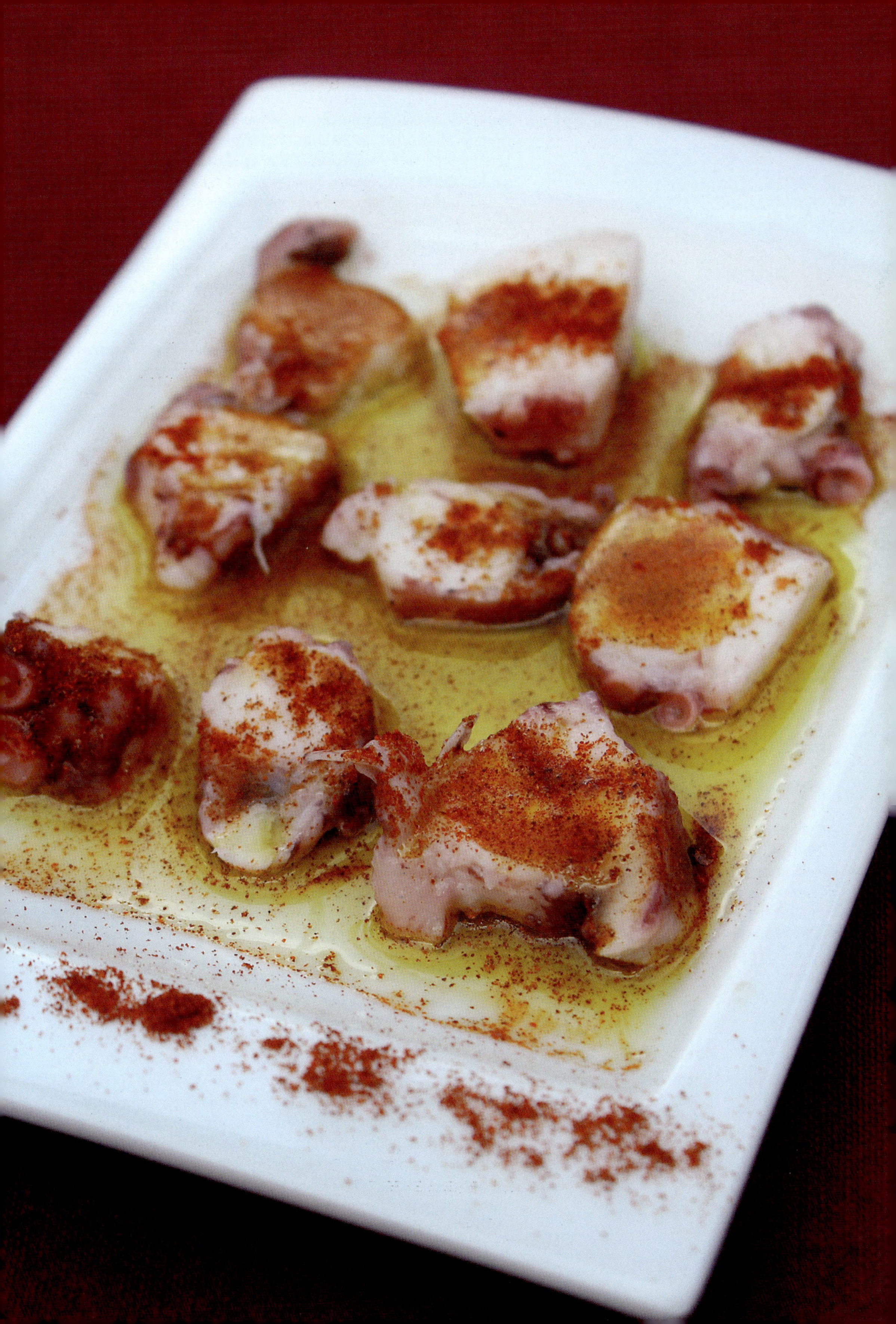

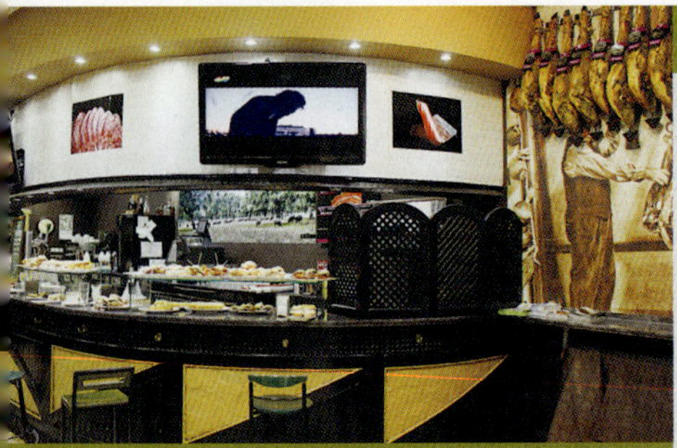

LA BELLOTTA

Aunque nació en Extremadura, **Carlos Rosco** vino con 4 años a Gipuzkoa y lleva **más de 25 años dedicándose al jamón que produce en su fábrica de Montánchez (Cáceres) y comercializa en todas sus formas desde su empresa, Jamones Rosco**: Bellota, recebo, paleta... En 2011, Carlos se hizo cargo del bar-restaurante La Bellotta, sito en el Centro Comercial Txingudi, local en el que se ofrecen raciones de jamón cortado a mano y en el que **casi todos los platos, ya sean de carta o menú, llevan jamón**, incluídas algunas ensaladas. El jamón también se encuentra presente en gran parte de los pintxos que se sirven en su barra. En La Bellotta podemos, además, adquirir todos los productos ibéricos de la casa Rosco, ya sea en entero o en prácticos sobres de 100 gramos envasados al vacío. También despachan en su almacén y tienda en la calle Dendaldegi nº 1 de Urnieta.

Centro Comercial Txingudi
IRUN
943 62 53 30
www.jamonesrosco.com

Otros pintxos:

- *Berenjena rebozada con jamón y huevo de codorniz*
- *Jamón ibérico, pimiento verde y antxoa*
- *Bacalao a la vasca*
- *Jamón ibérico y pato con Roquefort*
- *Jamón ibérico con pa amb tumaca*

Raciones:

- *Patatas fritas con jamón ibérico y queso fundido*
- *Tablón de lomo ibérico*
- *Surtido de ibéricos*
- *Bacalao frito con cebolla y pimiento*

Jamón ibérico rosco con tomate y champiñones rellenos

Ingredientes:

Jamón ibérico Rosco
Pimiento verde
Cebolla
Tomate
Reducción de Módena
Aceite de oliva
Pan

· Para el champiñón relleno:
Champiñón
Virutas de jamón Rosco
Queso Philladelphia
Harina

· Para la salsa de boletus:
Hongo
Nata
Sal
Pimienta negra

Elaboración:

Para la salsa de boletus: Picamos y salteamos los hongos en aceite de oliva. Cuando estén bien pochados, añadimos nata, y llevamos a ebullición dejando que hierva cinco minutos. Salpimentamos al gusto y pasamos la batidora.

Para los champiñones rellenos: Mezclamos el queso Philladelphia con las virutas de ibérico creando una pasta homogénea. Quitamos el pie a los champiñones dejando sólo las txapelas, y rellenamos éstas con la pasta de queso y jamón. Pasamos los champiñones por harina y los freímos en aceite de oliva hasta que se doren.

Cortamos la cebolla en juliana y la pochamos suavemente en aceite de oliva. Asimismo, cortamos una rodaja de pimiento verde y la freímos en aceite bien caliente.

Final y presentación: Cortamos una rebanada de pan sobre la que disponemos, primeramente, una rodaja de paleta de jamón. Sobre ella, colocamos la cebolla caramelizada, y sobre ella, una rodaja de tomate que podemos, optativamente, pasar por la plancha. Sobre el tomate colocaremos dos champiñones rellenos y sobre estos otra rodaja de jamón y la rodaja de pimiento verde frito. Acompañamos con la salsa de boletus y decoramos el plato con la reducción de Módena.

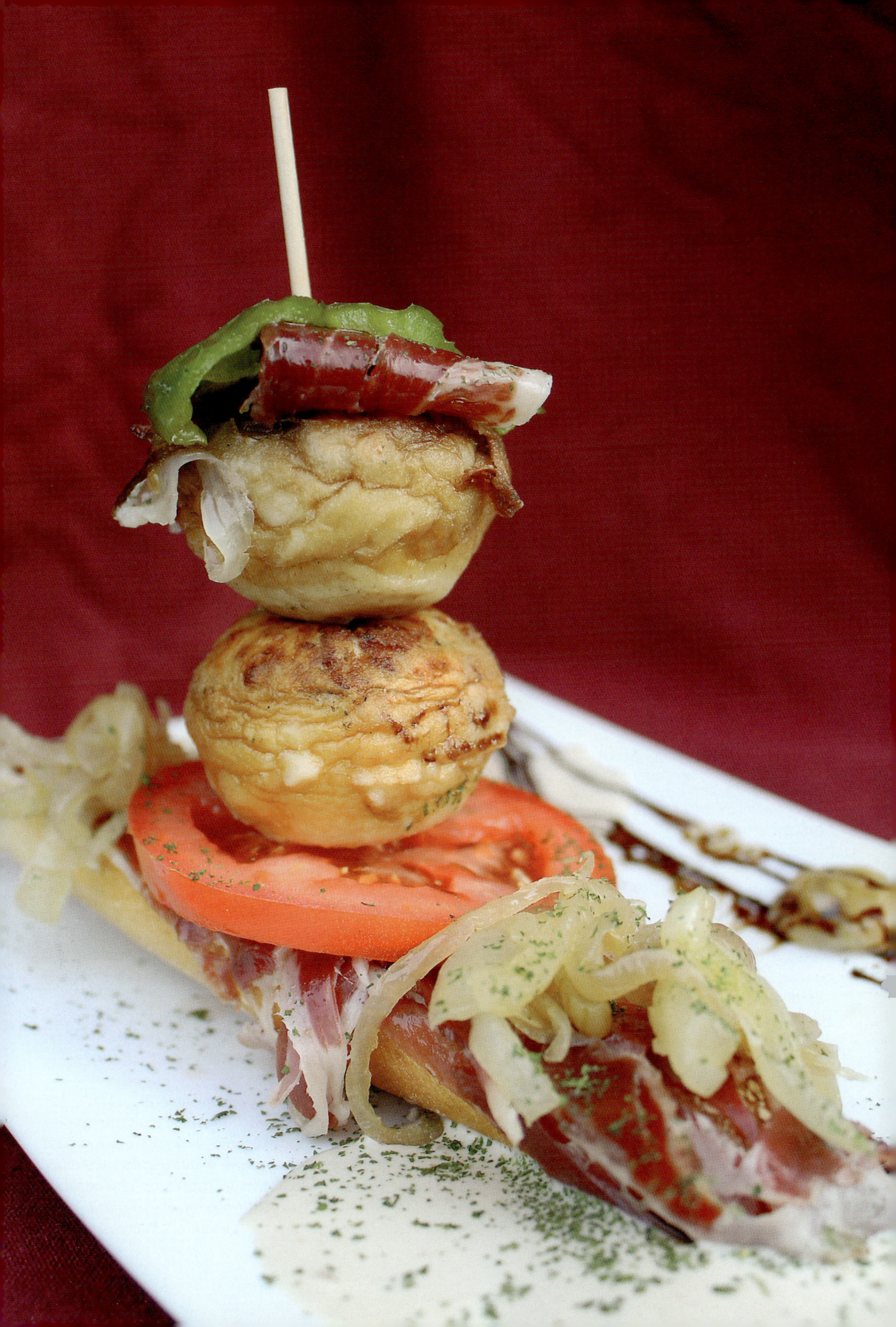

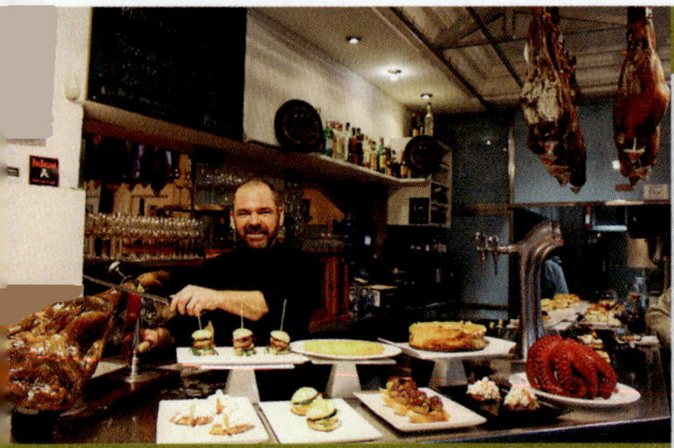

LA CEPA

Sin necesidad de pasar por ninguna academia de cocina, el propio bar La Cepa ha sido la escuela en la que desde su más tierna infancia se ha formado **Peio Balda**, al igual que hizo su padre, **Francisco Balda**, y su abuelo, **Pedro Antonio Balda**, que fundó este emblemático bar en 1940. Dedicado al 100% a dirigir el local desde los inicios de esta década, y con la impagable ayuda de su mujer, **Ana**, y su cuñada **Amaia**, Peio ha sabido mantener la identidad de este establecimiento, adecuándolo a los tiempos modernos. De hecho, Peio ha ganado en dos ocasiones (2010 y 2011) el **Premio a la Originalidad en el Campeonato de Pintxos de Gipuzkoa**, en el que quedó 2° en 2014, y también ganó el premio al Mejor pintxo con bacalao en uno de los primeros Campeonatos de Euskal Herria. **Las raciones, los pintxos y los bocadillos con pan recién horneado** son los fuertes de este local que también cuenta con un **txokito privado** para 6-8 personas en el que se sirven cenas por encargo.

Viteri, 26
ERRENTERIA
943 51 10 81

Otros pintxos:

- *Foie fresco sobre torrija de miel*
- *Cigalita asada sobre foie de marisco*
- *Carrillera de ibérico con reducción de sus jugos*
- *Migas de brownie con helado*
- *Lata de pulpo asado con ali-oli*

Raciones:
- *Jamón ibérico de bellota*
- *Atún rojo con berenjenas y shiitakes*
- *Presa ibérica al Oporto con papas y pimientos del Padrón*
- *Pulpo de barco a la gallega*

Torrija de brioche con espuma de natilla

Ingredientes:

Pan de brioche
Arroz con leche muy caldoso
Azúcar blanco
Cacao amargo
Natillas
Hoja de menta

- **Para el coulis de arándanos:**

Arándanos
Azúcar
Agua

Elaboración:

Para el coulis de arándanos: Cocemos los arándanos con agua y azúcar. Una vez el agua reduce, trituramos buscando la textura deseada.

Para la espuma de natilla: Metemos las natillas en el sifón y elaboramos la espuma.

Para el polvo de menta: Dejamos deshidratar la hoja de menta bien estirada durante un día encima del horno o en otra fuente de calor. Una vez seca, la trituramos a mano.

Para los "chococrispis" de arroz con leche: Freímos pequeñas porciones de arroz con leche, las pasamos por cacao amago y las tamizamos, para que adquieran apariencia de chococrispis.

Final y presentación: Empapamos el brioche en el arroz con leche, lo espolvoreamos por un lado con azúcar blanco y caramelizamos ese lado con la ayuda de un soplete. Colocamos dos porciones de brioche, tres montoncitos de espuma de natilla y unos círculos de coulis de arándanos. Terminamos decorando con los "chococrispis" de arroz y espolvoreamos con polvo de menta.

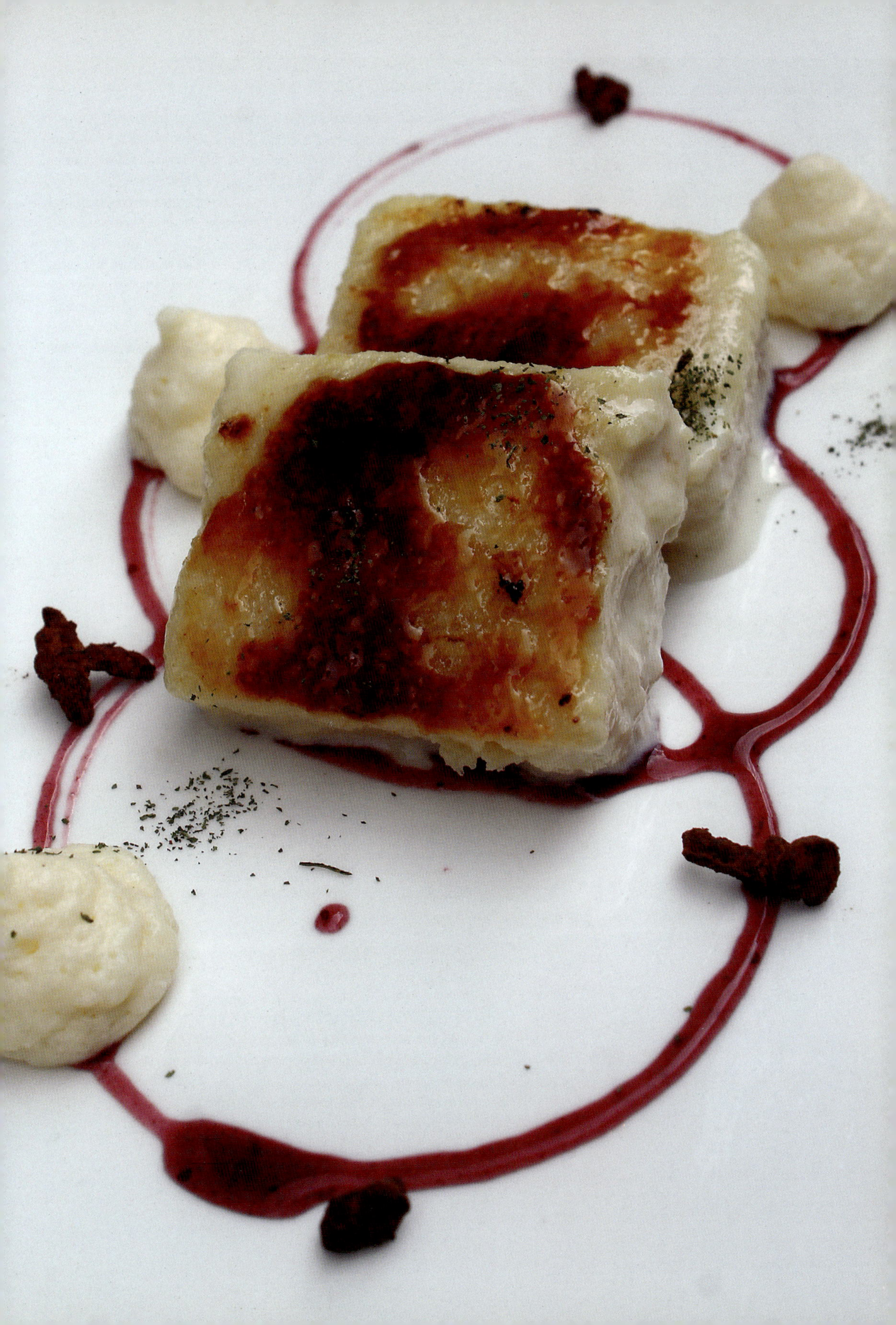

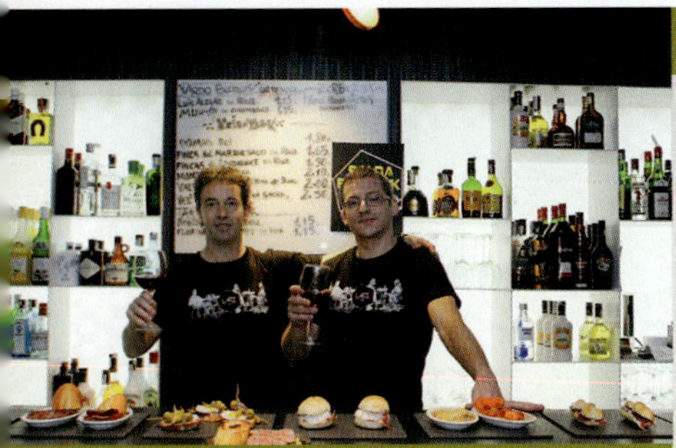

Kale Nagusia, 55
AZKOITIA
943 85 13 19

LATZ

Los azkoitiarras **David Iraundegi y Jon Ander Larramendi,** que dirigen desde 2006 el cercano **Zurt**, abrieron el Latz en agosto de 2013, convirtiendo un local que llevaba años y años en desuso en una de las referencias hosteleras de la villa. Y es que en Latz hay de todo y para todos, desde los cafés a partir de las 10 de la mañana hasta las **copas, la buena música y el ambiente nocturno** de última hora que los sábados se prolonga hasta las 6 de la mañana, pasando por su **amplia variedad gastronómica** enla que encontramos una extensa carta de **PIntxos, Raciones, Bocadillos y Pizzas artesanas** (hasta la masa se hace en casa) entre las que destacan la San Martín (Tomate, mozzarella, setas, gambas y ajos frescos) y la Kuku-Herri (Salsa de hongos, mozzarella, jamón y orégano), entre otras. Es de destacar en Latz **el cuidado y la variedad a la hora de tratar los vinos**, con 11 tintos y 11 blancos a elegir para tomar por copas. Los jueves, además, se ofrece pintxo-pote de 6:30 a 9.

Otros pintxos:

- *Morros en salsa*
- *Callos*
- *Manitas de cerdo rebozadas*
- *Lengua en salsa*
- *Bacalao a la plancha con pimientos*
- *Revuelto de champiñones*
- *Revuelto de bacalao*
- *Tortilla de patata*
- *Croquetas caseras*
- *Revuelto de espinacas con gambas*

Secreto ibérico a la plancha

Ingredientes:

Secreto ibérico
Patata
Sal gorda
Pimentón dulce de La Vera
Aceite de oliva
Pan
Perejil

Elaboración:

Haremos a la plancha la pieza entera de secreto ibérico. El tiempo de plancha por cada lado dependerá del grosor de la pieza, aunque es conveniente no hacerlo mucho para que quede bien jugoso por dentro.

Una vez hecho, con la ayuda de un cuchillo jamonero, filetearemos el secreto en lonchas finas.

Por otra parte, confitaremos unas patatas panaderas en aceite de oliva a fuego bajo.

Final y presentación: Dispondremos en un platillo 3 ó 4 porciones de patata panadera. Sobre ellas, colocaremos cinco filetitos de secreto ibérico y los espolvorearemos con pimentón de La Vera dulce, sal gorda y perejil fresco recién picado. Acompañaremos el pintxo de una rebanada de pan tostada al horno o en la plancha.

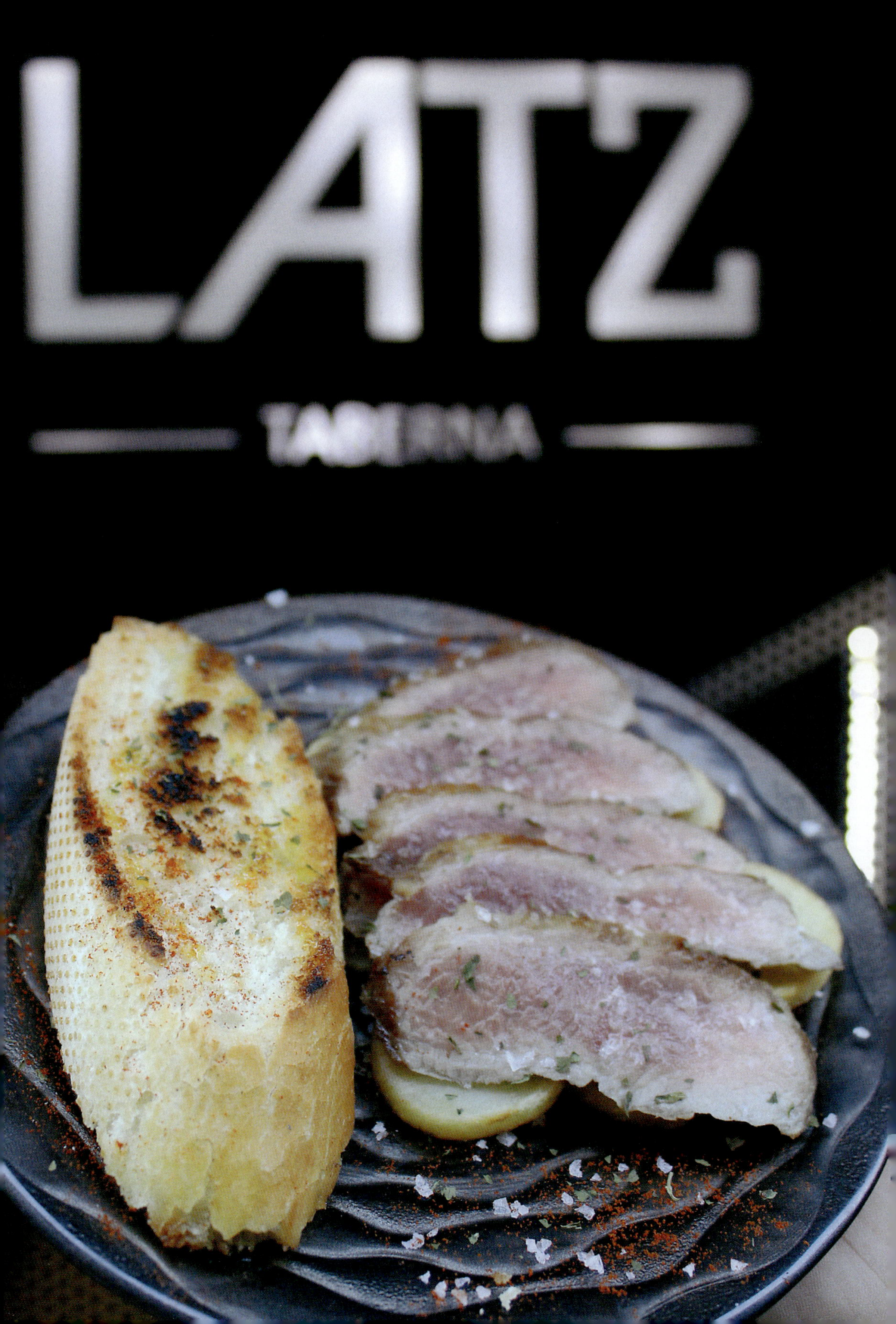
LATZ

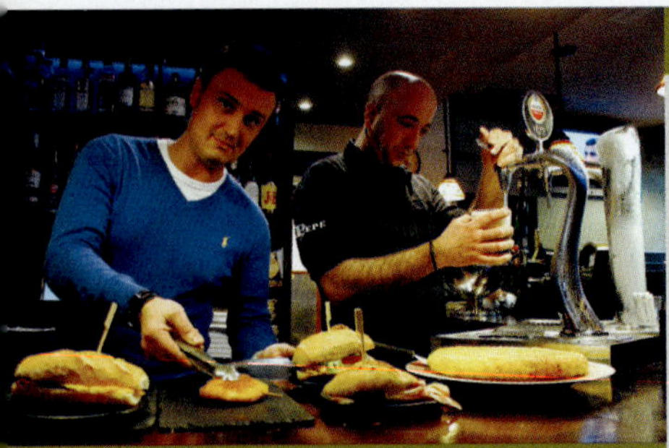

MANDRÁGORA

Plaza Jose Mª Sert, 9 (Benta Berri)
DONOSTIA
943 31 26 99

Lucas Rey, Javi Porto y Julián Melo, que también regentan el **Pepe** de El Antiguo (ver página 176), dirigen desde 2006 esta cervecería, frecuentada por un público joven y dinámico que acude atraído por su **amplia terraza** (una de las mejores de la zona) y su variedad de **Tortillas, Minis, Platos combinados, Raciones, Ensaladas, Bocadillos...** así como sus solicitadas **Tostas** elaboradas al momento.
Estos donostiarras, dotados de una gran experiencia en el mundo de la hostelería local, curtidos en establecimientos como Garagar, La Kabutzia, etc..., conocen igualmente las claves de la hostelería nocturna y ofrecen a sus clientes una amplia diversidad de **copas, combinados, buenas cervezas** y, ocasionalmente, presentaciones y degustaciones de diferentes marcas de cervezas y licores.
Mandrágora abre todos los días a las 9 de la mañana (fines de semana a las 10) y los miércoles ofrece **pintxo-pote** de 7 a 11.

Otros pintxos:

- *Minis de tortillas variadas*
- *Mini de bacon con queso y pimiento*
- *Mini de jamón serrano con tomate y aceite*
- *Croquetas de jamón*
- *Bola de carne picante*

Tostas:

- *Tosta de salmón ahumado con queso de cabra*
- *Tosta de carne picada estilo boloñesa con queso*
- *Tosta de mousse de canard*
- *Tosta de setas y bacon con queso*

Calabacín relleno de carne, bolognesa y jamón ibérico

Ingredientes:

Calabacín
Harina
Huevo
Aceite de oliva
Pan
Jamón ibérico

• Para la bolognesa
Cebolla
Zanahoria
Ajo
Carne picada
Tomate frito
Vino blanco
Sal
Pimienta

Elaboración:

Cortamos el calabacín en rodajas, las rebozamos en harina y huevo y las freímos en abundante aceite de oliva.

Para la bolognesa: Picamos finamente la cebolla, la zanahoria y el ajo y las dejamos pochar. Una vez pochadas las verduras, añadimos la carne picada y rehogamos todo junto hasta que la carne se dore. Adjuntamos tomate frito y un vasito de vino blanco y dejamos reducir el alcohol. Hervimos toda la mezcla un rato y le damos el punto de sal y pimienta.

Final y presentación: Sobre una rodaja de pan, colocamos una loncha de jamón ibérico crudo y una loncha de calabacín rebozado. Sobre el calabacín colocamos un par de cucharadas generosas de la salsa bolognesa y cubrimos todo con una segunda rodaja de calabacín. Ensartamos todo con un palillo.

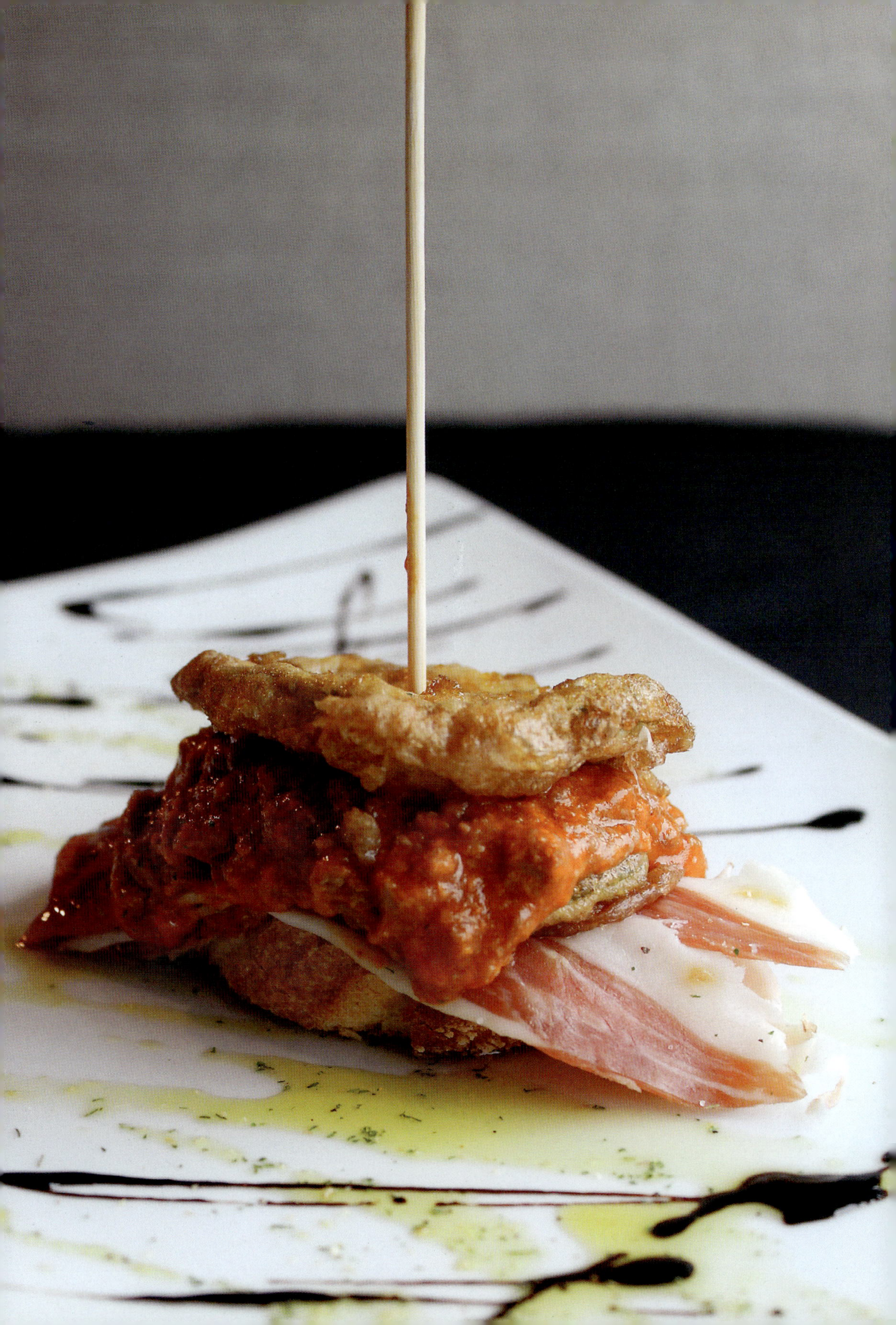

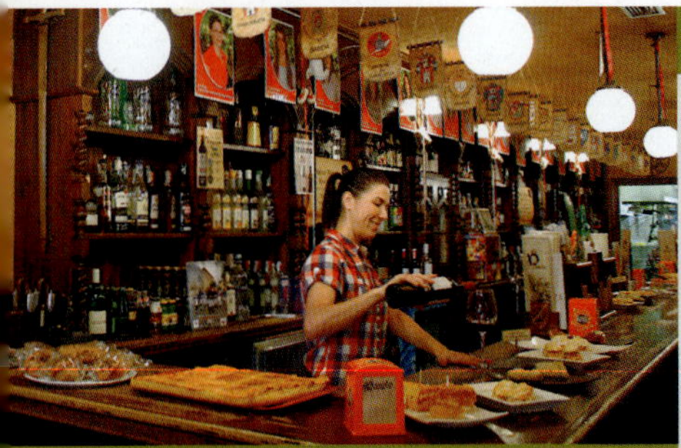

MANOLO

Este bar está dirigido por **Jose Mª Gonzalez Jiménez** y su mujer, **Raquel Jiménez**, aunque fueron los padres de Jose Mª, **Pepe y Mari** los que lo abrieron hace ya más de 50 años. En el Manolo nos encontramos con una **cocina muy casera, tradicional, sencilla y económica, así como con un amplio abanico de menús, ensaladas, bocatas, platos combinados...** Un comentario aparte merecen los **pintxos, con una gran variedad, desde los más tradicionales hasta los más modernos**, y la exquisita empanada, disponible sólo los viernes). Todos los meses, el Manolo ofrece un **pintxo recomendado** y un **vino recomendado**, y cuenta asimismo con una atractiva oferta de vinos y cervezas. Además, los jueves hay servicio de **pintxo-pote** y los viernes y sábados tarde, pintxos a precios populares. Por las noches, el Manolo cuenta con una carta de Gin-Tonics y buen ambiente de bar de copas.

Nagusia, 12
IRUN
943 62 11 95
www.barmanolo.net

Otros pintxos:

- *Empanada de bonito*
- *Ravioli de hongo con crema de carne al foie*
- *Bacalao con tomate*
- *Bola de morcilla*
- *Crêpes de espinacas con salsa de Roquefort*
- *Pimiento relleno de hongos con salsa de hongos*
- *Pintxo de champi*
- *Tosta de queso de cabra con frambuesa*
- *Tortilla de patata rellena*
- *Brocheta de langostino y queso en tempura*

Hamburguesa picante

Ingredientes:

Carne picada
PImiento verde
Pimiento rojo
Ajo
Leche
Huevo
Miga de pan
Guindilla cayena
Cebolla
Pan de hamburguesa
Patatas
Harina
Aceite
Sal

- **Para la salsa de mostaza:**

Mostaza
Miel
Nata

Elaboración:

Para la hamburguesa: Picamos el ajo, el pimiento verde y el pimiento rojo y lo pochamos bien junto a la guindilla cayena. Cuando esté todo bien pochado, añadimos la carne y le damos el punto de sal. Cuando esté hecha, añadimos la mezcla de miga de pan, huevo y leche, y cocinamos todo hasta que espese. Dejamos enfriar la mezcla y cuando alcance una temperatura manejable, boleamos las hamburguesas.

Para la salsa de mostaza: Mezclamos de manera homogénea la mostaza, la miel y la nata.

Final y presentación: Pasamos la hamburguesa por harina y la cocinamos con aceite. Mientras se está haciendo, pochamos la cebolla. Sobre el pan de hamburguesa colocamos la cebolla pochada y sobre ésta, la hamburguesa. Freímos unas patatas como acompañamiento, que serviremos junto a la hamburguesa, napadas con la salsa de mostaza.

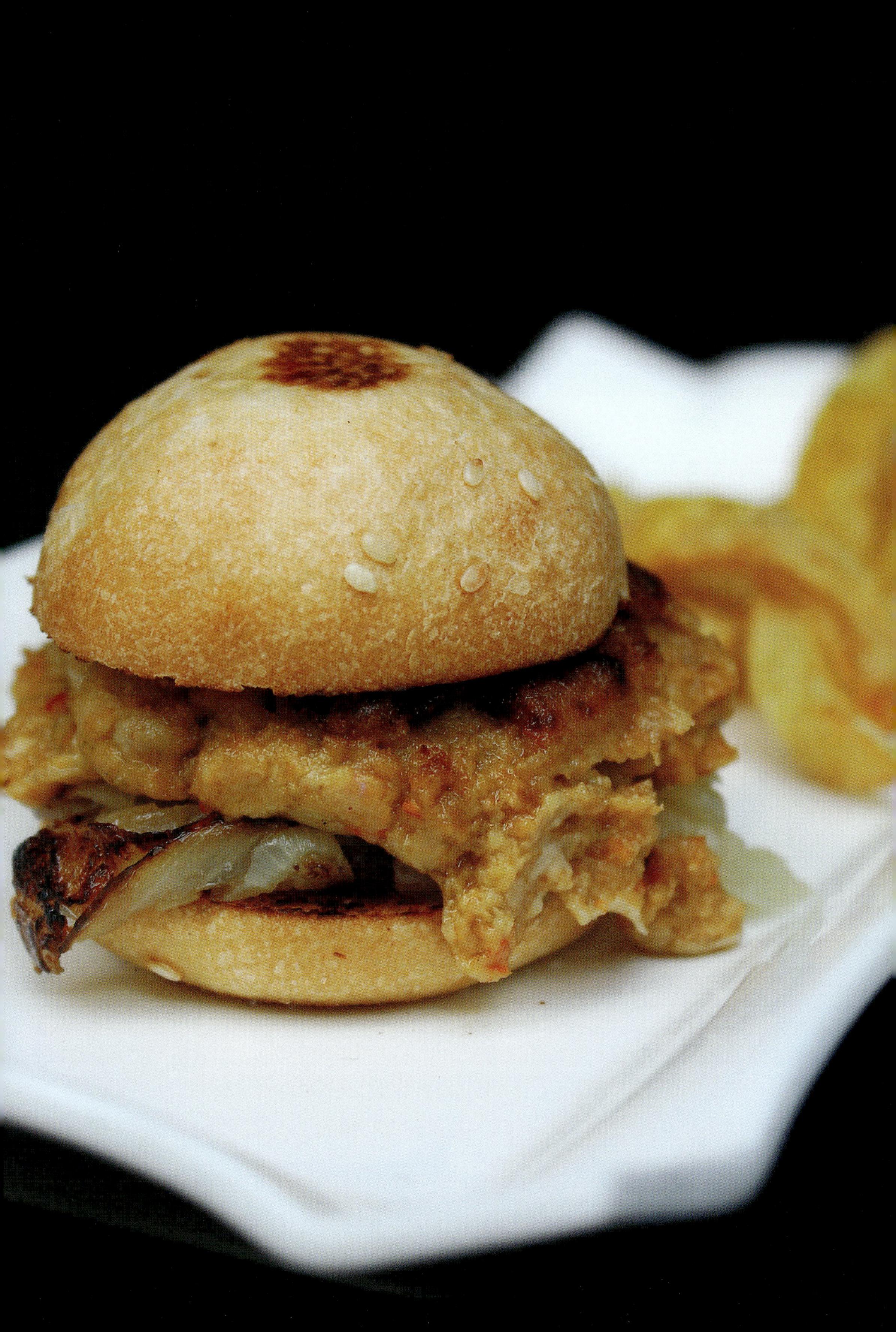

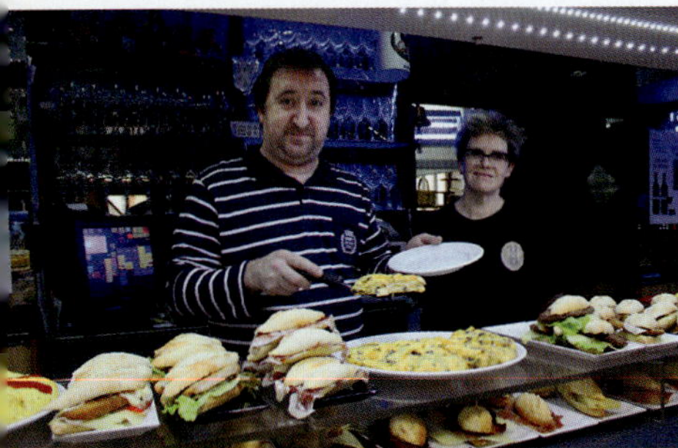

MAZZANTINI

Sokagin kalea, 7
DEBA
943 19 24 22

Fue a finales de los 90 cuando **Jesús Salegi Irureta** comenzó a dirigir este bar al que su anterior propietario, aficionado a los toros, había llamado así en homenaje a Luis Mazzantini, el famoso diestro de Elgoibar, protagonista de mil anécdotas. Jesús, con la ayuda de **Arrate Iriondo**, ha convertido este local en uno de los más frecuentados bares de pintxos de los contornos, con una **espectacular barra que alcanza su máximo esplendor los fines de semana**, en los que se sirven pintxos especiales como la Brocheta de langostinos, el Talo con jamón, el Talo con vegetal o el "Arrate", así como una variedad de **más de 40 bocadillos de generoso tamaño.** En temporada, también se ofrecen diversas raciones como Guindillas o Revuelto de hongos. En Mazzantini destacan también sus cervezas especiales como la Selecta Tostada o la Grimbergen que se sirve como caña o como zurito. Este bar abre todos los días a las 10 de la mañana y los jueves ofrece pintxo-pote de 7 a 9.

Otros pintxos:

- *Bocadillitos ibéricos (jamón, chorizo, cecina...)*
- *Ibérico con txaka*
- *Antxoillas con Roquefort y pimiento verde*
- *Antxoa, guindilla y pimiento verde*
- *Atún, antxoa y guindilla*
- *Lomo, queso y pimiento*
- *Tortillas variadas (patata, morcilla...)*
- *Jamón con mayonesa*
- *York con mayonesa*
- *Txaka, huevo y mayonesa*

"Euskal Burger"

Ingredientes:

Hamburguesa Eusko Label
Cebolla
Mayonesa
Lechuga
Queso Edam
Pan
Aceite de oliva

Elaboración:

Picamos la cebolla y la ponemos a pochar a fuego lento en aceite de oliva, durante al menos una hora.

Mientras se hace la cebolla, hacemos la hamburguesa, cuidando que nos quede jugosa por dentro.

Final y presentación: Abrimos un bollo de pan por la mitad y montamos el pintxo, disponiendo primeramente una cucharada de mayonesa. Sobre ésta, colocamos la lechuga, la rodaja de queso Edam y la cebolla recién pochada. Terminamos con la hamburguesa, de manera que con el calor de la cebolla y la hamburguesa se fundirá el queso Edam, adquiriendo una agradable textura.

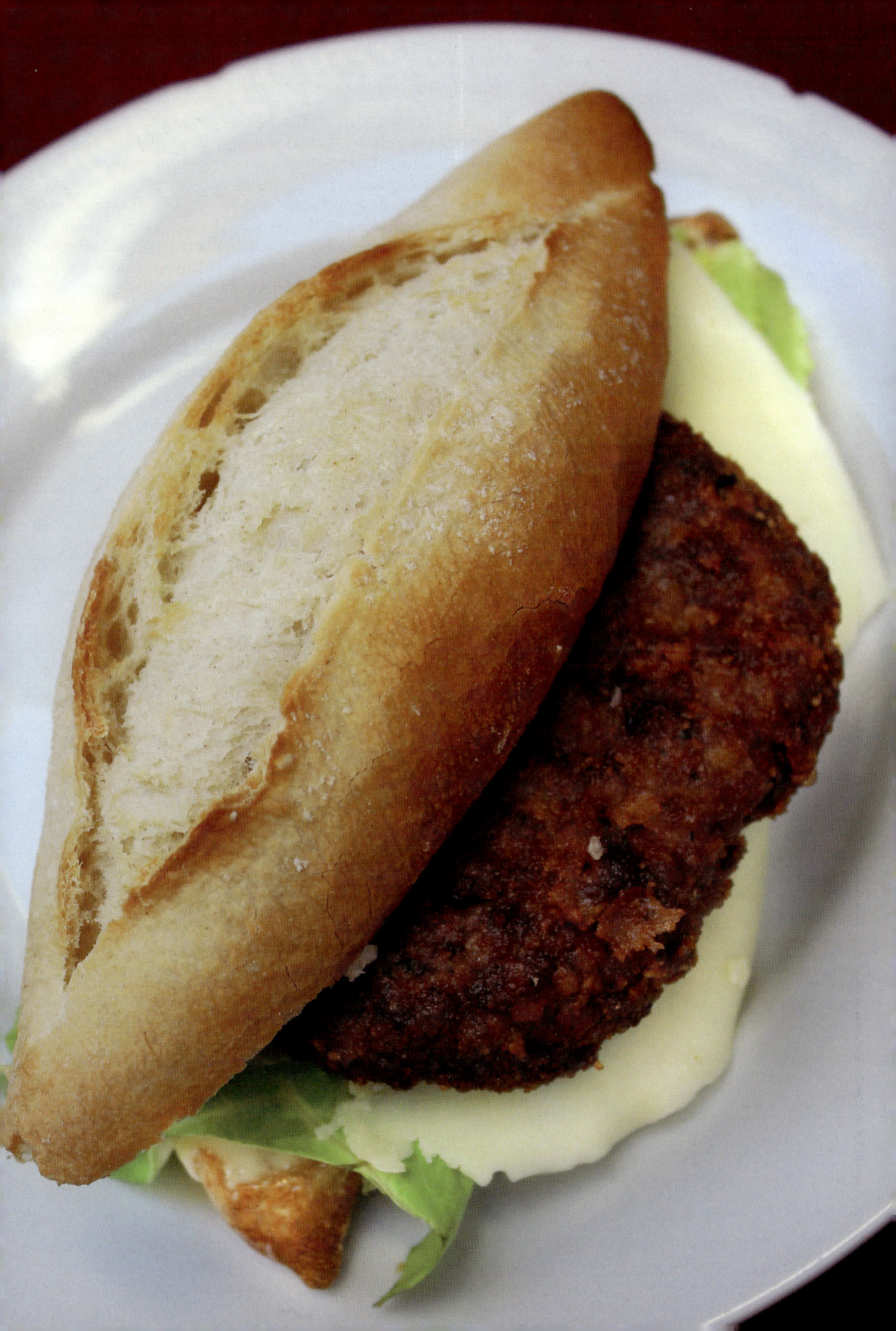

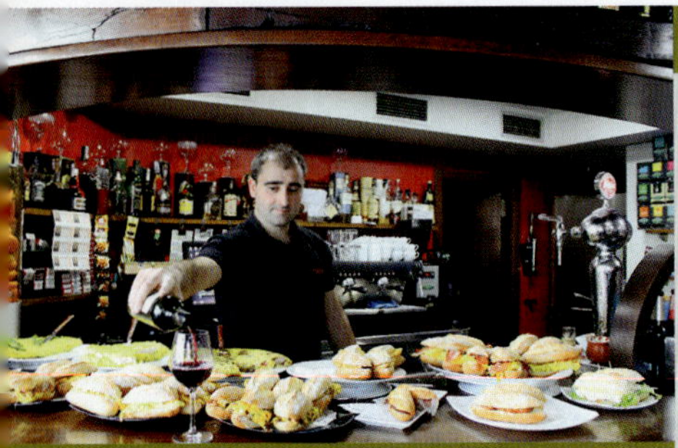

Landeta Hiribidea, 16
AZPEITIA
943 81 20 01

MENDIZABAL

Estratégicamente situado en la populosa y dinámica zona de Landeta, el asador Mendizabal fue bautizado así en 1976, cuando **Martín Mendizabal y Virtudes Uzkudun** se hicieron cargo de este establecimiento conocido hasta entonces como Casa Txintxokua. A cargo de su hijo Martín desde 2007, este asador **abre todos los días a las 6 de la mañana** para dar de desayunar a los cientos de trabajadores que acuden a las empresas de los alrededores. **En su oferta gastronómica sobresale la parrilla, siendo su especialidad los pescados** (Cogote, Sapo, Rodaballo, Besugo...) así como la chuleta de ternera. En temporada tienen gran éxito los hongos a la plancha, y es destacable el mantenimiento de un producto, **la Xexina** (carne de oveja conservada en sal) que se sirve todo el año con berza, y con morcilla en temporada. **Bocadillos, platos combinados, menú del día y menú especial** completan la oferta de este local también conocido en el mundo de las apuestas deportivas.

Otros pintxos:

- *Tortilla de Xexina*
- *"Miserable" (Tortilla de patata con bacon)*
- *Tortilla de patata con chaka y mayonesa*
- *Carne cocida con chorizo*
- *Pintxo "vegetal"*

Raciones:

- *Callos caseros*
- *Albóndigas en salsa o con tomate*
- *Morros en salsa*
- *Manitas de cerdo rebozadas*

Tortilla de patata, jamón y hongos

Ingredientes:

Huevo
Patata
Cebolla
Hongos
Jamón
Aceite de oliva
Sal

Elaboración:

Picamos finamente la cebolla y troceamos la patata en cuadritos. Asimismo, troceamos los hongos en trozos hermosos y picamos el jamón en tiras. Freímos todo en aceite de oliva, hasta que esté todo blandito y lo adjuntamos al huevo batido.

Cuajamos la tortilla cuidando de que quede jugosa en su interior.

Nota: Éste es el pintxo que más éxito tiene en la barra del Mendizabal. De hecho, hay cientes que acuden a este bar todos los días del año, sin excepción, a probarlo. El principal motivo de su éxito es que los hongos que se utilizan en el Mendizabal han sido embotados por ellos mismos, con lo que el producto es totalmente natural. Hay que subrayar también que la tortilla es de tamaño considerable (se hace con 14 huevos) y que se elabora dos veces a lo largo del día: a las 8 de la mañana y a las 5 de la tarde.

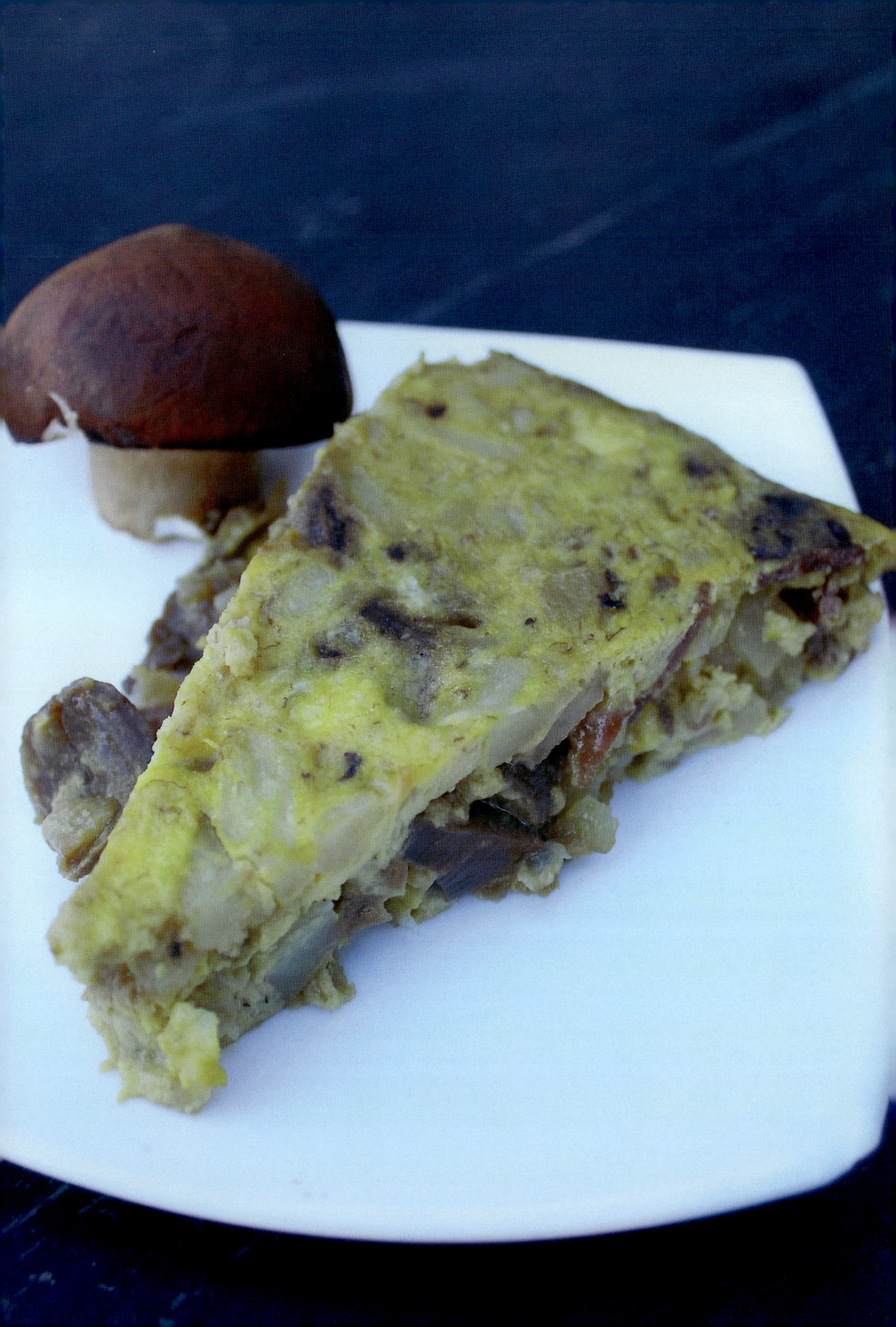

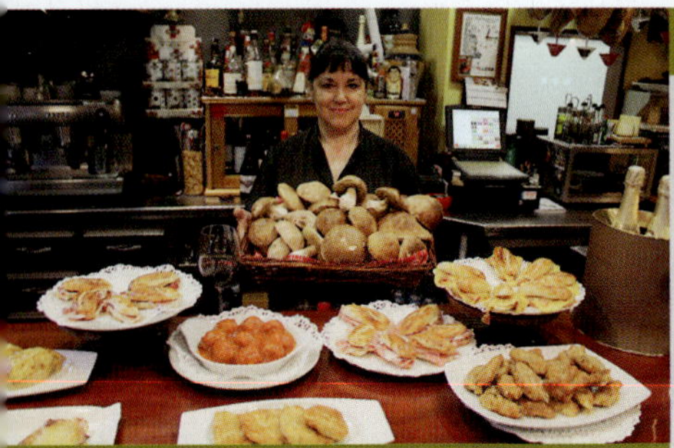

MESÓN LUGARITZ

Avda. Tolosa, 79 (El Antiguo)
DONOSTIA
943 21 85 03

Las hermanas **Mamen y Mertxe Beraiz**, naturales de Olazagutia, abrieron el Mesón Lugaritz en 2008 junto a **Antonio Cano**, pero anteriormente habían pasado **22 años en el bar Lugaritz, situado a escasos metros del local actual** y ahora rebautizado como Corner. **Las Beraiz trabajan el producto de temporada y prescinden de los menús**, al fin y al cabo su establecimiento no cuenta más que con cinco mesitas y los clientes están habituados a comer a base de raciones y cazuelitas. **La cocina de Mertxe Beraiz es eminentemente tradicional y casera, elaborada con productos de gran calidad adquiridos a proveedores de total confianza.** Son de destacar los embutidos ibéricos adquiridos directamente a un proveedor de toda la vida que realiza una cría casera de los cerdos en Los Pedroches (Córdoba). También llama la atención la gran variedad de vinos y Champagnes.

Otros pintxos:

- *Pa amb tumaca con jamón ibérico*
- *Presa ibérica de Los Pedroches*
- *Sardinas marinadas*
- *Lomo ibérico en aceite*
- *Chorizo criollo*
- *Tortilla de jamón*
- *Champiñón a la plancha*
- *Empanadilla de carne*
- *Croquetas caseras*
- *Vieiras gratinadas*

Manita "sin huesos" rebozada

Ingredientes:

Manitas de cerdo
Harina
Huevo
Hongos
Níscalos

- **Para el caldo de cocción de las manitas:**

Puerro
Zanahoria
Cebolla
1 hoja de laurel
Sal

- **Para la salsa:**

Cebolla
Puerro
Zanahoria
2 dientes de ajo

Elaboración:

Cocemos las manitas junto a las verduras a fuego lento por espacio de unas dos horas, hasta que estén blanditas. Una vez hechas, las sacamos del caldo, que reservamos, y las dejamos enfriar.

Deshuesamos las manitas y las ponemos en un molde para dejarlas con bonita forma.

Para la salsa: Picamos bien el ajo, la cebolla, el puerro y la zanahoria, y los doramos en una sartén. Una vez hecha la verdura, agregamos un poco de caldo de la cocción de las manitas. Dejamos que hiervaq durante unos minutos, trituramos con la batidora y pasamos por el chino.

Final y presentación: Cortamos las porciones de manita, las pasamos por harina y huevo y las freímos en aceite bien caliente. Acompañamos de la salsa y una guarnición de hongos y níscalos a la plancha.

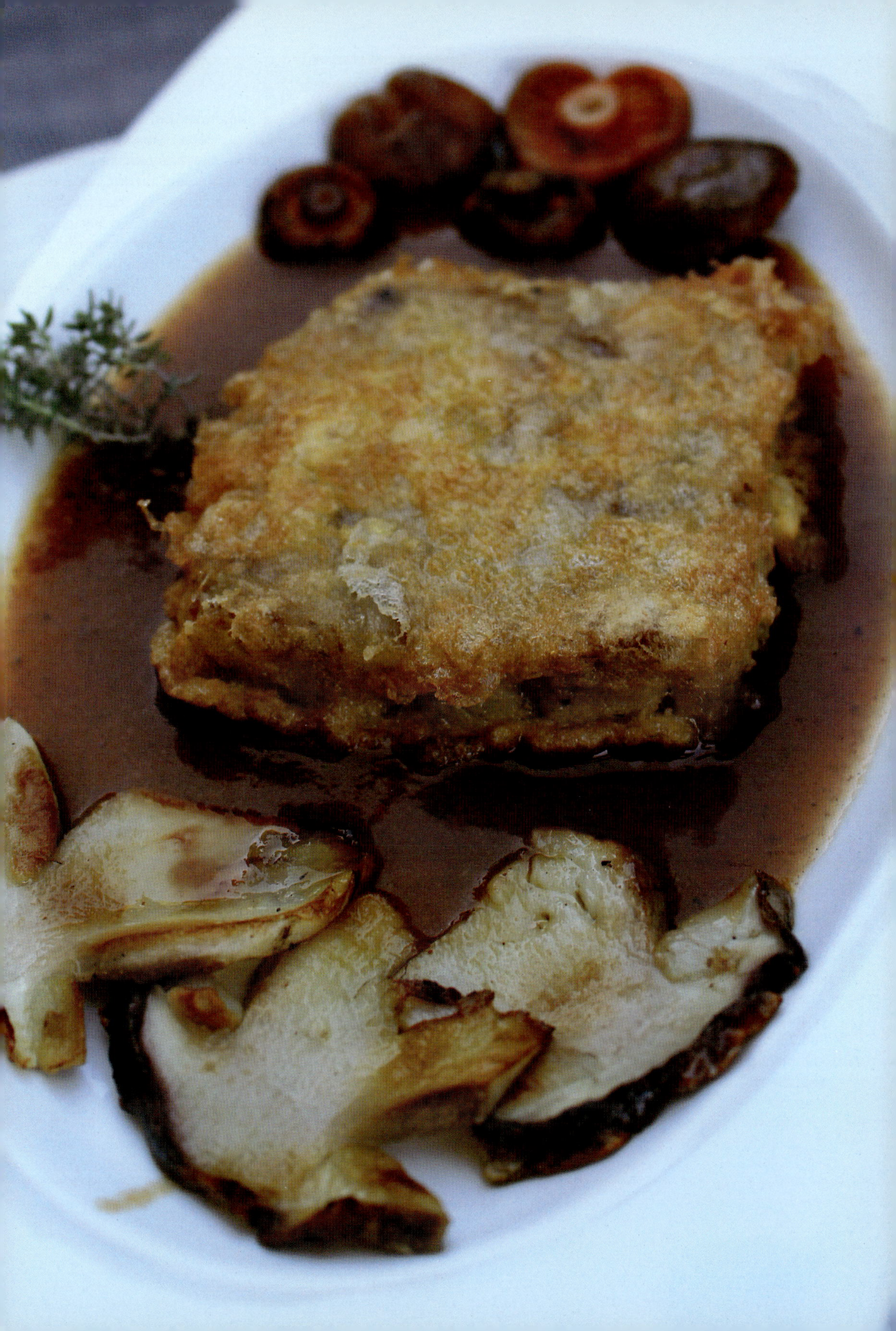

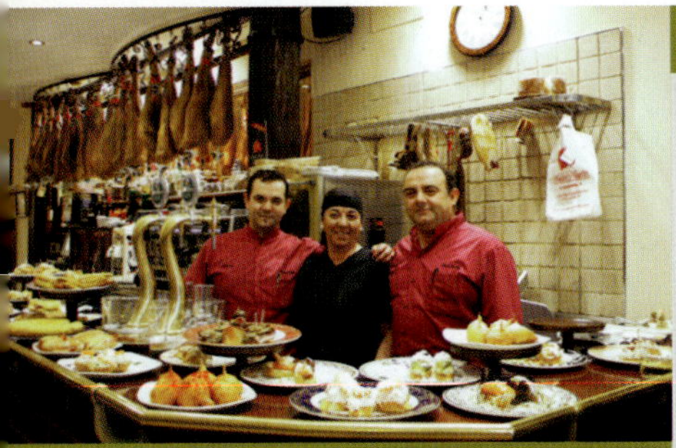

MESÓN MARTÍN

Los hermanos Martín se encargan de darle el nombre y el ambiente a este populoso local, estratégicamente situado en **una de las calles más transitadas de Donostia, entre el Boulevard y la Plaza de Gipuzkoa**. Abierto en 1996, cuenta con una agradable decoración rústica y elegante, con vistosas paredes de piedra. En su comedor, podemos disfrutar de **los mejores platos de la cocina tradicional vasca**. Además de sus pintxos, en el comedor podemos degustar especialidades como el Revuelto de txangurro y calabacín, la Ensalada templada de langostinos y gulas, el Panaché de verduras, las Kokotxas de bacalao en salsa verde, la Merluza con salsa de hongos, el Chuletón a la parrilla, las Manitas de cerdo rellenas de foie, hongos y trufa, el Arroz con leche casero y muchas más. Destacan también sus **excelentes embutidos Ibéricos**.

Elkano, 7 (Centro)
DONOSTIA
943 42 28 66
www.mesonmartin.com

Otros pintxos:

- *Trainera*
- *Croqueta*
- *Saquito*
- *Bola de carne*
- *Bola de queso*
- *Brick de txangurro*
- *Canelón de hongos y foie*
- *Gamba rebozada*
- *Pimiento relleno de bacalao o de morcilla*
- *Montadito de foie*

Milhojas de bacalao

Ingredientes:

Lascas de bacalao
Aceite de oliva
Tomate del país
Ajo
Vino blanco
Pimiento verde
Cebolla
Pimiento morrón
Patata
Patata de rejilla

- **Para la salsa de remolacha:**

Cebolla
Remolacha
Vino blanco
Agua

Elaboración:

Para la salsa de remolacha: Pochamos un poco de cebolla. Añadimos la remolacha en daditos y un poco de vino blanco. Dejamos reducir el vino y añadimos un poco de agua. Reducimos de nuevo y lo trituramos con la batidora.

Cortamos una rodaja de tomate y lo hacemos a la plancha con un poco de ajo picadito y vino blanco.

Picamos finamente la cebolla y el pimiento verde y lo pochamos a fuego muy lento.

Asamos el bacalao al vacío en el horno con un poco de aceite de oliva durante 5-7 minutos. Por otra parte, cocemos la patata. Una vez asado el bacalao, lo mezclamos con un poco de patata.

Salteamos los morrones en tiras en aceite de oliva.

Final y presentación: Ponemos como base la rodaja de tomate a la plancha y sobre ella la cebolla y el pimiento verde pochado. A continuación disponemos el bacalao con la patata y, coronando el pintxo, los morrones salteados. Decoramos el bocado con unas patatas de rejilla y unos hilos de salsa de remolacha.

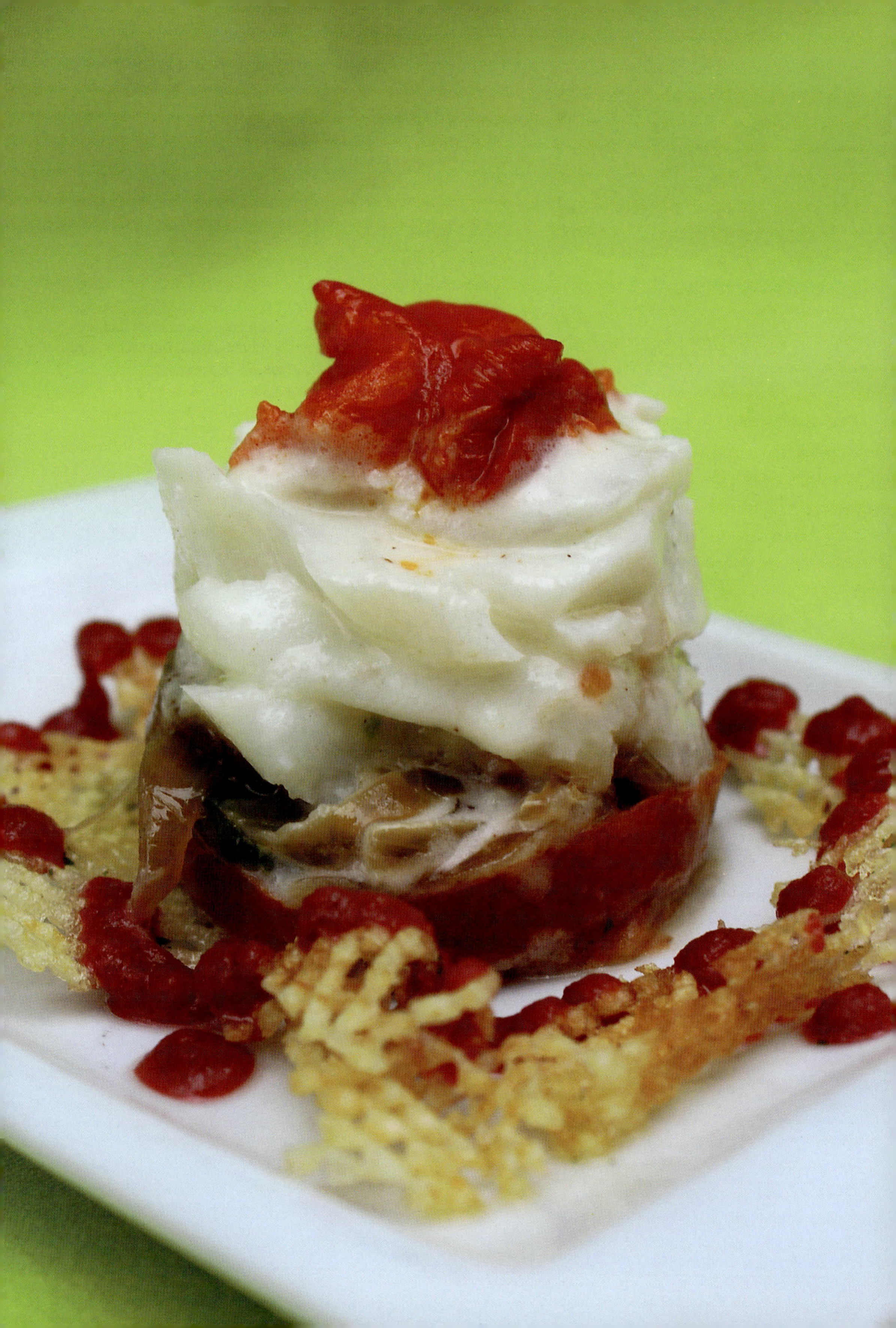

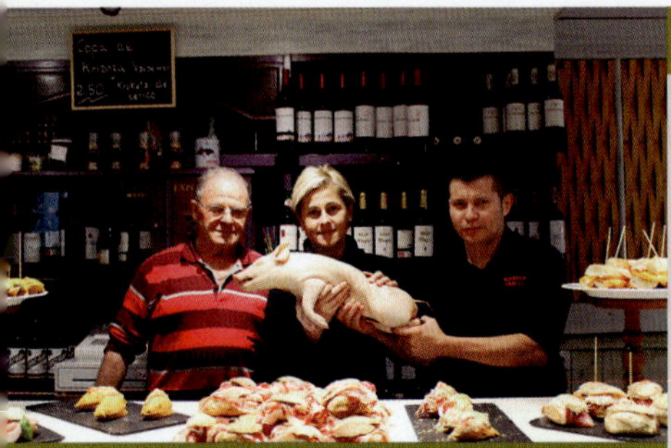

Barren Plaza, 1
ZARAUTZ
943 13 31 70

NAPARRAK

Agurtzane Onda Artetxe, conocida de siempre en la hostelería zarauztarra, abrió el Naparrak en 1994 y lo ha convertido en **uno de los más reputados bares de pintxos de Barren Plaza**. Además de los pintxos, que están disponibles desde las 9:30 de la mañana, en Naparrak puede disfrutarse de una variedad de platos y raciones en los que se le da mucha importancia al **producto de temporada** y al **pescado fresco** ("lo que nos trae el mar", según Agurtzane): Besuguito, Rodaballo, Rape, Txitxarro... servido además, a una buena relación calidad-precio. En Naparrak también se ofrecen otras tentadoras especialidades como Kokotxas de merluza pasadas por huevo de caserío, Colitas de cigala rebozadas, Solomillo al foie... Naparrak abre todos los días a las 8:30 y también cuenta con una cuidada oferta de **vinos** y una gran cantidad de **ginebras premium**.

Otros pintxos:

- *Croquetones de jamón ibérico*
- *Pintxo de kokotxa*
- *Pintxo de cigalita rebozada*
- *Ajoarriero*
- *Templadito de queso de cabra*
- *Txistorra de Arbizu*
- *Txipirón a la plancha*
- *Foie templado*
- *Solomillo sobre foie templado*
- *Tortilla de bacalao*

Risotto de hongos

Ingredientes:

Arroz bomba
Hongos
Caldo de pollo
Mantequilla
Nata
Sal
Cebolla
Agua
Puerro
Foie fresco
Pan
Aceite de oliva

Elaboración:

Rehogamos la cebolla con la mantequilla y los hongos. Una vez pochado, añadimos el arroz y lo rehogamos un poco.

Ponemos la cazuela a fuego medio y vamos añadiendo el caldo poco a poco hasta que el arroz tenga la consistencia que deseamos. Más o menos, nos harán falta unos 12 minutos.

Retiramos el arroz del fuego, le añadimos la sal y la nata y lo mezclamos bien para que quede un plato homogéneo y consistente.

Hacemos tiras de verde de puerro y las freímos en aceite de oliva virgen muy caliente.

Cortamos unas rodajas de pan y las freímos en aceite de oliva o las tostamos al horno.

Cortamos una rodaja de foie y la hacemos a la plancha, vuelta y vuelta.

Final y presentación: En un cuenco, servimos el risotto. y lo coronamos con el foie, las tiras de puerro y las rodajas de pan frito.

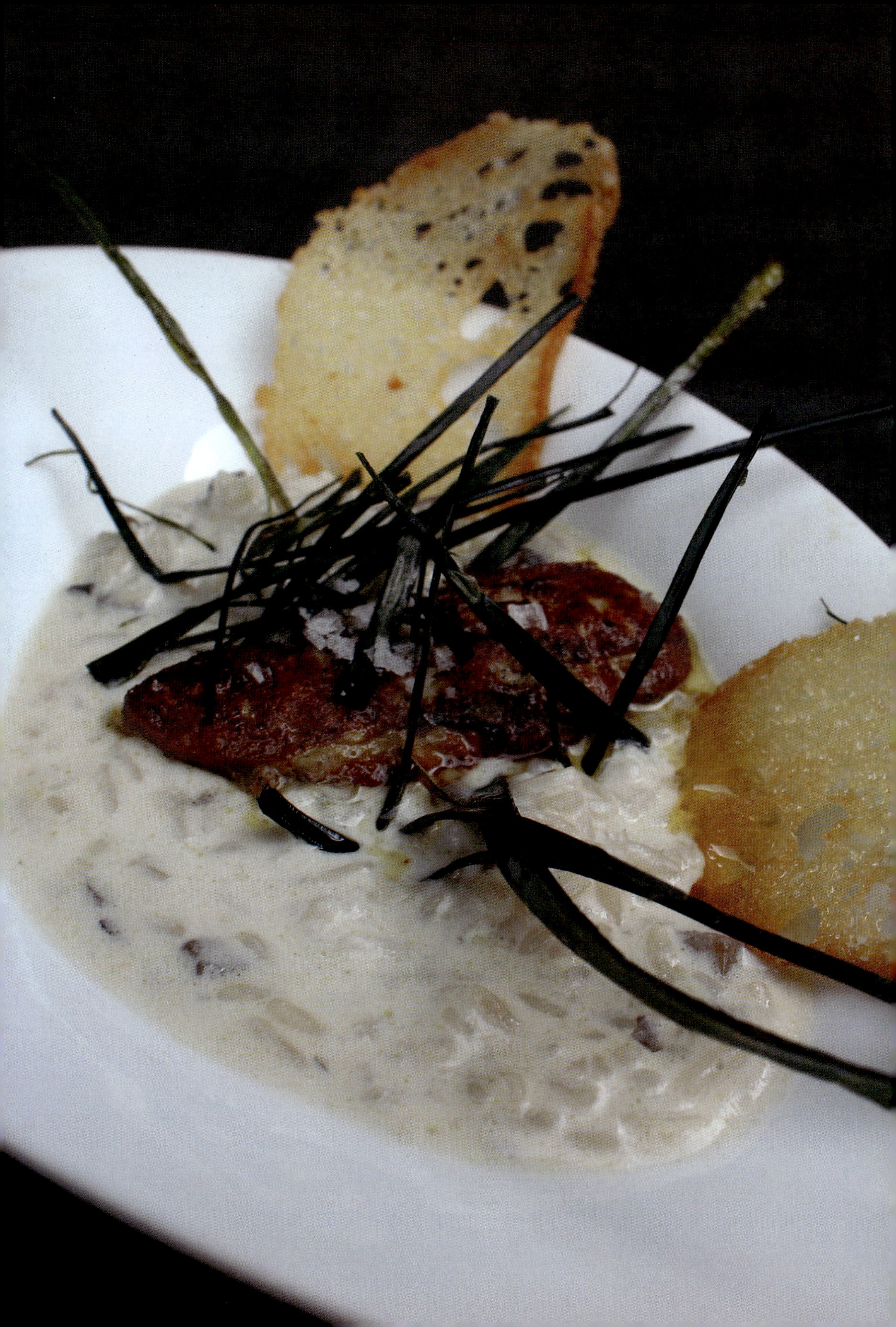

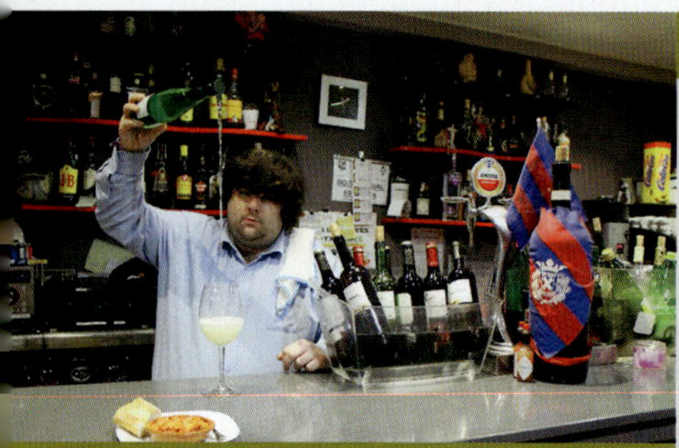

José Antonio Iturriotz, 1
EIBAR
943 56 70 36

NUEVO

José Luis Zurro y su hijo **Iraitz** se hicieron cargo del Nuevo en mayo de 2011, aunque este emblemático bar del barrio de Urki pasaba ya de los 40 años de vida. En el Nuevo, las tareas están claramente delimitadas: José Luis se ocupa de la cocina y de que no falten los **platos habituales que se sirven como pintxo o ración** (Champiñones, Callos, Riñones...) así como **Platos combinados y Pizzas**. Aparte de esta oferta básica, por encargo se preparan muchos más platos como Cochinillo, Cordero, Rape, Chuleta de viejo... Es muy apreciada también la Merluza con Kokotxas o la Brocheta de carne con langostinos, y entre las **cazuelas** que pueden encargarse para llevar o para tomar en el bar destacan las de Bacalao con piperrada o al pil-pil, Carrilleras, Guisote de rabo... También se preparan por encargo **Paellas y Pollos asados**. Iraitz, por su parte, se ocupa de la barra, aplicando en ella su amplia experiencia en hostelería, sector en el que lleva desde los 12 años y que, como dice él mismo, "lo lleva en la sangre".

Otros pintxos:

- *Chorizo*
- *Champiñones*
- *Riñones*
- *Callos*
- *Pulpo*

Raciones

- *Rabas*
- *Patatas bravas*
- *Chorizo ibérico*
- *Jamón ibérico*

Callos con chorizo

Ingredientes:

200 g de callos de ternera
50 g de chorizo para cocido
4 dientes de ajo
1 cebolla
20 ml de aceite de oliva
4 g de pimentón picante
4 g de harina
2 g de granitos de pimienta blanca
Una pizca de sal
1 hoja de laurel
Una pizca de guindilla seca
Clavo de olor

Elaboración:

Lavamos los callos en agua fría frotando bien. Los dejamos a remojo 2 horas cubiertos de agua fría con un chorro de vinagre. Transcurrido el tiempo, volvemos a lavarlos.

Disponemos los callos en una cazuela, los cubrimos de agua y la ponemos a cocer. Cuando comience a hervir, retiramos la cazuela del fuego, escurrimos y desechamos el agua. Volvemos a llenar con agua limpia la cazuela donde están los callos y agregamos el chorizo. Añadimos media cebolla y un clavo de olor, dos dientes de ajo, la hoja de laurel, un poco de perejil, pimienta y sal. Cuando comience a hervir, bajamos la potencia del fuego, tapamos la cazuela y mantenemos al mínimo unas tres horas. Una vez cocidos, troceamos los callos en cuadros y el chorizo en rodajitas, y reservamos el agua colada de la cocción.

Hacemos un sofrito con aceite de oliva, dos dientes de ajo y la cebolla, picados muy finos. Cuando la cebolla esté pochada, añadimos una pizca de guindilla, una cucharadita de pimentón y harina. Removemos rápidamente y mojamos con un poco de agua de la cocción. Agregamos los callos y dejamos a fuego suave 20 minutos.

Dejamos reposar de un día para otro en la nevera.

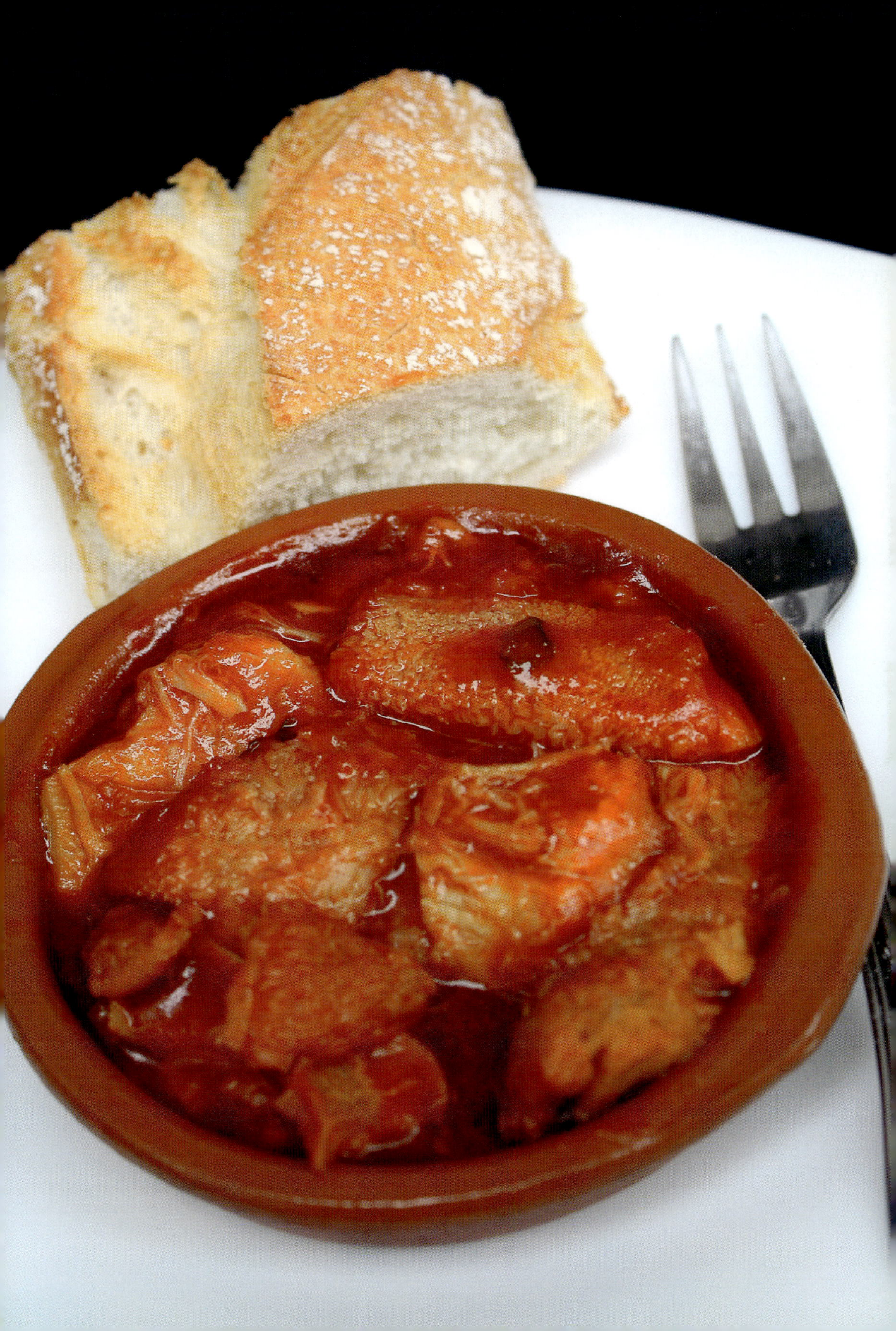

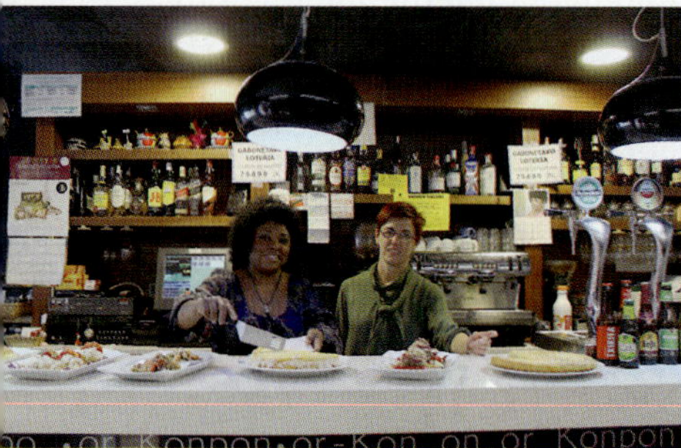

OR-KONPON

Kale Berria, 54
BILLABONA
943 01 91 00

El Or-Konpon es **uno de los más veteranos bares de Billabona**, con más de medio siglo de historia a sus espaldas. Desde diciembre de 2011 está dirigido por **Ángela Disla Castillo**, que también regenta el restaurante **Iturrigoxo** en el barrio de Amasa. Ángela ofrece desde las 7:30 de la mañana una gran cantidad de tortillas y pintxos en barra, sin olvidar las míticas bolas de marisco, elaboradas con la receta original de la señora que dirigía el bar en sus inicios. Entre sus raciones de **cocina tradicional** destaca el Bacalao en salsa verde, el Chorizo al txakoli, el Rabo en salsa de vino tinto, los Callos caseros y los Txipirones en su tinta. También se sirven **Platos combinados y generosos bocadillos**, destacando el "Especial Or-Konpon", compuesto de jamón ibérico, hongos y pimiento verde. Los jueves, de 6 a 10 de la tarde, se sirve **pintxo-pote**, y los fines de semana se sirven cenas (en verano, todos los días).

Otros pintxos:

- *Tortilla rellena de jamón, queso y chaka*
- *Setas a la plancha con jamón ibérico*
- *Chorizo al txakoli*
- *Piquillo, hongos y jamón*
- *Brocheta de gambas*
- *Pimiento verde relleno de gulas*
- *Piquillo, hongos, jamón y cebolla caramelizada*
- *Croquetas caseras*
- *Bacalao frito con pimientos rojos y verdes*
- *Espárrago a la plancha enrollado con jamón ibérico*

Rulo vertical de salmón y berenjena

Ingredientes:

Berenjena
Salmón ahumado
Harina
Huevo
Aceite de oliva
Gambas
Cebolla
Pimiento del piquillo
Gambas

· Para el aceite de perejil:
Aceite de oliva virgen extra
Perejil

· Para la salsa de miel:
Miel
Nata
Mostaza

Elaboración:

Para el aceite de perejil: Picamos muy finamente un ramillete de perejil y lo depositamos en un tarro o una botella. Llenamos el recipiente de aceite de oliva virgen extra y lo dejamos macerar. Esta operación deberá hacerse antes de elaborar los pintxos. De hecho, es interesante contar siempre con este aceite macerado pues nos puede venir bien para cualquier cosa.

Para la salsa de miel: En un cazo, calentamos la nata y disolvemos en ella la miel y la mostaza. Removemos bien.

Para el rulo de salmón y berenjena: Cortamos la berenjena en rodajas. Las rebozamos en harina y huevo y las freímos en abundante aceite de oliva. Una vez templadas, enrollamos con cada rodaja de berenjena una rodaja de salmón, formando tres rulos.

Salteamos las gambas. Cortamos en juliana la cebolla y la pochamos en aceite de oliva. Cortamos en tiras el piquillo y lo salteamos.

Final y presentación: Sobre una rebanada de pan, tostado al horno o a la plancha, disponemos los tres rulos en vertical. Vertemos en medio el piquillo y por todo la cebolla pochada. Coronamos cada rulo con una gamba y decoramos el conjunto con aceite de perejil.

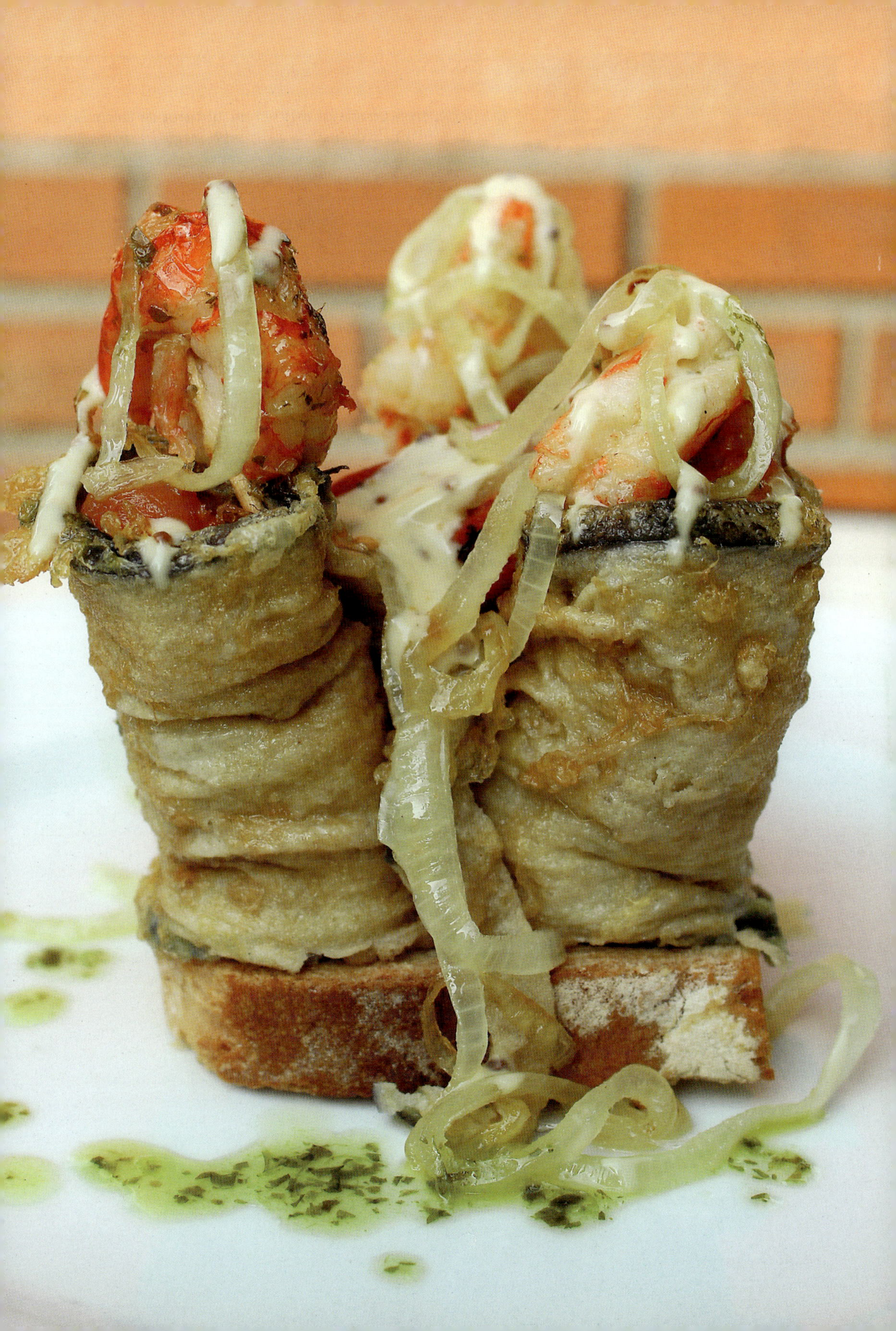

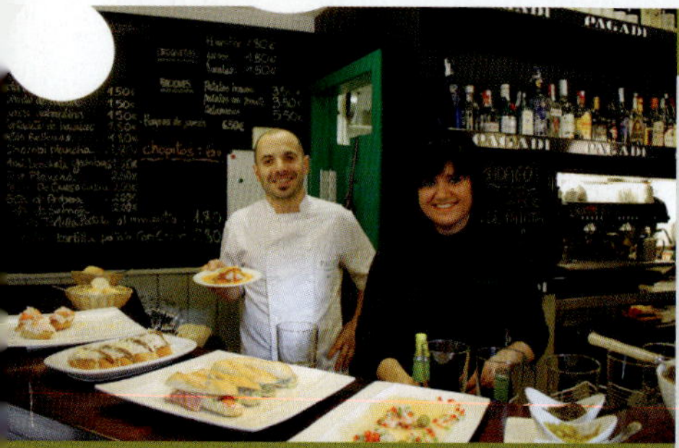

PAGADI

General Artetxe, 1 (Gros)
DONOSTIA
943 28 42 99
www.pagaditaberna.es

Igor Torre Mendizabal abrió en 1996 esta taberna, en pleno corazón de Gros, tras haberse formado en el Iturrioz, en el Aloña Mendi y, especialmente, en el bar Aiete, que dirigieron sus padres, Ángel y Manoli, durante 40 años. En Pagadi, además de sus pintxos, podemos disfrutar de un cuidado **Menú del día** de lunes a viernes, así como una amplia variedad de **Ensaladas, Hamburguesas, Bocadillos y Platos combinados.** En su carta, ocupan el puesto de honor las **croquetas, totalmente artesanales**, así como los **postres caseros**: Arroz con leche, Flan, Natillas, Tartaleta de queso fresco con frambuesa... todo ello elaborado por **Petri Sánchez**, cocinera que lleva con Igor desde el principio. Destacan también en Pagadi las excelentes **antxoas en salazón de Conserveras Gorostiaga**, elaboradas por el tío de Igor, que se limpian y preparan a mano en el propio bar. La terraza y una acogedora zona de mesas completan la oferta de este popular y concurrido bar.

Otros pintxos:

- *Tortilla de patata al momento*
- *Tosta de antxoa en salazón (preparada en casa)*
- *Buñuelo de bacalao*
- *Seta rellena de hongos y foie*
- *Tortilla de patata con callos (en invierno)*
- *Croquetas caseras (Hongos y foie, jamón, bacalao...)*
- *Bola de queso con Emmental*
- *Montadito de bacalao*

Raciones:

- *Pa amb tumaca*
- *Chopitos o calamares.*

Brocheta de gamba y bacon

Ingredientes:

3 gambas
2 trozos de bacon

• Para la vinagreta:
Cebolla
Pimiento verde
Pimiento rojo
Aceite de oliva virgen extra
Vinagre
Sal

Elaboración:

Para la vinagreta: Picamos finamente la cebolla, el pimiento verde y el pimiento rojo. Los mezclamos con aceite de oliva virgen extra, vinagre y sal y reservamos.

Ensartamos en un palillo intercalándolas las tres gambas y los dos pedazos de bacon formando una pequeña brocheta que haremos a la plancha hasta que se tueste el bacon.

Final y presentación: Disponemos en un platillo la brocheta de gambas y bacon y la cubrimos generosamente con la vinagreta de cebolla y pimiento.

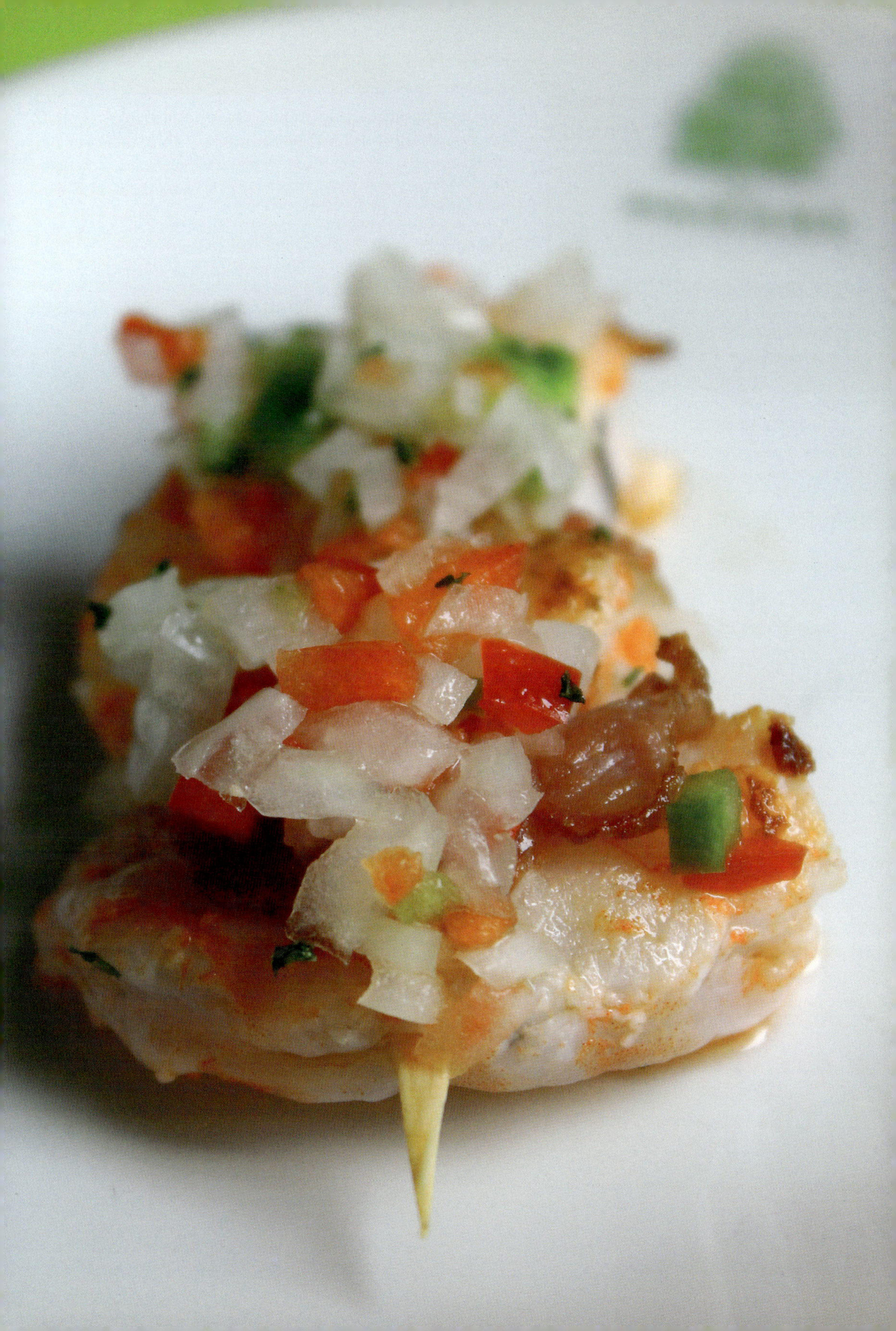

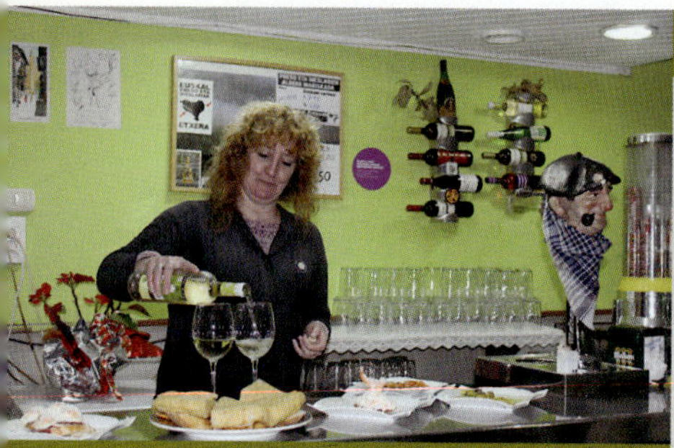

Santxoenea, 4
ORERETA
943 52 71 93

PARAÍSO

La oreretarra **Idoia Segurola**, que cuenta con una amplia experiencia en el mundo de la hostelería local dirige, desde el mes de diciembre de 2011, este **céntrico y veterano bar que se acerca al siglo de existencia.** Paraíso, que mantiene la apariencia clásica de los bares de antaño, abre sus puertas todos los días a las 8 de la mañana, y desde primera hora están disponibles los **callos y los morros**, sus dos especialidades más emblemáticas. A las 10:30 de la mañana hacen su aparición los pintxos de barra y las tortillas y los viernes y los sábados también se sirven cenas con especialidades como Ensalada templada de txipirones, Rabo en salsa, Cogote al horno, y las Manitas de cerdo con tomate, que cuentan con una gran aceptación. Paraíso cierra los domingos a partir del mediodía y los jueves a lo largo de todo el día.

Otros pintxos:

- *Tortilla de patatas*
- *Tortillas variadas*
- *Gildas*
- *Morros en salsa*
- *Chaka con mayonesa*

Raciones:

- *Txipirones en su tinta*
- *Manitas de cerdo con tomate*
- *Rabo en salsa*
- *Cogote de merluza al horno*

Callos con tomate

Ingredientes:

Callos
Cebolla
Pimiento verde
Pimiento rojo
Tomate triturado
Aceite de oliva
Chorizo
Jamón
PImentón picante
Sal

Elaboración:

Cocemos los callos por espacio de tres horas aproximadamente. Una vez cocidos y enfriados, los partimos en trozos y los reservamos.

Cortamos el chorizo en rodajas y el jamón en taquitos, y los reservamos.

Picamos finamente una hermosa cantidad de cebolla, un poco de pimiento rojo y un poco de pimiento verde. Lo pochamos todo en aceite de oliva y cuando esté todo bien pochado, añadimos los callos, el chorizo y el jamón. Rehogamos todo un rato y añadimos el tomate triturado. Rectificamos de sal y dejamos que se haga todo a fuego lento durante un par de horas.

Servimos los callos en un platito acompañados de un par de rodajas de pimiento verde que habremos freído previamente en la freidora.

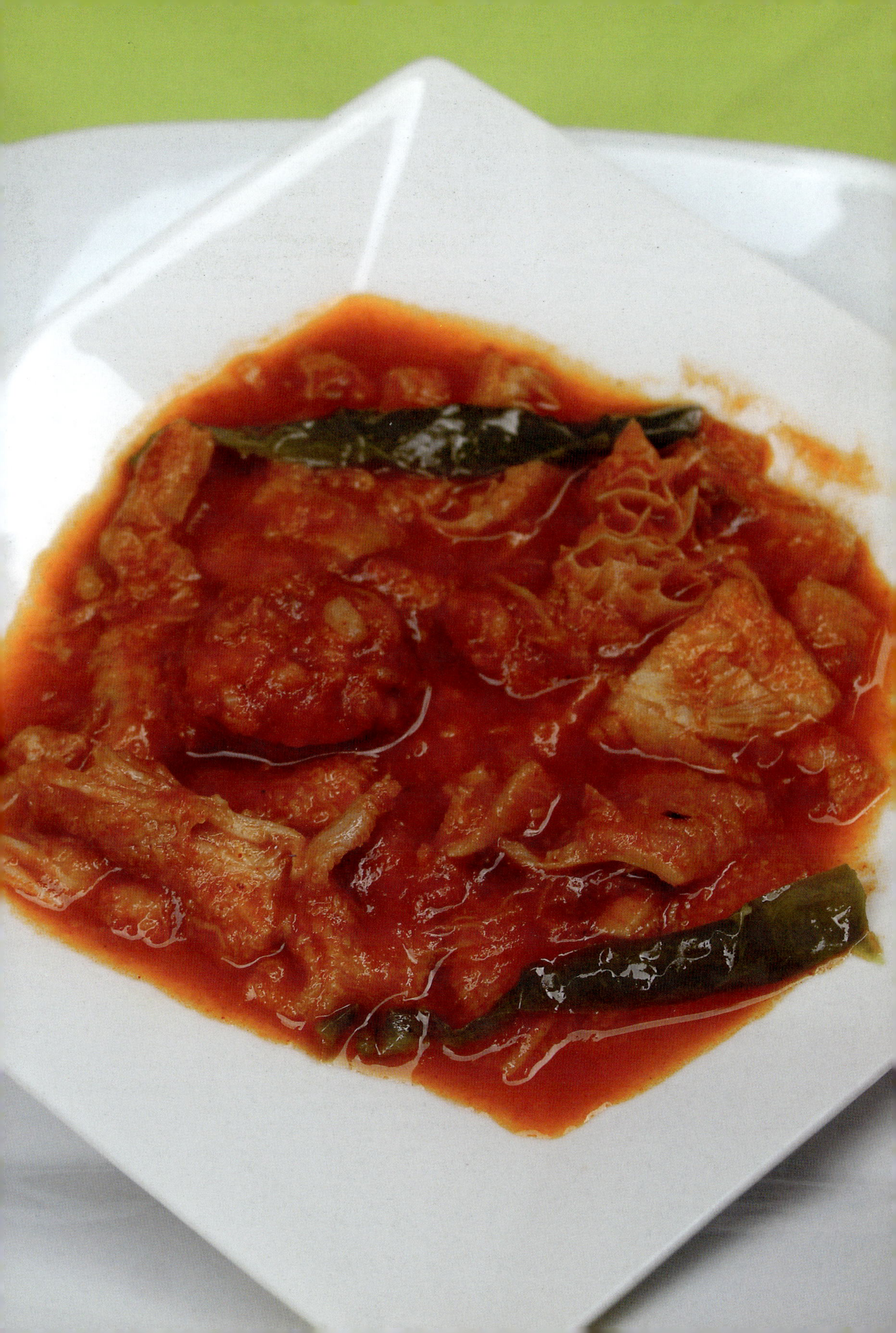

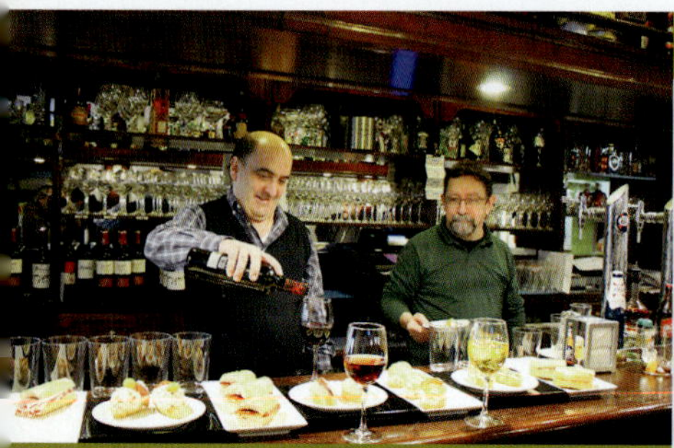

Patxiku Kalea, 5
ZARAUTZ

PATXIKU

Los hermanos **Juan Carlos y Manu Eizagirre** son dos viejos conocidos de la hostelería de Urola Kosta. Juan Carlos ha trabajado de siempre en el sector en locales como el Xoxoa, el Orbela o el Jai-Txiki, mientras que Manu ha atendido durante muchos años la barra del Itxas-Etxea en Getaria. En junio de 2014 se hicieron con este pequeño y estratégico bar que abre todos los días a las 9:30 de la mañana y que cuenta con el atractivo de estar dotado de un **terminal de apuestas hípicas "Turf"**, lo que permite que tomemos unos pintxos mientras jugamos en las diferentes carreras de caballos de todo el mundo, que se celebran entre las 11 de la mañana y las 9 de la noche. Además de sus pintxos, en Patxiku podemos optar por sus **raciones** de Jamón de Guijuelo, Lomo ibérico o sus Antxoas y Boquerones.

Otros pintxos:

- *Atún con antxoa*
- *Chorizo picante de Zamora*
- *Ensaladilla rusa*
- *Croissant relleno de chaka*
- *Atún con cebolla y antxoa*
- *Huevo de codorniz con gamba y txangurro*

Raciones:

- *Jamón de Guijuelo*
- *Lomo ibérico*
- *Antxoas y Boquerones*

Boquerón con txangurro

Ingredientes:

Pan tostado
2 boquerones de Getaria
Aceite de oliva

Para el txangurro:
Txangurro desmigado
Cebolla
Huevo duro
Sal

Elaboración:

Para el txangurro: Picamos muy finamente la cebolla y la clara del huvo duro y lo mezclamos todo con la carne de txangurro desmigado. Una vez todo mezclado le damos el punto de sal.

Final y presentación: Cortamos una rebanada de pan y la tostamos en la tostadora. Sobre ella disponemos dos boquerones de Getaria y sobre ellos el txangurro mezclado con la cebolla y el huevo. Terminamos con un chorrito de aceite de oliva.

Nota: Este pintxo se sirve en **tres variantes** en Patxiku taberna. Además del anteriormente descrito, puede servirse con puding de merluza y salsa rosa. Para ello se elaborará un puding clásico al horno con merluza desespinada y desmigada y un poco de nata, y una salsa rosa con mayonesa, zumo de naranja, ketchup y coñac. La presentación es la misma, sólo que en vez del txangurro se dispone un trozo de puding y se corona con la salsa rosa. Finalmente, la tercera variante es el mismo pintxo, colocando sobre los boquerones una mezcla de huevo duro, salmón ahumado y hierbas aromáticas.

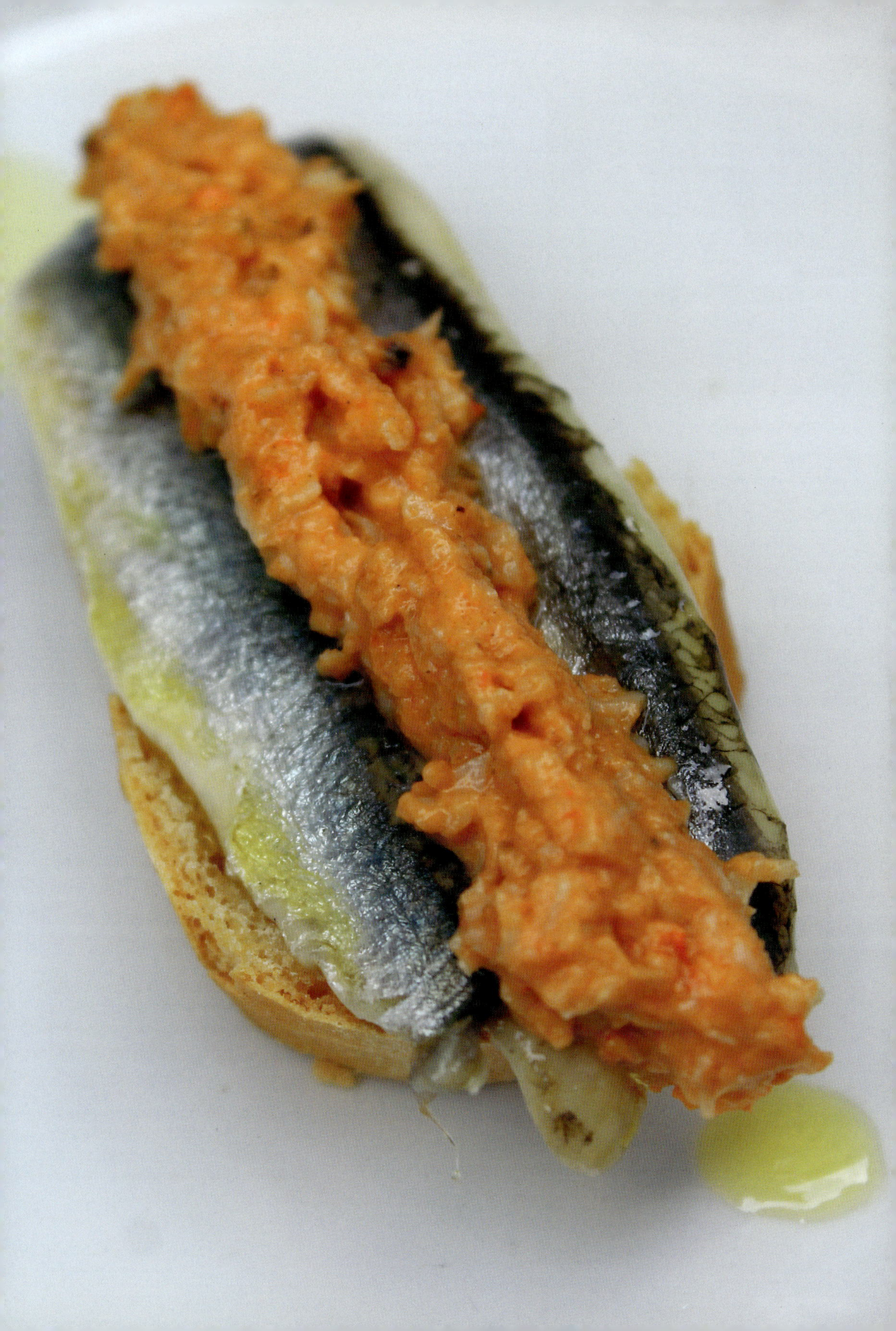

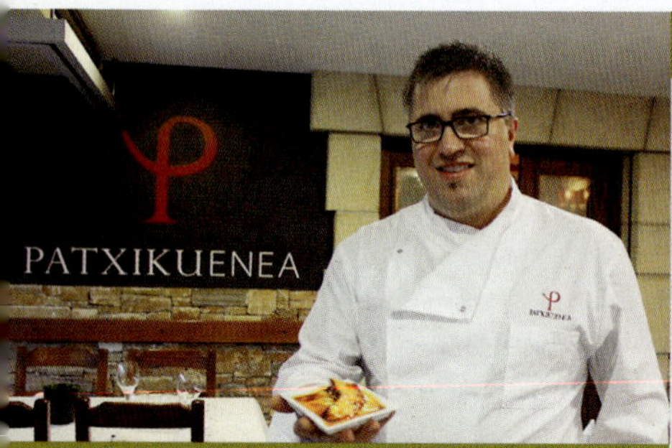

B° Gaintxurizketa
LEZO
943 52 75 45
www.patxikuenea.com

PATXIKU - ENEA

El Patxiku-Enea de Lezo no es, propiamente hablando, un bar de pintxos, pero cuenta con un servicio que está desapareciendo en los asadores de su categoría: una **barra de bienvenida** en la que los comensales pueden tomarse un vinito, una cerveza, un cóctel... y hasta un pintxito antes de pasar al comedor. Incluso, puede entrarse al Patxiku-Enea a tomar, sin más, algo en la barra atendida con gran profesionalidad por **Xabier Manterola**. Pasando al comedor, ya entramos en palabras mayores: un **caserío de más de 250 años**, carnes y pescados de excepción a la parrilla, una cocina tradicional elaborada con productos inmaculados, y **un trato cercano y familiar de la mano de los hermanos Aitor y Karmele Manterola, fieles seguidores de la filosofía de su padre, Emilio Manterola**, que fundara el restaurante en 1973. Patxiku-Enea es, sin duda, una cita obligada para los amantes de la buena mesa y la cocina con raíces.

Otros pintxos:

- *Chorizo a la sidra*
- *Croquetas caseras de jamón*
- *Bonito con guindilla y antxoa*
- *Pintxo de verdel con vinagreta de tomate (en temporada)*

Raciones:

- *Rabas*
- *Alcachofas fritas*
- *Ibéricos*

Pulpo a la brasa

Ingredientes:

Pulpo
Agua
Puré de patata
Pimentón de la Vera picante
Pimentón de la Vera dulce
Aceite de oliva virgen extra
Escamas de sal.

Elaboración:

Primeramente, congelamos 15 días el pulpo para que se rompan las fibras.

Llegado el día de prepararlo, lo cocemos en agua sin sal y lo vamos pinchando con un palillo. Como describe **Aitor Manterola**: "Debemos imaginar que el palillo es nuestro diente y hacernos a la idea del mordiente que queremos conseguir. Generalmente se cuece entre 20 y 25 minutos, pero cada pulpo es un mundo".

Sacamos el pulpo con cuidado de la olla y lo enfriamos en el abatidor. Le damos un corte longitudinal a una de las patas y cocinamos en la parrilla la parte interior del corte, es decir, la parte blanca. Bastará con dorar bien la parte interior comentada (si el pulpo es de calidad, se dora enseguida).

Final y presentación: Servimos el pulpo en un platillo con un puré de patata y una emulsión de aceite de oliva y pimentón de la Vera en proporción de dos partes de pimentón picante y tres de dulce. Finalmente, lo espolvoreamos con unas escamas de sal.

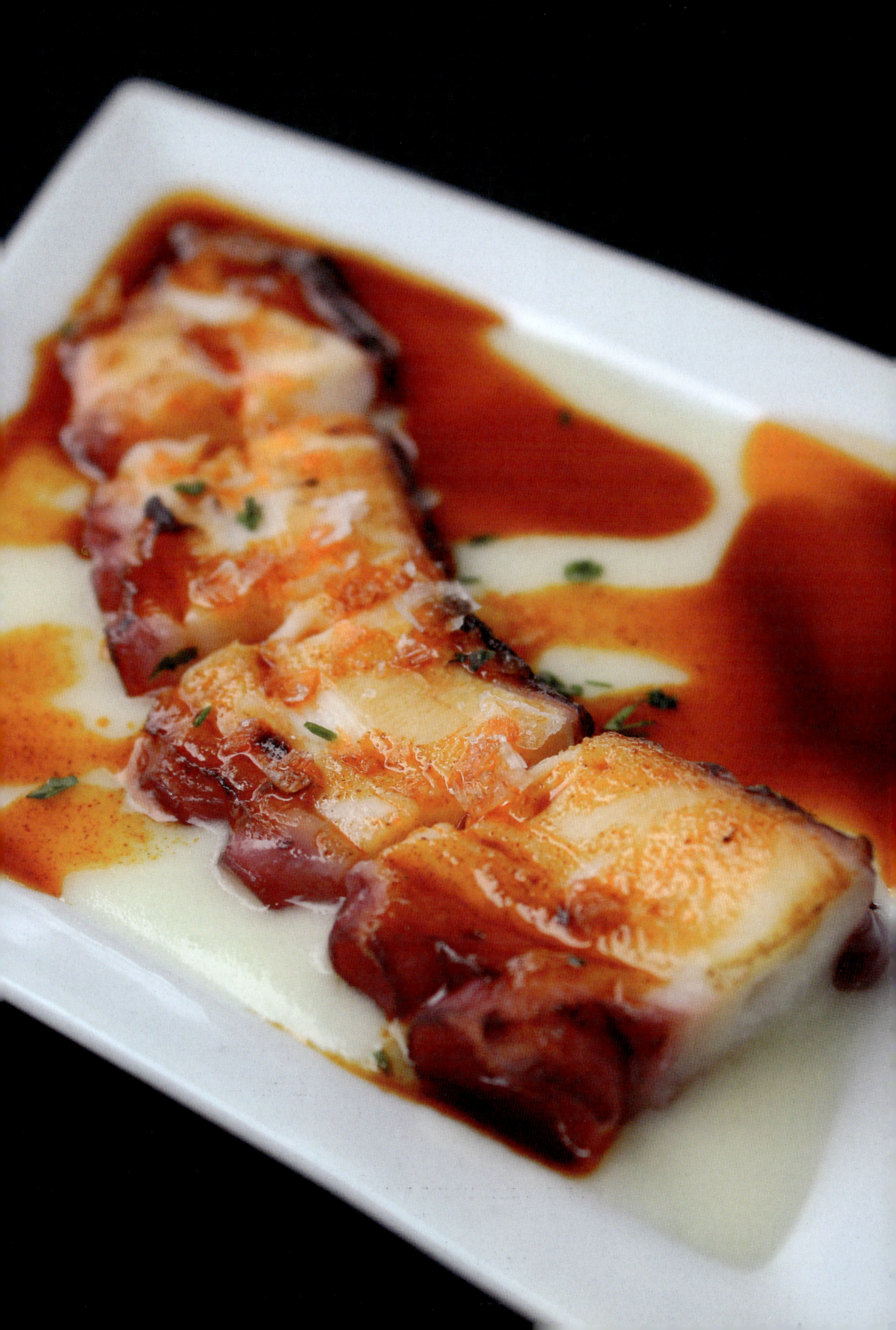

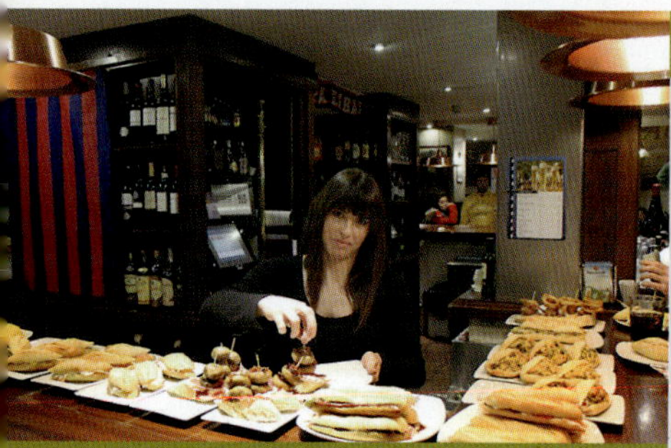

PAULANER

P° San Andrés 3, bajo
EIBAR
943 20 13 29
www.paulaner-eibar.com

Miguel Ángel Garzón dirige este amplio y acogedor establecimiento abierto en junio de 2005 y situado **en pleno centro de Eibar**, en el emplazamiento del antiguo bar Txorimalo, a un paso de la estación de autobuses, la Plaza Unzaga y el apeadero de Eusko Trenbideak. En este local encontraremos una **gran variedad de especialidades alemanas** como Codillo, Wurstchen (Surtido de salchichas alemanas) y buena cerveza de barril rubia, tostada y de trigo, así como diferentes cervezas de importación. Paulaner abre todos los días a las 8 de la mañana, y desde primera hora cuenta con diferentes pintxos en su barra. De lunes a viernes, además, se ofrece servicio de **menú del día**, y todos los días se ofrecen comidas y cenas. Paulaner-Eibar cuenta también con una amplia **terraza cubierta**, abierta todos los días del año.

Otros pintxos:

- *Tortillas variadas*
- *Ensalada de jamón y puerro*
- *Revuelto de bacalao con pimientos y cebolla*
- *Jamón con chatka*
- *Hojaldre de setas con gambas*
- *Revuelto de jamón serrano con champiñones*
- *Revuelto de langostinos con setas*

Raciones:

- *Paleta ibérica*
- *Rabas y Patatas bravas*

Pintxo de txipirón con aros de cebolla

Ingredientes:

1 txipirón
2 aros de cebolla
Ajo
Harina de tempura
Aceite de oliva
Pan

Elaboración:

Limpiamos el txipirón y lo salteamos junto con sus patitas en una sartén con un poco de ajo y aceite.

Una vez salteado lo salpimentamos, picamos e introducimos en su interior las patitas, lo rebozamos con harina de tempura y lo freímos en aceite de oliva.

Para los aros de cebolla: Cortamos un par de aros de cebolla, los pasamos por la harina de tempura y los freímos en aceite bien caliente.

Final y presentación: Cortamos una rebanada de pan, disponemos encima el txipirón y, encima del mismo, colocamos los dos aritos de cebolla. Atravesamos todo con un palillo.

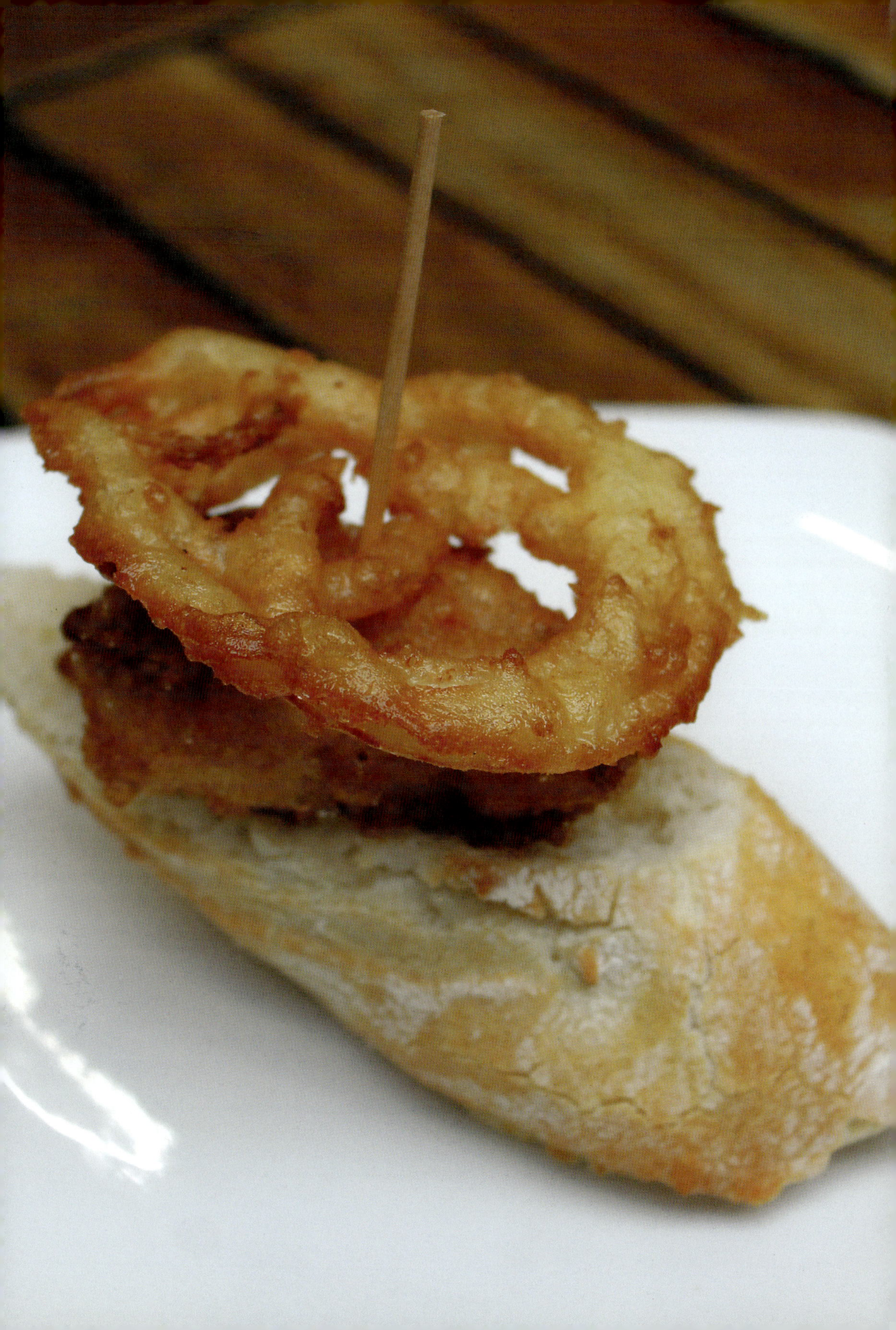

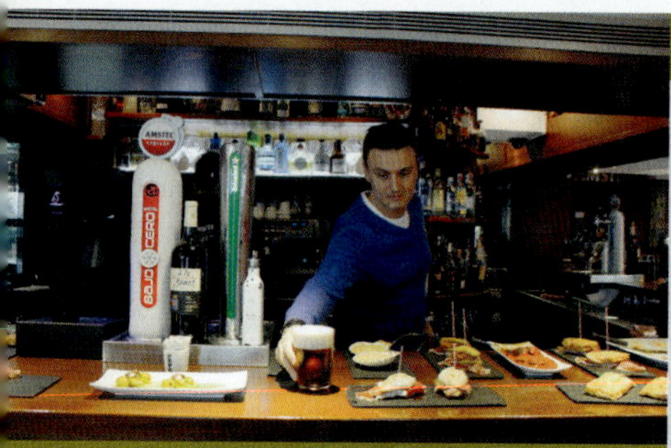

PEPE

Av. Zumalakarregi, 3 (El Antiguo)
DONOSTIA
943 11 67 33

Lucas Rey, Javi Porto y Julián Melo, que también regentan la cervecería **Mandrágora** de Benta Berri (ver página 148), dirigen desde 2009 este emblemático bar al que sometieron a una profunda reforma ampliándolo y convirtiéndolo en un local más de la ruta de poteo y pintxos de la Calle Matia. En Pepe hay una mayor variedad gastronómica, que se traduce en una **amplia carta de Bocadillos, Ensaladas, Raciones y Platos combinados**. Gozan de gran éxito las **Tostas**, como la solicitada Tosta de hongos, jamón y queso gratinado o la de 4 quesos y tomate natural, y otras **especialidades** como la Chuleta, el Centollo al horno, las Vieiras, las Nécoras, los Mejillones rellenos o con tomate... **Destaca también su variedad en vinos y su cuidada carta de ginebras premium**. Pepe abre todos los días a las 9 de la mañana (fines de semana a las 10) y cuenta con servicio de cocina continuo hasta las 11 de la noche. Los miércoles y jueves se ofrece pintxo pote de 7 a 11.

Otros pintxos:

- *Carrillera de ternera con piperrada*
- *Croqueta de jamón*
- *Berenjena rellena de mousse de canard, champi y jamón*
- *Berenjena rellena de carne picada y jamón*
- *Tortilla rellena de champis, langostino y tomate natural*
- *Tortilla rellena de setas y jamón*
- *Bacalao ahumado*
- *Salmón ahumado*
- *Gildas variadas*
- *Minis variados*

Champiñón a la plancha con gamba

Ingredientes:

2 champiñones hermosos
2 langostinos
Perejil

• Para la salsa de gambas:
Gambas
Ajo
Sal
Agua
Tomate frito

• Para el champiñón picado:
Champiñón
Cebolla
Zanahoria
Pimienta blanca

Elaboración:

Para la salsa de gambas: Salteamos unas gambas con un poco de ajo y sal. A continuación añadimos un poco de agua y tomate frito. Dejamos que hierva un ratito y trituramos con la batidora.

Para el champiñón picado: Picamos finamente la cebolla, la zanahoria y el champiñón y lo salteamos todo junto en la sartén. Añadimos un poco de pimienta blanca.

Final y presentación: Hacemos las txapelas de los champiñones a la plancha. Sobre el plato disponemos la salsa de gambas. Sobre ella, colocamos los champis boca arriba. Los rellenamos con el champiñón picado y los cubrimos con un poco más de salsa de gambas. Finalmente, coronamos cada champi con un langostino previamente hecho a la plancha y espolvoreamos con un poco de perejil recién picado.

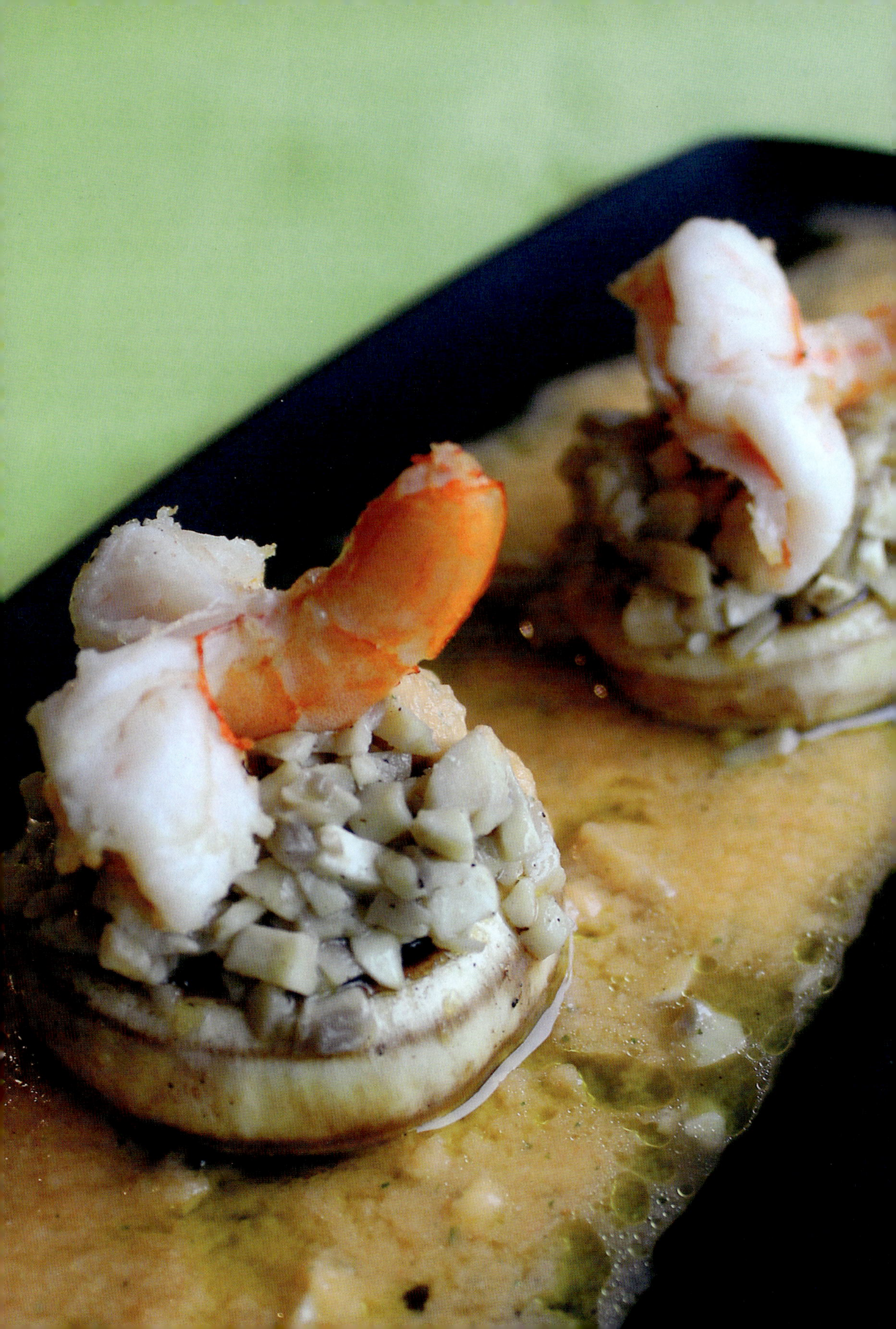

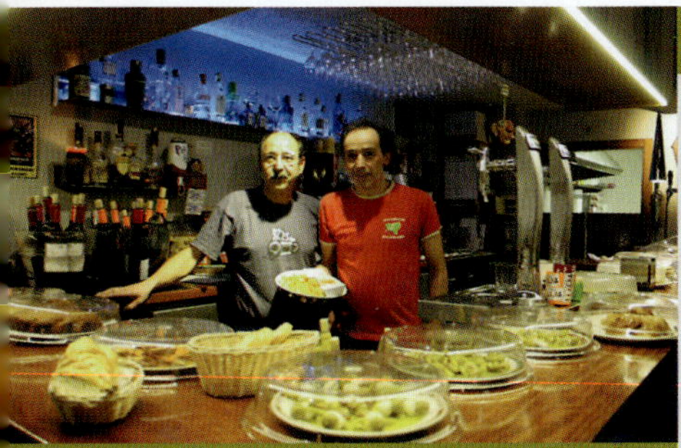

POL-POL

Domingo Irala, 16
BERGARA
943 76 30 01

El Pol-pol es un bar con historia. Inicialmente, en su emplazamiento original de la calle Komenio, perteneció a la asociación de montaña del mismo nombre, y en 1982 pasó a ser dirigido por **Dunixi Olabarria** junto a su hermano **Mikel Andoni**, encargado de la cocina. En aquellos años el bar fue un establecimiento dinámico en el que las exposiciones, los conciertos y las actividades culturales estaban a la orden del día. Tras verse obligados a cambiar de local, **el 16 de agosto de 2013, en pleno día de San Roke, fue inaugurado el actual Pol-pol**, más pequeño pero igual de dinámico y más céntrico que el anterior. Pol-pol abre todos los días a las 7 de la mañana para ofrecer desayunos y tartas caseras disponibles todo el día. A las 8 aparecen los primeros pintxos, aunque **su fuerte son los bocadillos del fin de semana y sus raciones de Croquetas** (de jamón, de hongos, de bacalao...) y otras especialidades como la Sopa de Ajo, que se prepara los lunes, y los Callos a partir de los martes.

Otros pintxos:

- *Brocheta de pulpo*
- *Gildas*
- *Tortillas variadas*
- *Vegetal*
- *Embutidos*

Raciones:

- *Pulpo a la gallega*
- *Bacalao al pil-pil*
- *Champiñones*
- *Albóndigas*

Patatas bravas con tres salsas

Ingredientes:

Patata
Aceite vegetal
Mayonesa
Sal

• Para el ali-oli:
Aceite de oliva virgen extra
Ajo

• Para la salsa de tomate:
Cebolla
Pimiento verde
Zanahoria
Cayena
Ajo
Tomate triturado
Sal

Elaboración:

Para la salsa de tomate: Picar finamente la cebolla, el pimiento verde, el ajo y la zanahoria y pochar a fuego suave. Añadir la cayena. Cuando esté todo bien pochado, añadir el tomate triturado, darle un hervor y dejar cocer a fuego suave unos minutos tras darle el punto de sal. Retirar la cayena y pasar la salsa por el pasapurés.

Para el ali-oli: Emulsionar con la batidora el ajo picado y el aceite de oliva hasta conseguir la consistencia deseada.

Para las patatas: Cortar las patatas en dados de 2 centímetros y freírlas en la freidora con aceite bien caliente hasta que cojan un tono dorado y una textura crujiente.

Final y presentación: Servir las patatas acompañadas de tres pequeños recipientes con las tres salsas: La mayonesa, el ali-oli y el tomate casero.

Nota: A pesar de no ser un pintxo, el precio popular de estas patatas hace que sean más solicitadas que cualquier pintxo de la barra. De hecho, en Pol-pol cuentan con una freidora destinada exclusivamente a freir las patatas para estas raciones.

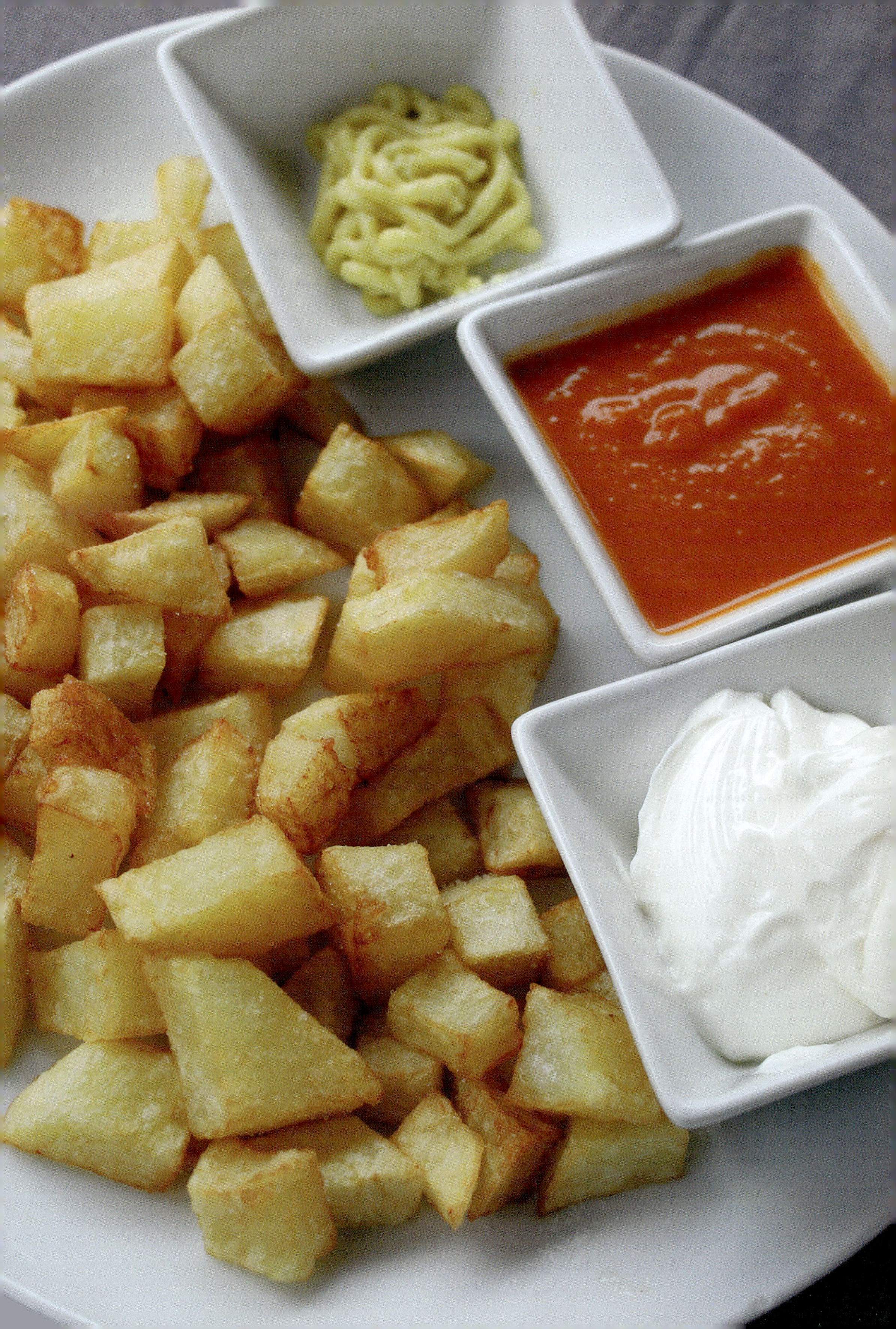

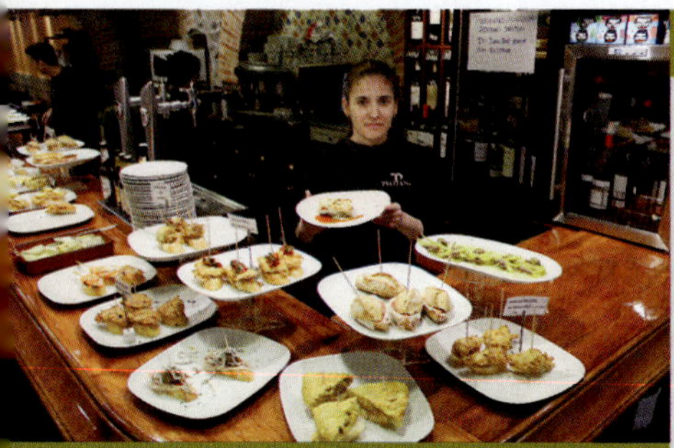

Nagusia kalea, 9
GETARIA
943 14 01 13
facebook.com/politena.getaria

POLITENA

Politena fue inaugurado como bar el 3 de agosto de 1968 por el difunto **Ángel Lazcano Lazcano** y su mujer **María Soledad Garmendia Bastida**. Ante el éxito del local y la demanda del público, dieron el paso a restaurante con parrilla en 1970, sirviendo una escueta pero cuidada carta limitada a Ensaladas, Sopa de pescado, Besugo y Chuleta a la parrilla. El local se reformó en 2001, y a día de hoy, con María Soledad merecidamente jubilada, son sus hijas, **Josune y Leire Lazcano Garmendia**, las que siguen al frente del negocio familiar. Las especialidades de Politena son su espectacular barra de pintxos, el **Menú del día con pescados frescos y el Menú de fin de semana que siempre incluye pescados a la parrilla**. En el bar, además de los pintxos, es de destacar el Pan de pita al grill, que se prepara al momento en la misma barra y las raciones de Rabas frescas (conocidas en Getaria como **"txibiarruak"**), así como el Pulpo a la gallega o a la plancha.

Otros pintxos:

- *Pintxo Politena (seta rellena de queso, bacon y pimiento verde)*
- *Hojaldre relleno de setas y gambas*
- *Alcachofa con jamón*
- *Pulpo a la gallega o vinagreta*
- *Penca de acelga rellena con jamón y queso*
- *Bacalao al pil-pil*
- *Foie a la plancha*
- *Queso de cabra con foie y manzana*
- *Croissant de cereales con ensalada de bogavante*

Lasaña casera de espinacas rellena de setas y gambas

Ingredientes:

3 placas de pasta fresca de espinacas (verde)
Cebolla
Ajo
Seta de cultivo
Gambas peladas
Aceite de oliva
Sal

- **Para la bechamel:**

Mantequilla
Harina
Leche
Sal
Queso Emmental rallado
Salsa de tomate casero

Elaboración:

Picamos la cebolla y la ponemos a pochar con un poco de aceite en una cazuela ancha. Le añadimos un poco de ajo picado y, a continuación, la seta picada. Después le añadimos las gambas picaditas, cocinamos el conjunto y sazonamos.

Para la bechamel: En otra cazuela, fundimos la mantequilla a fuego lento yañadimos la harina cocinándola un rato sin dejar de remover. Añadimos la leche y la sal removiendo constantemente, y lo terminamos de cocinar durante 10-15 minutos a fuego lento. De esta bechamel cogeremos una parte, un poquito para añadir al preparado anterior de las setas y gambas.

En una bandeja con fondo, que sirva para el horno, ponemos un poco de bechamel de base y a continuación una placa de pasta de espinacas y el relleno de setas y gambas, otra placa de pasta y el relleno, y terminamos con otra placa de pasta y toda la bechamel que nos queda, para cubrir bien toda la pasta de espinacas. Espolvoreamos con queso emmental rallado y lo introducimos unos 10 minutos al horno a 220-230°

Final y presentación: Servimos una porción de lasaña acompañada de un poco de salsa de tomate.

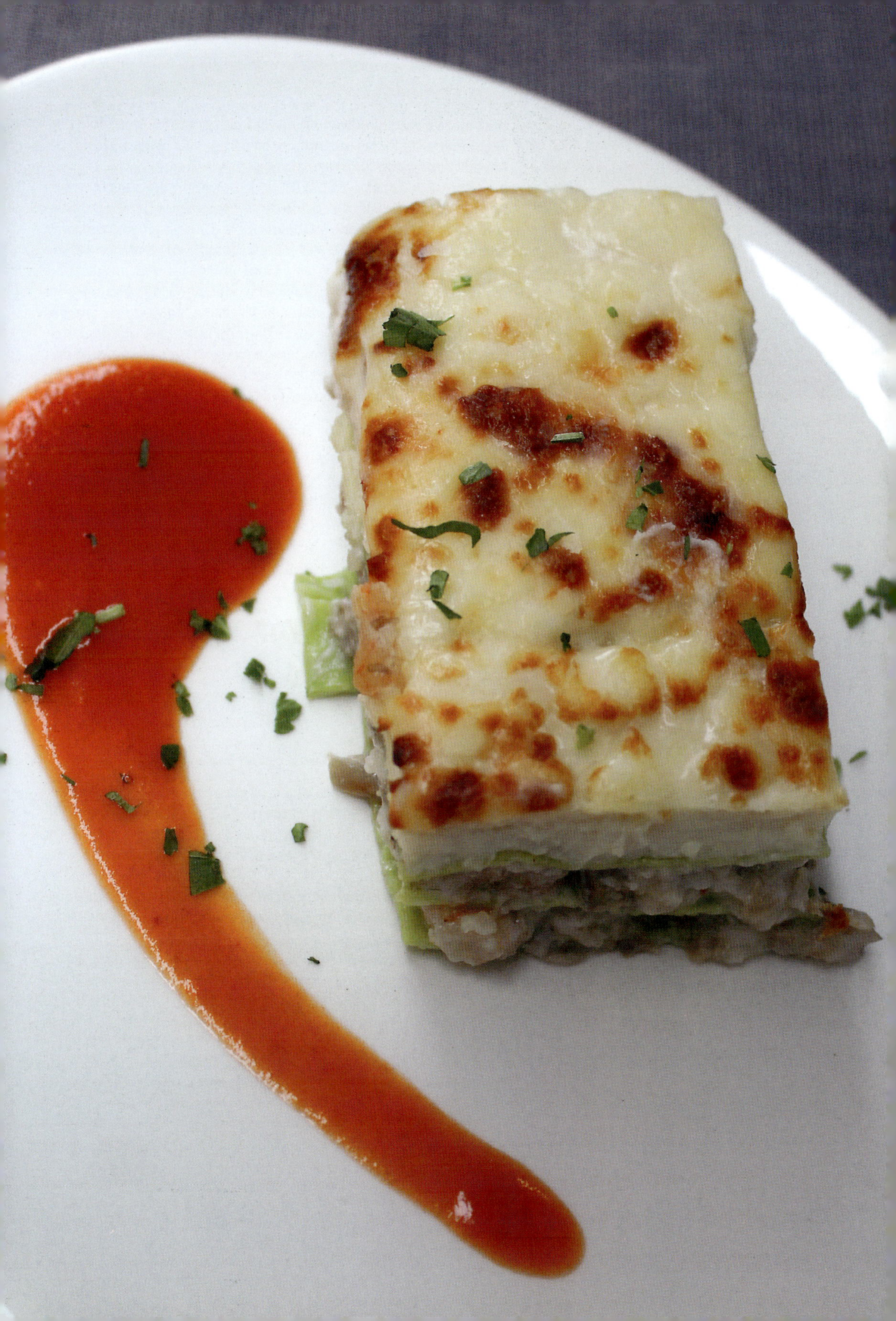

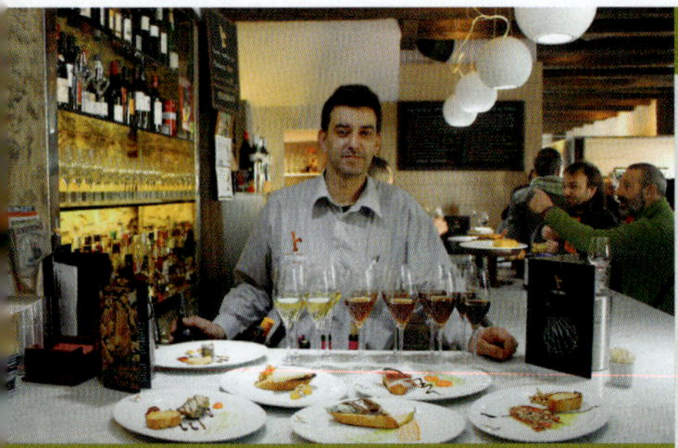

Nafarroa Etorbidea, 57
BEASAIN
943 88 98 88
www.dolareahotela.com

RK JATETXEA

Iban Mate y Arantxa Rancho, dos enamorados de los vinos, han conseguido que RK, el bar-restaurante situado en los bajos del **Hotel Dolarea**, cuente con una de las ofertas de pintxos y vinos más sugerentes de la comarca. En RK podemos optar por sus pintxos de barra, elegir un pintxo de cocina de su completa pizarra, o dejarnos seducir por la **pizarra de maridajes entre pintxos y vinos de Jerez**. Llama también la atención su tentadora **Tabla-degustación de pintxos**. La pizarra de vinos es, asimismo, una de las más interesantes de los contornos, con una completa y original oferta para todos los gustos y bolsillos, en constante actualización. Pasando al comedor, en RK podemos disfrutar de un cuidado menú del día, un completo y copioso menú de fin de semana y una carta de cocina tradicional puesta al día con platos como Carpaccio de pulpo sobre verduras confitadas, Terrina de cochinillo confitado y patata asada...

Otros pintxos:

- *Croqueta de morcilla de Beasain*
- *Brocheta de txipirón sobre salteado de habitas*
- *Foie plancha con mermelada de piquillos y puré de manzana*
- *Espárragos en tempura con ali-oli*
- *Huevo pochado con puré de patata trufado*
- *Brocheta de ternera con verduras y patatas*
- *Taco de pulpo con puré de patata y pimentón*
- *Crujiente de plátano con chocolate caliente*
- *Tiramisú*

Croqueta de txuleta del Goierri

Ingredientes:

1 trozo de txuleta (a ser posible, de lomo bajo)
Harina
Huevo
Pan rallado
Pimientos del piquillo
Aceite de oliva virgen extra

• Para la roux:
La grasa de la txuleta
Harina
Leche

Elaboración:

Para la roux: Elaboraremos una roux clásica, usando la grasa amarilla de la txuleta en vez de mantequilla. Para ello, trituraremos la grasa en la picadora, de manera que se volverá una pasta y, en la cazuela, se volverá líquida. Ponemos una cazuela al fuego, fundimos la grasa y añadimos la harina. Removeremos bien con una cuchara de madera y coceremos la mezcla bien cocida para que pierda el gusto de la harina. Finalmente, añadiremos la leche.

Picamos la carne de la txuleta y la salteamos 30 segundos contados. La mezclamos con la roux y hacemos bolas de croqueta de tamaño "Goierri". Las pasamos por harina, huevo y pan rallado y las freimos en aceite de oliva hasta que adquieran un atractivo color dorado.

Confitamos unos pimientos del piquillo en aceite de oliva con un poco de sal.

Final y presentación: Disponemos una pequeña cama de piquillo confitado y, sobre ésta, dos croquetas de txuleta por pintxo.

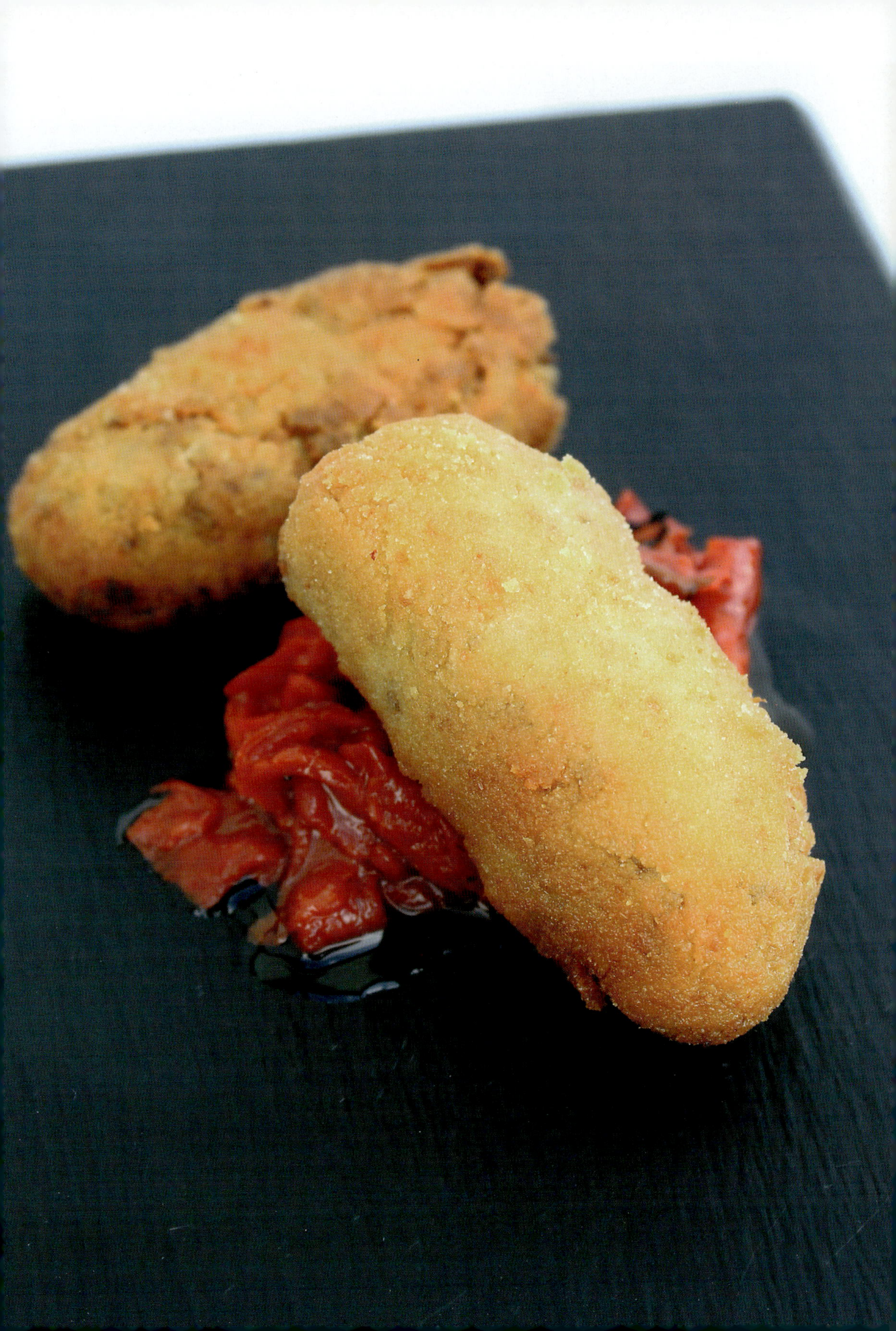

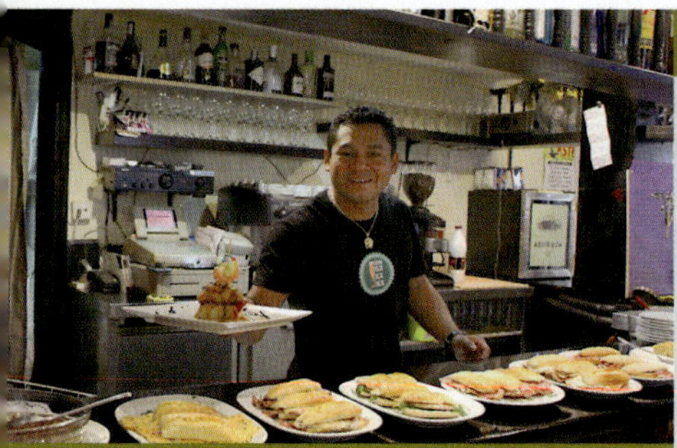

SAKANA

Roger Sosa, ecuatoriano que vive desde 2002 en Zarautz, dirige desde abril de 2013 este **bar con casi 50 años de historia que de siempre ha sido conocido por su tortilla de patata.** De hecho lo sigue siendo, pues Roger domina perfectamente este producto. Baste decir que anteriormente ganó en dos ocasiones el concurso de tortilla de Zarautz, cuando trabajaba en el Izaro y en el Orbela. En el Sakana, Roger abre a las 9:30 ofreciendo **pintxos, bocadillos, pizzas caseras, platos combinados, raciones y menú del día.** Goza de gran fama el enorme **Bocadillo vegetal** (lechuga, tomate, mahonesa, queso, jamón y huevo frito) al que la gente añade, además, pollo. También destaca la **Hamburguesa Sakana** (Carne, tomate, lechuga, mahonesa, jamón, queso, cebolla caramelizada y bacon), así como las **Empanadas artesanas al estilo sudamericano**, con clientes que vienen exclusivamente por ellas. Los miércoles, en Sakana se sirve **pintxo-pote con 7 variedades de pintxos** a elegir.

Zigordia, 33
ZARAUTZ
943 83 56 30

Otros pintxos:

- *Tortilla de patata (especialidad)*
- *Croqueta de ibérico*
- *Tigres*
- *Antxoa con boquerón y vinagreta con base de jamón*
- *Brocheta de langostinos*
- *Pechuga de pollo*
- *Merluza a la plancha*
- *Langostino empanado crujiente*
- *Pimiento relleno de bacalao*
- *Empanadas (carne, jamón y queso, pollo, bacalao...)*

Bacalao a la piperrada

Ingredientes:

1 taco de bacalao
Harina
Huevo
1 langostino cocido y pelado
Pan
Limón
Aceite de oliva

· Para la piperrada:
Aceite de oliva virgen extra
Cebolla
PImiento rojo
Pimiento verde

· Para la salsa de ajillo:
Aceite de oliva virgen extra
Perejil
Ajo

Elaboración:

Para la salsa de ajillo: Picamos muy finamente un ramillete de perejil y lo depositamos en un tarro o una botella. Llenamos el recipiente de aceite de oliva virgen extra y lo dejamos macerar. Esta operación deberá hacerse antes de elaborar los pintxos. De hecho, es interesante contar siempre con este aceite macerado pues nos puede venir bien para cualquier cosa.

Para la piperrada: Cortamos en Juliana la cebolla, el pimiento rojo y el pimiento verde y los pochamos a fuego muy suave en aceite de oliva hasta que las verduras estén bien blanditas.

Para el bacalao: Rebozamos el bacalao en harina y huevo y lo freímos muy suavemente en aceite de oliva hasta que coja un atractivo color dorado.

Final y presentación: Sobre una rodaja de pan colocamos una cama de piperrada. Sobre ella, el taco de bacalao rebozado y un chorro de salsa de ajillo. Coronamos el pintxo con un langostino cocido y pelado y una rodaja de limón, ensartando todo con un palillo.

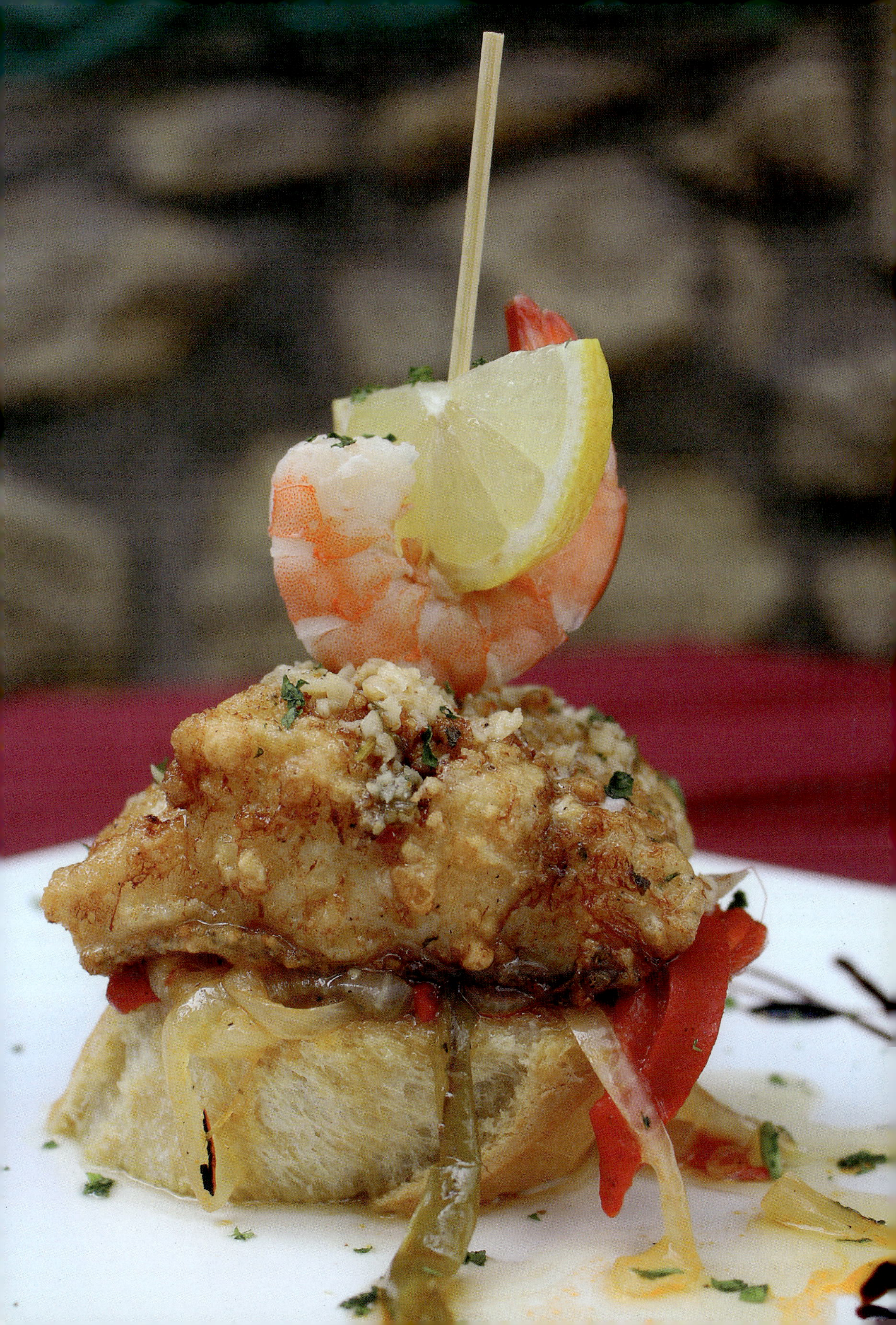

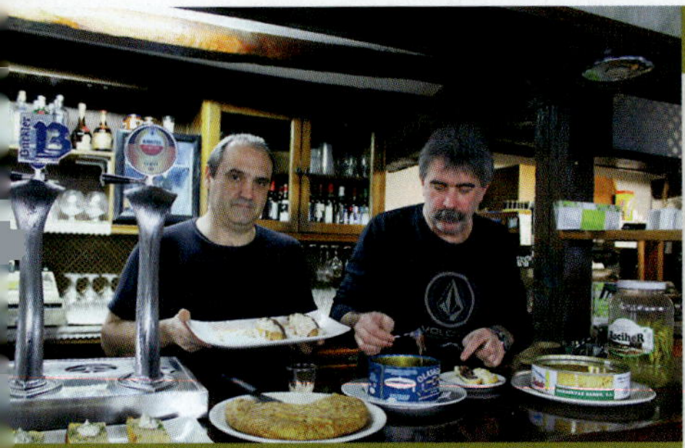

Madalena kalea, 38
ORERETA
943 34 61 83

SINDIKATO

Desde el 1 de mayo de 2014, **Javi Arenaza** se encarga de dirigir, con la ayuda en cocina de **Aitor "Reke"**, este céntrico bar que se acerca a los **50 años de existencia**. Este bar, "kasta" donde los haya, siempre había sido conocido por sus **cazuelitas**, a las que Javi se ha encargado de añadir una amplia oferta de **bocadillos y platos combinados**, aunque si por algo ha adquirido una merecida fama el Sindikato es por los **montaditos que se preparan a mano en la propia barra, delante del cliente, directamente de las latas**, con productos de gran calidad como guindillas de Ibarra, bonito del norte, antxoas de Olasagasti... Sindikato abre sus puertas todos los días a las 10 de la mañana y cuenta con pintxos disponibles desde primera hora entre los que no falta la solicitada Tortilla de patatas. También es de destacar la terraza del Sindikato, pequeña pero con un gran ambiente.

Otros pintxos:

- *Tortilla de patata*
- *Callos caseros*
- *Chorizo cocido*
- *Carne cocida*
- *Bola de queso o carne*
- *Croqueta*
- *Champis*

Raciones:

- *Txipirones en su tinta*
- *Pulpo*

Bacalao frito con pimientos

Ingredientes:

1 taco de bacalao
Cebolla
Pimiento verde
Pan
Aceite de oliva
Harina
Perejil picado
Sal

Elaboración:

Picamos la cebolla y la rehogamos pacientemente en aceite de oliva, a fuego muy suave, hasta que quede caramelizada.

Cortamos el pimiento verde en tiras y las freímos en aceite de oliva bien caliente.

Envolvemos el bacalao con una fina capa de harina y lo freímos en abundante aceite de oliva.

Final y presentación: Tostamos una rodaja de pan en el horno y colocamos sobre ella una cama de cebolla caramelizada. Sobre ella disponemos el taco o un par de tacos de bacalao frito y, sobre éste, las tiras de pimiento verde frito. Terminamos decorando con un chorrito de aceite de perejil que habremos elaborado macerando aceite de oliva virgen extra con perejil picado y sal.

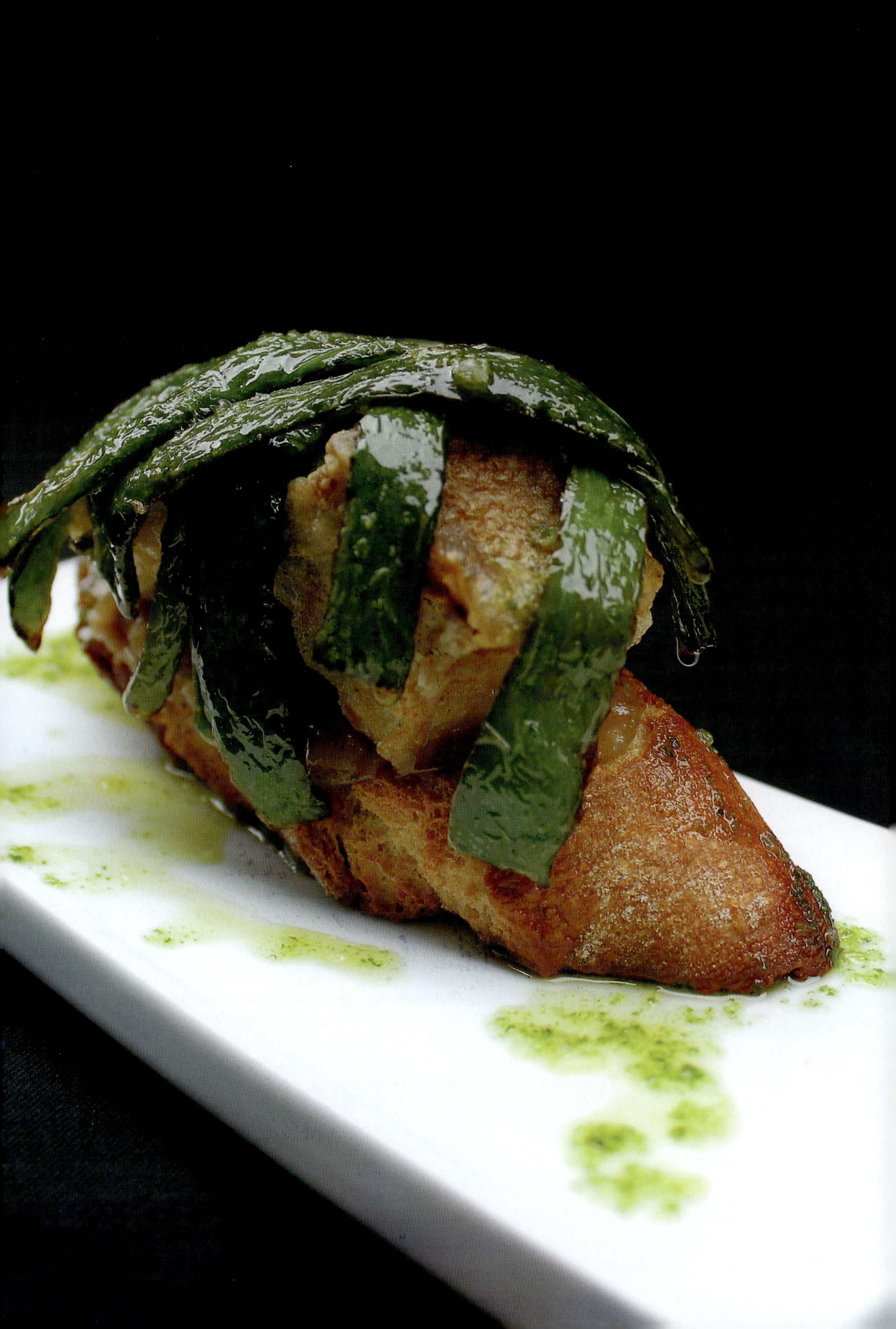

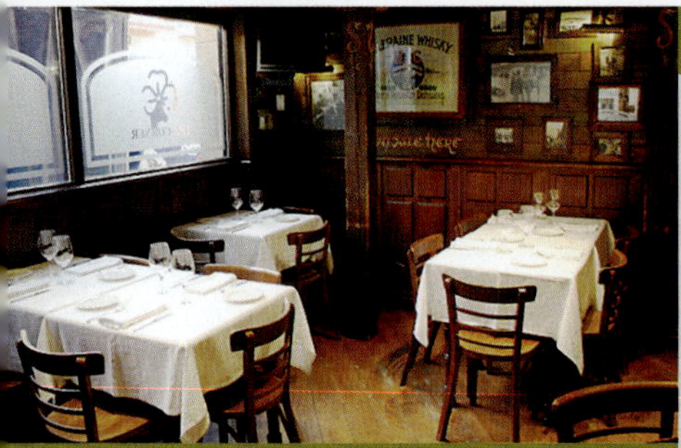

THE CORNER

Fueros, 2
IRUN
943 62 19 54

Este bar de estética irlandesa, situado en pleno centro de Irun, a dos pasos de la plaza del Ayuntamiento, es conocido por su **atractiva barra de pintxos y su cocina casera, sencilla pero servida con cuidadas presentaciones**, con especialidades como Merluza en salsa verde, Almejas en salsa verde, Ensalada de txipirones con langostinos, Postres caseros... Además de su menú del día, su menú especial y sus menús especiales para cuadrillas, The Corner ofrece una **amplia variedad de bocadillos y platos combinados**, y en los días de buen tiempo podemos comer o cenar en su terraza. The Corner abre todos los días a las 11 de la mañana ofreciendo pintxos en barra desde primera hora, y los fines de semana **por las noches, se transforma en un concurrido bar de copas** en el que podemos disfrutar de un gran ambiente y de la mejor música.

Otros pintxos:

- *Mini freidora de bravas con txistorra*
- *Brocheta de rape y langostino con confitura de tomate y albahaca*
- *Magret de pato con salsa de Oporto*
- *Bacalao "The Corner"*
- *Foie a la plancha*
- *Revuelto de hongos y mousse de foie*
- *Croqueta de bacalao*
- *Croqueta de hongos*
- *Croqueta de txipirón*

Risotto de hongos con nube de parmesano

Ingredientes:

Arroz
Hongos
Queso parmesano
Foie fresco
Cebolleta
Pimienta negra
Nata
Aceite de oliva virgen extra
Sal

Elaboración:

Cocemos el arroz y lo dejamos reservado a media cocción.

Picamos muy finamente la cebolleta, la pochamos y salteamos con ella los hongos.

Añadimos los hongos al arroz junto con un chorrito de aceite de oliva y seguimos cociéndolo mientras lo mezclamos. También le añadimos un poco de foie fresco troceado en trozos muy pequeñitos.

Añadimos a la mezcla un poco de sal, una migaja de pimienta negra y un poco de nata. Lo ponemos un momento a fuego vivo para que la nata se reduzca y se convierta en una crema.

Finalmente, espolvoreamos con queso parmesano rallado y coronamos el pintxo con una rodaja de foie a la plancha.

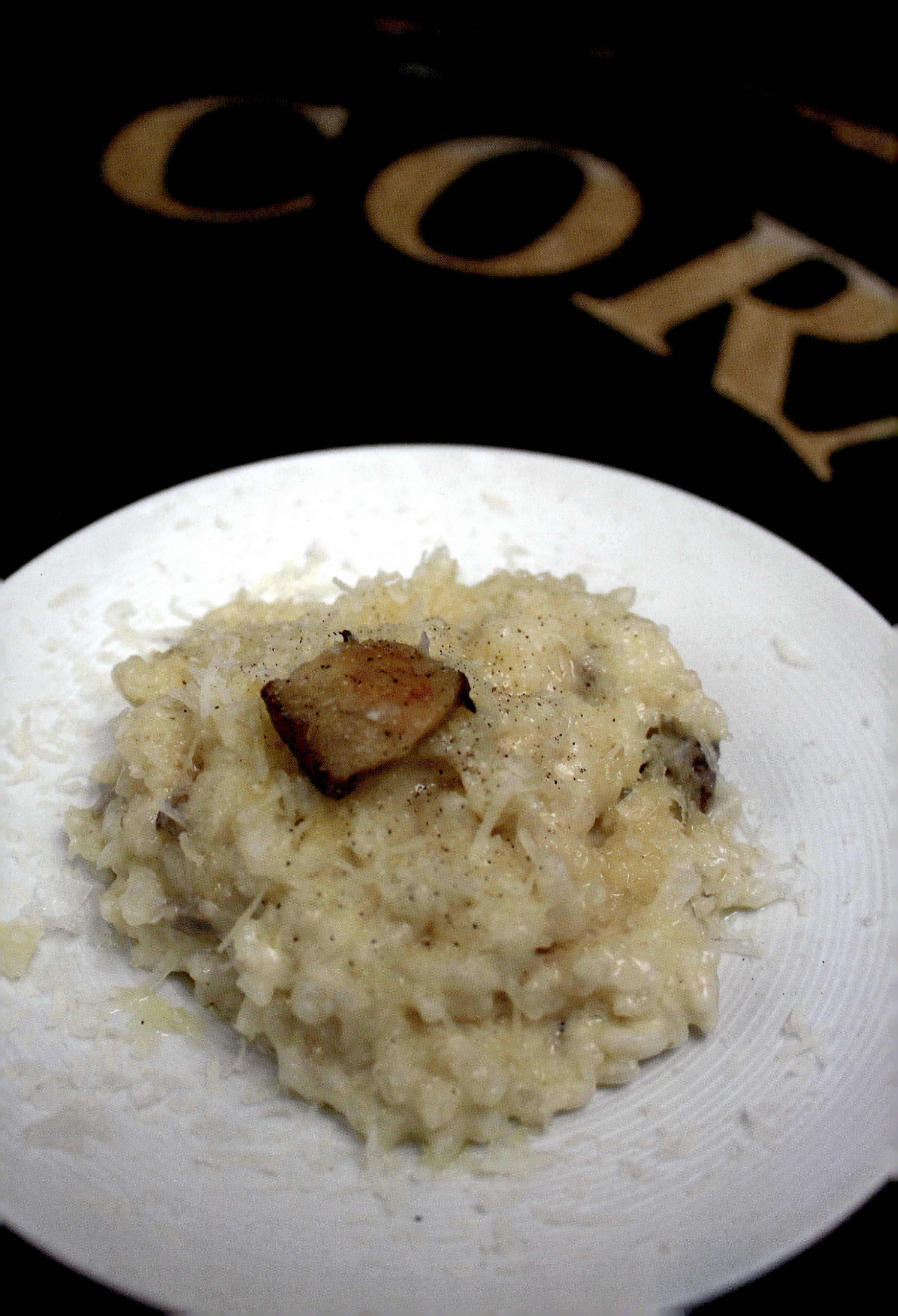
COR

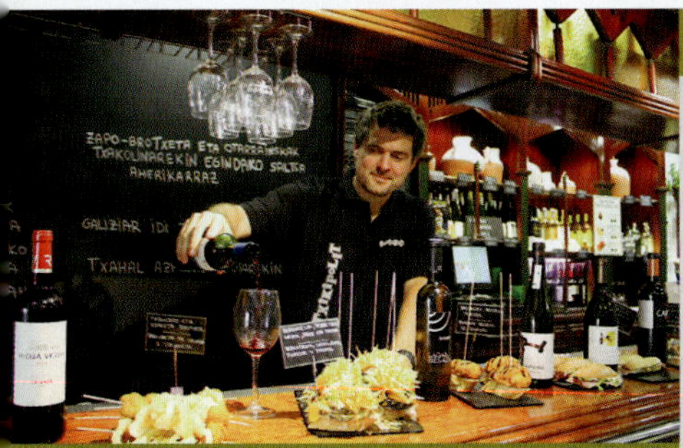

TXIKI POLIT

Musika plaza
ZARAUTZ
943 83 53 57
www.txikipolit.com

La **familia Aldalur** dirige desde mediados de los 80 este céntrico establecimiento que, tras una serie de reformas, incorporó al conjunto una acogedora pension de 36 habitaciones. En la zona de bar de Txiki Polit podemos disfrutar de sus pintxos de barra, o de lo que ellos denominan **"comida rápida de calidad"**, elaborada en casa con productos naturales sin utilizar congelados. Sus crujientes bocadillos (en baguette o txapata) con una carta que supera las 40 referencias, sandwiches, hamburguesas... Por otra parte, en su **amplio comedor con capacidad para más de 150 personas**, podemos degustar gran cantidad de **platos combinados, menú del día, menú de fin de semana, menú de sidrería, o platos de cocina tradicional vasca** como Revuelto de hongos, Ensalada templada de bacalao, Ensalada templada de txipirones, Bacalao frito, Chuleta de buey, Cordero (Por encargo), Postres caseros...

Otros pintxos:

- *Berenjena con setas e ibérico*
- *Crêpe de txipirón*
- *Croquetas caseras*
- *Brocheta de croqueta y calamar*
- *Pimiento relleno de bacalao*
- *Bacalao frito*
- *Brocheta de txipirones*
- *Tortillas variadas*
- *Brocheta de langostino y rape con salsa americana al txakoli*

Solomillo de ternera con foie

Ingredientes:

Solomillo de ternera
Foie fresco
Pan

- **Para la salsa de piquillos:**

Pimientos del piquillo
Aceite de oliva
Tomate
Cebolla

Elaboración:

Para la salsa de piquillo: Picamos finamente la cebolla y la ponemos a pochar en una sartén con aceite de oliva. Una vez pochada, añadimos los pimientos del piquillo y los confitamos un rato a fuego muy lento. Cuando estén blanditos, retiramos el aceite y añadimos unas cucharadas de tomate natural. Dejamos hervir un rato, lo trituramos todo con la batidora y lo pasamos por el chino.

Cortamos una rodaja de solomillo y la hacemos a la plancha, cuidando que quede jugoso.

Cortamos una rodaja de foie fresco y la hacemos a la plancha, vuelta y vuelta.

Final y presentación: Tostamos una rodaja de pan al horno o en la plancha. Sobre ella colocamos la rodaja de solomillo y, sobre ella o apoyada en ella, la rodaja de foie a la plancha. Servimos el pintxo en un platillo acompañándolo de la salsa de piquillos y unos hilitos de reducción de Módena.

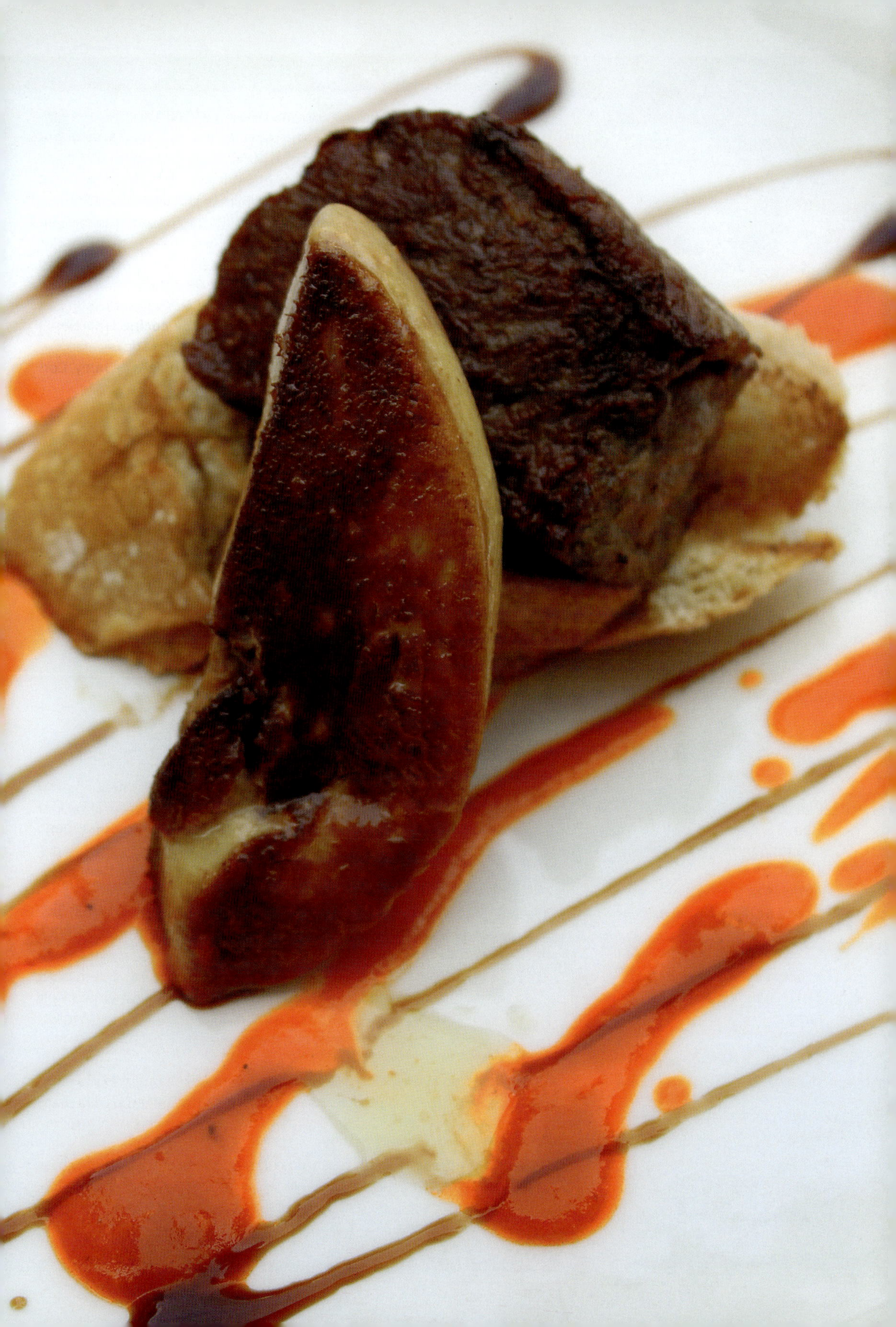

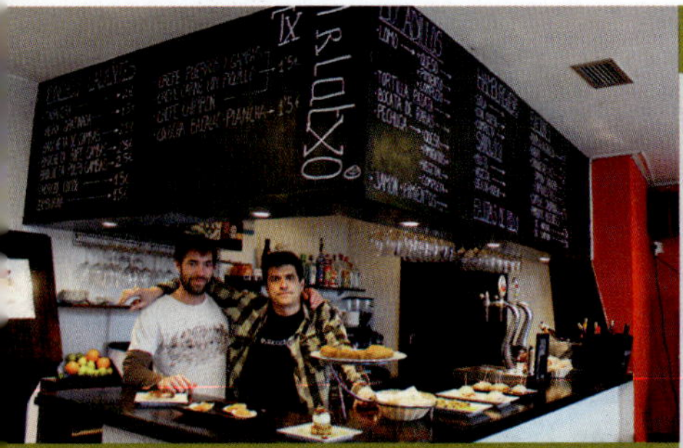

Muelle, z/g
MUTRIKU
943 19 50 70

TXIRLATXO

El dinámico **Mikel Lete** dirige desde mayo de 2012 este bar situado en pleno puerto de Mutriku, con la ayuda en barra y cocina de **Patxi Lasarte** y **Mikel Moroko**. Txirlatxo abre sus puertas todos los días a las 9 de la mañana y cuenta con una terraza con vistas directas al puerto. Los fines de semana es cuando más ambiente encontramos en este bar en el que además de sus pintxos y raciones se ofrecen todos los días **Pollos asados** y platos como Atún a la plancha, Cogote de merluza, Pulpo, Croquetas variadas, así como una variedad de **Bocadillos y Hamburguesas**. También, bajo encargo, se elaboran **Paellas** al momento. Es recomendable acudir a Txirlatxo en fechas emblemáticas como el Arrantzale Eguna (mediados de septiembre) o el Berdel Eguna (primeros de abril).

Otros pintxos:

- *Txistorras hojaldradas*
- *Jamón con chorreras*
- *Brocheta de carne*
- *Brocheta de gambas*
- *Txirlatxo (txirla rellena)*
- *Tortillas variadas (patata, queso, champis..)*

Raciones:

- *Ibéricos*
- *Pimientos rellenos de bacalao*
- *Antxoas de Mutriku*

Huevo escalfado sobre champiñón a la plancha

Ingredientes:

Confit de pato
Pan tostado
Huevo
Champiñón
Trufa
Almendras
Aceite de oliva virgen extra
Pan

- **Para la salsa de trigueros:**

Espárragos trigueros
Patata
Cebolla
Caldo de carne

Elaboración:

Para la salsa de trigueros: Pochamos la cebolla previamente picada y añadimos unas lascas de patata. Añadimos agua y caldo de carne y llevamos a ebullición. Cuando esté hirviendo añadimos los trigueros troceados en trozos pequeñitos y dejamos que hierva todo junto durante un rato. Trituramos todo con la batidora y pasamos la salsa por el chino.

Para el huevo escalfado: Colocamos un cazo con agua al fuego. Mientras se calienta el agua, disponemos un trozo de papel film en un vaso, dejando un hueco. Cascamos el huevo y lo vertemos en dicho hueco, añadiéndole un chorrito de aceite de oliva virgen y un poco de trufa rallada. Cerramos con un nudo el papel film y lo introducimos en el cazo, dejando que hierva durante 3 ó 4 minutos.

Resto de elaboración: Hacemos la txapela del champiñón a la plancha y troceamos y salteamos el confit de pato. Tostamos a la plancha o en el horno las almendras y las troceamos en el mortero.

Final y presentación: Cortamos una rodaja de pan y la confitamos a fuego suave en aceite de oliva. Encima disponemos el champiñón, el huevo escalfado y el confit. Espolvoreamos el conjunto con almendra rallada.

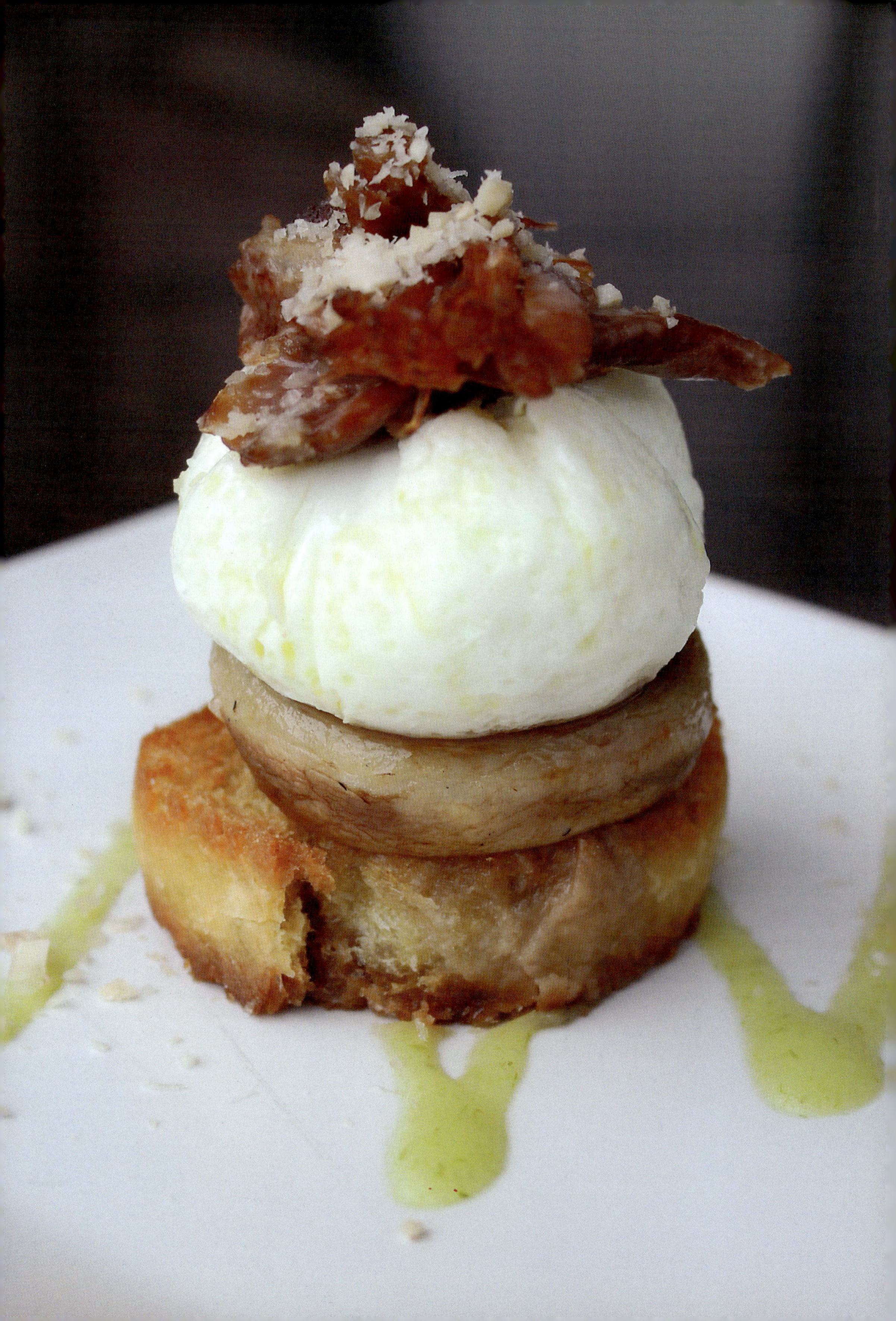

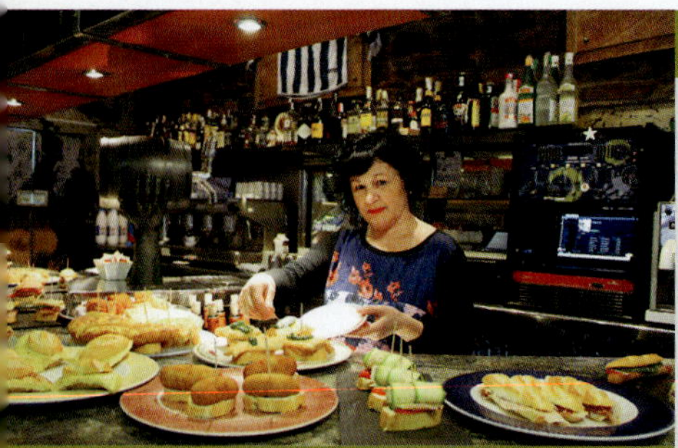

TXOKO

Mª Carmen Gullón y Aitor Bolinaga se hicieron en 1982 con las riendas de este bar situado en plena Plaza de Unzaga. Anteriormente había sido dirigido por Juanito Txoko, quien lo bautizó con su nombre actual, aunque originariamente su nombre era Arrate. Mª Carmen y Aitor se hicieron pronto con una amplia clientela que les permitió acometer una reforma entre 1998 y 1999, renovando el bar y dotándole de su aspecto actual. Txoko abre sus puertas todos los días a las 7:30 de la mañana ofreciendo **desayunos con bollería de la pastelería Antxon**, de Eibar, que ellos mismos se encargan de hornear. A partir de las 9 de la mañana empiezan a aparecer los primeros pintxos en la barra y puede disponerse asimismo de **raciones** como Pulpo, Paleta, Champiñones, etc... Txoko cuenta también con una pequeña carta de **bocadillos**, aunque su especialidad son las **Rabas**, que se sirven los fines de semana y festivos. Los jueves ofrecen pintxo-pote y los sábados las copas se sirven a precios populares.

Unzaga Plaza, 10
EIBAR
943 20 70 10

Otros pintxos:

- *Rollito de calabacín con jamón de york y queso*
- *Brocheta de pulpo*
- *Brocheta de bacon, queso y langostino*
- *Tortillas variadas (de espinaca, de pisto...)*
- *Croquetas caseras*
- *Champiñones*
- *Bola de carne o de marisco*
- *Empanada de atún*
- *Merluza rebozada*
- *Rabas (Ración) los fines de semana*

Penca rebozada

Ingredientes:

2 pencas de acelga
1 rodaja de jamón serrano duroc
1 rodaja de pimiento verde
Harina
Huevo
Aceite de oliva
Pan
Sal

Elaboración:

Cocemos las pencas en agua con sal durante media hora (o hasta que adquieran la consistencia que nos agrada), las sacamos del agua y las escurrimos.

Las rebozamos con harina y huevo, las freímos en aceite de oliva y las dejamos sobre un papel de cocina para que suelten el aceite sobrante.

Freímos la rodaja de pimiento verde en aceite de oliva.

Final y presentación: Sobre una rodaja de pan colocamos una penca. Sobre ella, disponemos una loncha de jamón duroc y la rodaja de pimiento verde frita. Coronamos el pintxo con otra penca y sujetamos todo con un palillo.

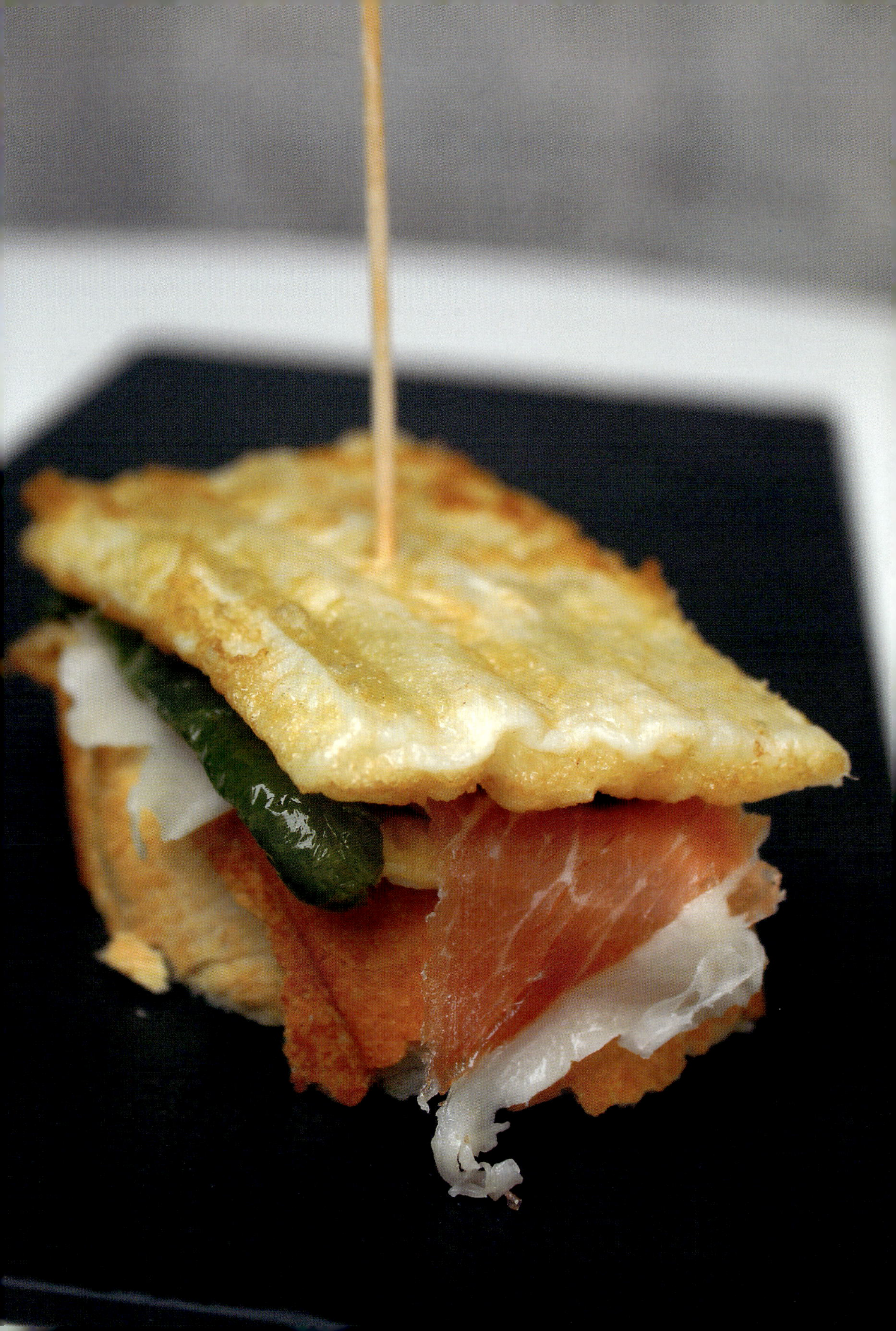

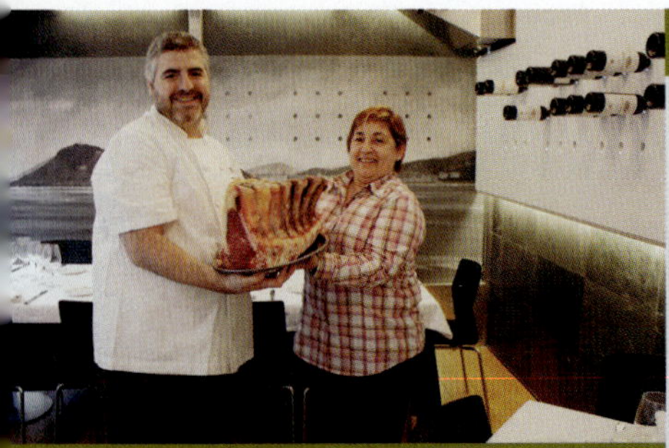

Pza. Trinidad, 2 (Parte Vieja)
DONOSTIA
943 44 10 07
www.txuletarestaurante.com

TXULETA

Aunque fue a finales de 2005 cuando **Ander Esarte y Marian Garmendia** se hicieron con el Txuleta, estos restauradores contaban con una amplia experiencia que incluye lugares tan diversos como París, el restaurante Akelarre de Pedro Subijana, el Hotel Aranzazu, la bodega Castillo de Monjardín en Navarra, La Rampa en el puerto donostiarra... Finalmente, pasaron 7 años en el asador Txistu de Madrid, propiedad de Pedro Abrego, tío de Ander, distinguido en su día con el Tambor de Oro. Durante su etapa en Madrid, Ander incluso trabajó de **cocinero para el Real Madrid** en los desplazamientos del equipo. En el Txuleta, esta pareja ofrece una **cocina de toda la vida basada en el producto de temporada**, cuidando especialmente los hongos y verduras de estación, los productos locales como la carne de **Euskal Txerri**, y principalmente las **carnes y pescados a la parrilla,** no en vano Ander ha sido distinguido como **Mejor Parrillero del estado en el Congreso San Sebastián Gastronomika de 2012 y 2013.**

Otros pintxos:

- *Croqueta de txuleta*
- *Bola de marisco o de carne*
- *Foie a la plancha*
- *Carrillera de ternera*
- *Codillo de pato*
- *Crujiente de morcilla*
- *Pimiento relleno de rabo de buey*
- *Espárrago relleno de espinacas y gambas*
- *Brocheta de pulpo y langostino*
- *Tortita de camarón*

Pintxo de txuleta

Ingredientes:

3 porciones de chuleta de la parte del lomo bajo
Aceite de oliva
Escamas de sal gruesa
Patata

Elaboración:

Tanto el Pintxo de txuleta que ilustra esta receta como la Croqueta de txuleta son dos opciones que ofrece Ander Esarte a quien no le apetezca comerse una txuleta entera, o a aquellos que quieran degustar el género antes de pasar a mayores.

En cualquier caso, el pintxo de Txuleta que se ofrece en este restaurante, está elaborado con el mismo género que las chuletas que se sirven en el comedor, concretamente de la parte del lomo bajo, la más jugosa.

Limpiamos bien el lomo bajo, lo deshuesamos y obtenemos una porción de txuleta para el pintxo, que dividimos en tres pedazos que atravesamos con un pequeño palo de brocheta para que el comensal pueda comerlo cómodamente.

Ponemos la plancha al fuego y, cuando esté bien caliente, hacemos la brocheta por los dos lados, tratando de que quede jugosa, pero que no nos quede fría por dentro.

Añadimos unas escamas de sal gorda y unas patatas fritas caseras para acompañar.

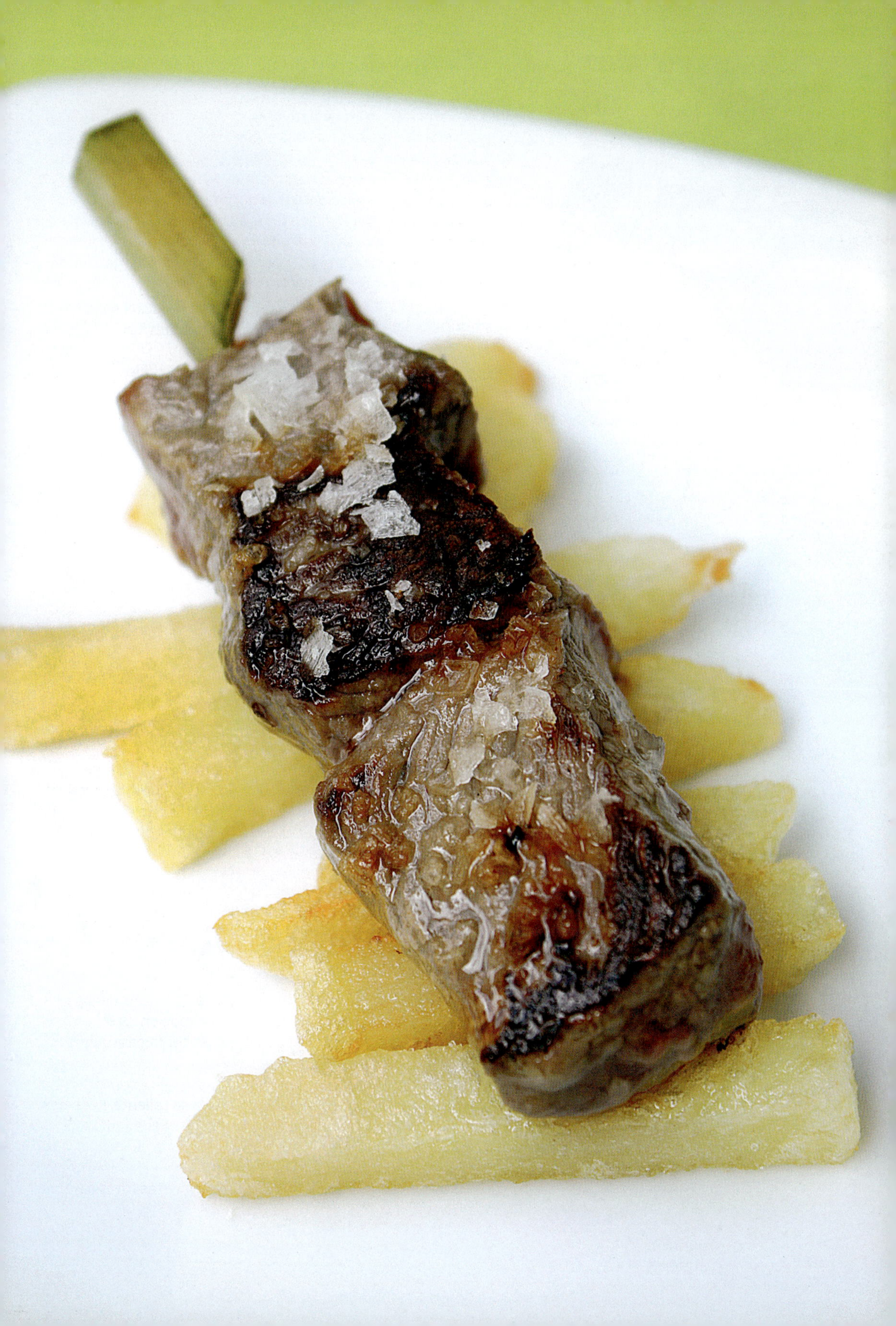

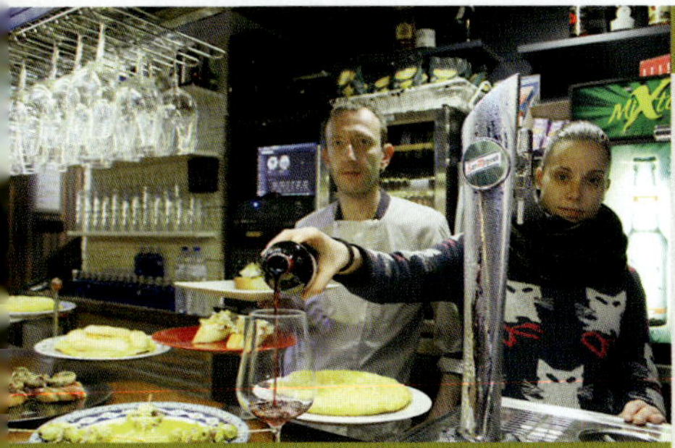

USUA

Giza Eskubideen parkea, 1
ELGOIBAR
943 25 60 28

José Agustín Alonso Muguerza, "Kaiser", ampliamente conocido en la hostelería de Elgoibar tras pasar más de 20 años en el Lanbroa, se hizo con las riendas de esta cafetería en mayo de 2012 y posteriormente, en julio de 2013, con las del anexo **asador Ibai-Ondo.** Usua destaca por su **excelente paleta ibérica** y su jamón, considerado por algunos como el mejor de los alrededores. Son también célebres sus callos caseros, y las rabas, que circulan a discreción los sábados, domingos y festivos, aunque **su plato estrella son los solicitados Huevos rotos con paleta ibérica de bellota**. También se ofrece una gran variedad de **Platos combinados, Hamburguesas y Sandwiches.** Usua abre sus puertas a las 9 de la mañana ofreciendo las primeras tortillas y en verano aumenta su capacidad con una **espectacular terraza** con 70 mesas que ocupa y da vida a todo el parque que circunda el establecimiento.

Otros pintxos:

- *Calabacín con cebolla pochada y bacon*
- *Berenjena rebozada con jamón y queso*
- *Croquetas caseras de Ibérico*
- *Txipirón a la plancha*
- *Rulo de cabra con tomate rebozado y frambuesa*
- *Pechuga-setas-gulas*
- *Tortillas variadas*
- *Brocheta de pulpo y langostinos*
- *Pimiento relleno de carne*
- *Merluza a la plancha o rebozada*

"Silviña"

Ingredientes:

1 lomo de rape
Pan casero

- **Para la vinagreta:**

Cebolla
Pimiento verde
Pimiento rojo
Zanahoria
Tomillo
Aceite de oliva virgen extra
Vinagre
Sal

Elaboración:

Para la vinagreta: Picamos finamente la cebolla, el pimiento verde, el pimiento rojo, la zanahoria y el tomillo. Disponemos todo en un bol y lo cubrimos con aceite de oliva virgen extra, vinagre y sal. Removemos todo y dejamos reposando.

Para el rape: Deshuesamos y troceamos el lomo de rape y lo hacemos a la plancha cuidando que no quede excesivamente hecho.

Final y presentación: Cortamos una rebanada de pan casero. Disponemos encima el rape a la plancha y cubrimos con la vinagreta que hemos reservado.

Este pintxo puede acompañarse, optativamente, de un puré de yuca.

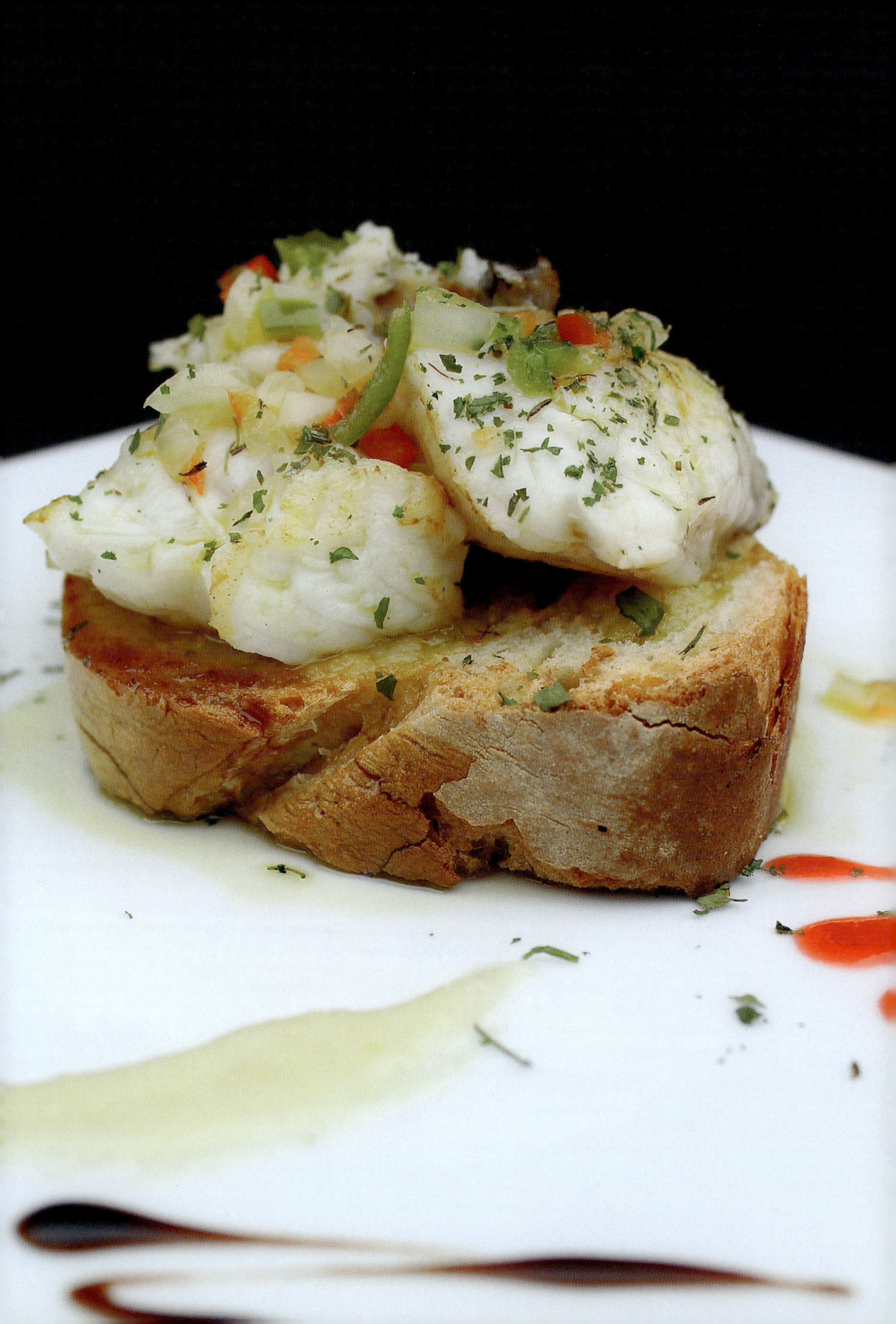

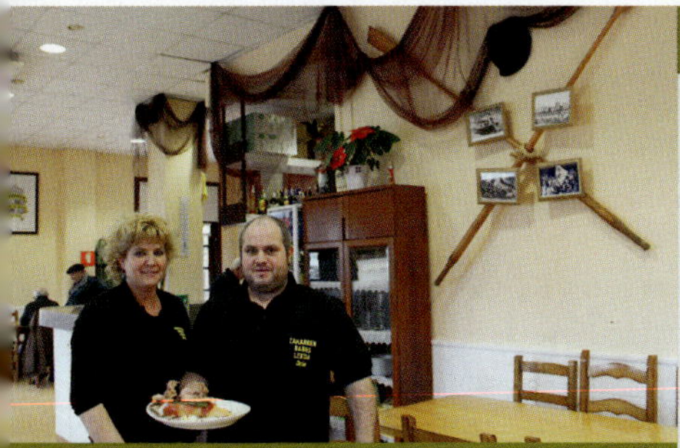

ZAHARREN BABESLEKUA

Herriko Enparantza, 1
ORIO
943 83 53 98

El Hogar de los Jubilados de Orio se encuentra en el punto más céntrico de la localidad costera, pero al contrario que ocurre en otros lugares, aquí **la entrada es libre para todo aquel que quiera entrar** a comer o a tomar un pote. Los hermanos **Juanjo y Mertxe Curiel Oliden** regentan desde octubre de 2010 este amplio establecimiento en el que ofrecen una gran variedad de **pintxos, platos combinados y bocadillos**, así como servicio de **menú del día**, siendo los Txipirones a la plancha y los Callos caseros las especialidades indiscutibles del lugar. Entre sus **cazuelitas** también encontramos platos caseros como la Lengua en salsa o las Albóndigas. Zaharren Babeslekua abre todos los días a las 10 de la mañana y cierra a las 9 de la noche, salvo los fines de semana en los que, habitualmente hay cenas. Eso sí, en los momentos de aglomeración, los mayores tienen preferencia en los espacios para sentarse, cosa que, dicho sea de paso, debería ser así no sólo en los hogares de jubilados.

Otros pintxos:

- *Tortilla de bacalao*
- *Tortilla de patata*
- *Tortilla de jamón*
- *Chorizo cocido*
- *Bacon*
- *Carne cocida*
- *Atún con antxoa*
- *Morcilla*
- *Manitas de cerdo rebozadas*
- *Callos*

"Trainera"

Ingredientes:

2 txipirones
1 loncha de jamón serrano
Una rodaja de pimiento verde
1 huevo
Harina
Pan

- **Para la salsa de caramelo:**

Azúcar
Agua

Elaboración:

Para la salsa de caramelo: Ponemos una sartén al fuego con azúcar. Cuando se empieza a fundir, añadimos un poco de agua y llevamos a la consistencia deseada.

Cortamos una loncha de pimiento verde y la freímos en aceite de oliva bien caliente.

Cocemos el huevo, lo pelamos y lo cortamos en dos como se aprecia en la fotografía.

Enharinamos los txipirones y los freímos en aceite de oliva.

Final y presentación: Sobre una rodaja de pan, disponemos la loncha de jamón serrano en crudo (también se podría hacer con el jamón frito), sobre ella la rodaja de pimiento verde frito, y coronando el pintxo los dos txipirones fritos. Decoramos con el huevo duro y unos hilos de salsa de caramelo.

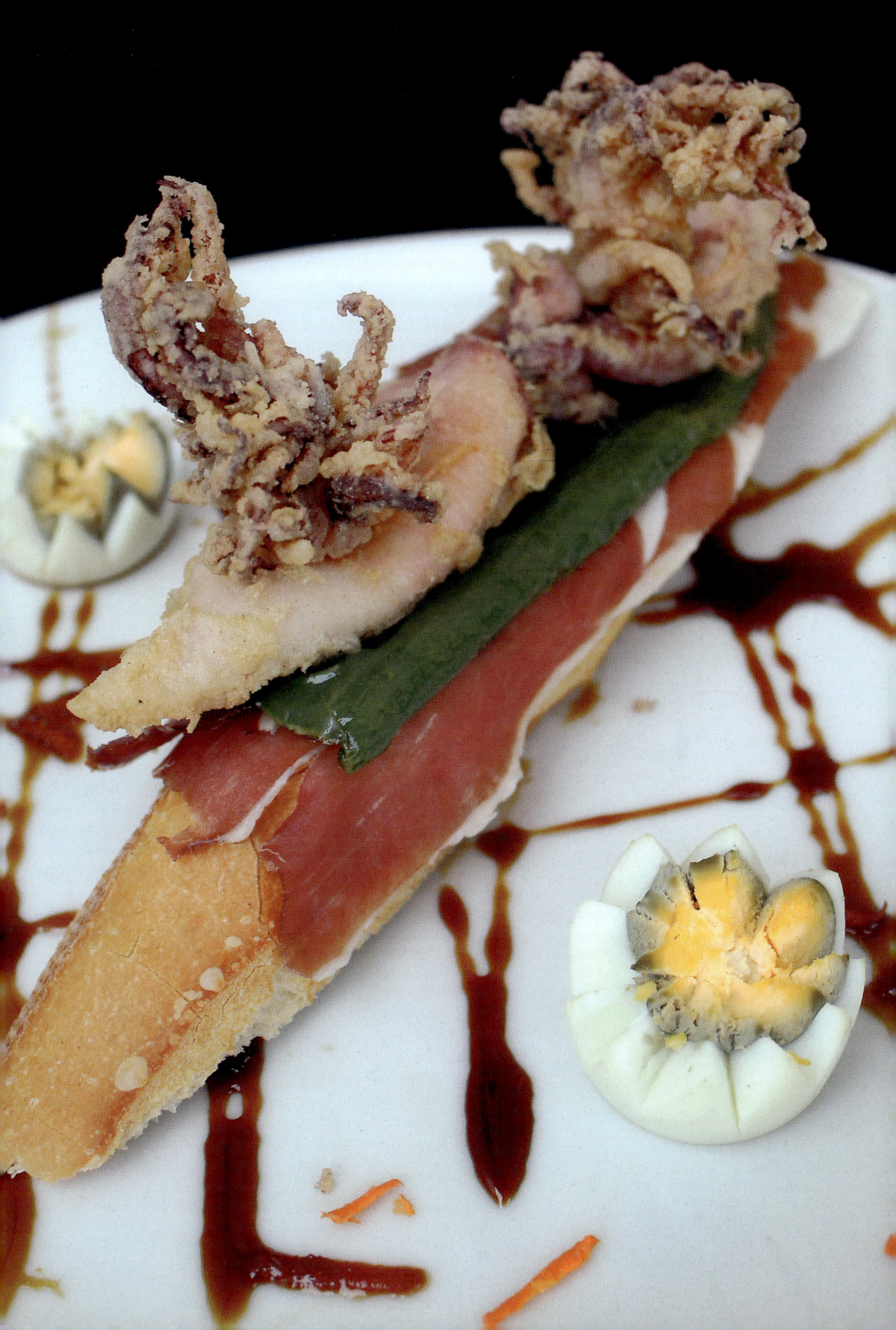

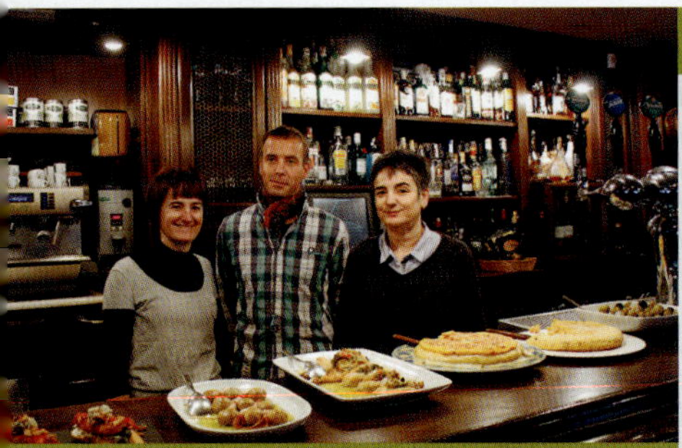

Uhaitz, 1
LAZKAO
943 88 24 85

ZELATA

Zelata es toda una referencia en Lazkao. Abierto en 1986, en 2001 acogió una profunda reforma que le dió la apariencia actual. Hoy en día está dirigido por **Unai Paredes Aldasoro** con la inestimable ayuda de **Karmele e Iñake Barandiaran** en la cocina y la barra respectivamente, y su mujer, **Diana Villar**, en la cocina. Zelata abre todos los días a las 8 de la mañana ofreciendo **desayunos con repostería, pan con aceite, tostadas con jamón, tortillas, sandwichs mixtos...** y durante todo el día, además de los pintxos que se reseñan más abajo, ofrece una gran variedad de **sandwiches, bocadillos, bizcochos artesanos, galletas caseras y raciones** como el solicitado Pulpo a la gallega o vinagreta, así como el Pastitxo, una suculenta lasaña que se ofrece el fin de semana, compuesta de calabacín, berenjenas, carne, ajo, pimiento verde, queso... Todo lo que se prepara en Zelata está hecho en casa. No en vano Karmele aprendió el oficio de su madre, **Maria Garmendia**, cocinera del Zelata original.

Otros pintxos:

- *Solomillo a la pimienta con foie*
- *Txipirones a la plancha*
- *Rollito cremoso de piquillo, bacon y jamón serrano*
- *Brick de hongos con langostino*
- *Chupito de crema de calabaza y txipirón en su tinta*
- *Croquetas*
- *Revuelto de bacalao o de hongos*
- *Tartaleta de hongos con foie*
- *Callos*
- *Caldo*

Pimiento relleno de txipirón

Ingredientes:

Pimiento del piquillo
Txipirón
Tinta de txipirón
Harina
Huevo
Aceite de oliva

· Para el relleno:
Txipirón
Ajo
Cebolla
Pimiento verde

· Para la bechamel:
Mantequilla
Harina
Leche
Nata

· Para la salsa de piquillo
Pimiento del piquillo
Cebolla

Elaboración:

Para la salsa de piquillo: Picamos finamente la cebolla y la ponemos a pochar en una sartén con aceite de oliva. Una vez pochada, añadimos los pimientos del piquillo y los confitamos un rato a fuego muy lento. Cuando estén blanditos, retiramos el aceite, lo trituramos todo con la batidora y lo pasamos por el chino.

Para la bechamel: Fundimos la mantequilla a fuego lento y añadimos la harina cocinándola un rato sin dejar de remover. Añadimos la leche, la sal y una pizca de nata, removiendo constantemente, y lo terminamos de cocinar durante 10-15 minutos a fuego lento.

Para el relleno: Picamos muy finamente el ajo, la cebolla y el pimiento verde. Lo ponemos a pochar suavemente en aceite de oliva. Mientras se hace picamos muy finamente el txipirón (salvo los tentáculos) y lo añadimos a la sartén. Seguimos rehogando y añadimos la tinta de txipirón. Mezclamos bien la tinta con la farsa y lo juntamos todo con la bechamel. Lo juntamos bien de manera que la mezcla quede bien negra y rellenamos el txipirón. Lo rebozamos en harina y huevo y lo freímos en aceite de oliva.

Final y presentación: Servimos el pimiento sobre la salsa de piquillo y junto a éste, los tentáculos del txipirón.

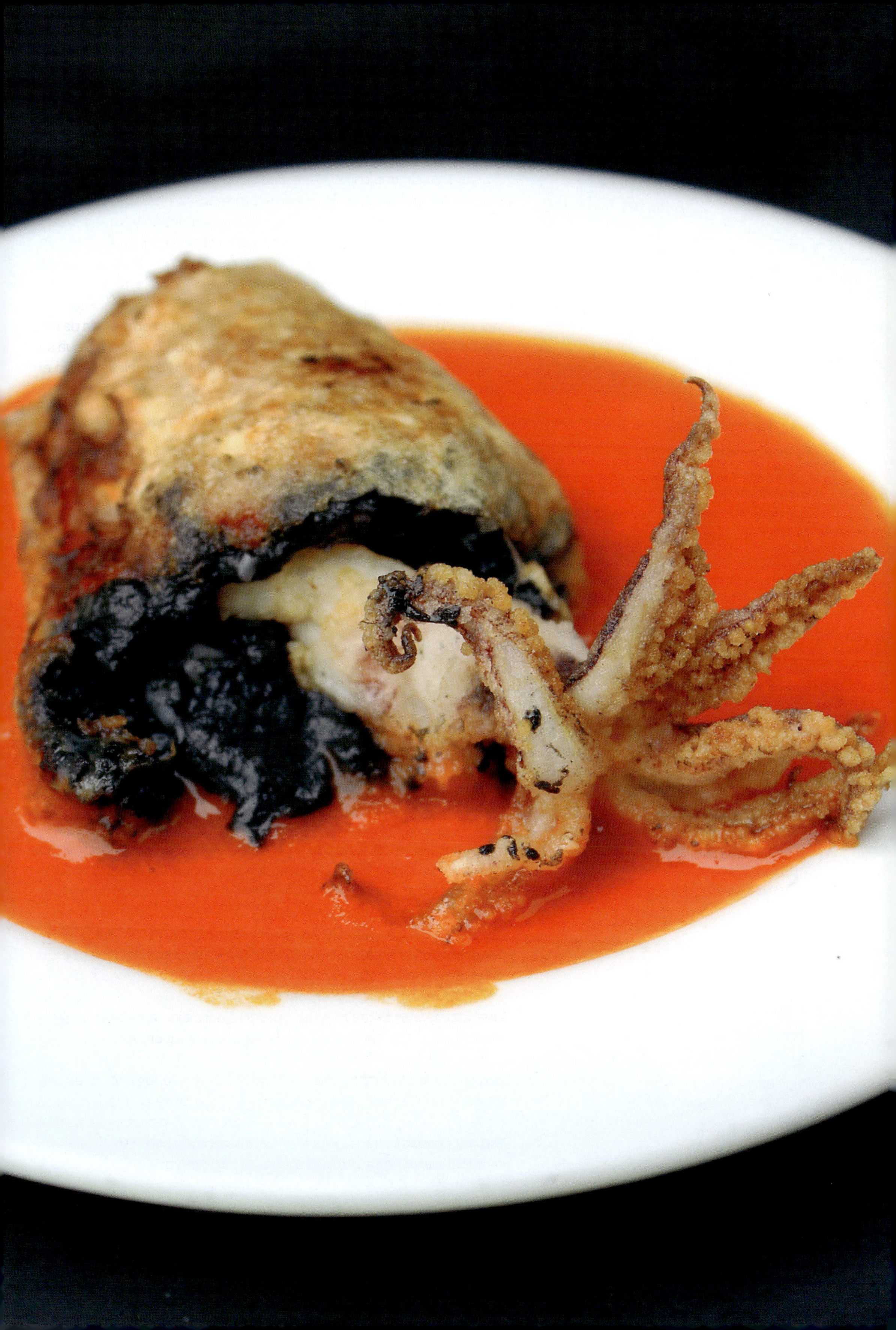

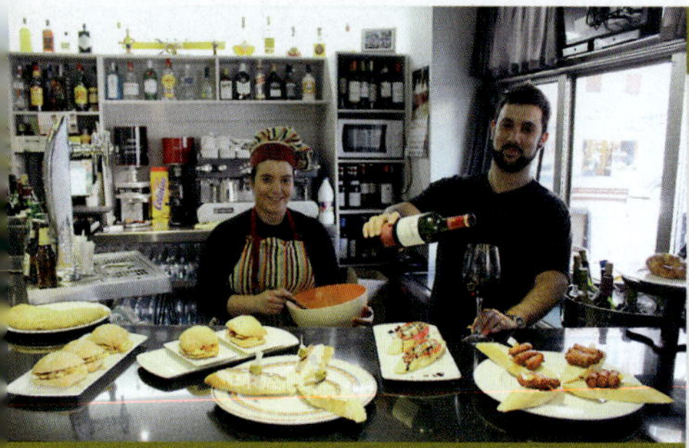

ZIABOGA

Nafarroa enparantza, 3
ZUMARRAGA
943 25 38 96

Abierto en noviembre de 2011, este céntrico asador dirigido por **Aitor Díaz de Arcaya** cuenta con la única **parrilla de carbón** de Zumarraga, en la que podemos degustar carnes de Cárnicas Goya, de Tolosa, y pescados como Rape, Lubina, Cogote de merluza, Muxarra, etc. En su carta, además, encontramos otras opciones como Revuelto de hongos con gulas y gambas, Revuelto de mar y tierra, Pulpo a la gallega, Fritos de ibérico y boletus, Ensalada de foie, ibérico y frutos secos, Ensalada Ziaboga (con hongos, gambas y gulas), Solomillo francés en salsa, Huevos rotos con jamón o txistorra... Ziaboga abre todos los días a las 8:00 de la mañana y además de buenos desayunos, desde las 10 podemos encontrar en su **barra pintxos** de todo tipo, desde una buena tortilla de patata hasta otras tentaciones como el solicitado pintxo de Brandada de bacalao, entre otros.

Otros pintxos:

- *Bola de marisco*
- *Brandada de bacalao*
- *Revuelto de hongos*
- *Tartaleta de txangurro*
- *Tortillas variadas*

Raciones:

- *Las famosas rabas del Ziaboga*
- *Pulpo a la gallega*
- *Gambas de Huelva a la plancha*
- *Patatas bravas*

Champiñón relleno

Ingredientes:

1 champiñón grande
Patata
Yema de huevo
Gamba
Perejil
Aceite de oliva
Pan

Elaboración:

Quitamos el tallo al champiñón y freímos la corona en la sartén con aceite de oliva.

Cocemos la patata. Cuando se enfría la despedazamos a mano y la mezclamos en un bol con yema de huevo y gamba pelada y triturada. Pasamos por la batidora y rellenamos el hueco del champiñón con esta masa.

Disponemos el resto de la masa encima y alrededor del champiñón.

Pelamos una gamba totalmente salvo la parte de la cola. Hacemos una incisión en la parte superior del champiñón y la introducimos dentro, dejando que la cola sobresalga hacia fuera.

Introducimos el champiñón relleno al horno y lo asamos cinco minutos a 180° aproximadamente.

Final y presentación: Colocamos el champiñón sobre una rodaja de pan tostado al horno o a la plancha.

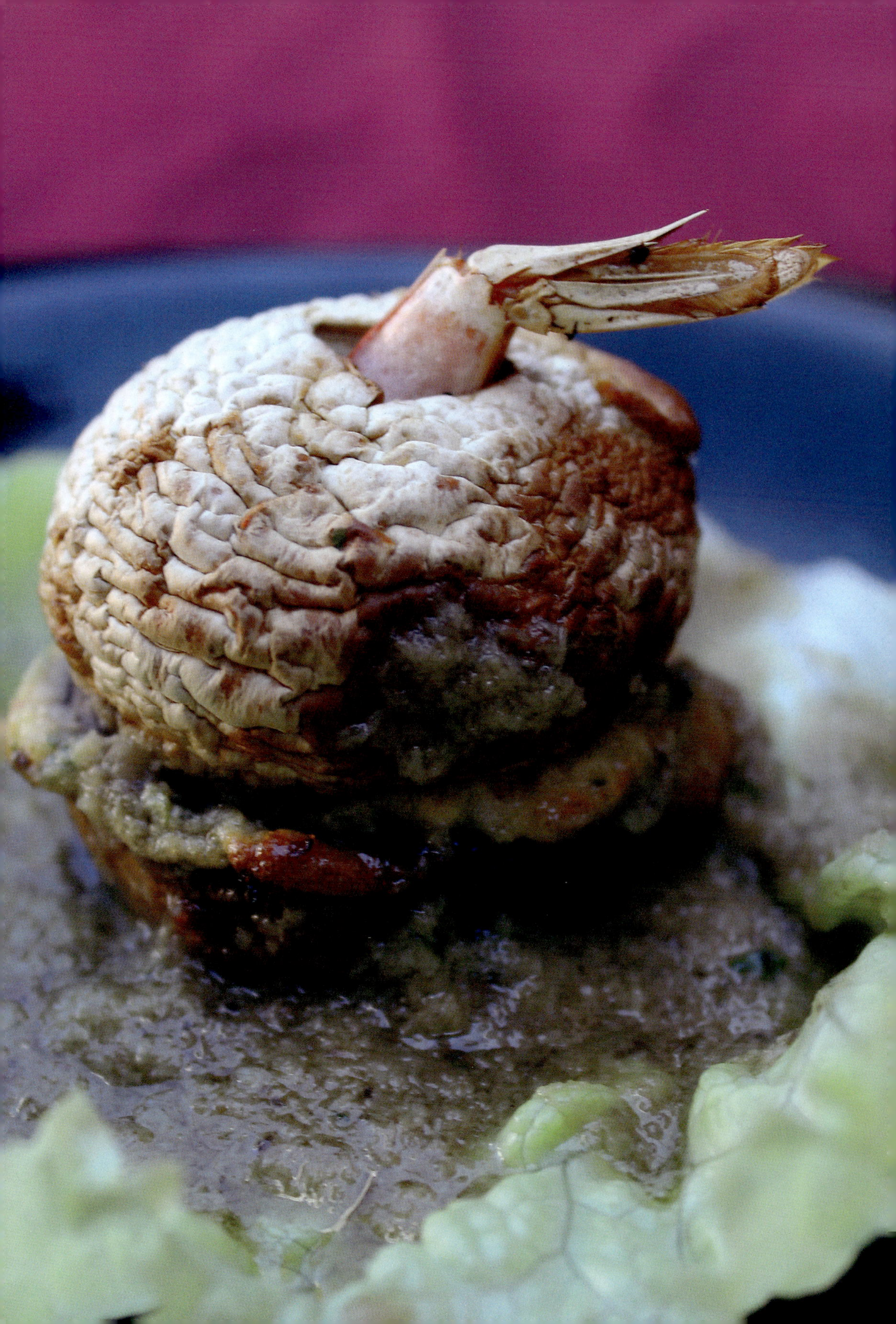

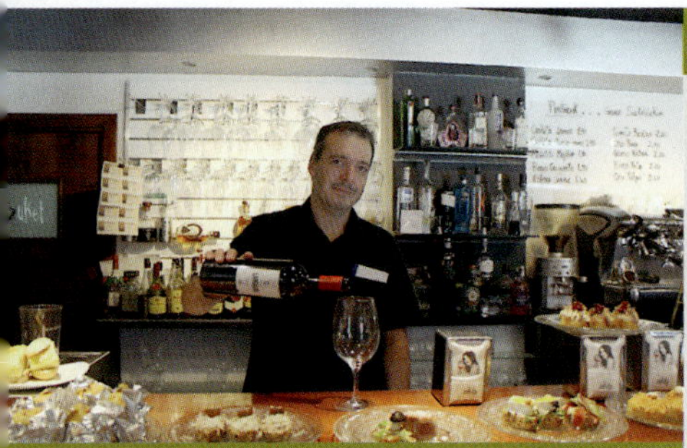

ZUKETZ

Pza. Koldo Mitxelena
ERRENTERIA
943 51 88 35
www.kafejatetxeazuketz.com

Inaugurado en 2006 y situado en pleno centro de Errenteria, Zuketz nos ofrece, de la mano del creativo chef **Jon Bizarro** y su socia **Larraitz Egilegor**, una **cocina contemporánea de base tradicional elaborada con productos sencillos trabajados de manera muy visual.** El resultado es una carta vistosa y colorista que cambia a menudo siguiendo el pulso de las estaciones. El conjunto se completa con un comedor decorado de manera sobria pero eficaz, acorde a la impronta culinaria del establecimiento, en el que adquiere una gran importancia el vino como elemento estético. Zuketz cuenta también con un **bar abierto desde las 8:30 de la mañana** en el que, además de desayunos, podemos degustar sus ricas croquetas cremosas y una gran variedad de pintxos entre las 9:30 y las 15:30. Los habituales de este establecimiento piden siempre, en una muestra de confianza, el **pintxo "Zuketz"**, un pintxo-incógnita elaborado por Jon en función del día, la temporada... o lo que tenga a mano.

Otros pintxos:

- *Croquetas cremosas de jamón ibérico o queso y nueces*
- *Filetitos de gallo en tempura sobre un licuado de espinacas y berberecho a la plancha (pintxo Zuketz)*
- *Carrillera de ibérico sobre tostita de queso de cabra y una salsa de turrón (pintxo Zuketz)*
- *Calamar napado en ceviche de bonito y un jugo de lima*
- *Falsa lasaña de solomillo con pringles, con emulsión de jugo de carne y escamas de Parmesano (pintxo Zuketz)*
- *Brick de txangurro y langostinos con crema de marisco*
- *Taquitos de salmón artesano*

Taco de toro de mar, ali-oli de almeja y mini bosque de temporada

Ingredientes:

1 lomo de atún rojo de 80-100 gr.
Bouquet de lechugas
Tomate cherry
Aceite de calabaza
Aceite de trufa
Tronco de hongo
1 hongo txiki
Aceite de oliva
Sal de escamas

- **Para el ali-oli de almejas:**

Almejas
Leche
Aceite de girasol
Ajo
Pimienta

Elaboración:

Para el ali-oli de almejas: Por una parte, cocemos unas almejas en agua. Por otra, elaboramos un ali-oli tradicional con aceite de girasol, ajo picado, leche, sal y pimienta. Lo mezclamos todo y lo pasamos por la batidora. Finalmente, mezclamos las almejas con el ali-oli y volvemos a batir. Quedará muy espeso, pero podemos rebajarlo a una textura más ligera mezclándole agua de la cocción de la almejas.

Confitamos el hongo txiki en aceite de oliva, al horno de vapor, a lo largo de 5 minutos a 90º. Cortamos una rodaja gruesa de tronco de hongo y la hacemos a la plancha.

Preparamos un pequeño bouquet de lechugas, le añadimos medio tomate cherry y lo aliñamos con aceite de calabaza y de trufa.

Marcamos el taco de atún a la plancha a punto de txuleta.

Final y presentación: Disponemos el taco de atún, coronado con unas escamas de sal. A su lado, el bouquet de lechugas y, sobre él, el tronco de hongo a la plancha y el hongo txiki. Terminamos de decorar el pintxo con unas gotas de ali-oli de almejas.

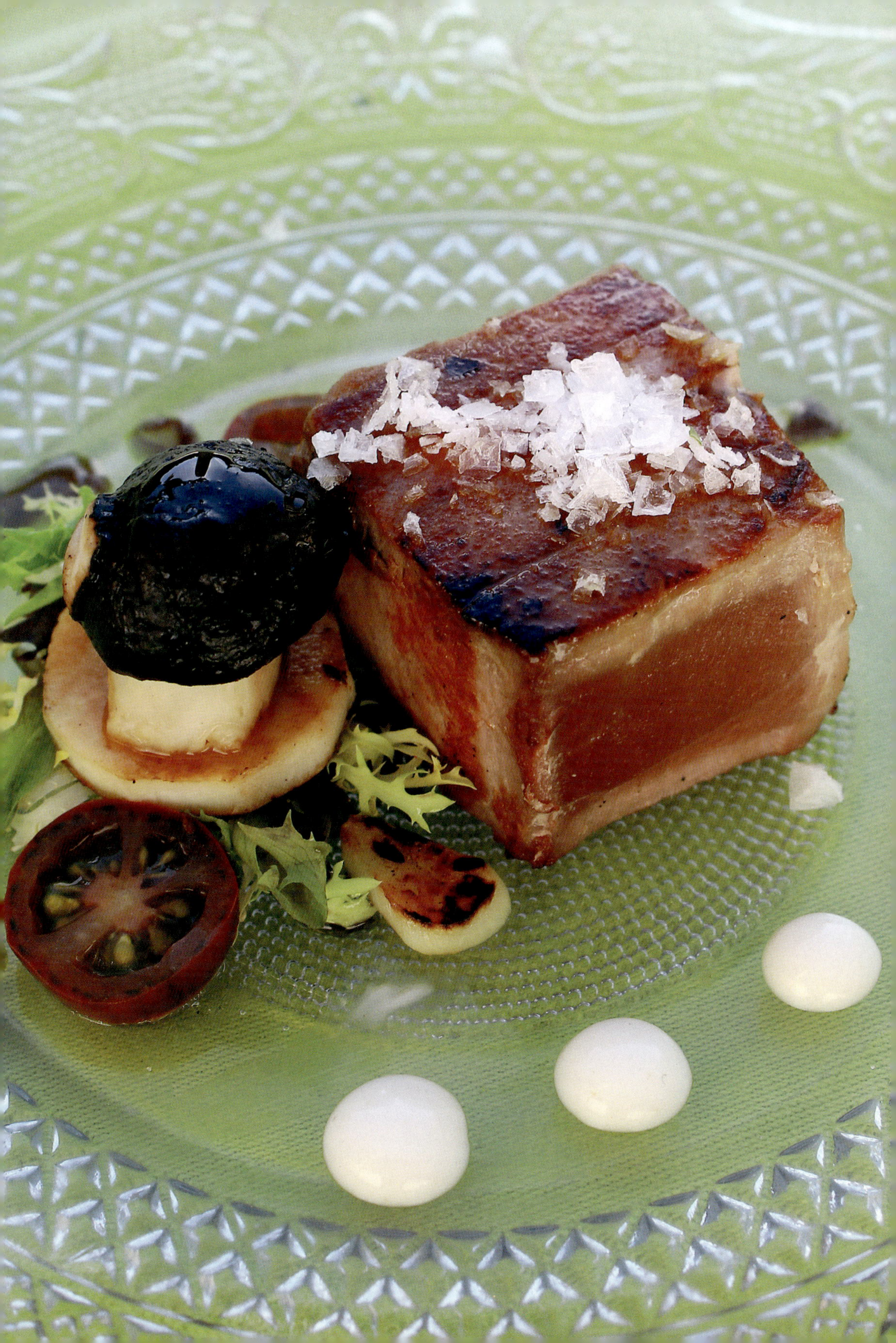

Publicado por:
ZUM Edizioak S.L.

Depósito legal:
D.L. SS-194-2015

ISBN:
978-84-940281-8-2

Idea original:
Juan Cintero
Josema Azpeitia

Textos:
Josema Azpeitia

Fotografías:
Ritxar Tolosa

Diseño y tratamiento de imágenes:
Ritxar Tolosa

Maquetación y tratamiento de textos:
Ritxar Tolosa
Josema Azpeitia

Prólogo:
Josema Azpeitia

Impresión:
Centro Gráfico Ganboa

Zum Edizioak S.L.
Patrizio Etxeberria 7, bis
20230 LEGAZPI (GIPUZKOA)
Tf. 943 73 15 83
E-mail: zum@zumedizioak.com
www.zumedizioak.com
www.ondojan.com
www.facebook.com/ondojan